BSAVA Manual of Small Animal Ophthalmology

Second edition

Editors:

Simon Petersen-Jones
BVetMed DVetMed PhD DVOphthal DipECVO MRCVS

Department of Small Animal Clinical Sciences
Michigan State University, D-208 Veterinary Medical Center
East Lansing, MI 48824-1314, USA

and

Sheila Crispin
MA VetMB BSc PhD DVA DVOphthal DipECVO FRCVS

Professor of Comparative Ophthalmology
Department of Veterinary Clinical Science, University of Bristol
Langford House, Langford, Bristol BS40 5DU

Published by:

British Small Animal Veterinary Association
Woodrow House, 1 Telford Way, Waterwells
Business Park, Quedgeley, Gloucester GL2 2AB

A Company Limited by Guarantee in England.
Registered Company No. 2837793.
Registered as a Charity.

Copyright © 2002 BSAVA
Reprinted 2006, 2008, 2010

All rights reserved. No part of this publication may be reproduced, stored in a retrieval system, or transmitted, in form or by any means, electronic, mechanical, photocopying, recording or otherwise without prior written permission of the copyright holder.

Figures 2.18, 2.20, 2.23, 2.27, 2.28, 2.29, 2.30, 5.9, 5.17c,d, 5.27, 5.42, 5.46, 5.51, 6.1, 6.2, 8.4, 8.16, 11.41 and 12.1 were drawn by S.J. Elmhurst BA Hons and are printed with her permission.

A catalogue record for this book is available from the British Library.

ISBN-10   0 905214 54 4
ISBN-13   978 0 905214 54 2

The publishers, editors and contributors cannot take responsibility for information provided on dosages and methods of application of drugs mentioned or referred to in this publication. Details of this kind must be verified in each case by individual users from up to date literature published by the manufacturers or suppliers of those drugs. Veterinary surgeons are reminded that in each case they must follow all appropriate national legislation and regulations (for example, in the United Kingdom, the prescribing cascade) from time to time in force.

Typeset by: Fusion Design, Wareham, Dorset
Printed by: Replika Press Pvt. Ltd, India
Printed on ECF paper made from sustainable forests

Other titles in the BSAVA Manuals series:

Manual of Canine & Feline Abdominal Imaging
Manual of Canine & Feline Abdominal Surgery
Manual of Canine & Feline Advanced Veterinary Nursing
Manual of Canine & Feline Anaesthesia and Analgesia
Manual of Canine & Feline Behavioural Medicine
Manual of Canine & Feline Cardiorespiratory Medicine
Manual of Canine & Feline Clinical Pathology
Manual of Canine & Feline Dentistry
Manual of Canine & Feline Dermatology
Manual of Canine & Feline Emergency and Critical Care
Manual of Canine & Feline Endocrinology
Manual of Canine & Feline Endoscopy and Endosurgery
Manual of Canine & Feline Gastroenterology
Manual of Canine & Feline Haematology and Transfusion Medicine
Manual of Canine & Feline Head, Neck and Thoracic Surgery
Manual of Canine & Feline Infectious Diseases
Manual of Canine & Feline Musculoskeletal Disorders
Manual of Canine & Feline Musculoskeletal Imaging
Manual of Canine & Feline Nephrology and Urology
Manual of Canine & Feline Neurology
Manual of Canine & Feline Oncology
Manual of Canine & Feline Rehabilitation, Supportive and Palliative Care: Case Studies in Patient Management
Manual of Canine & Feline Reproduction and Neonatology
Manual of Canine & Feline Thoracic Imaging
Manual of Canine & Feline Ultrasonography
Manual of Canine & Feline Wound Management and Reconstruction
Manual of Exotic Pets
Manual of Farm Pets
Manual of Ornamental Fish
Manual of Practical Animal Care
Manual of Practical Veterinary Nursing
Manual of Psittacine Birds
Manual of Rabbit Medicine and Surgery
Manual of Raptors, Pigeons and Passerine Birds
Manual of Reptiles
Manual of Rodents and Ferrets
Manual of Small Animal Fracture Repair and Management
Manual of Wildlife Casualties

For information on these and all BSAVA publications please visit our website: www.bsava.com

Contents

List of contributors   v

Foreword   vi

Preface   vii

1   Examination and diagnostic procedures

    1a   Ophthalmic examination   1
         John R.B Mould

    1b   Ocular imaging   13
         Elizabeth Munro and David T. Ramsey

    1c   Laboratory investigation of ophthalmic disease   23
         David J Maggs

2   Ophthalmic surgery and anaesthesia

    2a   Anaesthesia and analgesia   30
         Sheilah Robertson

    2b   Ophthalmic surgery: instrumentation   36
         David J Maggs

    2c   Ophthalmic surgery: basic principles   42
         David J Maggs

3   Ophthalmic drugs   50
    David Gould

4   The orbit and globe   60
    John R.B Mould

5   The eyelids and nictitating membrane   78
    Simon Petersen-Jones

6   The lacrimal system   105
    Sheila Crispin

7   The conjunctiva   124
    Sheila Crispin

8   The cornea   134
    Sheila Crispin

9   The sclera, episclera and corneoscleral limbus   155
    David T. Ramsey

10   The uveal tract   162
    Sheila Crispin

11   Glaucoma   185
    Peter Renwick

12	**The lens** *Simon Petersen-Jones*	204
13	**The vitreous** *Christine Heinrich*	219
14	**The fundus**	
	14a The canine fundus *Gillian McLellan*	227
	14b The feline fundus *Joan Dziezyc and Nicholas J. Millichamp*	247
15	**Neuro-ophthalmology** *Fabiano Montiani Ferreira and Simon Petersen-Jones*	257
16	**Rabbits** *David L. Williams*	276
17	**Exotic species** *Martin P.C. Lawton*	285

Appendices
- **Differential diagnosis** — 296
- **Ophthalmological emergencies and referrals** — 302
- **Eye schemes and hereditary eye disease** — 303

Index — 305

Contributors

Sheila Crispin MA VetMB BSc PhD DVA DVOphthal DipECVO FRCVS
Department of Veterinary Clinical Science, University of Bristol, Langford House,
Langford, Bristol BS40 5DU

Joan Dziezyc DVM DipACVO
Department of Small Animal Medicine and Surgery, College of Veterinary Medicine,
Texas A&M University, College Station, TX 77843, USA

David Gould BSc BVM&S PhD DVOphthal MRCVS
Department of Clinical Veterinary Science, University of Bristol, Langford House,
Langford, Bristol BS40 5DU

Christine Heinrich DVOphthal MRCVS
Willows Referral Services, 78 Tanworth Lane, Shirley, Solihull B90 4DF

Martin P.C. Lawton BVetMed CertVOphthal CertLAS CBiol MICiol DZooMed FRCVS
12 Fitzilian Avenue, Harold Wood, Romford, Essex RM3 0QS

David Maggs BVSc DipACVO
VM:SRS, 2112 Tupper Hall, University of California – Davis, Davis, CA 95616, USA

Gillian McLellan BVMS PhD DVOphthal MRCVS
Department of Veterinary Clinical Sciences, Veterinary Teaching Hospital, Iowa State University,
Ames, IA 50011–1250, USA

Nicholas Millichamp BVetMed BSc PhD DipACVO DVOphthal MRCVS
Department of Small Animal Medicine and Surgery, College of Veterinary Medicine,
Texas A&M University, College Station, TX 77843, USA

John R.B. Mould BVSc BA DVOphthal MRCVS
Department of Veterinary Clinical Studies, University of Glasgow, Bearsden Road, Glasgow G61 1QH

Fabiano Montiani Ferreira MV MSc CBOV Dipl.
Veterinary Medicine Department, Universidade Federal do Parana, Brazil
Currently at: Department of Small Animal Clinical Sciences, Michigan State University,
D-208 Veterinary Medical Center, East Lansing, MI 48824-1314, USA

Elizabeth A.C. Munro MA VetMB DVR CertVOphthal MRCVS
Department of Veterinary Clinical Studies, Royal (Dick) School of Veterinary Studies,
Hospital for Small Animals, Easter Bush Veterinary Centre, Roslin, Midlothian EH25 9RG

Simon Petersen-Jones BVetMed DVetMed PhD DVOphthal DipECVO MRCVS
Department of Small Animal Clinical Sciences, Michigan State University,
D-208 Veterinary Medical Center, East Lansing, MI 48824-1314, USA

David T. Ramsey DVM DipACVO
The Animal Ophthalmology Center, 412 Jolly Road, Okemos, MI 48864, USA

Peter W. Renwick MA VetMB DVOphthal MRCVS
Willows Referral Services, 78 Tanworth Lane, Shirley, Solihull B90 4DF

Sheilah Robertson BVMS PhD DipACVA DipECVA MRCVS
Department of Large Animal Clinical Sciences, University of Florida, Box 100136,
Gainesville, FL 32610-0136, USA

David L. Williams MA VetMB PhD CertVOphthal MRCVS
Department of Clinical Veterinary Medicine, University of Cambridge, Madingley Road,
Cambridge CB3 0ES

Foreword

The first BSAVA Manual of Ophthalmology was published in 1993. It has been one of the most successful manuals we publish and was reprinted in 1997, testament to the importance of the topic and the quality of the content.

This second edition calls on the services of the original editors, Dr Simon Petersen-Jones and Professor Sheila Crispin, both well known to BSAVA members and to their ophthalmological peers. The entire text has completely updated and several new authors have been recruited, resulting in what is, in effect, a new manual. As might be expected in a BSAVA Manual, the authors, many of whom will be familiar to regular visitors to the BSAVA Annual Congress, have been drawn from specialty practice and academia in both Europe and the United States.

Readers will be particularly pleased to see that the new manual now features sections on ophthalmic surgery, with analgesia, anaesthesia, instrumentation and basic principles included. All aspects of canine and feline ophthalmological disease are covered, and, in addition, the editors are to be congratulated on including a chapter on rabbit ophthalmology. As anyone in small animal practice will testify, the rabbit with an ocular discharge is a very common presentation.

BSAVA manuals are justly renowned for both content and presentation, with an easy-to-read layout and generous use of high-quality colour illustrations supplementing clinically relevant text. This manual delivers just that. The editors, authors, and the members of the BSAVA Publications Committee and the Publications team are to be congratulated.

Richard G Harvey BVSc PhD CBiol FIBiol DVD MRCVS
BSAVA President 2002/3

Preface

If the aims of clinical medicine – as of every aspect of science – can be summed up in the threefold object, 'to understand, to predict, to control,' it must be accepted that any scientific system of prognosis and treatment should depend upon complete and efficient means of diagnosis. In this respect ophthalmology is favoured above all other branches of medicine, for no other organ in the body offers the same facilities for minute and delicate examination as the eye. Elsewhere in the body the clinician reasons largely by inference; in the eye, because of its ready accessibility and the transparency of its structure, he can observe directly pathological processes as they occur in the living tissues. The opportunities for elaborating refined methods of investigation are obvious, and their application has undoubtedly made ophthalmology the most exact, and for that reason the most interesting, of all medical sciences.

Redmond J. H. Smith and Stewart Duke Elder (1962) In: *System of Ophthalmology*, *Volume VIII*, edited by Sir Stewart Duke-Elder, p. 233. Henry Kimpton, London

The first edition of this manual was very well received and we hope that the second edition will build on that success. Since the first edition was published in 1993, veterinary ophthalmology has grown into a vibrant specialty but this does not mean that veterinary surgeons in general practice can abandon all pretence of mastering the complexities of ophthalmic examination – quite the contrary.

Examination of the eye is an art, the practical aspects of which many veterinary surgeons find difficult to perform effectively. This is unfortunate, for the eye offers a unique opportunity for diagnosis, not just of ocular disease but of disease elsewhere in the body. Ophthalmic examination, performed with the aid of a few simple instruments, often yields an accurate diagnosis, and repeated meticulous observation and record-keeping enable accurate monitoring of the progression, or regression, of ocular disease. The confidence that comes with experience allows key decisions to be made with regard to the best way of managing the case and early referral to a specialist may be one of the options to be considered.

A clear and concise guide to the examination of the eye is provided in the first section of Chapter 1 and is essential reading for those veterinary surgeons lacking confidence in their ophthalmic examination technique. Using the techniques described and the lists of differential diagnoses provided in Appendix I, it should be possible for ocular lesions to be identified and localised with precision. The relevant chapters can then be consulted for more detailed information. The second section of Chapter 1 describes imaging techniques and the third section outlines some of the laboratory investigations that can be selected in an attempt to establish a specific aetiology.

Chapters 2 and 3 are new for this edition. Chapter 2 is in three sections covering anaesthesia, surgical instruments and surgical principles, while Chapter 3 is concerned with ophthalmic drugs. The twelve chapters that follow deal with specific ocular conditions of dogs and cats. Progressing from the adnexa (orbit and periorbital regions, eyelids and lacrimal system) to the eye itself and thence to the connections between the eye and the brain. Each chapter starts with a short section which considers the relevant anatomy and physiology of that portion of the eye. In most cases the conditions of the dog and cat are then considered separately, except where there are close similarities between them.

Hereditary eye diseases are included, particularly those listed by the British Veterinary Association/Kennel Club/International Sheep Dog Society (BVA/KC/ISDS) Eye Examination Scheme. Although the conditions listed under the scheme are up to date at the time of going to press, they are under constant review and the reader should refer to the latest published update, obtainable from the British Veterinary Association. Appendix II provides a brief overview of the BVA/KC/ISDS Eye Scheme, the European College of Veterinary Ophthalmologists (ECVO) Scheme and the Canine Eye Registration Foundation (CERF) scheme. Harmonization of the various eye schemes to produce an internationally acceptable certificate is under review.

The last two chapters of the Manual describe ocular conditions of rabbits and exotic animals, respectively, with emphasis both on the commoner disorders and those which differ markedly from the conditions already described for the dog and cat.

Colour photographs are used throughout the manual to illustrate both normality and disease. Numerous line drawings and relevant imaging photographs complement the colour illustrations. Each chapter includes key and recent references, as well as suggestions for further reading. No attempt has been made to make these lists exhaustive; nevertheless they should provide a useful guide to the reader.

The Manual is intended as a practical consulting room guide to small animal ophthalmology, with suggestions of which conditions require specialist management. The subject is, however, covered in sufficient detail to satisfy those who wish to study this fascinating specialty in greater depth.

Simon Petersen-Jones
Sheila Crispin
July 2002

1a

Ophthalmic examination

John R.B. Mould

'Diagnoses will not cluster around the ophthalmoscope like moths, just because we have switched on the light.'
Dr H.B. Chawla (1988)

Introduction

The essence of ophthalmology, as with all branches of veterinary medicine, is diagnosis which, in turn, depends on good clinical observation and interpretation. Without an accurate diagnosis, speculative treatment is rarely successful, nor is the use of 'polypharmacy' (a sure sign of diagnostic insecurity) and both will delay the start of specific therapy.

In the eye, more than in most systems, a diagnosis can often be made at the time of examination. Additional laboratory or radiographic investigations are not always necessary or helpful and will not make up for inadequate clinical observation. It follows, therefore, that much depends on the initial examination technique. The following points are particularly important in the examination of eye cases:

- It is crucial to be able to recognize what is normal. This can only be appreciated from personal experience gained from examining as many eyes as possible. Confidence in the examination of eyes will develop in time, but only if it is regarded as a process of continuous self-education, rather than a subject which is only taken up reluctantly when an abnormal eye is presented
- The most obvious clinical sign may not be primary but secondary. The objective should be to make a primary diagnosis whenever possible. Do not expect a diagnosis to appear immediately, but proceed methodically with the examination and then take time to assemble and evaluate all the information before reaching a conclusion.

This chapter will discuss equipment required and present a protocol for ophthalmic examination. Additional investigative techniques that may be performed at the time of initial examination are described. Differential diagnoses and suggested approaches for some common presenting signs are included in Appendix 1.

Equipment

The essential equipment for the proper examination of ophthalmic cases in general practice requires only a modest investment. Ophthalmic diagnosis is not a matter of expensive hardware but, rather, the careful use of readily available equipment. The first requirement is a room which offers good illumination and that can also be darkened as required.

Focal illumination
A bright focal light source is needed for examination of the adnexa and the anterior segment, and for testing pupillary light responses. The familiar penlight is satisfactory, but a focused beam can be more informative than a diffuse beam. The Finhoff rigid fibreoptic transillumination extension fits the ophthalmoscope handle and provides a simple beam; it is more expensive than a penlight, but is very durable.

Magnification
Simple head loupes have the advantage of leaving the hands free. Magnifications in the range 1.5–2.5X are typical. Spectacle-type examination loupes and operating spectacles are optically superior and offer magnification ranges up to 6X, but are more expensive. Hand lenses of various kinds are available, but both hands are then required to hold the lens and a light source. An otoscope with the speculum removed gives reasonable magnification and field of view, and has its own light source. The direct ophthalmoscope gives a good view of the anterior segment and external eye, but with much less magnification than for examination of the fundus. The most sophisticated instrument for examination of the anterior segment and adnexa is the slit lamp biomicroscope (see below).

Direct ophthalmoscopes
Direct ophthalmoscopes are relatively cheap, durable and portable, and are the most familiar instrument in veterinary ophthalmology. For some applications, however, they are not easy to use properly and it is likely that their value is not fully realised in the field. Clinicians wishing to improve their ophthalmic examination should first understand the features and capabilities of the instrument, as outlined in this section, and then practise the techniques for its use, as described later in the chapter.

Some modern ophthalmoscopes have numerous

functions and options, making them rather intimidating. Furthermore, the examiner may inadvertently use incorrect settings, with disappointing results. For veterinary work, some of these features are of limited use. The general clinician should look for a simple, well made instrument which gives a clear, wide angle view. There is no point in persisting with an outdated or faulty instrument giving an inferior image.

It pays to become fully familiar with the instrument before use, particularly where multiple options are available. Spectacle wearers are strongly advised to remove their spectacles to use a direct ophthalmoscope; this brings the instrument closer to the eye, improving the field of view, and the spectacles will not be damaged if the animal moves suddenly. The spectacle wearer will need to establish his/her dioptre correction and place a lens of the same value in the viewing path for examining the fundus.

Essentially, the direct ophthalmoscope can be used in three different ways:

- Distant direct ophthalmoscopy (see below)
- Fundic examination (close direct ophthalmoscopy (see below)
- Illumination/magnification for anterior segment and adnexal examination. High positive lenses (+10 to +20 D) are used to examine from the lens to the ocular surface. Magnification, however, declines sharply from the fundus (approximately 15X) to the ocular surface (2X).

Direct ophthalmoscopes offer a selection of the following features.

On/off switch
This incorporates a rheostat, allowing the light intensity to be varied. On full power, the light intensity would be uncomfortable for most patients.

Beam selector
This provides a choice of beam types for different applications:

- Small diameter beam. This is used for small diameter pupils, but consequently gives a narrower field of view than the larger beam. Where possible, dilate the pupil and use the largest beam available
- Large diameter beam. This is the routine beam for use with a pupil of adequate size
- Slit beam. This can indicate whether areas that are out of focus on the fundus are depressions or elevations by the way the slit moves over them
- Graticule. This projects a pattern on the fundus and is very occasionally of value as a rough means of measuring the extent of a fundic lesion, by comparing its size with the diameter of the optic disc
- Red-free light. The beam appears green and is used for specialized observation of the retinal or limbal vascular system, for the retinal nerve fibre layer and for distinguishing retinal haemorrhages from pigment
- Cobalt blue light. This is most commonly used to enhance fluorescence after the topical application of fluorescein to a corneal ulcer.

Lens magazine
Direct ophthalmoscopes contain a magazine of interchangeable lenses mounted on a disc or chain system. These start at zero (i.e. plain) and then move in plus dioptres, which can be accessed by moving the wheel clockwise, and minus dioptres, which are found by moving the wheel anticlockwise. Initially, they move in intervals of one dioptre (1 D) but at higher values the intervals may widen. An illuminated window indicates which lens is in the viewing path. The lens magazine is essential and serves three purposes:

- It allows the examiner to compensate for the refractive error in his/her eye. Myopic (short- or near-sighted) examiners require minus lenses and hypermetropic (long-sighted) examiners require plus lenses. If the refractive error is not known, it can be established by trial and error by looking through the instrument at a distant object and finding the lens that gives the sharpest image. Contact lens wearers and clinicians with normal refraction need not be concerned with this
- It allows the examiner to compensate for the refractive error in the patient's eye. This is important in people but animals' eyes tend to fall in a narrow range of refraction, which is near normal
- It allows the examiner to focus on structures at different depths in the eye. Like cameras, ophthalmoscopes have limited depth of field, and the whole eye cannot be seen in focus at once. Positive dioptre lenses are needed to focus through to the anterior eye and negative dioptre lenses are needed to focus into a depression such as a coloboma. It is also useful to know when examining the fundus that a difference of focus of 1 D represents a difference of level of 0.3–0.4 mm; this is important when assessing, for example, excavated colobomatous defects, or elevations caused by papilloedema.

Rapid lens-change switch
Some ophthalmoscopes have a rapid lens-change switch, so that the examiner can make a substantial change to the level of focus with a single movement without going through the lenses in the magazine one by one. Typically, the shift is 12–20 D, changing the level of focus from the plane of the retina to that of the anterior segment.

Indirect ophthalmoscopes
The direct ophthalmoscope gives a small, upright, highly magnified image. Indirect methods give an inverted, reversed image which is less highly magnified but covers a much wider angle of view. Binocular instruments give the additional benefit of stereopsis. Each type has its advantages and disadvantages and the direct and indirect methods should be regarded as complementary. The indirect method, however, has

been undervalued in veterinary work. The wide-angle view provides a great deal of information rapidly and the technique is not more difficult to learn. The high magnification of the direct method, although excellent, is often not needed for the diagnosis of fundus lesions in animals.

Binocular indirect ophthalmoscopes consist of a light source and prism system worn on the head in the form of either a headpiece or spectacles. After some simple adjustments the headpiece requires no attention in use. Binocular indirect ophthalmoscopes are several times more expensive than direct ophthalmoscopes and are only likely to be purchased by those with a special interest in ophthalmology. They have the advantages of a stereoptic view and a powerful, variable light source which is excellent for examination through opaque media such as inflamed eyes or immature cataracts.

All methods of indirect ophthalmoscopy require the use of a hand lens held in front of the eye. The examiner views an image formed by this lens rather than viewing the fundus directly, hence the term *indirect* ophthalmoscopy. There is a wide choice of lenses available, giving a range of magnification and field of view. Glass lenses from the major manufacturers are made to the highest optical standards and are expensive but give excellent image quality. Acrylic lenses are satisfactory for general use and cost much less than glass lenses.

Indirect lenses vary in terms of dioptre value and diameter. Low-dioptre lenses give higher magnification with a narrower field of view. The image is brighter and the working distance from the patient's eye is longer. Lenses below 20D are quite difficult to use and are not advised for general use. Higher-dioptre lenses in the region of 28–30D give a less magnified image with a wider field of view. The image is less bright but the working distance is closer and they are easier to use with a smaller pupil. For these reasons higher-dioptre lenses are probably easier for the beginner. Some higher-dioptre lenses have a restrictingly small diameter but the Volk 30D 43 mm-diameter lens is very suitable for animal use. The Volk 2.2 Pan-Retinal Lens offers something of the best of all worlds, with a wide-angle bright view of suitable magnification. Specialists are likely to have more than one lens available. Indirect ophthalmoscopy technique is described later in the chapter.

Tonometers

A tonometer is a device for measuring intraocular pressure (IOP; see Chapter 11). The IOP cannot be measured with any accuracy by digital tonometry; an objective reading is always preferable. Tonometry is not difficult and may provide crucial diagnostic information. The Schiøtz tonometer is a simple mechanical method which costs less than a direct ophthalmoscope. The Tonopen is an electronic instrument which is much more expensive, but it is simple to use and is probably the instrument of choice in animals. In view of the serious implications of glaucoma, veterinary practices with a large throughput of small animal cases should certainly consider purchasing a tonometer and learning how to use it.

Goniolenses

Glaucoma management often requires examination of the iridocorneal or drainage angle. Unfortunately, this cannot be seen by direct inspection in the dog and requires the use of a convex contact lens called a goniolens. Dedicated goniolenses are expensive and the method and interpretation are technically demanding, so goniolenses are likely to be used only by specialists.

Tonometry and gonioscopy provide different information in the evaluation of the glaucoma patient. Tonometry is the easier technique for the non-specialist, however, and provides immediate useful information about the IOP. Full details of the investigation and management of glaucoma are found in Chapter 11.

Lacrimal cannulae

Plastic and metal cannulae are available in a variety of materials, diameters and shapes (see Chapter 6). Essentially, the choice is between flexible plastic cannulae and more rigid, but malleable, metal ones. Some cannulae have a rounded bulb-type end which minimizes trauma to the tissues.

Disposables

The following are required:

- Slides for impression smears
- Swabs for bacteriology and virology sampling
- Transport medium for viral and chlamydial swab samples
- Schirmer tear test papers
- Fluorescein dye
- Proxymetacaine local anaesthetic drops
- Tropicamide 1%
- Sterile saline.

Rose bengal stain can be used to demonstrate the presence of devitalized tissue on the ocular surface (see Chapter 8). Pilocarpine 1% and phenylephrine 10% are used in the investigation of certain pupillary abnormalities (see Chapter 15).

Protocol for ophthalmic examination

With the eye, as with other body systems, the clinician needs a routine for examination that can be carried out quickly using standard equipment, but that will identify abnormalities and indicate what needs to be pursued with further tests, special equipment or referral. This section describes such a routine, beginning with taking the history. The method may be varied according to personal preference, the equipment available and the individual case. The description of such a protocol takes longer than the execution of it and may give the impression that examination of eyes is more complex or time-consuming than examination of other body systems, but this is not the case.

Good equipment and a standard protocol will minimize the chances of lesions being missed, but a familiarity with the range of normal appearances is paramount. This expertise will develop simply by examining more eyes and will, ultimately, be more important than the equipment or protocol used.

Signalment and history

Consideration of the breed of the patient can be very useful in the dog, as many conditions show strong breed associations. In taking a history, the same considerations apply as in other body systems; they do not need re-emphasizing. In addition, with ophthalmic problems, the following should also be established:

- The state of the patient's general health
- Whether vision is affected
- Whether the condition is painful
- Whether both eyes are affected.

With eye problems, the history should always be interpreted in the light of the clinical findings. When the patient has a painful eye, owners often assume a traumatic incident when none has been observed. In addition, owners are often poor judges of ocular pain.

Examination with normal illumination and without instruments

This is an important stage; it can be very informative.

1. Begin by observing the patient from a distance; assess for evidence of pain. This is the best time to do so, as the signs may be less apparent when the patient is being handled or subjected to bright lights. Evaluate the blink rate, checking for blepharospasm and photophobia.
2. Assess orbital and periocular conformation. Note particularly any asymmetry, by assessing the orbit, the globe size and position, and any strabismus.
3. Observe the lids more closely, still without manipulating the region, as it can be difficult to establish resting eyelid position once hands are restraining a moving head. In particular, examine the conformation of the upper and lower eyelids and the position of the nictitating membrane. Note the presence and nature of any discharge.
4. Now handle the patient (Figure 1.1). Examine the lids and conjunctiva. Retract the upper lid and examine the dorsal bulbar conjunctiva; evert the lid margin and check the upper palpebral conjunctiva and upper lacrimal punctum. Then apply pressure to the globe through the upper lid and protrude the nictitating membrane, checking its leading edge, its alignment and its outer surface. Finally, retract the lower lid and observe the lower lacrimal punctum and the conjunctiva as it enters the fornix. This can all be done in one almost continuous movement. The normal appearance of the conjunctiva shows regional variation, which must be borne in mind in diagnosing a 'red eye'.
5. Check the corneal reflex (Purkinje image), which in this instance is the smoothness and sharpness of the reflection of a light (from a window or an artificial light) on the corneal surface. This gives information as to the optical smoothness of the surface.
6. Note the resting pupil size in normal room light.
7. Attempt to repel the globes into the orbits by pressing through the upper eyelids.

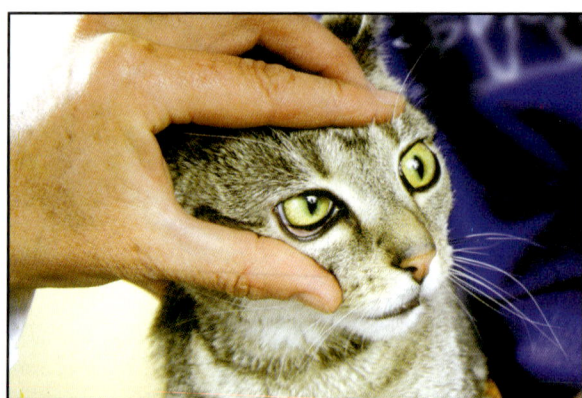

Figure 1.1 Handling the patient as part of the eye examination. (Courtesy of SM Crispin.)

Testing vision

Vision can be tested by various means:

- The menace response is tested by directing a finger towards the eye and observing a blink or retraction of the head. Causing a draught of air to contact the cornea may give a false normal result
- Vision may also be tested by the use of cotton wool balls (Figure 1.2). The ball is held high and

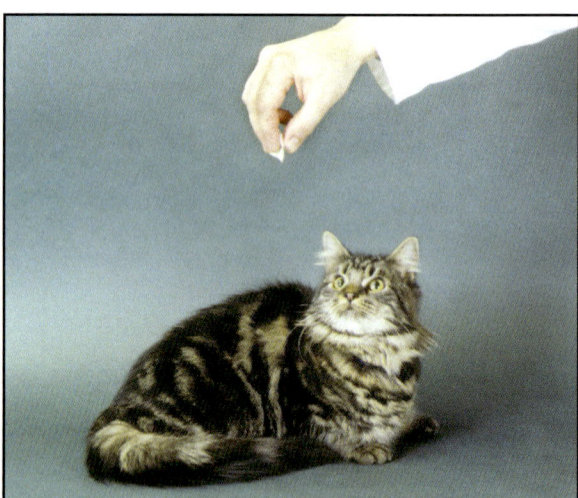

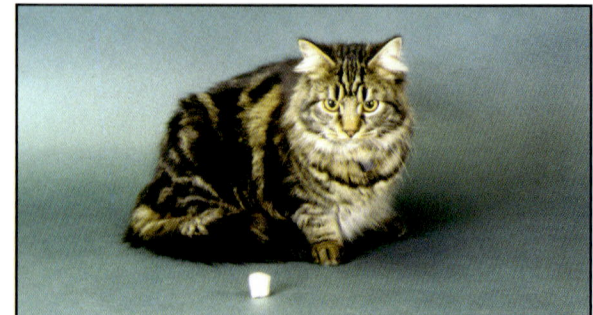

Figure 1.2 A cotton wool ball can be dropped as a test of vision. It should be noted, however, that some cats are indifferent to this test; it does not mean that they cannot see. (Courtesy of AH Sparkes.)

the animal's attention directed towards it by making a noise. The ball is then released in the animal's field of view and the animal is observed to see whether it follows its path
- Sighted animals, especially young ones, will readily follow the beam from the ophthalmoscope played on the examination table
- An obstacle course may be improvised from chairs, waste bins, etc. (Figure 1.3). The animal's performance may be assessed for both eyes or with one eye covered, and in full light or dim light.

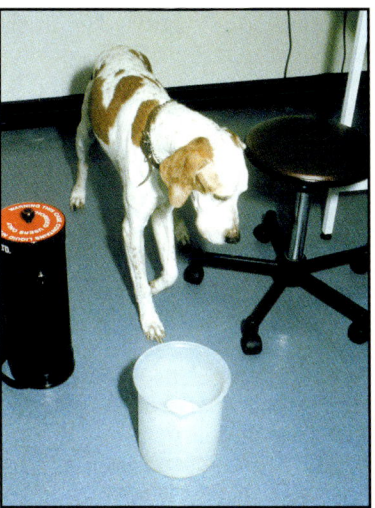

Figure 1.3 An obstacle course can be constructed easily for a maze test. (Courtesy of DJ Gould.)

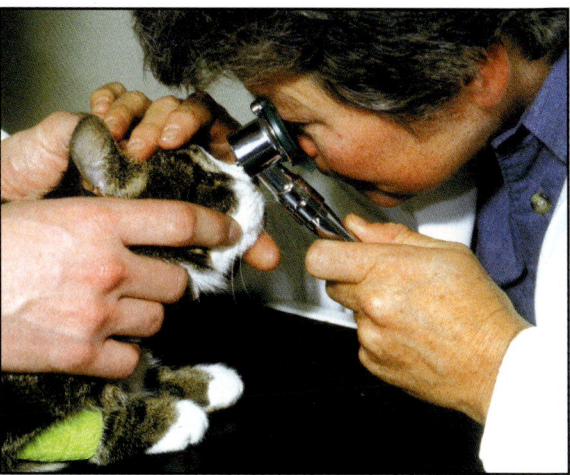

Figure 1.5 An otoscope is a simple means of providing both a light source and magnification. (Courtesy of SM Crispin.)

Examination in a darkened room, with focal illumination and magnification

The penlight or transilluminator should now be used with only a background light, or in darkness (Figure 1.4). This eliminates unwanted reflections and aids concentration on the features under study. If magnification is needed, this may be obtained using a head loupe or by using an otoscope (Figure 1.5).

1. Examine the adnexa, paying particular attention to the lid margins and conjunctival surfaces.
2. Examine the cornea, looking for lesions such as irregularities, opacities, vascularization, pigmentation etc., along with their depth and distribution.
3. Continue with the anterior chamber, noting its depth and any abnormal contents. When examining the anterior chamber; it is important to direct the light beam from various angles and also to look at it from different angles.
4. Examine the iris and pupil margin and then the lens. Mydriasis is usually necessary for full examination of the lens, but much may be learned from distant direct ophthalmoscopy (see below), which does not require the use of mydriatics.
5. Test the pupillary light reflexes. Observe the pupil size in normal room light initially. With the lights down, direct a bright light axially through the pupil in a distinct on/off fashion, observing the speed and extent of the pupillary constriction. In the 'swinging flashlight test', the light is directed at each eye alternately, with the observer noting the direct and consensual responses. Where there is a unilateral afferent pupillary defect, the affected pupil will dilate on stimulation.

The pupil size at rest and the light reflexes do vary between patients, as will the examiner's technique and the brightness of the light source used. Very anxious patients may have a larger pupil size and show a diminished response, due to raised circulating adrenaline. For these reasons, the test is difficult to quantify, but may be the best available indicator of afferent function, depending on the circumstances. A consistent method and repeated practice will aid interpretation. It is important to note that cataracts do not significantly affect the pupillary light reflex.

The dazzle reflex may be tested by shining a very bright light into the pupil. The normal response should be a rapid blink. This is a further test of afferent function (and should be normal in the presence of a cataract) but, unlike the menace response, the dazzle reflex is sub-cortical. Further details of neuro-ophthalmological testing and interpretation may be found in Chapter 15.

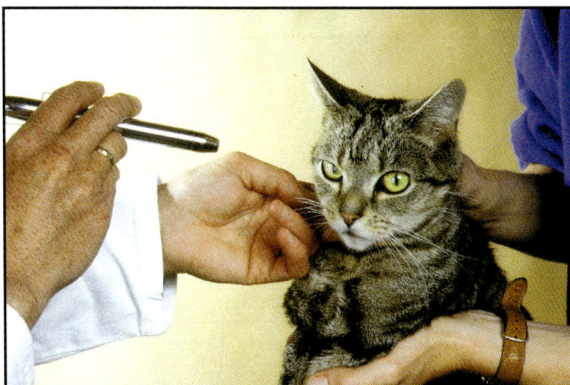

Figure 1.4 Penlight examination. The light should be used from as many different angles as possible. (Courtesy of SM Crispin.)

Ophthalmoscopy

Not all patients will require a full fundic examination (and of those that do, some will have pupils of adequate size) but, whenever necessary, the pupils should be dilated with tropicamide 1% and 20 minutes should be allowed for it to achieve its maximum effect. Examining the fundus through too small a pupil is a difficult and frustrating exercise, particularly for the beginner or non-specialist, and the experience will be a deterrent to ophthalmoscopy on the next occasion. Dogs and cats have potentially large pupils, and full advantage should be taken of this. Owners are not usually resentful that their time is being wasted; rather, they appreciate the thoroughness of the examination. Other patients can be seen while the drops are taking effect.

Nursing staff should be informed about what is required in restraint for ophthalmoscopic examination. Good handling can be very helpful. An assistant can hold the head steady with a hand under the angle of the jaw and the other hand holding the eyelids apart if necessary. The assistant's hands should not interfere with the clinician's access to the eye. With fractious animals, the risk of injury must always be minimized but, in general, only an appropriate level of restraint should be used. Some dogs resent having the muzzle held too tightly.

Distant direct ophthalmoscopy

This is a very useful technique, and strongly recommended. The room should be darkened, but mydriatic drops are not required. Set the ophthalmoscope to +1 to +2 D and find the tapetal reflex (the green or yellow light reflected from the tapetum) by looking into the pupil horizontally or slightly upwards. The examination is conducted at arm's length and there is no benefit in being closer (Figure 1.6).

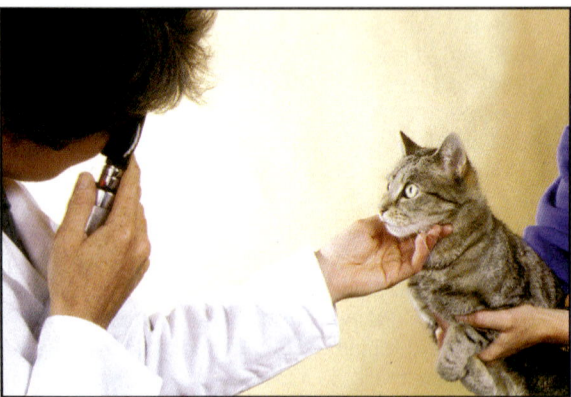

Figure 1.6 Distant direct ophthalmoscopy. (Courtesy of SM Crispin.)

The essence of the technique is that any genuine opacity in the path of the tapetal reflex will obscure it and appear black. This provides a very good rapid assessment of the degree and distribution of opacity in the visual axis. The method is of particular value with cataracts, but any opacity in the path of the light such as corneal and vitreous opacities will also appear black.

Nuclear (senile) sclerosis is a normal ageing change and gives the nucleus of the lens a hazy look in all older animals. It should not be confused with cataracts, and the two can be easily distinguished by distant direct ophthalmoscopy. Nuclear sclerosis shows as a refractile ring at the nuclear cortical interface, usually just inside the pupil margin, but there are no black areas and light is transmitted normally through the centre of the lens, even though it looks hazy in direct light. Nuclear sclerosis and cataracts may well be present in the same lens in older dogs. The clinician can also move from eye to eye to compare symmetry of gaze and pupil size (provided that no mydriatics have been used).

Lesions can be roughly localized in an anteroposterior direction, by taking advantage of the effect of parallax. As the observer moves to one side, the opacity may also appear to move. The direction of this movement can give an indication as to the location of the opacity. Opacities anterior to the plane of the pupil will appear to move in the opposite direction. Opacities in the plane of the pupil (i.e. anterior cataracts), will remain in the same position. Opacities posterior to the plane of the pupil will appear to move in the same direction as the observer. Posterior polar cataracts, for example, can be made to disappear completely under the side of the pupil towards which the observer has moved.

Close direct ophthalmoscopy

The fundus cannot be seen by direct inspection with a focal light. The direct ophthalmoscope is, therefore, a means by which a structure that could not otherwise be seen may be examined. The image is upright and highly magnified, but the field of view is very narrow.

The correct position may be assumed in one of two ways. One method is to start a little distance from the eye and to obtain a tapetal reflex. Keeping this in view, move closer until the fundus comes into focus. Alternatively, and more safely, the hands and ophthalmoscope may be positioned first and then the instrument is approached (Figure 1.7).

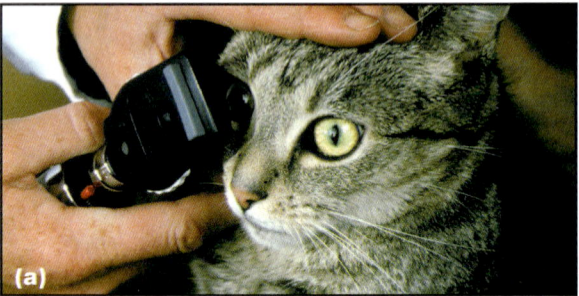

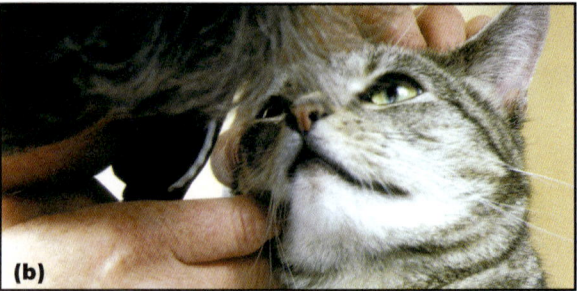

Figure 1.7 Close direct ophthalmoscopy. (a) Placing the ophthalmoscope. (b) Viewing the eye. Note that the fingers holding the ophthalmoscope are resting against the patient's head and that excessive restraint is unnecessary, unless the patient is dangerous if unrestrained. (Courtesy of SM Crispin.)

The ophthalmoscope should be held vertically, touching the examiner's orbital margin, and be close to the patient's eye, so as to maximize the field of view and eliminate distractions such as the iris (Figure 1.8). The ophthalmoscope should be set between −1 and +1 D for most patients. The light intensity should be sufficient for the purpose, but no more. Some animals understandably resent bright light settings and this is a particular risk with mains powered units.

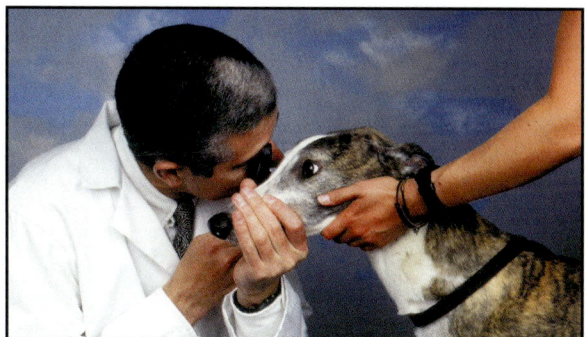

Figure 1.8 Close direct ophthalmoscopy. The head is being restrained correctly, with the hand under the mandible. The eye that is closer to the dog is being used for the ophthalmoscopy. The ophthalmoscope must be close to both the clinician's eye and the patient's eye.

1. Find the optic disc initially, as this is more or less at the posterior pole. Evaluate the disc for size, swelling, colour, blood vessels, etc.
2. Make a systematic examination of the fundus. One effective method is to divide it into quadrants and to examine each in turn. Avoid wide changes of direction, as the patient is probably doing the same, and areas may be missed. Indeed, the patient's own eye movements are often sufficient to allow the clinician to see most areas of the fundus. Attempt to see as far into the periphery as possible; this requires very positive movements of the head and neck on the examiner's part. Concentrate on keeping the light beam directed through the pupil when the angle of view is changed. Evaluate the retina for normal variation or changes in colour, reflectivity, pigment, haemorrhage, oedema and detachment.

    The direct ophthalmoscope gives a highly magnified image providing superb detail, but only a very small area of the fundus is seen at one time. The examiner, therefore, has to create a mental montage of the fundic appearance from a series of small images. As the patient inevitably moves its eyes, the examiner is moved to new fields which may be difficult to relate to the previous field. These are the most difficult aspects of direct ophthalmoscopy, but they do become easier with practice.
3. Then examine the fellow eye. Ideally, the examiner should always look through the ophthalmoscope with the eye closest to the patient (i.e. the left eye for the patient's left eye and the right for the patient's right). This gives the best access for examining the fundus as fully as possible. Some people find it difficult to use both eyes, though this can be practised. Whatever the technique, every effort should be made to cover as much of the fundus as possible in both eyes.
4. Finally, focus back through to the anterior eye, as required. It is, of course, equally acceptable to proceed from anterior to posterior. Unless the presence of vitreal abnormalities is suspected, it is usually simpler to select a setting of around +10 D to bring the lens into focus, the exact setting depending partly on the distance from the eye. This gives a good view of the lens, but with less magnification than for the fundus. Higher positive lenses of +15 to +20 D are required to examine structures anterior to the lens. With anterior structures, the examiner can simply retain the ophthalmoscope in position and then select progressively more strongly positive lenses until the features of interest are in focus. The absolute lens settings used are not significant and depend anyway on the distance from the eye.

Indirect ophthalmoscopy

All forms of indirect ophthalmoscopy require an adequately dilated pupil and a reasonably cooperative patient.

Binocular

Binocular indirect ophthalmoscopes offer various options and adjustments for the user according to the individual instrument. The light intensity can be varied but only an adequate level of light should be used, since indirect ophthalmoscopy is relatively bright for the patient. Some offer different beam types and settings for different pupil sizes. The user should be familiar with these options and the manufacturer's guidelines for their use before beginning. The instrument should be adjusted to give a clear view with the beam in or just above the centre of the field.

Essentially the lens is positioned in front of the patent's eye to form a wide-angle aerial image of the fundus. The lens is held between the index finger and thumb, and one or more of the other fingers should rest on the frontal sinus area for stability (Figure 1.9). Positioning of the lens is much the most important part of the technique and the most likely to be at fault if the image is poor.

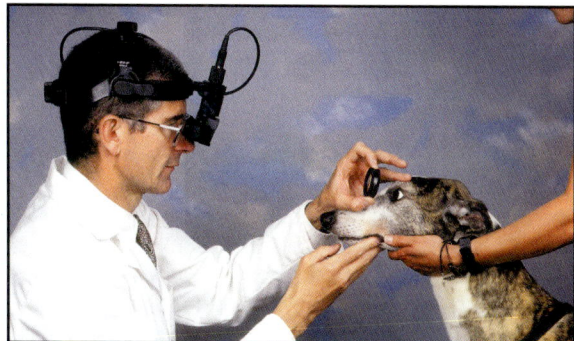

Figure 1.9 Binocular indirect ophthalmoscopy. This gives a wide-angle view of the fundus with stereopsis.

- The axis of the lens must lie on the same axis as the pupil (a relatively small movement away from this axis will lose the image)
- The lens must be at the correct working distance from the eye
- The lens must be parallel to the iris and not tilted
- In the correct position, the image of the fundus should fill the field of view of the lens.

One method for the beginner is to start with the lens close to the patient's eye (when iris and lids will still be visible) and then withdraw it along the axis of the pupil until the fundus image fills the field of view. A steady hand, making slow adjustments to position, is preferable to wide sudden movements. The technique requires practice, but no more than for the direct ophthalmoscope, and once acquired the correct positioning of the lens becomes rapid and instinctive. The wide-angle view can be very informative and adjusting to the inverted, reversed image is easier than might be imagined. Initially, the findings can simply be recorded 'as seen'.

Monocular

For those without a binocular instrument, a simple and effective form of indirect ophthalmoscopy may be carried out using only a hand lens and a focal light source such as a penlight or transilluminator and no apparatus on the head. Stereopsis is not possible and the examiner's second hand is now committed to holding the light source but these are minor disadvantages compared to the benefits of the wide-angle view at low cost. The light source is held against the examiner's temple or in front of the nose, making sure that the observer's eye, the light source, the lens and the patient's pupil all lie on the same axis as far as possible (Figure 1.10).

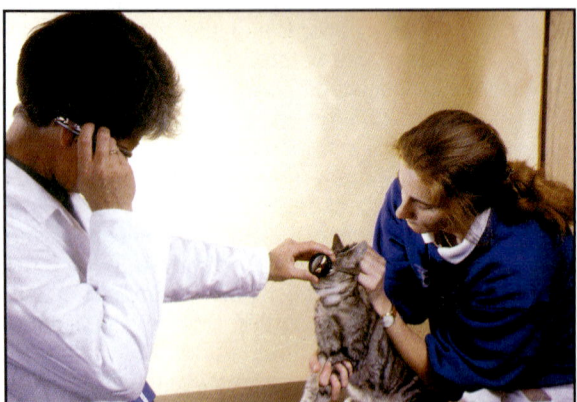

Figure 1.10 Monocular indirect ophthalmoscopy. Note that the fingers holding the lens are in contact with the patient's head. (Courtesy of SM Crispin.)

Further tests and examination techniques
Schirmer tear test

The Schirmer tear test uses standardized strips of filter paper to quantify aqueous tear production. The strips are supplied in sterile packs of two. Some manufacturers may include instructions for performing and interpreting the test in people, but different timings are used in animals. Where a deficiency in tear production is suggested by the clinical findings, the tear test should be carried out before any drops or irrigating fluids are used on the eye. The strips are notched near one end and should be bent slightly at the notch before removal from the pack. It is preferable to avoid touching the short end of the strip with the fingers, so as to maintain sterility and to avoid depositing cutaneous lipid on the paper, which might interfere with aqueous tear absorption.

The short end of the strip is then placed in the lateral half of the lower conjunctival sac so that the notch is at the level of the lid margin and the strip is in contact with the lower lid and the cornea (Figure 1.11). In most cases, it is best for the examiner to hold the lids closed, retaining the strip securely in position.

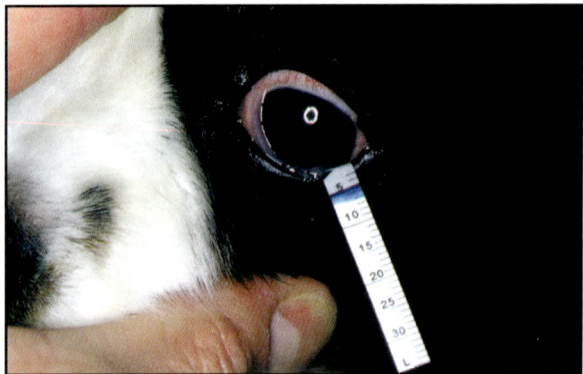

Figure 1.11 Schirmer tear test paper in position. In many dogs, it is best to hold the lids together during the test.

Schirmer I test: The Schirmer I test measures aqueous production over one minute in an unanaesthetized eye, and is therefore measuring basal and reflex tear production. At the end of one minute the strip is removed and the flow of aqueous tears recorded, either by measuring against the template on the box or from the graduations printed on the strip itself.

Normal values for the Schirmer I test in the dog are a mean of 20 mm and a minimum of 15 mm. The range 10–15mm is often referred to as borderline, but evidence of irritation and changes attributable to dry eye can usually be found in dogs with <15 mm. Lower normal values are usually quoted for the cat and the pattern of disease is often different.

The Schirmer I test has proved to be the most useful in veterinary ophthalmology and is the test on which most of the veterinary literature on deficient tear production is based.

Schirmer II test: The Schirmer II test measures basal tear production only, by eliminating reflex tear production induced by contact with the cornea and conjunctiva. One or two drops of local anaesthetic are applied to the eye, the excess is blotted away with a swab or cotton wool, and a few minutes are allowed to elapse. The test is then performed as above. Values will be lower than for the Schirmer I test but typically not lower than 50% of the Schirmer I reading and, in cats, about 80% of the value. The Schirmer II test is used in human patients, where high reflex tear production may mask low basal tear production. This situation probably does arise in animals but the test is not commonly performed. Diagnosis of dry eye in cats and dogs is described fully in Chapter 6.

Fluorescein

Fluorescein is an orange dye that changes to green in alkaline conditions such as contact with saline solution or the tear film. It is highly lipophobic and hydrophilic. Thus, when it is applied to the surface of the eye it does not remain in contact with the lipid-containing cell membranes of the corneal epithelium but adheres to, and is absorbed by, any exposed corneal stroma. It is, therefore, of great value in the diagnosis of corneal ulcers, where the epithelium is absent and stroma is exposed. Fluorescein is detectable in minute concentrations, especially when viewed in blue light. Only disposable sources should be used, such as impregnated strips or single dose vials, since multi-dose bottles are readily colonised by *Pseudomonas aeruginosa*, a potentially serious corneal pathogen.

The strip should be wetted with sterile saline or water (this may not be necessary in patients with ample tear production) and touched to the dorsal or ventral bulbar conjunctiva (Figure 1.12). Alternatively, one drop of fluorescein solution can be applied to the eye. The eye is then irrigated with further saline to flush excess fluorescein from the ocular surface.

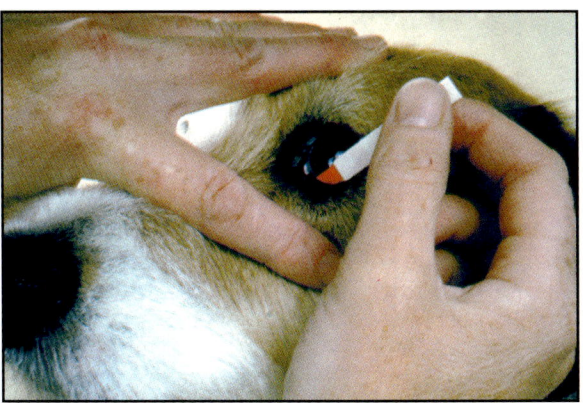

Figure 1.12 Fluorescein application using a strip in the lower conjunctival sac. (Courtesy of SM Crispin.)

Interpretation does not usually present problems. Positive staining indicates a defect in the epithelium and, hence, an ulcer. Fluorescein will not stain healed ulcers that have re-epithelialized, even if there is still an obvious concavity as a result of stromal loss. Irrigation is important in flushing fluorescein from such surface defects, in order to prevent a false impression of dye uptake. Irrigation will not flush dye from exposed corneal stroma in the case of genuine ulcers. Under-run epithelium at the edge of ulcers is well demonstrated by fluorescein. If interpretation is difficult, especially where minute punctate staining is suspected, then the use of magnification and a blue light source may be helpful. Descemet's membrane does not stain with fluorescein, so a clear area in the centre of a deep ulcer may be an ominous, rather than an encouraging, sign.

Fluorescein is a valuable tool in the diagnosis of ulceration and should be used routinely. It usually gives unequivocal results and there are no contraindications. Corneal ulcers cannot always be diagnosed on simple appearance alone and so it is often said that every red painful eye should receive a fluorescein test and an IOP measurement. Even in the presence of corneal perforations, sterile fluorescein is not harmful to intraocular tissues. Indeed, fluorescein may be applied to the eye in the Seidel test, when a small leaking hole in the cornea is suspected. When a hole is present, aqueous humour can be seen running through the film of fluorescein on the corneal surface, turning it a bright apple green (see Chapter 8). Fluorescein is easily seen by owners, and this aids in client understanding of the patient's problem.

Fluorescein test for nasolacrimal patency: Where tear overflow is suspected to be due to poor drainage, rather than increased lacrimation, fluorescein can be used in a simple functional test of nasolacrimal drainage. Further details of nasolacrimal disease can be found in Chapter 6.

Fluorescein angiography: This provides additional information about fundic lesions that are not visible by simple ophthalmoscopy. However, this test is used infrequently in veterinary medicine. Fluorescein is injected intravenously and then the passage of the dye is visualized as it passes through the fundic vasculature and associated tissues. The fundus is viewed via a camera fitted with exciter and barrier interference filters which, respectively, stimulate fluorescence by the dye and filter out other wavelengths of light reflected from the fundus. The result is that the film (or other recording medium) effectively only records the fluorescein. This provides valuable information about the retinal and choriocapillaris vascular systems through which the fluorescein travels and also indicates areas of ischaemia, sites of vascular leakage and hyper- and hypofluorescence in a variety of lesions.

It is usual to take rapid sequential photographs within a few seconds of injection as the dye enters the arterial system, and then to follow its passage through the venous system. The frequency of photography reduces, until finally so-called late stage appearances are recorded after several minutes.

The method may also be used in the investigation of the anterior segment, for example if there is an iris lesion, but is less informative with dark irises, which excludes most dogs.

The injection can cause allergic reactions and even anaphylactic shock, and appropriate precautions must be in place before the start of the procedure.

Fluorescein angiography is very widely used in human patients and there is a wealth of medical literature on the subject. The technique has been limited in the veterinary field by problems of restraint of the patient and the cost of the necessary equipment, as well as problems associated with differences of anatomy such as the degree of pigmentation and the presence of a tapetum.

The patient must be effectively immobile for the crucial initial seconds of the passage of the dye, as this cannot be repeated. Deep sedation or general anaesthesia is therefore required. Even where the facilities are available, the clinician must weigh the likely usefulness of the information against the difficulties of obtaining it. Oral fluorescein avoids some of the technical problems, but the dye accumulates more slowly in the tissues, allowing for only late stage photographs.

Posterior segment vascular and inflammatory disease is common in both the dog and the cat. Vasculopathy associated with systemic hypertensive disease in particular is now recognized as an important veterinary problem. Fluorescein angiography would add considerably to the understanding of some of these diseases in animals and, notwithstanding the technical difficulties, the method may become more widely used in specialist centres in the future.

Rose bengal

Rose bengal is a dark magenta dye that stains dead and devitalized tissue. It is slightly irritant on application. Rose bengal is widely used in human patients to demonstrate ocular surface damage in cases of dry eye (see Chapter 6). It is also a particularly useful diagnostic aid in the diagnosis of some forms of herpetic keratitis in the cat, where the damaged area may not stain with fluorescein. It is likely that rose bengal is undervalued in veterinary work and could be more widely used in the management of ocular surface disease.

Cannulation and flushing of the tear drainage system

The anatomical patency of the nasolacrimal drainage system may be investigated by cannulation and flushing via the lacrimal puncta as described in Chapter 6.

Ocular ultrasonography

Ultrasonography of the eye is useful in the same circumstances as in other organs: namely, in providing good soft tissue detail when this is not visible clinically or radiographically. There is the additional benefit of the production of a dynamic image. Opacity of the cornea, anterior chamber, lens or vitreous may impede visual examination of intraocular tissues, making ultrasonography very useful in these cases. Furthermore, ultrasonography may be useful in cases of anterior iris displacement (iris bombé or iris thickening), intraocular tumours (to assess their size and extent), preoperative cataract assessment, vitreous opacity and detachment, possible sub-retinal masses and posterior scleral lesions. Ultrasound is also very sensitive in identifying retinal detachment.

Ultrasonography is safe and painless. Sedation is optional, depending on the individual patient and the operator's preference. General anaesthesia is not usually necessary and the ventral rotation of the globe under general anaesthesia may be a problem.

Local anaesthetic drops are applied repeatedly to the cornea. The probe, with adequate amounts of ultrasound gel, is then applied directly to the cornea, which avoids the problems inherent in using hairy skin. Excessive pressure should not be used. Deep tissue penetration is not required for the globe alone, so it is best to use the highest frequency probe available, commonly 7.5–10.0 MHz, to maximize tissue resolution. The probe is applied to the cornea and then moved vertically and horizontally across the eye to cover the entire globe. For the orbit, a lower frequency probe may be preferable; the orbit can be imaged obliquely though the region of the orbital ligament. The technique is described in detail and images shown in Chapter 1b.

Slit lamp biomicroscopy

The slit lamp biomicroscope is the best instrument for examining the anterior segment and adnexa, combining higher magnification (at least 10X) with bright focused illumination and a choice of full or slit beams (Figure 1.13). It derives its name from its ability to illuminate tissues with a slit beam of light, showing an optical section of transparent structures such as the cornea, aqueous, lens and anterior vitreous.

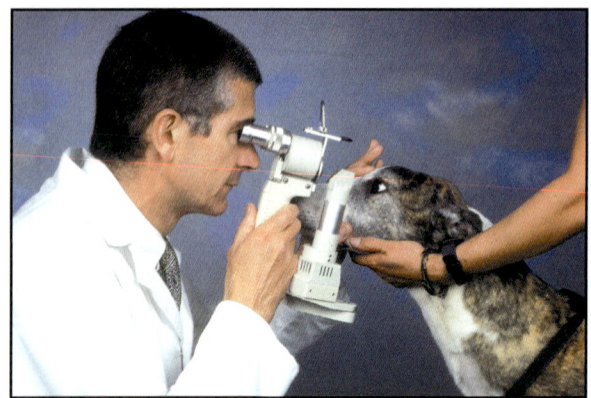

Figure 1.13 Slit lamp biomicroscopy. The portable slit lamp gives an excellent magnified view of the adnexa and anterior segment. It is not a difficult technique, but cost has been the main limitation for general use.

The full beam is also useful for examination of fine detail in the adnexa. With the use of a special fundic hand lens, an excellent wide angle stereoptic view can be obtained of the posterior vitreous and retina. Portable slit lamp biomicroscopes are most commonly used in veterinary work; cordless models are especially useful (Figure 1.14). They are relatively easy to use but are expensive, and tend to be limited to those with a special interest in ophthalmology.

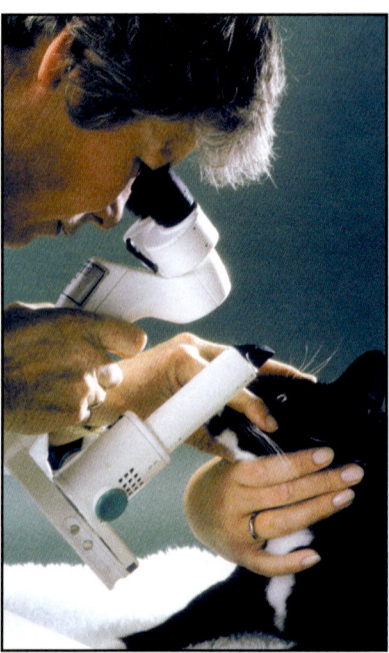

Figure 1.14 Slit lamp biomicroscopy using a rechargeable cordless model. (Courtesy of SM Crispin.)

Specular microscopy

The corneal endothelium is a monolayer of cells forming the deepest layer of the cornea; it is in contact with the aqueous humour in the anterior chamber. The main action of the endothelium is in maintaining the cornea in a state of relative dehydration by pumping water into the aqueous.

The specular microscope provides a highly magnified image of the endothelial cells. The cells can then be evaluated for their density in each area and variations in their size and shape.

Specular microscopes for veterinary use are currently found in only a few specialist centres. Endothelial disease is not rare in animals, particularly in the dog, where chronic endothelial degeneration can lead to bullous keratopathy and painful refractory ulcers. The use of specular microscopy is, therefore, likely to increase in time.

Retinoscopy

A retinoscope is a handheld instrument, similar in size and cost to an ophthalmoscope, which provides a means of objectively measuring the refractive power of an eye (i.e. how accurately light rays are focused on to the plane of the retina). Historically, refractive error, i.e. long and short sight, has not been a significant part of veterinary ophthalmology, for various reasons:

- Most animals' refraction is probably near normal
- Refractive error is effectively not treatable
- The most familiar method of measuring the refraction of the eye in people requires responses from the patient and is therefore not possible in animals.

The refraction of canine eyes is now of interest, however, as a result of the increasing use of intraocular lenses to correct the large refractive error resulting from cataract and lens luxation surgery. Use of the retinoscope is, therefore, likely to increase among veterinary intraocular surgeons.

Ocular centesis

There are situations where it is potentially informative to analyse a sample of cells or fluid from within the eye. Examples would include the differential diagnosis of inflammatory, infectious or neoplastic disease. Ocular centesis avoids more invasive diagnostic procedures and may lead to earlier or more specific diagnosis and, hence, treatment.

Technique: Samples may be obtained from the anterior or the vitreous chamber. General anaesthesia may be required. Using a 25 gauge needle, or finer, the anterior chamber is entered via the conjunctiva and scleral shelf dorsally, where there is a relatively elongated zone of overlapping cornea and sclera overlying the anterior chamber and anterior to the drainage angle. The needle is introduced into the aqueous, taking care to avoid the deep cornea, the iris and the lens, and sample material is aspirated. The vitreous may be entered via the sclera overlying the pars plana. The needle is advanced into the vitreous, avoiding the lens and retina.

When ocular centesis is undertaken in the differential diagnosis of an iris tumour, it may be useful to run the needle carefully over the iris surface while applying a slight negative pressure, in order to sample surface cells.

In all cases, material aspirated can be submitted for cytology and/or culture, according to the circumstances of the case.

The wound is self-sealing; it is usual to apply antibiotic ointment and one drop of atropine to the eye after the procedure.

The procedure requires some expertise and familiarity with ocular anatomy, and should only be used where its potential contribution to the management of the case is clearly understood.

Complications and problems:

- The consequences of cornea, iris and, particularly, lens trauma during the procedure could be serious
- As with many investigative techniques, there remains the possibility of inconclusive or false negative results
- Tumour cells shed into the aqueous may be unrepresentative of the main tumour mass, which may contain a mixed population, or the aspirate may consist only of cell debris
- Intraocular bacterial infection is much more likely to establish in the vitreous than the aqueous, regardless of the route of entry
- Lens rupture may recruit large numbers of polymorphonuclear neutrophils to the area, even when the eye is sterile.

Cytology should, therefore, always be interpreted by a pathologist with appropriate experience.

Electroretinography

Electroretinography (ERG) records electrical discharges from the retina in response to external light stimulation. General anaesthesia is usually necessary. An electrode is applied to the cornea in the form of a contact lens and reference and ground needle electrodes are applied to the skin of the head. Under standardized conditions, the eye is stimulated by flashes of light and the responses recorded. The output consists of a wave form composed of a-, b- and c-waves, which can then be interpreted in terms of different aspects of retinal function. Other electrophysiological techniques such as visual evoked potentials (VEPs) are less commonly employed.

ERG is valuable in canine ophthalmology in particular, as there are several circumstances in which retinal function cannot be interpreted from the ophthalmoscopic appearance alone (see Chapter 14a). ERG is used in the preoperative assessment of retinal function in dogs with advanced cataracts.

There are also situations in which dogs may be showing poor vision in the presence of a normal fundic appearance. In these cases, ERG can indicate whether the retinal function is normal and, hence, whether the possibility of optic nerve or intracranial disease should be considered.

Retinal photography

Good quality photographs of the fundus can be valuable in the documentation of lesions, in research and in education. Modern fundus cameras are very sophisticated, with the addition of numerous features and options, producing high quality images.

For various reasons, it is difficult for veterinary surgeons to be able to take full advantage of these instruments. They are expensive (and photography in itself does not usually generate income) and they are table mounted, making patient access and positioning difficult. Hand-held fundus cameras have, therefore, traditionally been used for animals. They give much better access to the patient, but only give a relatively narrow field of view, and they cannot be used for fluorescein angiography without additional equipment. However, they are very good for anterior segment photography, giving high resolution images.

During the early use of a fundus camera, the operator can expect to undergo a learning curve. Common mistakes include having the camera too far from the patient's eye, resulting in a white mark on the photograph, or photographing obliquely through the pupil, resulting in black or out-of-focus areas.

There may also be problems with the exposure. The high proportion of light reflected from the tapetum easily leads to overexposure of fundus photographs in animals. In contrast, much more light is required for correct exposure of the anterior segment. Ideally, the lowest and highest settings of the camera will be able to cope with these two extremes, but it will be necessary for the operator to experiment with film speeds and light settings to determine the optimum protocol.

Further reading

Ballantyne AJ and Michaelson IC (1970) Methodical investigation of the fundus. In: *Textbook of the Fundus of the Eye, 2nd edn*, pp. 1–52. Livingstone, Edinburgh and London

Duke-Elder S and Smith RJH (1962) Clinical methods of examination. In: *System of Ophthalmology, Volume VII. The Foundations of Ophthalmology*, ed. S. Duke-Elder pp. 233–458. Henry Kimpton, London

Strubbe DT and Gelatt KN (1999) Ophthalmic examination and diagnostic procedures. In: *Veterinary Ophthalmology, 3rd edn*, ed. KN Gelatt pp. 427–466. Lippincott, Williams and Wilkins, Philadelphia

1b

Ocular imaging

Elizabeth Munro and David T. Ramsey

Introduction

During the last 20 years, there have been many innovations in diagnostic imaging, including the development of a variety of new imaging modalities that have improved the clinician's ability to diagnose ocular and orbital disease. However, conventional radiography and B mode ultrasonography remain the most widely used forms of imaging, because the advanced diagnostic imaging methods have restricted availability and are relatively expensive for use in private veterinary practice.

B mode ultrasonography is indicated in the assessment of intraocular structures when direct visualization is not possible. It should be the initial imaging technique used for all animals with signs of orbital disease, as general anaesthesia is not required. A suggested protocol for the investigation of orbital disease (adapted from Dennis, 2000) is shown in Figure 1.15.

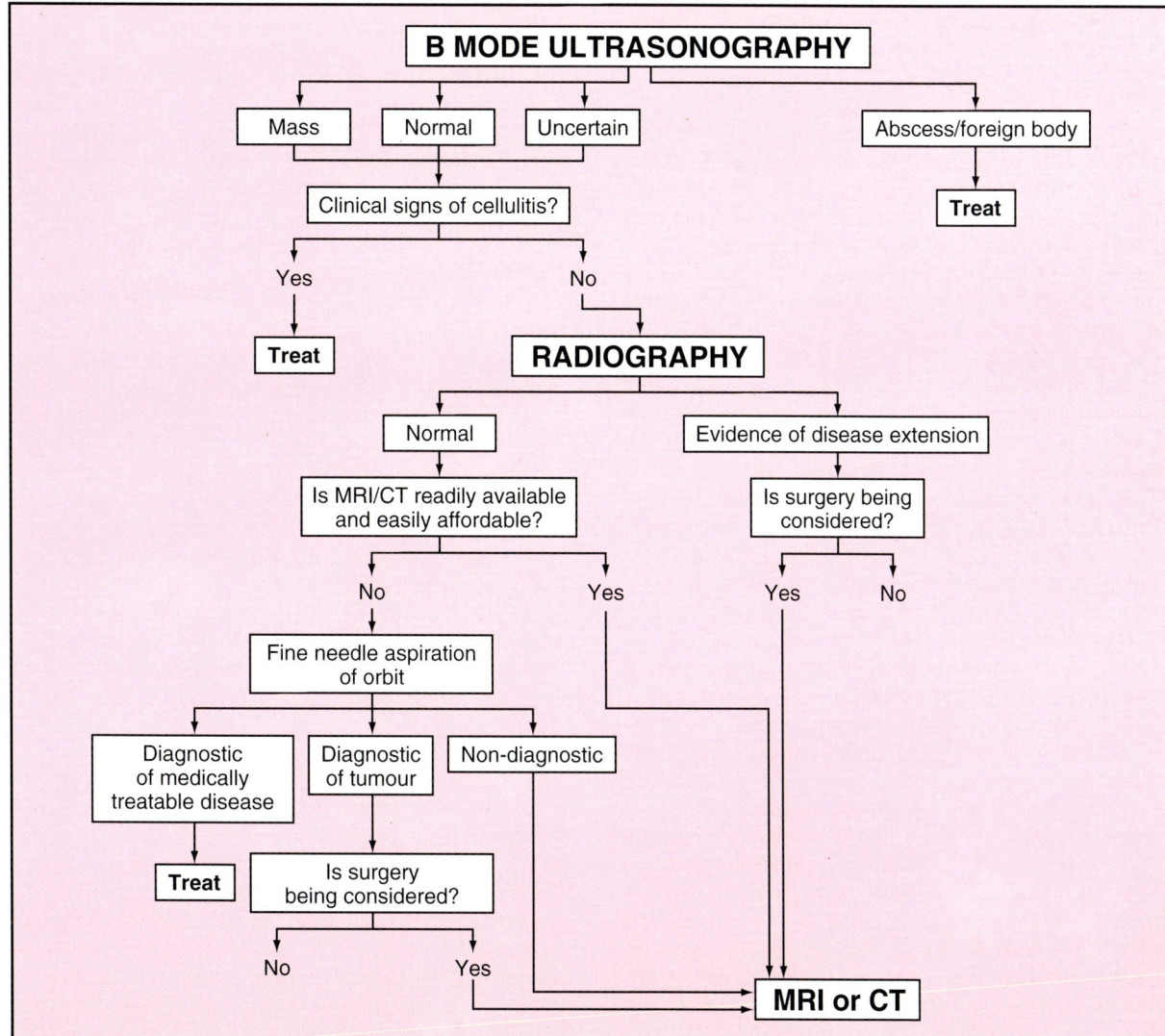

Figure 1.15 A suggested protocol for the investigation of orbital disease (adapted from Dennis, 2000).

14 Ocular imaging

Further imaging techniques are computed tomography (CT) and magnetic resonance imaging (MRI). The image quality provided by MRI is superior to that of CT in most animals, except in cases of orbital trauma. However, longer scanning times are required with MRI, and there is restricted access for animal monitoring; these factors should also be considered when selecting the most appropriate technique for a particular animal. With the limited availability of both MRI and CT to the veterinary profession, however, a choice between the two rarely exists.

Radiography

Plain film radiography

Plain film radiography is only diagnostic for conditions involving alterations in architecture of the bony orbit, and in the detection of radiopaque foreign bodies within the orbit or globe. Use of alternative imaging modalities (cross-sectional imaging) is recommended for soft-tissue imaging.

Radiography is used to investigate retrobulbar mass lesions, in order to detect the presence of bone lysis in osseous orbital, or neighbouring, structures. Lysis is most readily appreciated when the destruction of bone involves the nasal chamber and paranasal sinuses.

Dental disease

Apical lysis of caudal maxillary dental structures (e.g. tooth root, alveolus) attributable to dental disease also occurs and is one of the most common causes of inflammatory orbital disease (abscess and cellulitis) in dogs. When inflammatory orbital disease is suspected and the results of orbital echography (ultrasonography) are inconclusive or are normal, dental radiographs are indicated.

Orbital neoplasia

When orbital neoplasia is suspected, the appropriate views should be taken; general anaesthesia is required. These include the intraoral and open-mouth views of the nasal cavity, and the skyline view of the frontal sinuses. The intraoral view of the nasal cavity is the most sensitive for the detection of subtle nasal turbinate lysis. High definition intraoral film should be used, and the film placed, corner first, as far back into the mouth as possible. This view will not include the bony orbit, however, which is best assessed with a ventrorostral–dorsocaudal view of the nasal cavity.

To obtain the open-mouthed ventrorostral–dorsocaudal view, the animal is positioned in dorsal recumbency. The jaws are opened maximally and secured by separate lengths of crepe bandage, or similar material, around the upper and lower canine teeth. The beam is directed toward the cranium through the open mouth at an angle of approximately 20 degrees, i.e. parallel to the mandibles. The abbreviated description, V20°R–DCdO, describes the direction of the beam from entry to exit point (V = ventro; 20° = beam angle; D = dorso; Cd = caudo; O = oblique). Regardless of positioning, superimposition of bone in the orbital region and the breed variation seen in canine skull shape or conformation hinder interpretation, but as malignant orbital disease is asymmetrical, careful scrutiny may reveal loss of bone on one side (Figure 1.16).

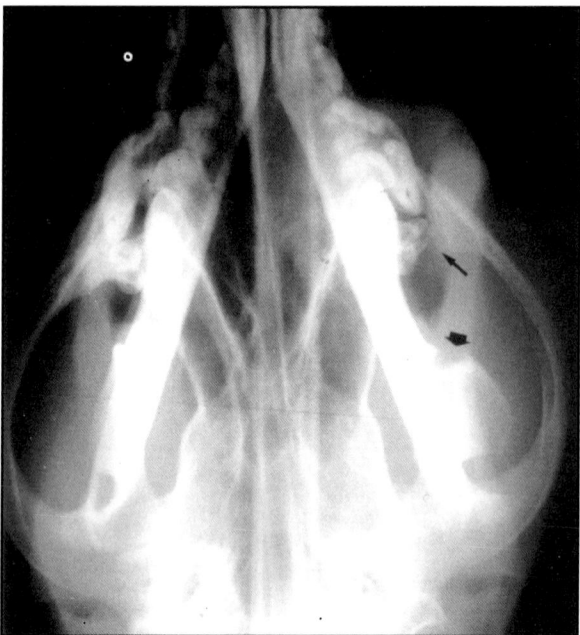

Figure 1.16 Dorsoventral radiograph of the head of an 18-month-old Rottweiler with a poorly differentiated sarcoma of the orbit. Bone lysis is identified around the alveolus of M1 (long arrow), and the rostral border of the vertical ramus of the mandible (short arrow). There is soft tissue opacification of the nasal cavity on the affected side, and soft tissue swelling over the rostral zygomatic arch.

Frontal sinuses

The frontal sinuses should be evaluated using a rostrocaudal view, obtained by positioning the animal in dorsal recumbency with the atlanto-occipital joint in flexion, until the hard palate is at right angles to the film. The beam is directed through the frontal sinuses and parallel to the hard palate.

In animals with orbital disease, opacification of the frontal sinuses may be attributable to neoplastic infiltration or, more commonly, to fluid accumulation caused by a mass obstructing the drainage of the sinus(es) through the nasal cavity.

In some cases, oblique lateral projections may be rewarding. Thoracic and abdominal radiographs, to look for evidence of metastatic disease, should also be considered when malignant disease is suspected.

Bone lysis

Radiographic evidence of bone lysis involving the bony orbit and/or the nasal cavity generally indicates malignancy or deep mycotic osteomyelitis, and a poor prognosis. If surgery is considered in these animals, further assessment of the anatomical extent of the disease process should be performed with CT or, preferably, MRI.

However, radiographic evidence of bone destruction is not a feature of all malignant orbital neoplasms. When evidence of bone lysis is not apparent, orbital malignancy cannot be distinguished radiographically from benign inflammatory orbital disease.

Contrast techniques

Dacryocystography

Dacryocystography is occasionally performed in the diagnostic investigation of epiphora and ocular discharge, to evaluate the anatomical course of the nasolacrimal system. The technique is straightforward, but rarely performed. It is indicated in animals with obstruction of the nasolacrimal system, when the cause of obstruction is not apparent on plain film radiography, or when an intraluminal foreign body is suspected.

Technique: Under general anaesthesia the upper lacrimal punctum is cannulated with an appropriate size of cannula (21 G for dogs, 26 G for cats). A small volume (1–2 ml) of water-soluble iodinated contrast material is gently injected via the cannula, while the lower punctum is gently occluded using fine mosquito forceps. In the rabbit, the sole lower punctum is cannulated. Lateral and ventrodorsal views should be obtained immediately after or during injection so that leakage from the nasal ostium does not interfere with visualization of the duct.

Cranial sinus venography

This technique was developed to demonstrate mass lesions, either in the orbit or in the region of the cavernous sinuses, at the floor of the cranial vault. The cavernous sinuses lie close to the pituitary gland and to the second, third, fourth and sixth cranial nerves. Masses adjacent to the vessels can alter the course of the vasculature, or create filling defects by extramural compression. CT and MRI, if available, are superior to this technique.

Technique: General anaesthesia is required. The technique is safe and applicable to the practice situation, but it is time-consuming and interpretation can be difficult. A plain film dorsoventral view of the skull is obtained, following the induction of general anaesthesia. A large roll of gauze is placed longitudinally over the jugular furrow lateral to the trachea on each side of the neck. The rolls of gauze are secured with tape around the neck to occlude the jugular veins, but to spare occlusion of the airway. The angularis oculi veins can be visualized through the skin at the medial canthus. The skin on both sides overlying the angularis oculi veins is clipped and scrubbed. A catheter is then placed transcutaneously into the angularis oculi vein on each side, and secured to the overlying skin with glue or a suture. Approximately 5 ml of a water-soluble iodinated contrast agent (420 mg iodine per ml (mg I/ml)) is injected simultaneously into both angularis oculi veins. Dorsoventral and lateral radiographs are then made and the tape encircling the neck is removed (Lee and Griffiths, 1972).

Contrast orbitography

Positive or negative contrast orbitography may be used to image specific intraorbital compartments. Under general anaesthesia, air (negative contrast) or water-soluble iodinated contrast agent (420 mg I/ml) (positive contrast) is injected into the intraconal space, and radiographs are then made, in both dorsoventral and lateral views. This technique is used infrequently, because of the increased resolution afforded by cross-sectional imaging techniques.

Sialography of the zygomatic salivary gland

This technique is indicated for suspected zygomatic sialocoele, which is a rare cause of orbital disease (Schmidt and Betts, 1978). The zygomatic salivary gland forms part of the floor of the orbit, and may cause exophthalmos when sialocoele or sialoadenitis occurs.

Technique: A blunt 25 G cannula is introduced into the zygomatic papilla, which is found in the buccal mucosa above the first molar tooth, about 1 cm caudal and ventral to the parotid papilla. Then 1–2 ml of iodine-based water-soluble contrast agent (420 mg I/ml) is slowly injected via the cannula. If the duct is ruptured, a lateral radiograph will reveal contrast leaking into the mucocoele.

Cross-sectional imaging

Cross-sectional imaging comprises the powerful diagnostic tools of ultrasound, CT and MRI. The two-dimensional image correlates with the selected two-dimensional 'slice' through the animal. The advantages of cross-sectional imaging include the ability to obtain images in multiple sequential planes, and the absence of tissue superimposition and summation that is inherent in conventional plain-film radiography.

CT and MRI can greatly facilitate the diagnosis of orbital and intracranial disease. Although certain conditions of the globe, such as lens luxation or vitreal haemorrhage, may also be identified with these modalities, they are rarely used for this purpose, as the globe can be adequately assessed with direct visualization and ultrasonography.

Ultrasonography

Ultrasonography is valuable in the investigation of both ocular and orbital disease. It is safe, non-invasive, rapidly performed and relatively inexpensive.

It is most frequently employed in ocular disease when the cornea, lens or ocular media have lost transparency, and direct visualization of intraocular structures is compromised. It is also useful for the evaluation of the orbit. Whenever it is available, it should be used in all animals that have signs of orbital disease.

Image production and display

The principle underlying diagnostic ultrasonography is that part of the incident sound beam is reflected to its source when an interface between two tissue types is encountered. Two kinds of echo are produced to form the image on the screen:

- Specular echoes originate from interfaces at right angles to the beam, and produce boundaries between tissues that appear similar to those seen in a gross anatomical cross-section
- Scattered echoes usually combine with others to produce a detectable echo. These echoes are responsible for producing a visible texture within tissues. They do not depend on the orientation of the small structures that produce them.

A and B modes: The earliest reports of ocular ultrasonography described the use of A (amplitude) mode. In this mode, a single fixed beam of ultrasound is directed through the eye, and returning echoes are shown as spikes on a horizontal line. Biometric measurements can be reliably obtained with this method, although it is not in common usage.

Real-time B (brightness) mode, on the other hand, is both widely used, and more readily interpreted. Multiple sound beams are directed through the eye, and the returning echoes are shown as dots on the screen. The position of the dots corresponds to their anatomical locations, and their brightness corresponds to the strength of the returning echo.

Resolution: In general, the higher the frequency of sound produced by a transducer, the higher will be its resolution. This improvement in image quality is at the expense of tissue penetrance, although the technological advances applied to the latest equipment have overcome this problem to some extent. A 5 or 7.5 MHz transducer may be suitable for imaging the orbit, whereas a 10 or 12.5 MHz transducer is ideal for the globe. Both regions may be imaged with a 7.5 MHz transducer, but it is impossible to differentiate the retina from the choroid or the sclera with transducers of less than 10 MHz.

Technique

The globe and orbit should be imaged in both the horizontal and vertical planes. The beam should be swept from top to bottom in the horizontal plane, and from side to side (e.g. left to right) in the vertical plane. It is very important that the ultrasonographer is aware of the image orientation on the screen at the time of conducting the scan, otherwise the spherical nature of the globe, and the lack of distinguishing features in the orbit, may cause confusion when localizing lesions.

Gel should be removed by careful irrigation of the eye with sterile eyewash after completing the ultrasound examination.

Placement of the transducer: The transducer (and standoff, if used) is best placed directly on to the anaesthetized cornea, after manually parting the eyelids. Acoustic gel is applied directly to the cornea. Alternatively, the transducer may be placed against the upper eyelid, when more liberal use of gel is required. This technique is easier, but the image quality is inferior. Imaging of the orbit may also be achieved through the lateral periorbital tissues in the region of the orbital ligament. The transoral approach may be used, but this requires general anaesthesia.

Standoffs: A standoff is required to image the cornea, anterior chamber and iris, and will improve the visualization of the ciliary body and lens. A built-in standoff, available for some machines, is ideal. Failing this, the finger of an examination glove may be filled with acoustic gel and knotted, or a comercially available gel pad may be trimmed to a less cumbersome size. These are both ways of producing a home-made standoff. Alternatively, a generous amount of sterile acoustic gel may be applied to the surface of the globe, and may act as a standoff. The posterior globe and orbit are scanned without a standoff.

Patient behaviour: Most animals tolerate the procedure well, following topical anaesthesia of the ocular surface. The animal is scanned standing, sitting or in sternal recumbency, with an assistant holding the head steady. Occasionally, sedation is required.

Normal appearance

Anterior view: The cornea, iris and anterior lens capsule may only be visualized if the globe is scanned using a standoff and high frequency transducer in direct contact with the cornea. Under ideal conditions, the cornea appears as two parallel curvilinear lines separated by an anechoic (black) stroma (Figure 1.17). The iris may occasionally be seen as an echoic structure in close contact with the anterior lens capsule, but it is difficult to image consistently.

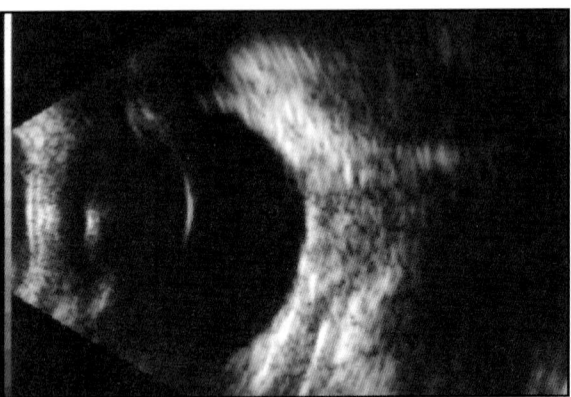

Figure 1.17 Ocular ultrasound image of the anterior aspect of a normal globe, obtained using a 10 MHz transducer and a large amount of scanning gel as a standoff. The gain has been adjusted to maximize resolution in the near field. The cornea appears as two hyperechoic lines at the left of the image. Reverberation artefacts are evident directly posterior to the corneal reflections. The anterior and posterior lens capsule are represented as biconvex focal curvilinear reflections. The retina, choroid and sclera cannot be differentiated from each other in this image. The intraconal orbit appears as a roughly triangular area posterior to the globe.

The anterior lens capsule is echogenic, but its convexity causes peripheral echo dropout due to refraction of the sound beam. It is, therefore, not possible to image its entire surface in any one scan plane. The equatorial lens capsule and the echogenic ciliary body are best imaged with the beam oriented at right angles to their surfaces. The anterior chamber, vitreous and lens (apart from its capsule) are normally anechoic.

Posterior view: The posterior lens capsule appears as a concave curvilinear echo (see Figure 1.17). The posterior wall of the globe produces a readily visualized composite curvilinear echo that represents the retina, choroid and sclera, when using a 7.5 MHz transducer. The optic disc appears as a slightly brighter region that may be either raised or depressed, relative to the posterior globe, in normal eyes. When a 10 or 12.5 MHz transducer is used, the retina, choroid and sclera can be clearly differentiated. The retina appears as a single thin hyper-reflective curvilinear echo directly adjacent to a thicker hyporeflective curvilinear echo, representing the choroid (Figure 1.18). The posterior sclera appears as a hyperechoic curvilinear echo, located parallel and directly posterior and adjacent to the hyporeflective choroid.

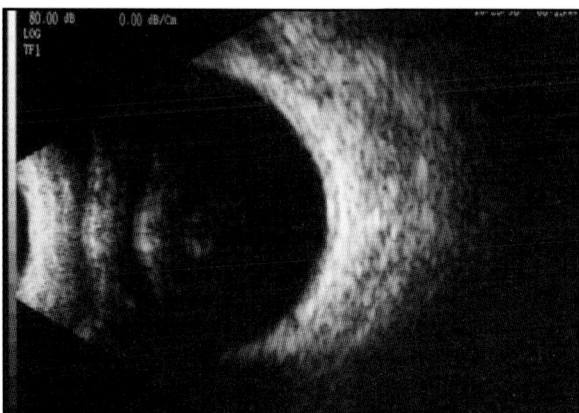

Figure 1.18 Ocular ultrasound image of the posterior aspect of a normal globe, obtained using a 10 MHz transducer. The retina appears as the first hyperechoic curvilinear density apposed against the hypoechoic choroid. The sclera appears as another hyperechoic density, posterior to the choroid. Reverberation artefacts are evident in the area of the crystalline lens.

The optic nerve and extraocular muscles are hypoechoic, relative to the echogenic retrobulbar fat separating them. These structures converge toward the posterior orbital apex near the optic canal, forming a cone shape, with the base at the posterior wall of the globe.

Extraocular structures: The temporalis muscle is seen laterally in the horizontal plane, and dorsally in the vertical plane. The zygomatic salivary gland may occasionally be identified, when scanning in the vertical plane, as a hypoechoic structure adjacent to the ventral extraocular muscles.

Any interface between the soft tissues within the orbit, and the adjacent bones, will create an echogenic boundary with acoustic shadowing (e.g. the appearance of the frontal bone medially when scanning in a horizontal plane). It is useful to have a specimen skull for reference and orientation.

Abnormalities

Intraocular disease: Abnormalities within the globe appear as mass lesions, membranous lesions, multiple point-like echoes, or changes in echogenicity of tissues. Disorders of the lens may be identified: lens luxation can be recognized readily, and cataract formation is associated with increased echogenicity of the normally anechoic lens material.

Mass lesions: Neoplasia and organized haemorrhage are the most commonly identified intraocular masses. Primary intraocular neoplasms are most frequently localized at the anterior uveal tract, and may be seen to displace the lens. Their association with the uveal tract will distinguish neoplasms from organized vitreal haemorrhage, which appears as a hyperechoic or heterogenous mass in the vitreous.

Choroidal granulomas, attributable to oculomycoses and aberrant parasite migration, can produce a similar appearance (Figure 1.19), though they are more frequently located in the choroid or subretinal space. Such conditions are rare in the UK but may be common in some countries.

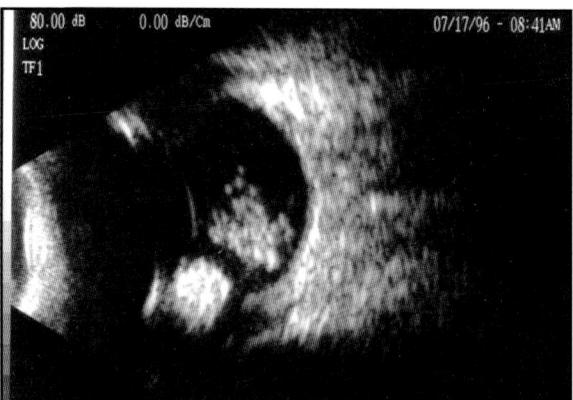

Figure 1.19 Ocular ultrasound image of a 5-year-old mixed breed dog. Note the hyperechoic mass arising from the ventral ciliary body located ventral to the posterior lens capsule reflection. There are numerous point-like opacities throughout the vitreous body that represent asteroid hyalosis. (10 MHz transducer; no standoff.)

Retinal detachment may be associated with any of the above.

Intraocular foreign bodies are identified as a bright interface associated with acoustic shadowing.

Mass lesions of the optic nerve head (prelaminar optic neuritis/papillitis, papilloedema and neoplasms) and the peripapillary retina and choroid are detected infrequently. Papillitis and papilloedema cannot be differentiated, based on their ultrasonographic appearance, because they share characteristic ultrasonographic features. In both cases, the optic papilla is raised, protrudes into the vitreous chamber, appears hyperechoic, and may have an associated peripapillary retinal detachment. Retinal detachment is more likely to occur with inflammatory and neoplastic lesions of the optic papilla, than with papilloedema.

Multiple point-like echoes: Multiple point-like echoes (see Figure 1.19) may be produced by inflammatory cells or erythrocytes within the vitreous, and by degeneration of the vitreous humour (Mattoon and Nyland, 1995). In one study, vitreous degeneration was identified in 23% of eyes of 147 dogs with cataracts (van der Woerdt et al., 1993).

Membranous lesions: Ultrasonography has an important role to play both in the identification of retinal detachment in the opaque eye and in the differentiation

18 Ocular imaging

of retinal detachment from posterior vitreous detachment. Total bullous retinal detachment has a characteristic appearance. The retina balloons forward, producing a V or 'seagull' shape, by virtue of its remaining attachments at the ora ciliaris retinae and optic disc (Figure 1.20). The detached retina will display slow and sinuous after-movements. It is very important to identify the attachment to the disc (Figure 1.21) in order to distinguish retinal detachment from the other membranous lesions that may mimic this appearance. These include vitreous membranes, which frequently follow intravitreal haemorrhage, and posterior vitreous detachment. Posterior vitreous detachment demonstrates 'serpentine' after-movements and, unlike retinal detachment, does not attach to the optic disc (Figure 1.22).

Partial retinal detachment produces a curvilinear echo bowing forward from its points of attachment to the posterior globe (Figure 1.23). The demonstration of subtle after-movements of this echo will differentiate partial retinal detachment from local choroidal detachment, which can appear similar but is less commonly recognized (Mattoon and Nyland, 1995). The simultaneous use of A and B mode imaging may permit easy differentiation between vitreous detachment and retinal detachment (Figure 1.24).

Cataract: Because of the high association of retinal detachment and cataracts in dogs, ocular ultrasonography is indicated as part of the pre-surgical diagnostic testing whenever substantial opacification of the crystalline lens is evident. In one study, retinal detachment was detected in 4% of eyes with immature cataracts, in 6.5% of eyes with mature cataracts, and in 19% of eyes with hypermature cataracts (van der Woerdt et al., 1993).

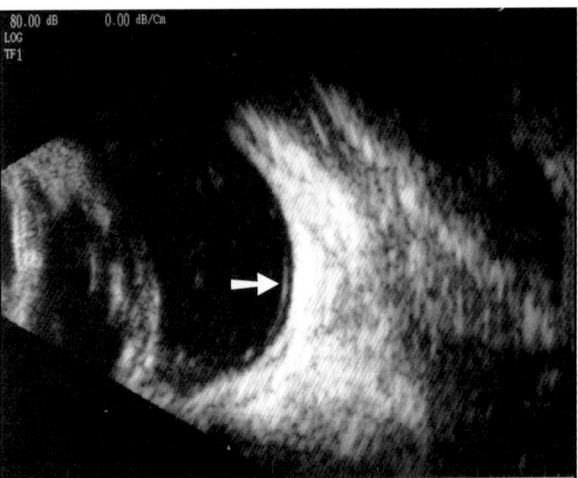

Figure 1.22 Ocular ultrasound image of a 12-year-old mixed breed dog with a posterior vitreous detachment. Note the curvilinear hyperechoic density (arrowed) located in the vitreous cavity, which is parallel to the posterior globe and does *not* attach to the optic papilla. (10 MHz transducer; no standoff.)

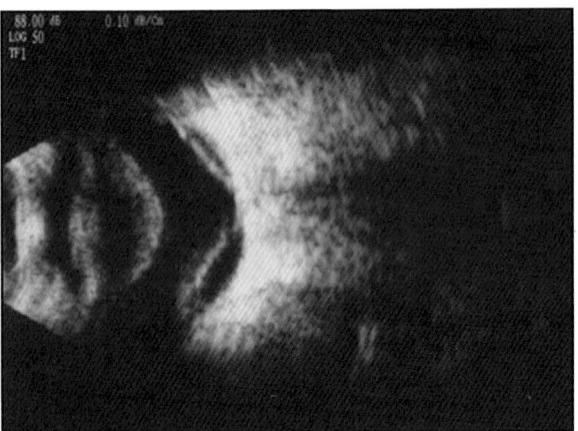

Figure 1.20 Ocular ultrasonography was performed as part of the pre-surgical diagnostic testing in a 10-year-old American Cocker Spaniel with mature cataracts. Note the two hyperechoic linear densities arising from the area of the optic papilla, and coursing anteriorly toward the ora ciliaris retinae. This finding indicated the presence of concurrent retinal detachment and, therefore, precluded cataract surgery in this dog. (10 MHz transducer; no standoff.)

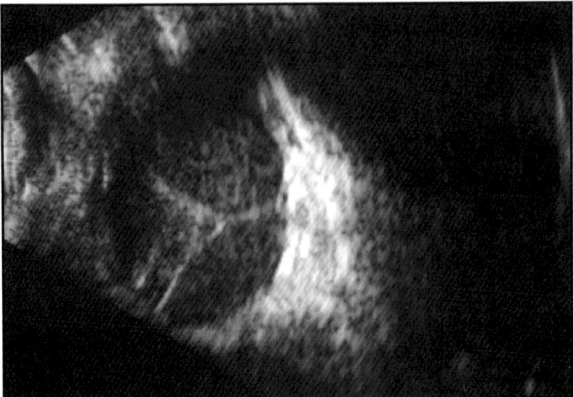

Figure 1.21 Ocular ultrasound image of the left eye of a 9-year-old Miniature Poodle that suffered an acute onset of blindness. A total retinal detachment appears ultrasonographically as a hyperechoic line arising from the area of the optic papilla and branching in the mid-vitreous cavity. The homogeneous hypoechoic appearance in the subretinal space represents haemorrhage in the subretinal space. (10 MHz transducer; no standoff.)

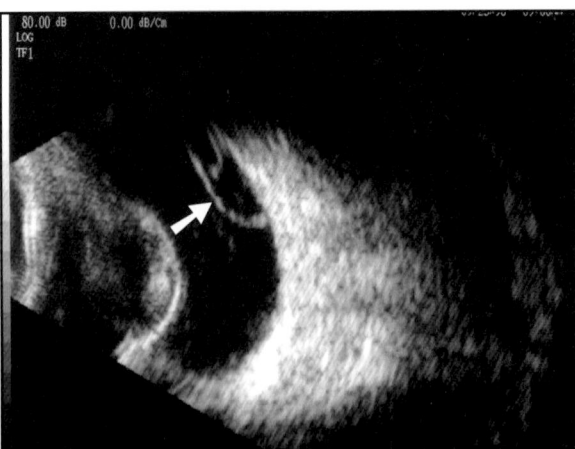

Figure 1.23 Ocular ultrasound image of a 6-year-old Samoyed with cataracts. There is a bullous retinal detachment (arrowed), characterized ultrasonographically as a well delineated hyperechoic line arising from the area of the optic papilla. (10 MHz transducer; no standoff.)

Ocular imaging 19

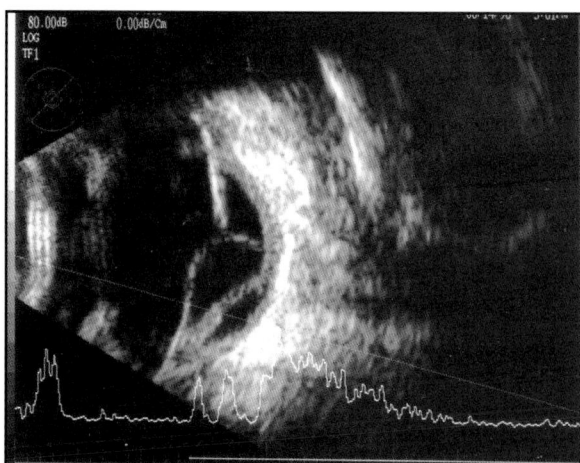

Figure 1.24 Ocular ultrasound image, obtained using simultaneous B mode and A mode imaging, of a 7-year-old Springer Spaniel with an exudative retinal detachment and choroidal detachment. (10 MHz transducer; no standoff.)

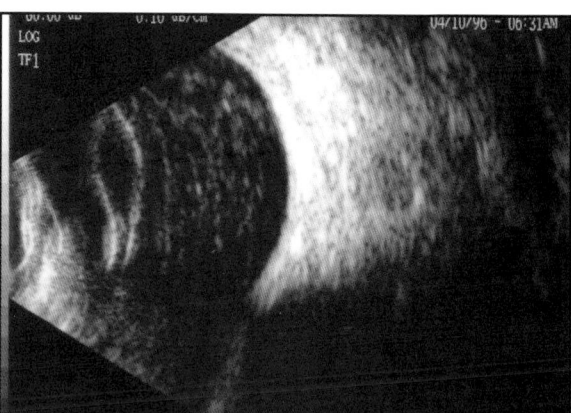

Figure 1.26 Ultrasound image of the left eye of the dog in Figure 1.25, showing a hypermature cataract. Note the small axial diameter of the resorbing lens. Vitreous degeneration is characterized ultrasonographically by multiple point-like opacities throughout the vitreous cavity. (10 MHz transducer; no standoff.)

When the lens develops an opacity, it appears hyperechoic instead of anechoic, and the entire lens becomes evident on ultrasonography. Diabetes mellitus often results in the uptake of fluid by the lens, resulting in an intumescent cataract and an increased axial diameter of the lens (Figure 1.25). The resorption of lens material is characteristic of a hypermature cataract, and is typified ultrasonographically as a decrease in the axial diameter of the lens (Figure 1.26).

Retrobulbar disease: Ultrasonography is an invaluable aid in the diagnosis of retrobulbar orbital disease, and can be used to identify the presence of orbital mass lesions and foreign bodies. It provides relatively little information about the nature of soft tissue masses, however, and a distinction between inflammatory, neoplastic and cystic disease may not be possible.

The accuracy of collecting fine-needle aspirates or non-surgical biopsies to enable precise diagnosis may be increased when this is performed under ultrasonic guidance although, surprisingly, a recent study of orbital neoplasia found no significant increase in the diagnostic yield acquired when samples were obtained with guidance compared to without (Hendrix and Gelatt, 2000). A thorough knowledge of orbital anatomy, and some practice, are required to master this technique.

Diffuse orbital cellulitis produces a generalized loss of definition of the orbital tissues, rendering the optic nerve and extraocular muscles difficult to visualize when compared with the opposite eye. Cellulitis may also produce focal mass lesions, that may be mistaken for neoplasms (Dennis, 2000). Abscesses are variable in appearance, but most are recognized as a hypoechoic area within a well defined hyperechoic wall (Figure 1.27) (Mattoon and Nyland, 1995). The abscess wall may not be seen in all cases.

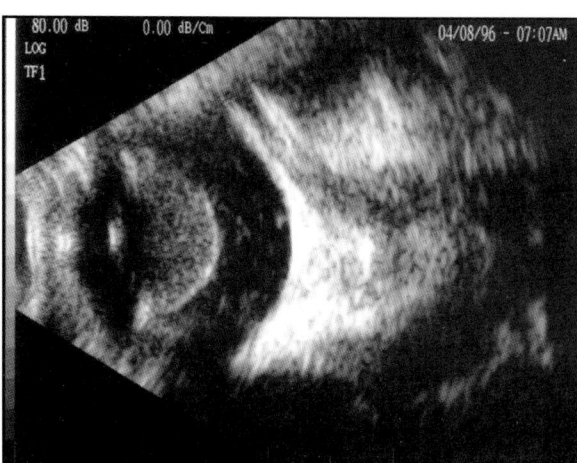

Figure 1.25 Ultrasound image of the right eye of a 4-year-old diabetic Miniature Schnauzer, showing an intumescent cataract. Note the large axial diameter of the lens. There are also numerous point-like opacities in the vitreous chamber that are consistent with vitreous degeneration. (10 MHz transducer; no standoff.)

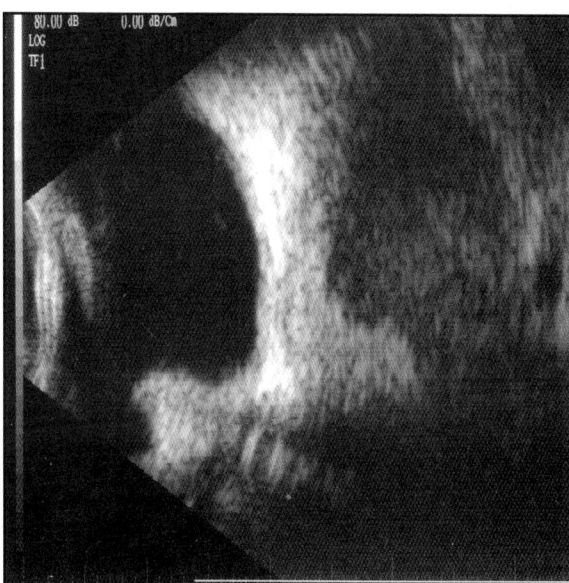

Figure 1.27 Orbital ultrasound image from a dog with acute-onset exophthalmos. Note the hypoechoic area of homogeneous density posterior to the globe. An orbital abscess was surgically drained. (10 MHz transducer; no standoff.)

20 Ocular imaging

Orbital ultrasonography reveals evidence of a mass in 70–80% of animals with orbital neoplasia (Dennis, 2000; Hendrix and Gelatt, 2000). The majority of orbital neoplasms are hypoechoic, relative to orbital fat (Figure 1.28), although osteogenic tumours and chondrosarcomas of the skull that are invading the orbit will appear strongly echogenic. Interpretation of bone involvement is difficult, as only the soft tissue–bone interface can be imaged. The anatomical extent of masses invading the bony orbit will be underestimated when ultrasonography is used as the sole imaging modality.

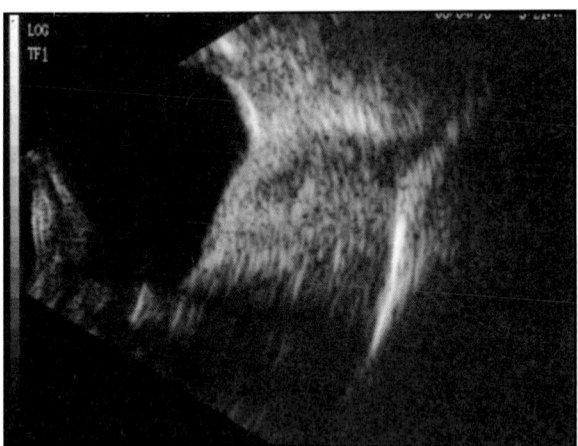

Figure 1.28 Ultrasound image of the left orbit of an 8-year-old Labrador Retriever with slowly progressing exophthalmos. Note a homogeneously hypoechoic mass, causing posterior indentation of the globe. Ultrasound-guided fine-needle aspiration and cytology of the mass revealed a soft tissue sarcoma. (10 MHz transducer; no standoff.)

Cystic orbital disease is characterized ultrasonographically by a well delineated structure with a hypoechoic or anechoic centre, relative to the surrounding orbital soft tissue echodensity (Figure 1.29).

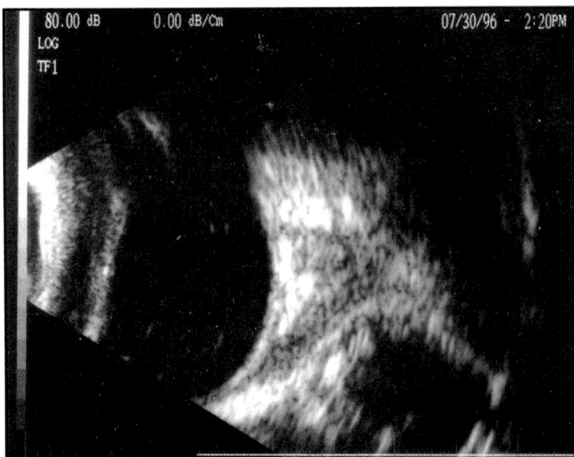

Figure 1.29 Orbital ultrasound image of a 3-year-old German Shepherd Dog that presented for evaluation of progressive exophthalmos of 1 week's duration. Note the well delineated anechoic area in the caudoventral orbit. Ultrasound-guided fine-needle aspiration revealed a viscous material consistent with saliva. A zygomatic sialocoele was removed surgically. (10 MHz transducer; no standoff.)

Polymyositis of the extraocular muscles is a rare cause of exophthalmos in young dogs (Carpenter et al., 1989). Ultrasonographically, the rectus and oblique muscles appear markedly enlarged and well delineated (Figure 1.30).

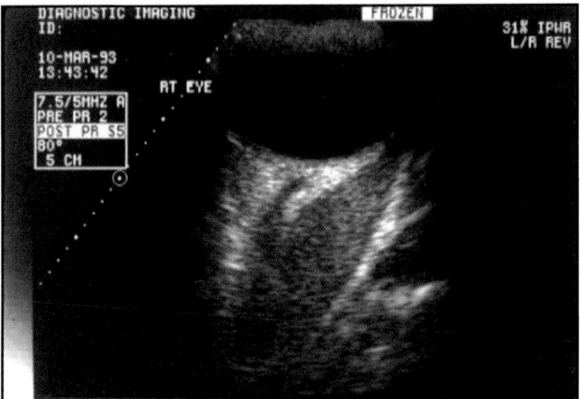

Figure 1.30 Orbital ultrasound image of a young female Golden Retriever with bilateral exophthalmos. Note the prominent hypoechoic lateral rectus muscle. A diagnosis of bilateral extraocular polymyositis was made.

High-frequency ultrasound biomicroscopy

Increasing the frequency of ultrasound used to examine the eye to 40–100 MHz will produce images of the structures within the anterior 4–5 mm of the globe with much greater resolution than conventional B mode scanning. The resulting images appear similar to histological preparations viewed with low power microscopy. They also allow assessment of the iridocorneal angle and ciliary cleft. This technology is not widely available for diagnostic purposes, as the cost of the ultrasound biomicroscope is usually prohibitive in private practice.

Computed tomography

CT provides a computer-generated image of a cross-sectional 'slice' through an animal, at the level at which it is being examined. A thin collimated X-ray beam is rotated around the animal, and monitors register the exiting photon doses. The computer then generates an image, based on the output of these monitors. Sequential images are obtained along the area of interest. The latest generation of CT scanners now have acquisition times of a few minutes. As it is essential that the animal remains still during scanning, general anaesthesia is always required.

Appearance of scans

As in conventional radiography, tissues that absorb X-ray energy will appear lighter in a grey scale image, and areas where there is little attenuation of the beam will appear darker. The range of contrast in soft tissues is much greater than that of conventional radiography. The orbit is well suited to imaging by CT, given the inherent high contrast of the tissues in the region. The bony orbit is clearly visualized, and the optic nerve, extraocular muscles, globe and zygomatic salivary gland contrast well with the relatively radiolucent orbital fat. Intravenous injection of an iodinated radiographic contrast agent improves visualization of many lesions (contrast enhancement) but is not an accurate means of finding out which tissue type is (or are) involved, or of diagnosing the presence of a specific orbital neoplasm.

Indications

CT imaging is a valuable tool in the investigation of orbital diseases, including neoplasia, optic neuritis, foreign bodies and cystic or inflammatory orbital disease. It is superior to MRI in the detection of orbital fractures, haemorrhage and proliferation of bone, and is the imaging modality of choice in orbital trauma. As with MRI, CT offers considerable advantages over ultrasonography in its ability to demonstrate tissues beyond the confines of the bony orbit (Figure 1.31).

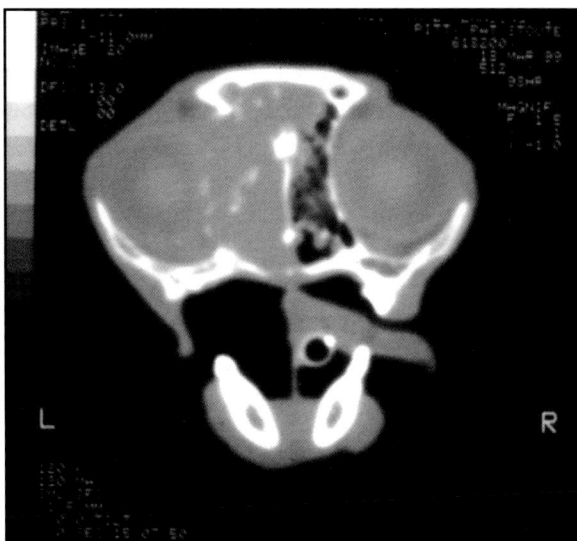

Figure 1.31 CT image of an 11-year-old cat with exophthalmos of the left eye and severe distortion of the side of the face. Lysis of the pars orbitalis of the frontal bone is evident, with proliferation of bone matrix in the frontal sinus and left nasal passage. There is an area of soft tissue density extending from the orbital space into the left frontal sinus and nasal passage.

Reformatted images

Obtaining images in different planes requires the repositioning of the animal within the gantry. Reformatted CT images of the sagittal plane may be used to provide a three-dimensional location of intraconal, extraconal, or extraendorbital masses, by viewing sequential cross-sectional images in succession. However, reformatted images lose considerable image resolution, compared with images obtained in the primary scan plane. Reconstructed three-dimensional images can also be used to demonstrate proliferative and lytic bone lesions by eliminating soft tissue images from bone (Figure 1.32).

Detection of neoplasia

CT imaging has been used to evaluate orbital neoplasms in cats and dogs. Lysis of bone was present in 82% of malignant orbital neoplasms in cats (Calia *et al.*, 1994). However, images obtained by CT may not clearly delineate the extent of a neoplasm within the orbit or calvarium in cats (Ramsey *et al.*, 1994).

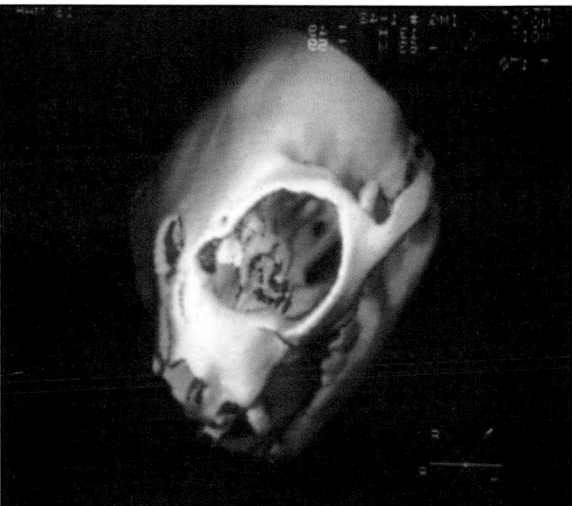

Figure 1.32 Reformatted CT image of the cat in Figure 1.31, showing lysis of the left frontal bone at the anterior orbital rim and of both nasal bones along the midline. Osteosarcoma was the final diagnosis.

Guidance for diagnostic tests

CT imaging can also be used to guide the placement of a needle precisely within pathological tissue for fine needle aspiration and biopsy.

Magnetic resonance imaging

Magnetic resonance images are generated by placing the animal within a gantry containing a powerful magnetic field that determines the direction of the angular momentum of nuclei (particularly hydrogen). A small surface coil is then placed within the magnetic field, and pulsed radio wave sequences are delivered to the surface coil to disturb the alignment of tissue protons. Electromagnetic energy released from proton realignment is then detected by computer sensors and analysed with regard to tissue-specific properties, to generate an electron-dense image.

The animal must remain still during image acquisition and therefore general anaesthesia is required. However, repositioning the animal within the gantry is not necessary to obtain images in multiple planes. Volumetric acquisition of signals with direct multiplanar MRI, in combination with different surface coil techniques, provides very detailed anatomy and high resolution of intra- and extraorbital tissues. Acquisition times are longer for MRI than for CT, usually about 45 minutes.

Ferrous metals are not permitted in the scanner room, and this must be considered when designing anaesthetic protocols, or when ferrous intraorbital or intraocular foreign bodies are suspected. MRI is contraindicated when the differential diagnosis includes a metallic foreign body, as this could migrate under the influence of the magnetic field and induce serious damage to ocular tissues.

Resolution and contrast

The resolution of images produced by MRI is superb, and soft tissue differentiation is superior to that provided by CT. Image contrast sensitivity can be manipulated by selection of different pulse sequences, or by the intravenous injection of a paramagnetic contrast agent (gadolinium-diethylenetriamine penta-acetic acid, DTPA). Bone is not imaged directly but bone destruction in orbital neoplasia is, nevertheless, recognized as loss of the normal signal void.

Indications

MR images provide detailed anatomy of soft tissues, with greater spatial and soft tissue resolution and contrast than CT images (Figure 1.33). However, when detailed images of bony structures are required, MRI is less specific than CT. MRI may not show the extent of mineralization within soft tissues, but it is better than CT imaging when soft tissue detail and resolution are necessary. Thus, the two are complementary.

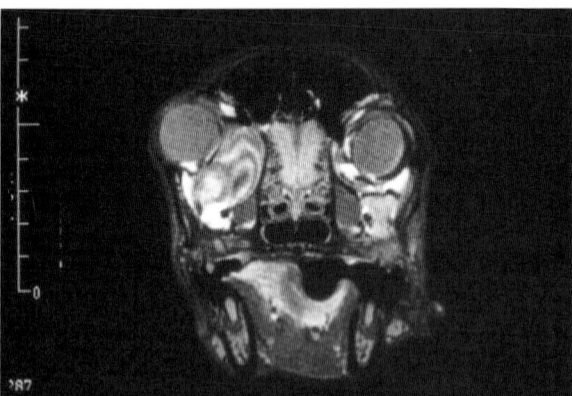

Figure 1.33 MR image of a 4-month-old Brittany Spaniel with intermittent exophthalmos of the right eye, attributable to a congenital orbital arteriovenous malformation (AVM). Note the dilated orbital venous structure ventral and medial to the globe. Laminar flow of blood within the dilated vascular structure appears as different electron-dense layers within the AVM.

By altering components of the pulse sequence, such as repetition time (TR), interpulse delay (T1) and echo time (TE), the operator can maximally differentiate the electron density signals of many different soft tissues, thereby maximizing the differentiation of soft tissues.

MRI is more sensitive than CT in the detection of intracranial disease, and is, therefore, the imaging technique of choice in animals with clinical signs of chiasmal or retrochiasmal disease, or orbital neoplasms with suspected intracranial extension. In a recent study, MRI demonstrated abnormalities in 25 out of 25 dogs with orbital disease (Dennis, 2000).

As with all imaging techniques, tissue type may not be reliably determined in all cases, and distinguishing between malignant and benign neoplastic disease may not always be possible. Inferences about the likely tissue type can, however, be made from the extent of the disease process (which is clearly demonstrated) and by assessing the signals produced with different pulse sequences: these alter, according to certain tissue characteristics.

For these reasons, MRI is the imaging technique most likely to provide a definite diagnosis in orbital disease.

References

Calia CM, Kirschner SE, Baer KE and Stefanacci JD (1994) The use of computed tomography scan for the evaluation of orbital disease in cats and dogs. *Veterinary and Comparative Ophthalmology* **4**, 24–30

Carpenter JL, Schimt GM, Moore FM, Albert DM, Abrams KL and Elner VM (1989) Canine bilateral extraocular polymyositis. *Veterinary Pathology* **26**, 510–512

Dennis R (2000) Use of magnetic resonance imaging in the investigation of orbital disease in small animals. *Journal of Small Animal Practice* **41**, 145–155

Hendrix DVH and Gelatt KN (2000) Diagnosis, treatment and outcome of orbital neoplasia in dogs: a retrospective study of 44 cases. *Journal of Small Animal Practice* **41**, 105–108

Lee R and Griffiths IR (1972) A comparison of cerebral arteriography and cavernous sinus venography in the dog. *Journal of Small Animal Practice* **13**, 225–237

Mattoon JS and Nyland TG (1995) Ocular ultrasonography. In: *Veterinary Diagnostic Ultrasound*, ed. JS Mattoon and TG Nyland, pp.178–197. WB Saunders, Philadelphia

Ramsey DT, Gerding PA, Losonsky JF, Kuriashkin IV and Clarkson RD (1994) Comparative value of diagnostic imaging techniques in a cat with exophthalmos. *Veterinary and Comparative Ophthalmology* **4**, 198–202

Schmidt GM and Betts CW (1978) Zygomatic salivary mucocoeles in the dog. *Journal of the American Veterinary Medical Association* **172**, 940–942

Van der Woerdt A, Wilkie DA and Myer W (1993) Ultrasonographic abnormalities in the eyes of dogs with cataracts: 147 cases (1986–1992). *Journal of the American Veterinary Medical Association* **203**, 838–841

1c

Laboratory investigation of ophthalmic disease

David J. Maggs

Introduction

No other body structures lend themselves to more complete visual examination than the eyes and adnexa. Therefore, laboratory examination is not always necessary in ophthalmic disease. Laboratory investigations tend to be required when neoplastic, genetic, immune-mediated or infectious disease is suspected. It is, therefore, essential that the clinician is well informed with regard to the appropriate laboratory tests for the suspected disease process, the correct method of sample collection and handling, and the interpretation of the laboratory results. In all cases, close communication with the laboratory is essential to define these three aspects further.

In this section, sample collection and handling techniques are discussed. Laboratory tests and their interpretation are then considered under the broad categories of cytological/histopathological, microbiological and genetic assessment. For further information regarding recommended tests and their interpretation, the reader is also referred to chapters of this manual dealing with individual disease processes.

Sample collection and handling

Conjunctival and corneal swabs

A sterile swab may be rolled gently through the conjunctival fornix or across the cornea to collect surface samples. The technique is simple, and conjunctival swabs can be taken without topical anaesthesia in compliant patients. Although cellular integrity is well preserved with this technique, the number of cells collected is typically too small for complete cytological assessment (Bauer et al., 1996). The technique is used more commonly for collection of microbial samples. It is tolerated better, and is more likely to yield viable organisms, if the swab is pre-moistened with appropriate culture media or sterile saline. Samples may be collected by applying the swab directly to the area to be sampled. However, samples with higher numbers of cells can be harvested through scrapings or aspirates (see below) and these can be applied in a sterile manner to a pre-moistened swab. These techniques yield more organisms, particularly obligate intracellular pathogens.

Because a normal flora exists on the ocular surface, care must be taken not to contaminate the swab by inadvertently touching it on tissues or regions without obvious pathology. Mini-tip swabs are available for obtaining samples from focal or delicate ocular surfaces such as deep corneal ulcers (Fig 1.34).

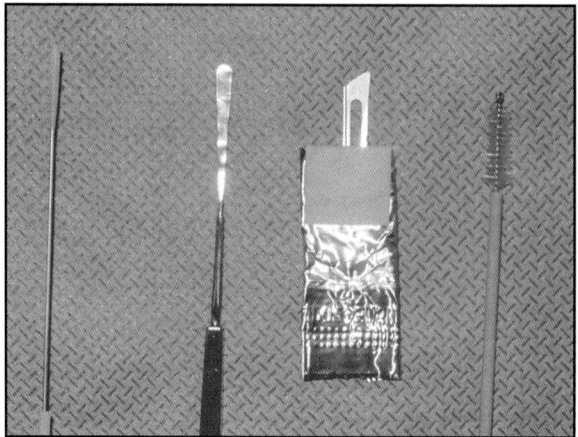

Figure 1.34 Instruments suitable for collecting cytological and microbiological samples from ocular surface tissues. From left to right: mini-tip swab; Kimura platinum spatula; Bard–Parker scalpel blade with the handle end exposed but the blade sheathed; cytobrush.

Eyelid, conjunctival and corneal scrapings

Superficial cells may be collected by gently scraping the epithelium and superficial connective tissue of the cornea, conjunctiva, or periocular skin. When conducted properly, this technique is safe, well tolerated and particularly useful for the assessment of inflammatory or neoplastic cells, and/or infectious organisms involving these surface tissues. Assessment of pathology involving deeper sites usually necessitates surgical biopsy (see later).

Periocular skin scrapes are performed using a scalpel blade in the same way as they are elsewhere on the body. Care must be taken to avoid abrading specialized tissues of the eyelid margin. Gentle squeezing of the skin and eyelid margin will cause expression of material from hair follicles and glandular structures; this technique is particularly important for the detection of *Demodex* species. Collection of corneal or conjunctival samples requires administration of topical anaesthetic and adequate physical or chemical restraint to avoid injury to the eye. Corneal anaesthesia can be rapidly achieved by applying one or two drops of topical anaesthetic, such as proxymetacaine. The highly vascular nature of the conjunctiva may necessitate a more sustained application of a topical local anaesthetic. This is achieved by soaking a cotton-tipped applicator in proxymetacaine and applying it to the conjunctival surface for 20–30 seconds. Care should be taken not to abrade surface cells that may be diagnostically important; however, surface mucus and debris should always be removed prior to collection of cytological samples. Furthermore, samples for culture should be collected before performing any procedure that could alter or affect the microorganisms present.

Corneal and conjunctival samples are best collected using a Kimura platinum spatula or the blunt end of a scalpel blade (see Figure 1.34). A brisk scraping movement, with pressure sufficient to abrade cells, is used to harvest enough cellular material for assessment. Cells collected in this manner may be gently spread on to a clean dry microscope slide for cytological or immunofluorescent antibody (IFA) assessment, applied to a sterile swab for culture, or suspended in a sterile solution for testing by polymerase chain reaction (PCR).

Cytobrushes

The use of small, nylon-bristled gynaecological cytobrushes (see Figure 1.34) for collection of conjunctival cytology specimens has been described in veterinary patients (Bauer et al., 1996; Willis et al., 1997). The brush is gently rolled in the conjunctival fornix or across the corneal surface. Cells are then very gently rolled out on to a glass slide before being air-dried. Samples collected using cytology brushes tend to be less cellular but to form more even monolayers than those acquired by scraping. Other advantages of this technique are safety and patient tolerance. Cytobrushes are designed for single use.

Impression cytology

This technique relies on cells that exfoliate easily and is, therefore, most readily applied to investigation of superficial conjunctival disease. A clean glass slide or specially prepared cellulose acetate filter paper is pressed firmly against the area to be sampled, and exfoliated epithelial cells (including goblet cells) and surface inflammatory cells are then examined cytologically. This technique has received some use in keratoconjunctivitis sicca (KCS) research, but does not usually provide clinically significant advantages over cytological scrapings or brush samples, both of which tend to collect more cells from deeper in the epithelium and from superficial stroma.

Impression smears may also be made by lightly pressing biopsy specimens on to a glass slide prior to fixation. This technique is not intended to replace histopathological assessment of tissue specimens but, rather, to provide information more rapidly.

Aspirates

Fine-needle aspiration is an extremely useful technique for assessment of masses involving the eye, adnexa or orbit. This technique provides an excellent yield from tissues that shed cells relatively freely, especially round cell neoplasms, such as mast cell tumours and lymphoma, granulomas and abscesses. Cystic masses tend to be less cellular unless there is marked associated inflammation. Eyelid and conjunctival masses may be aspirated using identical techniques to those used for skin masses at other sites. Care should be taken to ensure that ocular penetration does not occur. This can usually be assured with adequate physical (or, less commonly, chemical) restraint and always by directing the needle away from the globe. Where possible, the mass should be isolated between the fingers, and the needle inserted into the mass without a syringe attached. The needle should be redirected within the mass a number of times in order to ensure that adequate and representative cellular material is collected.

Prior to aspiration of orbital masses, imaging techniques are usually performed to define mass location, extent and nature, and because aspiration is likely to disrupt tissue architecture, or cause haemorrhage. Orbital ultrasonography may also be used to direct the needle during aspiration. Because of the need for imaging techniques, and because orbital aspirates carry a relatively high risk of globe perforation if not performed correctly, they are best carried out by a specialist familiar with the technique. Oral, transconjunctival, transpalpebral and lateral approaches are possible, depending on the location of the mass. All are usually performed under general anaesthesia.

Intraocular aspirates are indicated for investigation of intraocular masses, uveitis and retinal detachment. They are necessary when less invasive techniques have not yielded a diagnosis. Typical targets for aspiration are aqueous humour, intraocular masses, vitreous, and subretinal fluid. Intraocular aspiration is performed under general anaesthesia, and frequently with ultrasound guidance. Due to the risk of intraocular haemorrhage, lens capsule rupture and retinal detachment, these are specialist procedures.

Orbital, adnexal, and intraocular aspirates may be submitted for cytological or microbiological assessment. For cytological assessment, aspirated material should be expressed on to a clean glass slide, using a syringe. A second slide is then used to spread aspirated cells gently. The aim is to create areas of cellular monolayer on the slide; these may be examined by the cytologist. However, this must cause minimal mechanical disruption of harvested cells. Less cellular aspirates, such as those obtained from the anterior chamber, require centrifugation to yield sufficient cells for a diagnosis. Cellular and fluid aspirates can also be applied in a sterile manner to a pre-moistened swab, for microbiological assessment. Cytological interpretation can be difficult and is best performed by pathologists experienced in cytology.

Biopsy

Biopsy is performed on tissues that are too deep to be sampled using the cytological methods already described, or when tissue architecture, rather than individual cellular morphology, is likely to be diagnostically important. Biopsy is routinely performed for investigation of conjunctival, eyelid, corneal and orbital disease.

Biopsies of intraocular structures are performed infrequently, and usually only by specialists. Because biopsy is likely to involve sedation or general anaesthesia, it is often deferred until a cytological technique has already been attempted.

Ocular tissues are very delicate, and special care must be taken to handle them gently and as little as possible, during the biopsy procedure. Samples for histopathology should be placed immediately in an adequate volume of fixative. Small samples can be placed on filter paper or gently stretched over a tongue depressor, prior to immersion in formalin to maintain tissue orientation and to avoid loss during processing. Before fixation, biopsy samples can be divided in a sterile manner and a small section submitted for culture. Samples for culture should be placed in a sterile container and transported immediately to the bacteriology laboratory. Where necessary, impression smears can be prepared from a cut surface, prior to fixation.

Conjunctiva

Conjunctival biopsy is readily performed on an unsedated patient and may provide valuable information that is not always available from cytological examination. The area of conjunctiva to be sampled is anaesthetized, using the same technique described for conjunctival cytology. While an assistant restrains the animal's head and everts the eyelid, a small piece of conjunctiva is delicately elevated using a fine-toothed instrument, such as Bishop–Harmon forceps. A small snip biopsy of conjunctiva and subconjunctiva is harvested by cutting across the base of the tented conjunctiva using small tenotomy scissors (Figure 1.35). No sutures are required, and haemorrhage is usually minimal. Gentle pressure may be applied to the conjunctival wound, if necessary.

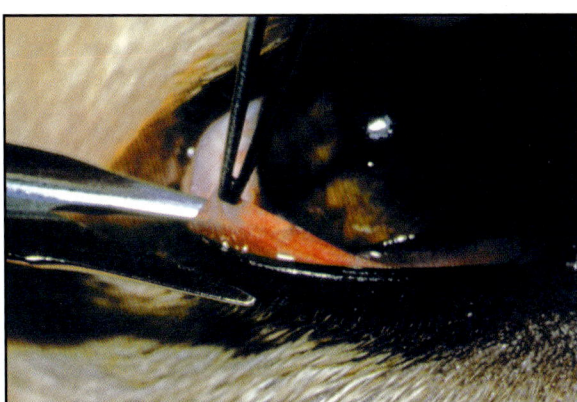

Figure 1.35 Conjunctival biopsy technique.

Eyelid

Eyelid skin biopsies may be obtained using a scalpel or skin biopsy punch, as would be done elsewhere on the skin, and usually require local anaesthesia only. The eyelid margin should be avoided unless there is significant pathology at that site. If the margin must be used, then the biopsy site should be closed using the figure-of-eight technique described in Chapter 2c. Careful attention should be paid to realignment of the margin, to avoid distortion, ectropion, entropion, trichiasis and corneal ulceration.

Cornea and orbit

Corneal biopsy is performed by lamellar keratectomy. This requires general anaesthesia and magnification. Due to the need for special equipment and expertise, this procedure is routinely performed by specialists. Biopsy of the orbital contents also requires advanced knowledge of orbital anatomy, and is best left to a specialist.

Cytological and histological assessment

The methods used for collecting cytological samples are described above. Once collected, cells should be spread as thinly as possible on glass slides, with minimal disruption of cellular morphology. The three techniques commonly used for collecting surface cells have been compared, and their relative advantages are shown in Figure 1.36 (Bauer et al., 1996; Willis et al., 1997). Samples collected by swab tend to contain insufficient cells for diagnosis, but those cells that are collected are well preserved and spread in an even monolayer. Samples collected by spatula are highly cellular but tend to clump together, making cytological interpretation more difficult. Samples collected using cytobrushes tend to have high cellularity, integrity and distribution on the slide.

Characteristic	Swab	Spatula	Cytobrush
Total cellularity	+	+++	+++
Cellular integrity	+++	+	+++
Cellular distribution	+++	+	+++

Figure 1.36 Comparison of three methods for collecting surface cells from the cornea or conjunctiva. Topical anaesthesia is necessary with all techniques for corneal specimens, though conjunctival sampling by swab or cytobrush may be performed without.
+ = poor; +++ = good

Cytological specimens can be examined following application of a Romanowsky-type stain, such as Diff-Quik®. This allows rapid 'in-house' assessment of the disease process, and immediate initiation of the appropriate treatment. However, in most cases, samples should also be sent to a cytologist for review. If possible, two or three slides should be left unstained until after initial assessment, in case special stains are suggested. Cytology is particularly useful for confirmation of suspected neoplastic or immune-mediated diseases. It should also be performed for any refractory or unusual disease processes. Frequently, a predominantly suppurative (neutrophilic) inflammatory response is seen in a cytology specimen collected from the ocular surface. This must be interpreted cautiously, since it may simply represent non-specific inflammation in response to the overgrowth of flora. Further investigation should be carried out to determine the primary pathology.

Good samples for histopathological assessment provide more, and frequently better preserved, cells than does cytology. They also retain cellular relationships and tissue architecture, and are more likely to permit a definitive diagnosis. Numerous special stains and immunohistochemical techniques are available to characterize cellular details further.

Microbiological assessment

Microbiological diagnoses are arrived at either by direct identification of the organism, or by demonstration of a specific host response. Methods of organism detection used commonly in investigation of ophthalmic disease include direct microscopic examination, culture, PCR and IFA. Host responses are assessed by using antibody titres, usually within serum, although intraocular antibody production can also be measured.

There are many tests available and each has distinct advantages and disadvantages. The preferred test will vary with many features, including abundance of organism being tested for, stage of disease, and biological behaviour of individual organisms. Figure 1.37 compares the features of four tests commonly employed for investigation of feline herpesvirus-1 (FHV-1).

Regardless of the test modality or the organism, the distinction must be made between simply detecting the organism, or the host response to it, and *proving* that the organism is the cause of the disease being investigated. This is particularly relevant for ocular surface tissues, which have a normal flora, and for organisms such as *Chlamydophila* spp. and FHV-1 for which a carrier state is established. The composition of normal conjunctival and eyelid flora has been surveyed for dogs and cats and comprises principally Gram-positive bacterial species (Gerding and Kakoma, 1990). Some variation occurs in specific composition due to geographical, climatic, seasonal and other factors; however, *Staphylococcus* and *Streptococcus* spp. tend to predominate. Bacterial cultures from normal cats' eyes tend to yield organisms approximately half as frequently as those from dogs' eyes. Anaerobic species are isolated very rarely from either species. Identification of fungal and mycoplasmal species from healthy ocular surface tissues is possible.

Direct microscopic examination

Microscopic examination of scrapings, smears, aspirates and biopsy specimens often permits direct observation of organisms, as well as associated host cellular responses. Larger organisms, such as fungi and yeasts, can be observed directly in routinely stained specimens. The periphery of a moderately sized clump of epithelial cells is frequently a rewarding place to look in cytological preparations (Figure 1.38). Smaller organisms, such as bacteria, may also be observed with stains routinely used for histology, or cytology stains; however, Gram's stain makes identification easiest and most specific. The presence of bacteria within cells is generally considered to be more relevant than the observation of extracellular organisms only. Results of cytological examination and bacterial culture have been compared, and found to be complementary (Massa *et al.*, 1999). Cytological examination provides rapid and reliable identification of the organism type and permits the initiation of therapy, pending culture results. Therapy can then be modified, if necessary, when susceptibility data become available.

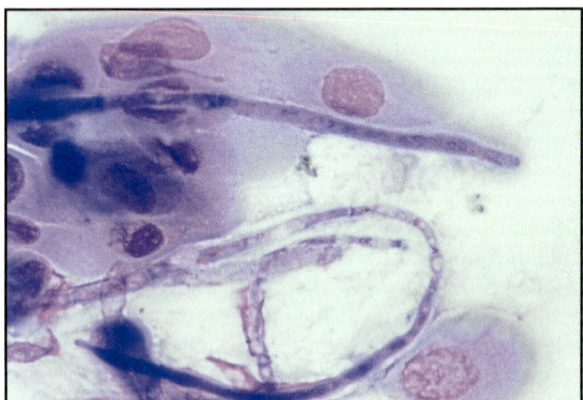

Figure 1.38 Cytological specimen revealing fungal hyphae adjacent to numerous corneal epithelial cells. Wrights–Giemsa staining (Courtesy of R. Marrion.)

Although viruses, *Mycoplasma* spp. and *Chlamydophila* spp. are too small to be seen by routine light microscopy, occasionally, characteristic inclusion bodies may be seen, particularly in acute infections. The help of an experienced pathologist is valuable in distinguishing inclusion bodies from pigment granules. However, inclusion bodies are not a frequent finding, and failure to detect them should not be considered proof that these organisms are not present. IFA assays have also been used as a diagnostic aid. The technique involves addition of a fluorescently labelled antibody to an air-dried cytological preparation. The antibodies are directed at microbial epitopes that are expressed on host cell surfaces. Prior use of topical fluorescein will produce a false-positive IFA test result. Currently, IFA assays exist for canine distemper virus, FHV-1 and *Chlamydia* spp. These tests are most likely to give positive results in acute infections.

Feature	Virus isolation	Polymerase chain reaction	Indirect fluorescent antibody test	Serology
Detection of virus (V) or host response (H)	V	V	V	H
Viable virus necessary	Yes	No	No	No
Prior use of vital stains affects test result	Yes	No	Yes	No
Collection and transport techniques	Detailed	Detailed	Simple	Simple

Figure 1.37 Comparison of testing modalities for FHV-1.

Culture and susceptibility (sensitivity) testing

Ocular surface tissues may be cultured using swabs, scrapings or brushings. Cultures of deeper tissues may be obtained from aspirates or biopsy specimens. In all cases, better results are likely when sufficient material is submitted for culture. Refrigeration (not freezing) of the sample will assist in maintaining viable organism numbers if a delay in testing is anticipated. Bacteria, chlamydiae, mycoplasmas, fungi and viruses have different culture requirements. Attention must, therefore, be given to swab type, transport medium and storage and transport conditions. This requires close communication between the practitioner and the laboratory to which the sample will be sent. In some cases, specialized laboratories need to be contacted for culture of certain organisms. The following are general guidelines.

Bacteriology

Cultures from ocular surface tissues are usually submitted for aerobic culture, while aspirates and deeper biopsies, particularly from orbital masses, may require anaerobic culture. *Chlamydophila* and *Mycoplasma* spp. must be collected into, and transported in, special media. Bacteriological samples should, ideally, be collected prior to the start of antibiotic administration; however, organisms that persist in the face of antimicrobial use are also relevant. The application of topical anaesthetics is essential prior to collection of corneal samples, due to the extreme sensitivity of this tissue. Although topical anaesthetic preparations contain preservatives, it is unlikely that they alter cultures in a clinically relevant way (Champagne and Pickett, 1995). Topical anaesthetic is not usually necessary prior to the collection of conjunctival or eyelid specimens. Differentiation of pathogens and normal flora may be difficult; however, cultures of normal flora tend to be represented by more than one isolate, and usually appear in light growth, often only in enrichment media.

Susceptibility testing of aerobic bacteria is highly recommended. Most laboratories will conduct a minimum inhibitory concentration (MIC) determination. This technique determines the viability of bacteria at various concentrations of each antibiotic tested. This method is generally considered to provide more clinically relevant data than the Kirby–Bauer agar disc-diffusion test. However, there are some important considerations specific to the treatment of ocular surface pathogens. First, the clinician should verify that the laboratory is able to test antibiotics that are applied topically, since these are not routinely included in all test panels. Secondly, topical application achieves a higher drug concentration at the corneal surface than is possible with systemic administration. Therefore, it is possible that frequent topical administration of an antimicrobial agent may produce a perfectly adequate clinical response, even if MIC testing suggests that the isolate is only moderately susceptible to that drug.

Susceptibility testing of anaerobic isolates is not commonly performed, but their susceptibility patterns tend to be more predictable than those of aerobic bacteria.

Virology

The most frequent ophthalmic application for viral culture or virus isolation (VI) has been the diagnosis of FHV-1. A number of steps are important to maximize the chances of collecting, transporting and culturing viable virus. Dacron- or cotton-tipped swabs should be used, since calcium alginate swabs can be inhibitory to some herpesviruses. Swab tips should be pre-moistened with viral transport medium. The conjunctival fornix, cornea, or sometimes the oropharynx, should be swabbed aggressively enough to harvest cells, since FHV-1 is an obligate intracellular organism. Following collection, the swab should be broken into a vial of viral transport medium. Testing prior to application of stains, such as fluorescein and rose Bengal, is essential, since these stains are toxic to herpesviruses. Refrigeration and shipping of samples on ice are usually recommended. The sample should be rapidly frozen if an extended delay in shipping or testing is likely. The laboratory will adsorb the sample on to monolayers of a permissive cell line, and observe cells for characteristic viral cytopathic effects. This is usually rapid, but can take up to 10 days. While VI does detect FHV-1 reliably, viral presence within the eyes of cats does not correlate with disease in all cases, since FHV-1 can be isolated from the conjunctival fornix of up to 11% of normal cats using this technique (Maggs *et al.*, 1999).

Mycology

Other than eyelid dermatophytosis, ocular fungal infection is uncommon in the UK, but this should be considered in animals from geographical regions where orbital, intraocular, systemic or keratoconjunctival mycosis is possible. Fungal involvement is suggested by inadequate response to appropriate antibacterial agents, or following systemic or local immunosuppression or prolonged use of antimicrobial drugs that may have altered bacterial flora. Material harvested by orbital or intraocular aspirates, deep biopsies, swabs, scrapings, or by plucking hairs from the periorbital area, can be submitted for fungal culture. Dermatophytes may be identified more rapidly by culturing plucked hairs on an agar slope. Fungal susceptibility testing is available at specialist laboratories, but tends to be expensive. Although fungi can be found as part of the normal flora in dogs and cats, detection of these organisms in a diseased eye may prompt the clinician to consider treatment with an appropriate antifungal agent.

Polymerase chain reaction (PCR)

PCR technology has revolutionized microbiological testing. The technique can be performed only if a 'target' section of DNA from the organism in question has been sequenced. Multiple copies of this region of DNA are then constructed *in vitro*, by the repeated cycling of sample DNA and nucleic acid 'building blocks' with *Taq* polymerase enzyme, under highly regulated conditions. This is done in an automated fashion, and each cycle approximately doubles the previous number of copies made. The result is an exponential increase in copy number of target DNA, to levels at which it can be visually detected when appropriately stained or labelled. PCR is, thus, an exquisitely sensitive (and specific) test. Sensitivity is primarily dependent on the number of test cycles performed.

This creates new dilemmas for clinicians and laboratory personnel, regarding sample collection and handling, and test interpretation. In the past, the principal problem was that of ensuring adequate sensitivity. By contrast, PCR requires great care at all stages of collection, transport and testing, to guard against contamination, since minute quantities of DNA may be detected. Similarly, the chance of truly positive, but clinically irrelevant, test results is dramatically increased, particularly for diseases in which a carrier state develops, or for those organisms that are part of the surface flora. It is also important to recognize that PCR detects DNA: it does not require viable organisms to be present.

Because relatively large numbers of bacteria tend to be present in ocular surface disease, and because they can usually be readily cultured, PCR has infrequent application in detection of conjunctival or corneal bacteria; however, it has been used to diagnose endophthalmitis.

The major ophthalmic application for PCR at this stage is diagnostic testing for *Chlamydia psittaci*, *Mycoplasma* spp. and FHV-1. A number of techniques have been reported, and some are available commercially. Although special laboratory protocols may be necessary, any tissue sample, theoretically, can be tested for the presence of DNA from these organisms. Because they are obligate intracellular pathogens, highly cellular samples are more likely to yield positive results. This means that biopsy samples are more likely to yield a positive result than scrapings, which, in turn, are more likely than swabs to yield positive results. Because *C. psittaci* and FHV-1 can be detected in the conjunctival fornix of cats with healthy eyes, it is also important to know the expected number of positive test results in unaffected cats, for each laboratory's test protocol. PCR tests have also been developed for feline coronaviruses, feline leukaemia virus (FeLV) and feline immunodeficiency virus (FIV). Due to the existence of reliable serological assays for FeLV and FIV, PCR testing for these organisms is not widely used at this stage. A PCR assay that reliably differentiates enteric coronavirus from the virus responsible for feline infectious peritonitis (FIP) has yet to be developed. Due to the frequency with which the feline coronaviruses mutate, identifying reliable genomic targets is challenging.

Serology

Serology is frequently used to assess the host response to an organism. It gives evidence that the host has been exposed (at some time in the past) to the organism being tested for, or to any other organisms (including vaccine variants) that cross-react in that assay with the organism that is being sought. This highlights two features of serological testing that must be considered when interpreting results:

First, organism exposure and disease are not automatically correlated. An example is the serological assay for FHV-1. Approximately 97% of the feline population shows serological evidence of exposure to FHV-1. Mere detection of an antibody response to this virus is therefore not sufficient proof that FHV-1 is likely to have caused the disease being investigated. Secondly, serological assays vary in their specificity. For example, no serological assay currently differentiates the coronavirus that causes FIP from enteric forms of coronavirus. Provided that these limitations are borne in mind, serological tests may provide useful confirmatory evidence of disease in some instances. Specific serological assays and their interpretation are discussed in the relevant chapters.

The comparison of intraocular and circulating (serum) antibody titres has been used to indicate local (intraocular) antibody production. This ratio is called the Goldmann–Witmer coefficient or *C*-value:

$$C\text{-value} = \frac{\text{organism-specific antibody titre in aqueous humour}}{\text{organism-specific antibody titre in serum}} \times \frac{\text{total antibody concentration in serum}}{\text{total antibody concentration in aqueous humour}}$$

This has been used to assess aetiological agents in uveitis. In theory, a *C*-value greater than 1 suggests intraocular antibody production and, therefore, a specific and local response. However, interpretation of this test is confounded by information suggesting that a *C*-value greater than 1 can also be caused by non-specific immune stimulation.

Genetic assessment

Although phenotypic evidence of inherited ophthalmic disease has been monitored for a long time, the recent introduction of genotype testing promises to advance the goal of selective breeding against inherited traits. There are currently two types of test available.

Tests for specific mutations

Testing for a specific causal gene mutation is preferred because it is highly specific; however, it requires knowledge of the mutation responsible for the genetic defect. Tests of this type exist for five diseases of ophthalmic importance:

- Rod/cone dysplasia (*rcd*) in Irish Setters (*rcd1*) (Clements *et al.*, 1993) and Cardigan Welsh Corgis (*rcd3*) (Petersen-Jones and Zhu, 2000)
- Progressive retinal atrophy in Miniature Schnauzers and in Sloughis
- Congenital stationary nightblindness in the Briard.

It is likely that several other tests will be developed over the next few years.

Tests for marker alleles

These tests target a marker allele that is closely linked to the gene of interest and, therefore, is highly likely to be inherited with it. So-called *marker* or *linkage tests* are available for progressive rod/cone degeneration (*prcd*) – a form of progressive retinal atrophy. This test has currently been validated for English Cocker Spaniels, Portuguese Water Dogs, Labrador Retrievers and Chesapeake Bay Retrievers.

Because this is a marker test, its value lies in its ability to identify homozygous normal dogs unequivocally. However, some dogs identified by the test as 'homozygous affected' are actually heterozygous, and some dogs identified by the test as heterozygous may actually be homozygous and normal. This is due to what has been termed a 'false allele'. The important point for breeders to understand is that the identification of homozygous normal dogs is reliable, and that these dogs can be bred with all other dogs.

These tests have been introduced only recently and are affording new information as test results are accumulated. One predicted difficulty in test interpretation is that there appear to be gene pool differences between large groups within the same breed. This has reinforced the need for continued annual examinations by a veterinary ophthalmologist, regardless of test results.

All these tests require canine DNA and, therefore, necessitate the submission of highly cellular samples. In most cases, DNA may be provided by a venous blood sample collected into EDTA or citrate tubes. Occasionally, laboratories utilize buccal mucosal scrapings. As always, direct correspondence with the laboratory to which the sample will be submitted is essential.

References

Bauer GA, Spiess BM and Lutz H (1996) Exfoliative cytology of conjunctiva and cornea in domestic animals: a comparison of four collecting techniques. *Veterinary and Comparative Ophthalmology* **6**, 181–186

Champagne ES and Pickett JP (1995) The effect of topical 0.5% proparacaine HCL on corneal and conjunctival culture results. *Proceedings of the 26th Annual Meeting of the American College of Veterinary Ophthalmologists* **27**, 144.

Clements PJM, Gregory CY, Petersen-Jones SM, Sargan DR & Bhattacharya SS (1993) Confirmation of the rod cGMP phosphodiesterase ß-subunit (PDEß) nonsense mutation in affected rcd-1 Irish Setters in the UK and development of a diagnostic test. *Current Eye Research* **12**, 861–866

Gerding PA and Kakoma I (1990) Microbiology of the canine and feline eye. *Veterinary Clinics of North America – Small Animal Practice* **20**, 615–625

Maggs DJ, Lappin MR, Reif JS, Collins JK, Carman J, Dittmer DA and Bruns C (1999) Evaluation of serological and viral detection methods for diagnosing feline herpesvirus-1 infection in cats with acute respiratory or chronic ocular disease. *Journal of the American Veterinary Medical Association* **214**, 502–507

Massa KL, Murphy CJ, Hartmann FA, Miller PE, Korsower CS and Young KM (1999) Usefulness of aerobic microbial culture and cytologic evaluation of corneal specimens in the diagnosis of infectious ulcerative keratitis in animals. *Journal of the American Veterinary Medical Association* **215**, 1671–1674

Petersen-Jones SM and Zhu F-X (2000) Development and use of a polymerase chain reaction-based diagnostic test for the causal mutation of progressive retinal atrophy in Cardigan Welsh Corgis. *American Journal of Veterinary Research* **61**, 844–846

Willis M, Bounous DI, Hirsh S, Kaswan R, Stiles J, Martin C, Rakich, P and Roberts W (1997) Conjunctival brush cytology: evaluation of a new cytological collection technique in dogs and cats with a comparison to conjunctival scraping. *Veterinary and Comparative Ophthalmology* **7**, 74–81

Acknowledgements

The author gratefully acknowledges William Fales PhD Hon DipACVM for helpful discussions in preparing this chapter.

2a

Anaesthesia and analgesia

Sheilah Robertson

Introduction

Eye disease requiring surgery is common in companion animals, and practitioners often perform procedures ranging from basic entropion correction in healthy young animals, to advanced intraocular surgery in geriatric animals that may also have concurrent diseases. Because of the wide variety of procedures and clinical status of patients, the anaesthetic protocol will be different for each individual patient, but a good outcome is not difficult to achieve if the following are considered carefully and understood:

- Pain associated with eye disease
- Special handling of ophthalmic patients
- Special handling of blind animals
- Special handling of animals with elevated intraocular pressure (IOP)
- The type of surgery to be performed.

It is also important to be knowledgeable about ocular physiology e.g intraocular pressure, the oculocardiac reflex, the influence of concurrent and intraoperative medications, and the influence of concurrent disease (e.g. diabetes mellitus).

It should be remembered that older animals may have impaired cardiac, renal or hepatic function. There may also be unique requirements of the surgeon and difficulties associated with the anaesthesia of an ophthalmic patient including patient positioning, complete immobilization of the globe, and difficulty in monitoring a patient when access to the head is limited. The patient may have ophthalmic pain.

Pain and pain relief

Ocular pain is often severe and requires prompt treatment. Signs of ophthalmic pain are not always obvious; for example, animals with glaucoma may become quiet and subdued. An animal with painful or irritated eyes may rub and scratch vigorously, leading to worsening of the original disease. Corneal foreign bodies and erosions produce superficial pain, which is acute and sharp. Keratitis, iritis and glaucoma result in a dull, deep pain that may often be caused partly by inflammation. It is important to determine the cause of pain and to treat the primary disease; for example, once glaucoma has been confirmed, therapy is aimed at reducing the intraocular pressure. In some cases, enucleation may be the only way to relieve the animal's pain. If pain is associated with bright light (photophobia), placing the animal in a darkened room may bring substantial relief.

Local anaesthetics

For relief of corneal pain, topical local anaesthetics such as tetracaine, procaine and proparacaine are excellent, but cannot be used frequently because they inhibit corneal re-epithelialization, interfere with lacrimation and may produce corneal swelling and increased permeability. Topical local anaesthetics should be used only for ocular examination, minor procedures, such as removal of a foreign body, or as an adjunct to general anaesthesia. The effects of topical morphine sulphate on corneal sensitivity in both rabbits and humans have been reported (Peyman et al., 1995). This drug is rapid acting and provides excellent analgesia for corneal abrasions without delaying epithelial wound healing. However, the efficacy of this treatment has not been studied in dogs or cats.

Anti-inflammatory agents

Inflammatory pain may respond well to corticosteroids or non-steroidal anti-inflammatory drugs (NSAIDs) (see Chapter 3). NSAIDS can be used short term or long term. In recent years, several new drugs in this category have become available for use in cats and dogs. The newer agents such as carprofen and meloxicam are more specific inhibitors of the cyclo-oxygenase (COX) - 2 enzyme that is initiated in the inflammatory process. In theory, these agents cause less disruption of the COX-1 pathway and prostaglandin production that is critical for gastrointestinal protection, renal perfusion and platelet aggregation. NSAIDs should not be used in animals with pre-existing renal disease. If NSAIDs are used preoperatively, renal perfusion must be maintained by providing adequate intravenous fluids and maintaining adequate systemic blood pressure. Gastrointestinal bleeding and/or renal and hepatic dysfunction can occur with chronic NSAID use, and these should be monitored on a regular basis. Compared to dogs, cats are more susceptible to the unwanted side-effects of NSAIDs but, with care, these agents can be used in cats over long periods of time. Dosing must be accurate, and both the owner and veterinary surgeon should monitor the cat's health closely. Meloxicam is particularly useful in cats because of its palatability, and reports from practice indicate few problems (Lascelles, 1999). A loading dose of 0.3 mg/kg orally, followed by 0.1 mg/kg for the next 4 days, is recommended for the management of acute pain. If chronic therapy is indicated, treatment may be continued with lower doses; 0.1 mg/cat/day or 0.2–0.3 mg/cat two or three times a week have been suggested.

Opioids

Opioid analgesics are most commonly used for short periods of time to relieve surgical pain. Oral morphine can be used for longer periods of time and may be useful in an animal when surgery is not an option and medical treatment of the ophthalmic condition does not fully alleviate the pain. The pure opioid agonists, such as morphine and pethidine, may cause miosis in dogs and mydriasis in cats, and these side-effects should be considered when formulating an analgesic plan. Although unusual in animals that are in pain, morphine may cause vomiting with resultant increase in IOP (see below for details). The partial agonist, buprenorphine, is ideal in ophthalmic patients because it has fewer effects on the eye, does not cause vomiting and is relatively long acting (4–8 hours). Oxymorphone is also a good choice.

Special handling of ophthalmic patients

Blind patients may become quite distressed when removed from their familiar surroundings. Care should be taken to ensure they cannot injure themselves in a cage or run, and that they can find their water bowl. It is important to talk to these patients when approaching them and to maintain physical contact when working with them.

Increased venous pressure raises the intraocular pressure, so patients with elevated IOP or serious ocular diseases such as deep corneal ulcers or penetrating foreign bodies should not be restrained with neck collars or leashes (Figure 2.1a). A leash can be placed around the front of one shoulder and behind the other (Figure 2.1b) or a harness may be used.

Aspects of ocular physiology

Intraocular pressure

The balance between aqueous humour production and removal, the volume of vitreous humour, the blood volume within the uveal vasculature and extraocular muscle tone determines intraocular pressure. Sudden increases can have disastrous consequences including compromised retinal blood flow in a closed globe, or lens and vitreous prolapse in an open globe. The IOP is influenced by several factors, which include:

- Venous pressure
- Direct pressure on the globe
- Endotracheal intubation
- Ventilation
- Blood pressure
- Drugs.

Venous pressure

As previously mentioned, elevation of the venous pressure causes elevation of the IOP. Venous pressure will increase if the jugular veins are occluded to obtain a blood sample, or by a collar around the neck (see Figure 2.1a). Careless positioning of an animal for surgery, or pressure from equipment lying on the neck will have the same effect (Figure 2.2). The head and neck should be elevated to avoid venous congestion. Airway obstruction also causes dramatic increases in venous pressure in addition to the obvious consequences of not being able to inhale or exhale. Endotracheal tubes can become occluded when animals are positioned in a flexed neck position for intraocular surgery. To prevent this, special spiral-embedded (armoured) tubes that do not kink should be used (Figure 2.3).

Vomiting also raises the IOP, so potentially emetic drugs such as morphine, xylazine and medetomidine should not be used in animals when increases in IOP must be avoided. Coughing has a similar effect, and if the animal is known to be coughing, this should be treated aggressively; the agonist–antagonist opioid

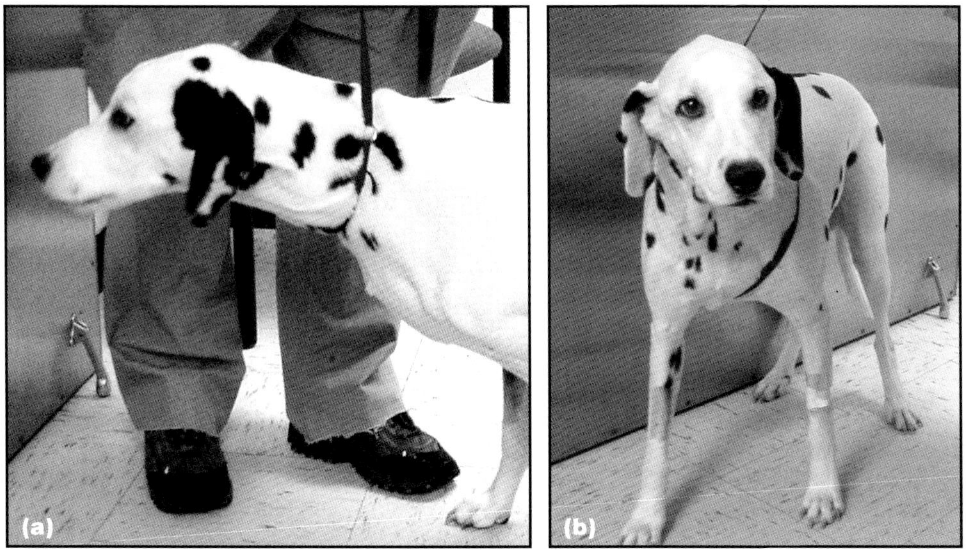

Figure 2.1 (a) Animals with eye injuries or increased intraocular pressure should not be restrained with collars or leashes around their neck. (b) Correct placement of a leash when increases in intraocular pressure must be avoided.

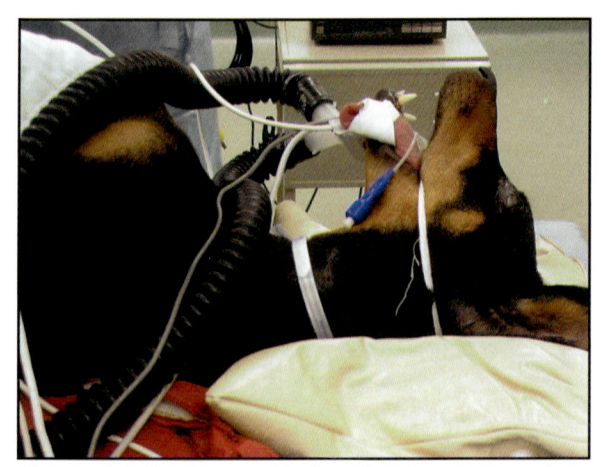

Figure 2.2 Careless positioning of equipment can raise jugular venous and intraocular pressure. When pulse oximeter probes are placed on the tongue of ophthalmic patients they must be well secured.

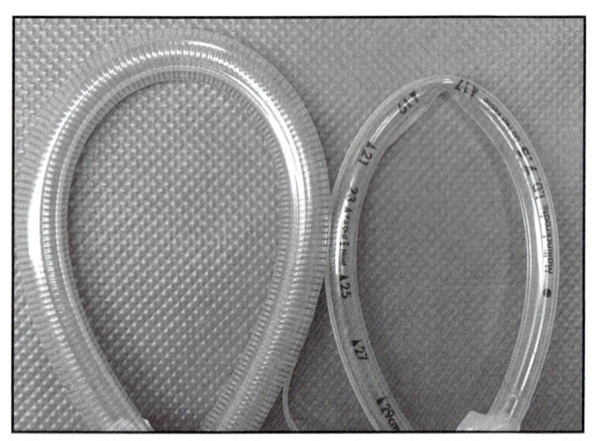

Figure 2.3 Special reinforced endotracheal tubes should be used to prevent airway occlusion when the neck is flexed; positioning of the patient for ocular surgery involves flexion of the neck.

butorphanol is an effective antitussive agent. Attempting endotracheal intubation under a light plane of anaesthesia will induce coughing and should be avoided.

Direct pressure on the globe
Accidental pressure on the globe will raise the IOP. This can happen with careless placement of facemasks and positioning of an anaesthetized patient.

Endotracheal intubation
Coughing, laryngeal reflexes and blood pressure changes all increase IOP during endotracheal intubation. As previously mentioned, coughing occurs when attempting to intubate lightly anaesthetised animals. Laryngeal reflexes and changes in systemic blood pressure can be minimized by touching (of) the larynx as little as possible. In animals with a perforated globe, where sudden increases in IOP could be disastrous, topical lignocaine (lidocaine) can be sprayed on the larynx before intubation. Alternatively, intravenous lignocaine (2 mg/kg) or fentanyl (1–2 μg/kg) given 2–3 minutes before intubation will greatly decrease laryngeal reflexes.

Blood pressure
IOP is stable over a wide range of systemic blood pressures, but sudden increases will cause transient changes. Ensuring an adequate plane of anaesthesia and good analgesia can alleviate sudden changes associated with any surgical stimulus.

Ventilation
The adequacy of ventilation plays an important role in controlling blood flow in ocular vessels. Hypercapnia causes vasodilation and increased IOP; therefore, arterial, venous or end-tidal CO_2 should be monitored during anaesthesia and the anaesthetist should aim for normocapnia (pCO_2 40–45 mmHg) or mild hypocapnia. Monitoring is discussed later in this chapter.

Drugs
The choice of anaesthetic drugs is important when changes in IOP are of concern. The only specific drug that is absolutely contraindicated is succinylcholine, a rarely used depolarizing neuromuscular blocking agent, because it produces an initial increase in skeletal muscle tone, including the extraocular muscles before resulting in a longer period of muscle relaxation.

The commonly used premedicant agents acetylpromazine and the benzodiazepines cause either no change, or a decrease in IOP. The opioids have little effect on IOP, unless emesis occurs. Analgesia is important for ophthalmic surgery; good choices of opioids are discussed above. Ketamine alone is not recommended, because nystagmus may occur and the palpebral reflex remains strong. The increased muscle tone associated with ketamine includes the extraocular muscles and this will elevate IOP. A rough emergence from anaesthesia, which is common if ketamine is used alone, is undesirable in ophthalmic patients. Fortunately, many of these problems can be counteracted with the prior use of acetylpromazine or the benzodiazepine agents (diazepam and midazolam), making ketamine, if given subsequently, a useful agent for many ocular procedures. However, ketamine should be avoided when the eye is already perforated or likely to perforate, for example in an animal with a penetrating foreign body or deep corneal ulcer.

Thiopentone and propofol can be used safely for induction of general anaesthesia for ophthalmic surgery. For short procedures, anaesthesia can be maintained with propofol, but more commonly, inhalant agents such as halothane, isoflurane and sevoflurane are used. Isoflurane and sevoflurane are preferred because they cause less sensitization of the heart to catecholamines than does halothane; this is relevant in ophthalmic surgery when adrenaline may be instilled into the eye and absorbed systemically.

Oculocardiac reflex
The oculocardiac reflex (OCR) occurs when a stimulus to the eye (pressure, manipulation or traction) is transmitted centrally through the ciliary nerves to the ophthalmic branch of the trigeminal nerve and continues to the trigeminal sensory nucleus. Here, connections continue through the visceral motor nucleus of the vagus to the vagus nerve itself, finally reaching the

heart. Initiation of the reflex can result in profound bradycardia, arrhythmias or asystole, which are well documented and not uncommon in humans during ophthalmic surgery. In dogs, the OCR appears to be of minor clinical importance (Clutton et al., 1988), but the effects can be dramatic when it does occur. The incidence of the OCR in cats has not been reported.

Theoretically, the reflex can be blocked on the afferent side by retrobulbar injection of local anaesthetics, or by anticholinergic agents such as atropine and glycopyrrolate, which act on the vagal component of the reflex. Neither of these techniques guarantees complete inhibition of vagally induced slowing of the heart, and both carry risks. Performing a retrobulbar block (see later for full description) can in itself initiate the reflex and other inherent dangers of this technique include puncture of the globe and retrobulbar haemorrhage. Atropine can promote arrhythmias, and in animals with cardiac disease the resultant tachycardia and increased myocardial oxygen demand can be detrimental. For these reasons, the best policy is to monitor the heart rate closely during ocular surgery and if significant bradycardia occurs, stop the initiating stimulus and give atropine (0.02 mg/kg i.v.).

Use of anticholinergic drugs in dogs with glaucoma is controversial and is not recommended by all authors. A well designed study (Frischmeyer et al., 1993) measured changes in IOP after systemic administration of anticholinergic drugs in normal dogs and those with pre-existing glaucoma. This study concluded that the risks of inducing angle-closure glaucoma were very low and that the decision to use these drugs should be based on other criteria.

Preoperative evaluation

Influence of concurrent disease

Preoperative evaluation of ophthalmic patients must include a thorough history and clinical examination. A cause for any abnormal heart rate or rhythm should be investigated. Each individual will warrant its own preoperative work-up, but in older animals the cardiac, renal and hepatic systems should be carefully evaluated. Depending on current medication and health status, acid–base and electrolyte analysis may be justified.

A significant number of animals presented for cataract removal have diabetes mellitus that may or may not be well regulated. Various protocols have been suggested; the recommended dose of insulin on the morning of surgery ranges from zero to 100% of the animal's normal dose. These protocols have not been critically evaluated in dogs until recently. Kronen et al. (2000) compared the effect of giving 25% or 100% of the normal insulin dose on the morning of surgery and concluded that the former group was usually hyperglycaemic and ketotic prior to surgery and that a full dose of insulin was more likely to reduce glucose to the normal range. These authors cautioned that neither protocol consistently produced normoglycaemia and that most animals were ketoacidotic. It is advisable to monitor blood glucose every 30–45 minutes in these patients and make adjustments according to the results; additional insulin or intravenous dextrose may be required. Profound hypoglycaemia must be prevented because the clinical signs of sleepiness and coma are masked by general anaesthesia.

Influence of concurrent and intraoperative medication

Ophthalmic patients often have a history of multiple previous and/or current drug therapies, which may be relevant to their anaesthetic management. As with all patients, it is important to obtain a detailed history. These patients may receive drugs for their ocular condition or for other, unrelated, reasons. For example, an older dog that is to undergo cataract removal may be on corticosteroids or NSAIDs for arthritis, and on cardiac medication such as angiotensin-converting enzyme (ACE) inhibitors or ß-blockers for cardiac disease. Reviewing the implications of all concurrent medication is outside the scope of this chapter, but those specific and relevant to the ophthalmic patient will be discussed.

Chronic administration of topical or systemic corticosteroids often causes an elevation of liver enzymes, and may result in iatrogenic hypoadrenocorticism. These patients should not be abruptly withdrawn from corticosteroids and some may require additional corticosteroids in the perioperative period (Court et al., 1988).

Mannitol (given intravenously) and glycerine (given orally) reduce the IOP by their osmotic actions and may be given to animals preoperatively. The benefits of these agents must be weighed against the potential problems they cause, which include increases in plasma osmolarity, circulating blood volume and central venous pressure. These effects are detrimental to animals with pre-existing cardiac disease.

Systemic carbonic anhydrase inhibitors such as acetazolamide reduce production of aqueous humour, but their effects are not confined to the eye. Their renal actions result in metabolic acidosis, hypokalaemia and hyperchloraemia. If respiratory acidosis occurs during anaesthesia, the problem is compounded. This, combined with abnormal potassium balance, can lead to compromised cardiac function. Newer topical carbonic anhydrase inhibitors should have fewer undesirable side-effects.

The anaesthetist should be aware of pilocarpine treatment in glaucoma patients, because systemic absorption of cholinergic drugs can cause bradycardia. Conversely, the topical use of adrenergic agonists such as adrenaline, phenylephrine and dipivefrin may lead to systemic hypertension and tachycardia, and predispose the patient to arrhythmias during anaesthesia. ß-Blockers may be used as a component of glaucoma therapy, but side-effects that need to be monitored include bradycardia and bronchoconstriction.

It is always wise to anticipate which drugs may be used by the ophthalmic surgeons so that one is prepared, or can take preventive measures against potential side-effects. For example, if the use of adrenaline is likely, the inhalant agents isoflurane or sevoflurane are preferred over halothane.

The anaesthetic plan

Much of the information needed to formulate a plan has been discussed above. A quiet recovery following delicate ocular surgery is of paramount importance and this is achieved with adequate sedation and analgesia. Figure 2.4 summarizes the preanaesthetic, induction and maintenance agents that can be used in these patients. If the surgical procedure involves the cornea, applying topical local anaesthetic a few minutes before the surgeon begins is very beneficial. This provides additional analgesia, decreases the initial surgical stimulus and the sympathetic responses, and prevents sudden changes in the plane of anaesthesia.

Preanaesthetic agents
Acetylpromazine
Midazolam
Diazepam
Pentobarbitone
Buprenorphine
Oxymorphone
Induction agents
Thiopentone
Propofol
Ketamine [a]
Maintenance agents
Propofol
Halothane
Isoflurane
Sevoflurane
Adjunct agents
Topical proparacaine
Intravenous lignocaine [b]
Intravenous fentanyl [b]
Neuromuscular blocking agents:
Pancuronium
Atracurium

Figure 2.4 Commonly used anaesthetic agents for ophthalmic patients.
[a] Ketamine should not be used alone – see text for details.
[b] May be given prior to intubation to decrease laryngeal reflexes – see text for details.

Special techniques

Retrobulbar block

This technique involves injecting local anaesthetic behind the globe (Skarda, 1996). It can only be performed safely in cats and dogs after induction of general anaesthesia. To perform the block, lignocaine (lidocaine) and bupivacaine are mixed in a ratio of 1:4, not exceeding a total dosage of 3 mg/kg for the combined drugs. This mixture results in fast onset (<10 minutes) and long duration of action (2–3 hours). One of several described techniques is to deposit local anaesthetic behind the globe by sliding a needle, which has been slightly bent, along the inside of the orbit, on the lateral side (Figure 2.5). Possible complications include retrobulbar haemorrhage, injection into the cerebrospinal fluid, penetration of the globe and initiation of the oculocardiac reflex. Although intra- and postoperative analgesia are excellent, this technique is reserved for enucleation and evisceration surgery.

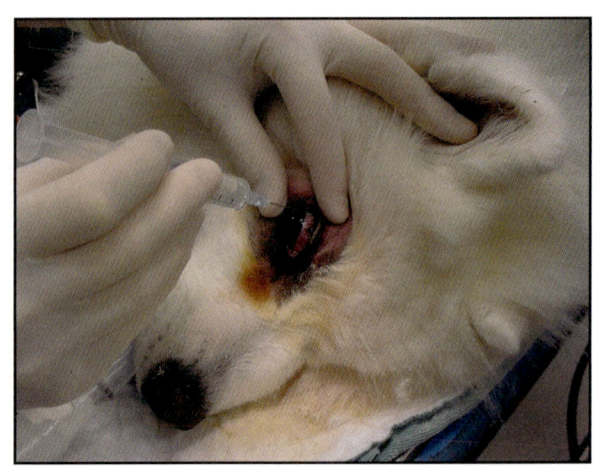

Figure 2.5 A retrobulbar block with local anaesthetics provides good analgesia for enucleation. The procedure involves a long curved needle being inserted close to the wall of the bony orbit and then being advanced gently.

Immobilization of the globe for intraocular surgery

A central, immobile eye is essential for delicate corneal or intraocular surgery. The eye is central in a deep plane of anaesthesia, but the inherent dangers associated with this are cardiopulmonary depression and a prolonged recovery. Ideal conditions can be achieved by using non-depolarizing neuromuscular blocking agents (Young et al., 1991), such as pancuronium, vecuronium and atracurium. These agents cause paralysis of all skeletal muscle; therefore, the animal must be manually or mechanically ventilated. The extent and duration of neuromuscular blockade is highly variable between individuals and a peripheral nerve stimulator is strongly recommended to monitor the degree of muscle relaxation. Using a low dose of pancuronium to paralyse the ocular muscles but 'spare' the respiratory muscles has been shown to be a dangerous practice (Lee et al., 1998). It is essential to ensure there is no residual muscle weakness when the animal recovers and is extubated, otherwise potentially fatal respiratory depression may occur. These techniques are most commonly reserved for use in specialist practices and the reader is directed to a recent review by Martinez (1999).

Monitoring the ophthalmic patient

Monitoring a patient during eye surgery can be a challenge because the anaesthetist cannot test jaw tone and palpebral reflexes, which are commonly used to assess the depth of anaesthesia. In addition, it may not be obvious that the endotracheal tube has become disconnected when it is hidden beneath the drapes.

Doppler flow probe

The peripheral pulse can be monitored with an inexpensive Doppler flow probe placed over the digital or dorsal pedal arteries. With the addition of a cuff, this set-up can also be used to measure systemic blood pressure. The Doppler reflects the systolic blood pressure and, as a general guide, this should be > 80 mmHg. This system is ideal because it produces an audible sound and when there is a problem, operating room personnel respond to audible monitors more quickly than to visual ones. An ECG is useful in the event of arrhythmias, but it must be emphasized that it does not reflect the mechanical activity of the heart.

Pulse oximetry

Pulse oximeters have become very popular in practice and are useful, if their limitations are understood. They measure haemoglobin saturation, the normal value being >95%. They are commonly placed on the tongue (Figure 2.2), and must be well secured in ophthalmic patients. Alternatively, a hind toe web or a rectal probe can be used. Pulse oximeters detect the peripheral pulse, and usually emit an audible beep. These monitors measure haemoglobin desaturation, but give no indication of adequacy of alveolar ventilation, which is reflected by end-expired, or arterial carbon dioxide levels. In an anaesthetized animal breathing 100% oxygen, a pulse oximeter will not detect serious respiratory depression. The following example from a dog undergoing cataract removal serves as an example (normal values for dogs are given in parentheses):

Pulse oximeter reading 98%
Arterial blood gas results:
    pH   6.944 (7.400)
    p_aO_2 454 mmHg (4–5 times inspired concentration)
    p_aCO_2 114 mmHg (40–45)
    Base excess 12.2 mEq/l (–4 to + 4)

This dog had a severe respiratory acidosis that had gone undetected. Severe hypercapnia may lead to prolonged recoveries and contribute to arrhythmias. The cause of the problem in this case was discovered to be a partially occluded endotracheal tube caused by extreme flexion of the neck. For these reasons, the value of monitoring carbon dioxide is obvious.

End-tidal carbon dioxide usually mirrors arterial CO_2 levels and can be measured by a capnograph. It may not be suitable for very small patients because of the added dead space, and is inaccurate when used with non-rebreathing systems (T-piece, Bain circuit). Alternatively, a blood gas analyser may be used. Venous samples are sufficient for measuring CO_2, but give no indication of oxygenation status. With the advent of affordable portable blood gas machines, this option has become more feasible for practitioners.

Regardless of the monitoring equipment available, the peripheral pulse should be palpated frequently and an oesophageal stethoscope with extension tubing can be used to auscultate the heart and monitor breath sounds.

References and further reading

Clutton RE, Boyd C, Richards DL and Schwink K (1988) Significance of the oculocardiac reflex during ophthalmic surgery in the dog. *Journal of Small Animal Practice* **29**, 573–579

Court MH, Dodman NH, Norman WM and Seeler DC (1988) Anaesthetic management of small animal patients with endocrine disease. *British Veterinary Journal* **144**, 323–341

Frischmeyer KJ, Miller PE, Bellay Y, Smedes SL and Brinson DM (1993) Parenteral anticholinergics in dogs with normal and elevated intraocular pressure. *Veterinary Surgery* **22(3)**, 230–234

Kronen PW, Moon PF, Erb NH, Ludders JW, Gleed RD, Kern TJ and Randolph JF. (2000) Comparison of two insulin protocols for diabetic dogs undergoing cataract surgery. In: *Proceedings of the Association of Veterinary Anaesthetists, Spring Conference, Cambridge, MA, March 26–28*

Lascelles BD (1999) Analgesia in cats and the results of a field study examining the use of meloxicam in cats. In: *Recent Advances in Non-Steroidal Anti-Inflammatory Therapy in Small Animals*, Paris, June 11–13 pp.75–79

Lee DD, Meyer RE, Sullivan TC, Davidson MG, Swanson CR and Hellyer PW. (1998) Respiratory depressant and skeletal muscle relaxant effects of low-dose pancuronium bromide in spontaneously breathing isoflurane anesthetized dogs. *Veterinary Surgery* **27**, 473–479

Martinez EA (1999) Newer neuromuscular blockers, is the practitioner ready for muscle relaxants? *Veterinary Clinics of North America: Small Animal Practice* **29 (3)**, 811–817

Peyman GA, Rahimy MH and Fernandes MI (1994) Effects of morphine on corneal sensitivity and epithelial wound healing: implications for topical ophthalmic analgesia. *British Journal of Ophthalmology* **78**, 138–141

Skarda RT (1996) Local and regional anesthetic and analgesic techniques: Dogs. In: *Lumb and Jones' Veterinary Anesthesia*, 3rd edn, ed. JC Thurmon et al., pp.426–447. Williams and Wilkins, Baltimore

Young SS, Barnett KC and Taylor PM (1991) Anaesthetic regimens for cataract removal in the dog. *Journal of Small Animal Practice* **32**, 236–240

2b

Ophthalmic surgery: instrumentation

David J. Maggs

Introduction

Although instruments used for general surgery can also be used for certain ocular procedures, instruments intended specifically for ophthalmic procedures will reduce the frustration of the surgeon and the length of the procedure, and improve surgical outcome and client satisfaction. These benefits justify the purchase of some dedicated ophthalmic instruments. These instruments can be assembled in surgical packs and preserved in excellent condition for delicate ocular surgery. Ophthalmic instruments for procedures that are commonly performed in general practice may be conveniently divided into:

- Those required for enucleation and exenteration
- Those required for eyelid and third eyelid procedures
- Those required for corneo-conjunctival surgery.

Suggested minimum contents for these three surgical packs are described in Figures 2.6, 2.7 and 2.8. In each case, a list of additional instruments is provided for veterinary surgeons with special interest or expertise in ophthalmic surgery.

Because fine instrument control is essential when operating on or near the eye, ophthalmic instruments are designed to be manipulated with minimal movement

Suggested minimum set of instruments for enucleation or exenteration	
Bishop–Harmon tissue forceps (fine)	1
Brown–Adson tissue forceps	1
Hartman mosquito haemostatic forceps	2 straight; 2 curved
Kelly haemostatic tissue forceps	2 straight; 2 curved
Barraquer wire eyelid speculum	1
Bard-Parker scalpel handle	1
Stevens straight tenotomy scissors	1
Metzenbaum curved scissors	1
Storz pattern enucleation scissors	1
Derf needle holder with lock	1
Jones cross action towel forceps	2–4
Additional optional instruments	
0.3 Castroviejo fixation forceps	1
Castroviejo eyelid speculum	1
Allis tissue forceps	2
Metzenbaum straight scissors	1
Stevens curved tenotomy scissors	1

Figure 2.6 Suggested instruments for a surgical pack for enucleation or exenteration.

Suggested minimum set of instruments for surgery of eyelids and the third eyelid	
Bishop–Harmon tissue forceps (fine)	1
0.3 Castroviejo fixation forceps	1
Hartman straight mosquito haemostatic forceps	2
Desmarres chalazion forceps	1
Brown–Adson tissue forceps	1
Barraquer cilia forceps	1
Barraquer wire eyelid speculum	1
Jaeger stainless steel lid plate	1
Bard-Parker scalpel handle	1
Stevens straight tenotomy scissors	1
Westcott wide-handled curved tenotomy scissors	1
Meyerhoefer chalazion curette	1
Harms–Tubingen curved tying forceps	1–2
Derf Needle holder with lock	1
Barraquer curved tapered jaw needle holder (non-locking)	1
23 gauge curved anterior chamber irrigating cannula	1
Jones cross action towel forceps	2–4
Additional optional instruments	
Hartman curved mosquito haemostatic forceps	2
Castroviejo eyelid speculum	1
Stevens curved tenotomy scissors	1
Westcott wide-handled straight tenotomy scissors	1

Figure 2.7 Suggested instruments for a surgical pack for procedures involving the eyelids and the third eyelid.

Suggested minimum set of instruments for corneal and conjunctival procedures	
Bishop–Harmon tissue forceps (fine)	1
Colibri type corneal utility forceps	1
0.3 Castroviejo fixation forceps	1
Hartman straight mosquito haemostatic forceps	2
Barraquer wire eyelid speculum	1
Martinez double-ended corneal dissector	1
10cm Beaver hexagonal scalpel handle	1
Stevens straight tenotomy scissors	1
Westcott wide-handled curved tenotomy scissors	1
Harms–Tubingen curved tying forceps	1–2
Derf needle holder with lock	1
Barraquer curved tapered jaw needle holder (non-locking)	1
Small (4cm) serrefine	2
23 gauge curved anterior chamber irrigating cannula	1
Jones cross action towel forceps	2–4
Additional optional instruments	
Bishop–Harmon tissue forceps (extra delicate)	1
Hartman curved mosquito haemostatic forceps	2
Castroviejo eyelid speculum	1
Storz pattern straight iris scissors	1
Stevens curved tenotomy scissors	1
Westcott wide-handled straight tenotomy scissors	1

Figure 2.8 Suggested instruments for a surgical pack for corneal and conjunctival procedures.

of the surgeon's upper arms. Microsurgical instruments are further refined to limit movement of the forearms and wrists.

The major differences between instruments used in general surgery and those intended for ophthalmic applications are:

- Their weight: many ophthalmic instruments have holes in their handle shafts to minimize weight
- The need for tactile feedback with ophthalmic instruments. This is usually provided via ridges, flattened surfaces, or the knurling of handles
- Ophthalmic instruments are often sprung, so that changes in hand or wrist position are not required to reopen the instruments.

The following is a brief description of ophthalmic instruments that might be used regularly by veterinary surgeons in general practice, along with important features of each instrument. The reader is referred to the further reading list for description of microsurgical instruments for corneal and intraocular use. Instruments are grouped into those intended for stabilizing or grasping tissues, those for separating and incising tissues and those for reuniting or suturing them. Brief discussions of disposable items and drapes, and care of instruments, are also included.

Instruments for stabilizing tissues

Tissue and cilia forceps

Forceps are commonly used in ophthalmic surgery for grasping eyelid skin, conjunctiva and corneal edges, and for the epilation of cilia. Since it is essential to minimize ocular tissue trauma, tissue forceps with delicate teeth are common. A 1 × 2 intermeshing tooth pattern (one tooth on one arm and two teeth on the other) is typical. Forceps should be light enough to cause minimal damage to the tissue grasped, without being so delicate that they are bent by the tissue. Fine tissue forceps should not be used to handle suture needles. Tissue forceps should not be used to grasp suture material, unless they have tying platforms incorporated into their design, since fine suture material is easily damaged by instrument teeth. As a rule:

- Eyelids may be grasped using Brown–Adson or Bishop–Harmon forceps
- Conjunctiva is best grasped using more delicate Bishop–Harmon, Castroviejo or Colibri-style forceps
- Cornea should be grasped with 0.3 Castroviejo fixation forceps or Colibri-style forceps only
- Barraquer cilia forceps have finely finished blades and are specifically indicated for the removal of distichia (abnormal, inwardly growing eyelashes)
- Serrefines are attached to the end of the conjunctival stay sutures to help position the globe for surgery.

Examples of commonly used ophthalmic forceps are shown in Figure 2.9.

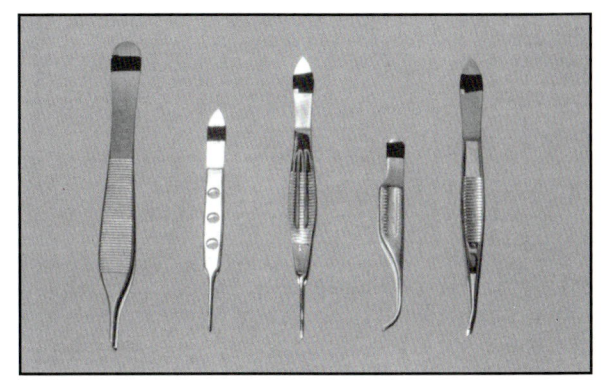

Figure 2.9 Forceps commonly used in ophthalmic surgery. From left to right: Brown–Adson tissue forceps; Bishop–Harmon tissue forceps; 0.3 Castroviejo fixation forceps; Colibri-style corneal utility forceps; Barraquer cilia forceps.

Eyelid specula

Eyelid specula are inexpensive and of enormous value in ophthalmic surgery, yet are frequently not owned by veterinary surgeons in general practice. The Barraquer wire eyelid speculum (Figure 2.10) is a versatile, light instrument that ensures ready visualization of the conjunctiva, the cornea, and the third eyelid. Its degree of opening may be manually adjusted prior to insertion, so as to provide adequate exposure. It should be placed with its open end facing medially, by gently elevating the eyelid margins using fine forceps (Figure 2.11).

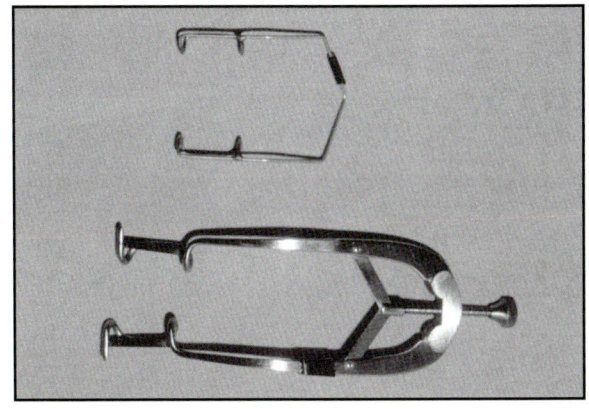

Figure 2.10 (top) Barraquer wire eyelid speculum. (bottom) Castroviejo eyelid speculum.

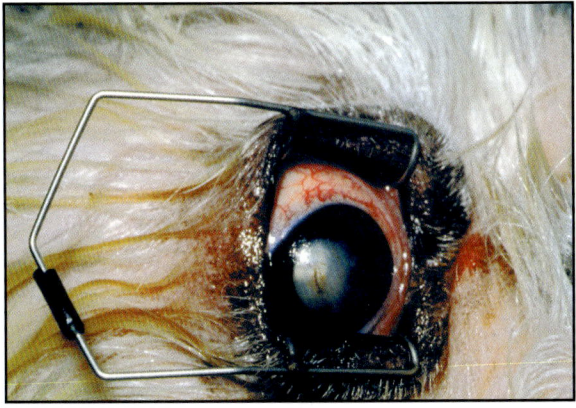

Figure 2.11 The correct positioning of a Barraquer wire eyelid speculum.

38 Ophthalmic surgery: instrumentation

The Castroviejo eyelid speculum (Figure 2.10) is heavier, and is opened and closed using a small threaded screw. This speculum tends to be too heavy and cumbersome to place, retain in position and to work around in small animal patients.

Desmarres chalazion clamp

Desmarres chalazion clamps or forceps consist of a stainless steel base plate and an opposing circular or oval steel ring (Figure 2.12a). This clamp provides ideal stabilization of the eyelid margin, while still permitting surgical access to one side of the lid, usually the conjunctival surface (Figure 2.12b). It is indispensable for surgical resection of ectopic cilia or curettage of eyelid masses, especially chalazia. It also aids with haemostasis, which improves intraoperative visualization, and, during cryosurgery, facilitates rapid freezing and slow thawing of tissue retained within the clamp. Numerous sizes are available, but a medium oval clamp is appropriate for most patients and procedures.

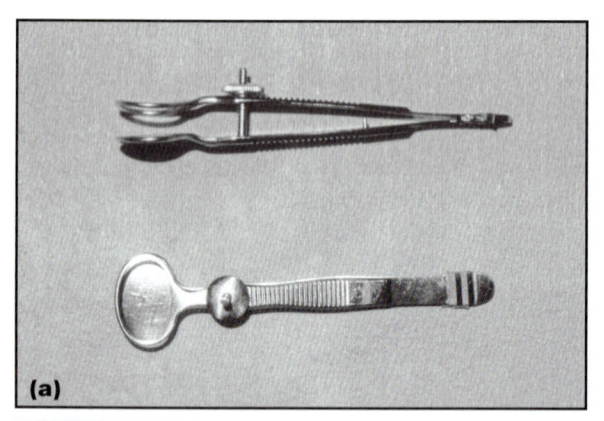

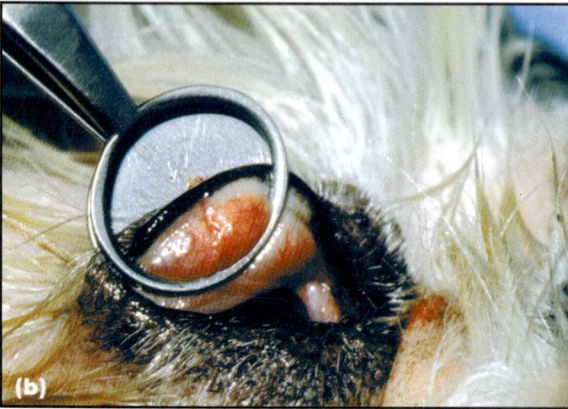

Figure 2.12 (a) Desmarres chalazion clamp: (top) side view; (bottom) front view. (b) The correct positioning of the Desmarres chalazion clamp on the upper eyelid of a dog.

Jaeger eyelid plate

The smooth stainless steel surface of the Jaeger lid plate provides a means of elevation and stabilization of eyelids, a firm surface for incising against, and protection of the underlying globe from inadvertent penetration (Figure 2.13). The instrument is inexpensive and will be frequently used in most general practices. Its use is described more fully in Chapter 2c.

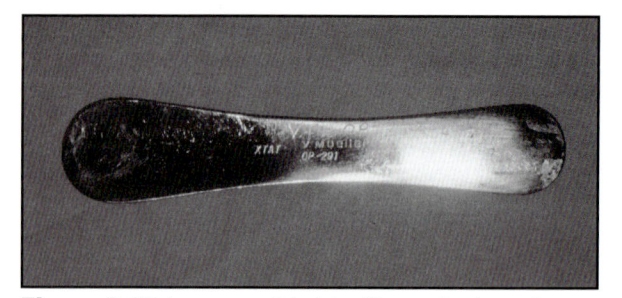

Figure 2.13 Jaeger eyelid plate. (Its use is shown in Chapter 2c.)

Instruments for separating tissues (incisions)

Scalpels and blades

Bard–Parker and Beaver scalpel handles and matching blades are commonly used in ophthalmic surgery (Figure 2.14). The number 3 Bard–Parker handle is familiar to general surgeons and is the primary instrument for adnexal surgery. The number 15 Bard–Parker blade permits the surgeon to exert excellent control of the depth and of the direction of the incision. Corneal incisions are best made with the lighter and smaller Beaver handle and number 64 Beaver blade. The number 65 Beaver blade has a sharp point and is useful for stab incisions preparatory to intraocular surgery. A variety of Beaver handles is available. While all are similar to each other, it is essential that they provide adequate tactile feedback to the surgeon, thereby permitting accurate blade control.

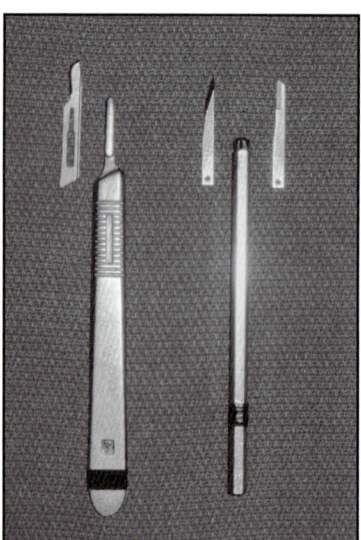

Figure 2.14 Scalpel handles and blades commonly used in ophthalmic surgery. Number 3 Bard–Parker scalpel handle with number 15 Bard–Parker blade. Hexagonal Beaver scalpel handle with number 64 (right) and 65 (left) Beaver blades.

Scissors

A number of different types of blunt-tipped scissors are used in ocular and periocular surgery. Stevens tenotomy scissors (Figure 2.15) are excellent general purpose scissors. Their major use is the undermining of conjunctiva during conjunctival graft harvesting or transconjunctival enucleation. They may also be used to undermine or to complete incisions in skin that have been initiated with a scalpel blade. Scissors with sprung handles, such as Westcott tenotomy scissors (Figure 2.15), are ideal for more delicate incisions, as they may be operated using only the fingers, and active motion is necessary only for the closing action. Larger straight or curved, blunt-tipped scissors, such as Mayo or Metzenbaum designs, are used for surgery involving the periocular skin, and for enucleation and exenteration. Specialized enucleation scissors that have sharply curved blades, but blunt tips, are recommended to facilitate the final retrobulbar dissection during enucleation.

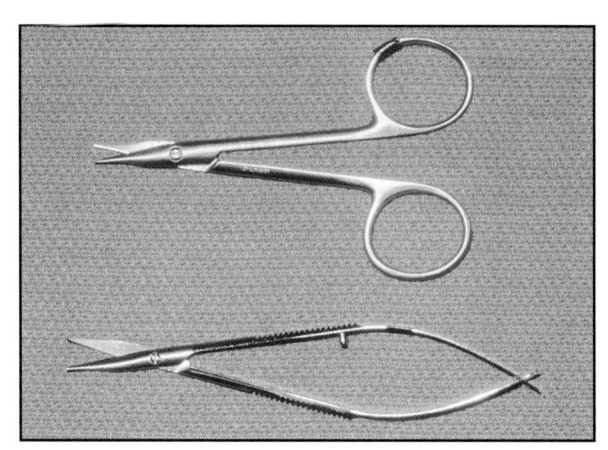

Figure 2.15 (top) Stevens tenotomy scissors. (bottom) Westcott tenotomy scissors.

Meyerhoefer chalazion curette

The Meyerhoefer chalazion curette is a small, sharp curette on a light handle (Figure 2.16). It is designed for curetting inspissated material from within a chalazion or lipogranuloma of the eyelid glands. Ideally, the eyelid is grasped using a Desmarres chalazion clamp, and the chalazion is incised through the conjunctival surface. All inflammatory and secretory material is then removed with the Meyerhoefer curette, using a firm sweeping action. A number of sizes, either with straight or curved shafts are available; however, a straight, medium instrument is usually all that is required.

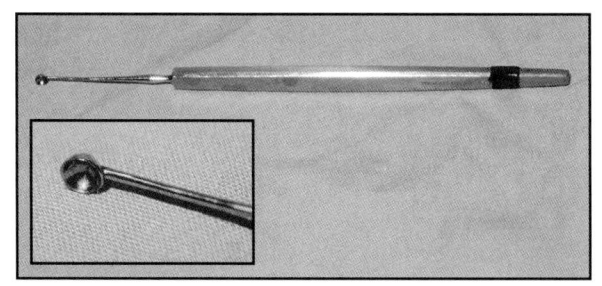

Figure 2.16 Meyerhoefer chalazion curette. The inset shows the curette at higher magnification.

Instruments for uniting tissues (suturing)

Needle holders

Needle holders used in ophthalmic applications fall into two broad groups based on the size of the needle that they are intended to grasp. Small needles should be grasped with small-tipped microsurgical needle holders, while Derf needle holders are practical for larger needles (Figure 2.17). Microsurgical needle holders may be damaged if they are used to grasp large needles, and microsurgical needles are likely to be damaged if they are grasped with Derf needle holders. Opinions regarding the needle size at which one needle holder is considered appropriate, and the other inappropriate, vary. However, it is generally recommended that microsurgical needle holders are used for needles with a diameter of 0.203 mm or less (Troutman, 1974). These are generally used with 6-0, or smaller, suture material, although the needle size can vary for a given suture material.

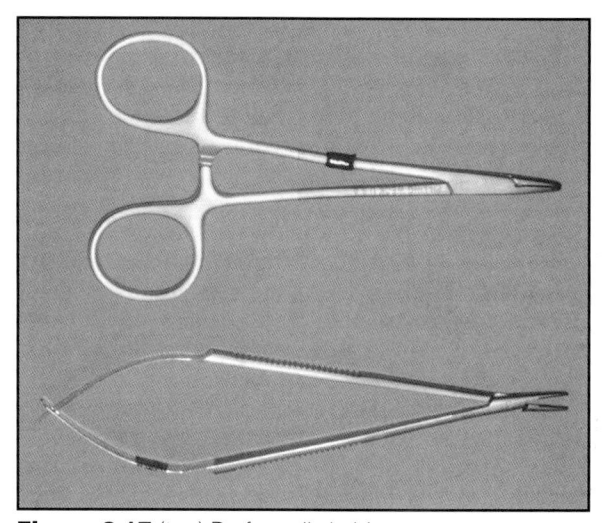

Figure 2.17 (top) Derf needle holder. (bottom) Microsurgical needle holder.

Locking mechanisms are standard (and desirable) for larger needle holders, and are optional on microsurgical needle holders. Their use in microsurgical operations should usually be avoided, as they inevitably cause the instrument tips to jump when the locking mechanism is unlatched, and this can cause significant damage, or needle misdirection.

Fine suture material should not be grasped using needle holders with serrated tips or with toothed forceps, as these can significantly damage suture material. Specialized forceps, such as Harms–Tubingen tying forceps, are available for this purpose, and are recommended for the handling of fine suture material. This is discussed more fully in Chapter 2c.

Suture material

A multitude of suture materials and needles is now available to the veterinary surgeon. A full description of each suture material, its characteristics, advantages, and disadvantages goes beyond the scope of this chapter. An excellent review of suture and needle types for ophthalmic surgery is available in Ethicon's online catalogue. Further details of suture materials may also be obtained from the relevant chapters of this book; however, some general comments regarding suture and needle selection are appropriate here.

40 Ophthalmic surgery: instrumentation

There are three specific considerations when suturing eyelid skin:

- Needles and suture material should be of small gauge, and the sutures should be closely spaced. The reasons for this are discussed in Chapter 2c. However, this can make suture removal challenging in some non-compliant patients
- Periocular suture ends may, occasionally, abrade the cornea
- A good cosmetic result is essential for surgery involving periocular skin.

As in many biological situations, each of these factors may suggest a different 'ideal' suture material. For example, placement of an absorbable suture may obviate the need for suture removal, a braided suture material may be less likely to ulcerate the cornea than a monofilament one, but fine non-absorbable monofilament suture may cause less tissue reaction and provide a better cosmetic result. With all of these features in mind, suture materials that are commonly used in adnexal surgery are fine braided nylon, polyglactin 910 or silk.

Fine, absorbable suture material is always used in conjunctival incisions. Polyglactin 910 (6-0 or finer) is an excellent choice. Corneal incisions in human patients are usually closed using very fine (9-0 to 10-0) monofilament nylon, because it stimulates minimal tissue reaction. Nylon must be removed from the cornea, and this requires general anaesthesia in veterinary patients. Therefore, polyglactin 910 is commonly used to close corneal incisions in animals. Ideally, 8-0 or smaller should be used; however, this requires adequate magnification, and is, therefore, more commonly selected by specialists than by general practitioners.

Suture needles

The choice of the correct suture needle is critical for ophthalmic surgery. The major consideration is needle tip design. There are four commonly available designs: taper point, cutting, reverse cutting and spatula tip (Figure 2.18). Each leaves a different tissue tract, and they cause different amounts of tissue damage. In general, taper point needles are ideal for conjunctiva, since they cause little tissue trauma. They are, however, not sharp enough for use in skin or cornea. Cutting, or reverse cutting, needles are necessary for suturing skin but should not be used for the cornea, due to the increased tissue trauma that they cause, and the difficulty experienced in accurately directing their depth within tissue. Spatula-tipped needles are specifically designed for use in lamellar tissues such as cornea and sclera, because they are more likely to remain in the desired tissue plane and their depth can be accurately regulated by the surgeon.

Disposable materials and drapes

Although many standard drapes and disposable items used in routine surgery will be applicable to ophthalmic surgery, a number of specialized items warrant special mention. It is critical that gauze swabs and cotton wool, which may be used routinely in adnexal procedures, do not contact the cornea, as these materials can cause corneal ulceration. The cornea should be blotted using special cellulose foam sponges.

Although the eye and adnexa may be draped using normal towels or disposable drapes, special fenestrated drapes with pre-cut oval windows and adhesive posterior surfaces provide a far more convenient alternative. Some of these drapes also have a foam patch that provides an area of increased friction, for the retention of instruments during surgery. Rectangular, clear plastic adhesive drapes are also available. These permit the surgeon to cut a window of the desired size and shape for individual patients and surgical procedures.

Care of instruments

The delicate nature and the expense of many ophthalmic instruments dictate that great care is taken in their use, sterilization and storage. Routine steam sterilization of ophthalmic instruments is satisfactory, but can dull instrument edges, after multiple applications. Where available, ethylene oxide gas sterilization is preferred. The removal of organic material prior to sterilization is essential. This is best accomplished using distilled

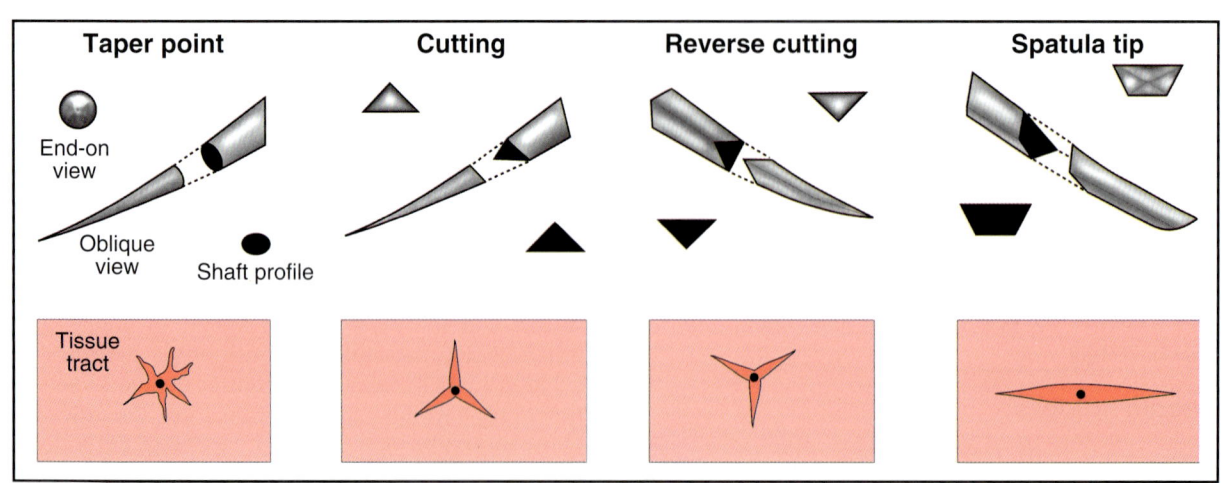

Figure 2.18 Suture needle tip designs and the tissue tracts they create. (Redrawn after Eisner (1990) with permission.)

water and, where necessary, gentle brushing with a toothbrush. Larger scrubbing brushes should not be used. Instruments must not be allowed to damage each other when being cleaned or stored. Special fenestrated plastic caps that protect instrument tips, but permit passage of the sterilizing agent, are available. Instrument trays provide an ideal method for keeping instrument damage to a minimum, at all points of the process. If instruments are damaged, they can often be repaired at a cost that is lower than the cost of replacing them; this should be done by a certified repairer, usually the manufacturer.

References and further reading

Eisner G (1990) *Eye surgery. An Introduction to Operative Technique.* Springer-Verlag, Berlin

Nasisse MP (ed.) (1997) Surgical management of ocular disease. *Veterinary Clinics of North America – Small Animal Practice* **27**, 963–1010

Troutman RC (1974) *Microsurgery of the Anterior Segment of the Eye. Vol. 1. Introduction and Basic Techniques.* CV Mosby, London

Acknowledgements

The author gratefully acknowledges the assistance of Ms Lisa Boland, RVT in preparing this chapter.

2c

Ophthalmic surgery: basic principles

David J. Maggs

Introduction

Due to the delicate nature of ocular tissues, marked variability in anatomy and physiology of various structures and the need for the best possible cosmetic and functional result, ophthalmic surgery requires different and specialized knowledge, instrumentation and techniques from those commonly used in general surgery. The optimal approach to ophthalmic surgery begins with a thorough knowledge of surgically relevant anatomy and physiology, followed by adequate attention to surgical technique, including surgeon and patient positioning, sterile preparation of the eye and adnexa, and fine control of instrument position, particularly depth. This chapter includes a general discussion of these basic principles, along with their practical application for each ocular tissue. Specific surgical techniques are discussed in chapters devoted to individual disease conditions.

Perhaps one of the most critical differences between general and ophthalmic surgery is the need for adequate magnification. This may be provided by binocular head loupes (Figure 2.19), or an operating microscope. Head loupes vary widely in their optical quality, magnification (2–8 X) and working distance. Some surgeons are, initially, uncomfortable with the fixed working distance dictated by loupes, particularly at higher magnification. Therefore, loupes that offer lower magnification (2–5 X) are more practical for most adnexal procedures. Operating microscopes provide optimal magnification and resolution but are expensive and tend to be used only by specialists.

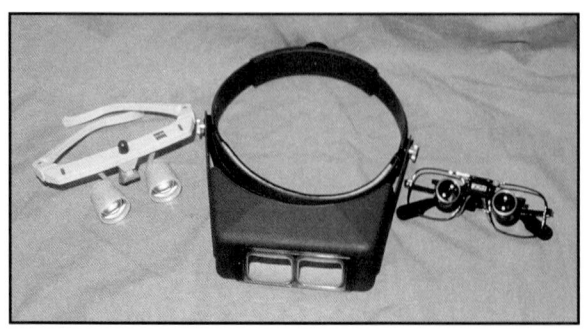

Figure 2.19 Binocular head loupes of variable quality, magnification and working distance are available for adnexal and some corneal procedures.

Patient and surgeon positioning

Maximizing the comfort of the surgeon and his or her manual control is a critical first step in optimal surgical technique. In most cases, this is facilitated if the surgeon is seated, with the forearms or wrists comfortably stabilized on the patient, operating table, or platforms created by vacuum beanbags (see below). The height of the table and position of the patient should be arranged so as to increase the comfort of the surgeon. A mental checklist of items to consider during preparation is recommended:

1. Adjust the chair height so that the positions of your legs and body are comfortable
2. With the patient approximately in the required position, adjust the table height so that a comfortable arm position is attained
3. Make final, small adjustments to the position of the patient, so that surgical access and visualization are maximized
4. Recheck that the height of the chair and the position of the patient permit an adequate working distance, and focus, if you are wearing binocular loupes that have a fixed focal distance.

The patient is usually best positioned so that the surface to be operated upon is parallel with the table surface. In most cases, lateral recumbency with the nose raised provides adequate positioning. Ventral or dorsal recumbency provides the opportunity to view both eyes, which can be advantageous, if a symmetrical surgical result is required. Vacuum beanbags are an excellent means of firmly retaining a patient's position throughout the surgery. A rectangular bag is useful for restraint of the patient's body, and a U-shaped bag provides excellent head restraint. These bags can also be adjusted to form platforms for stabilizing the surgeon's wrists or forearms.

Sterile preparation

There are two important considerations when preparing the ocular surface for a sterile surgical procedure:

- The conjunctival fornix is an external surface with a normal flora (see Chapter 1c). This is composed primarily of Gram-positive bacteria, but may also include fungi and viruses

- Ocular surface structures must be handled gently during preparation for surgery, to avoid excessive swelling, bruising, corneal trauma, or chemical injury. The choice of ocular disinfectants and method of surgical preparation are therefore very important.

Clipping periocular hair

The minimum amount of periocular hair should be carefully trimmed, using electric clippers with sharp, fine blades. Clipped hair should then be removed with a dry gauze and a vacuum, before being rinsed from the eye and the surrounding skin, during sterile preparation. Cilia may be trimmed, when necessary, using small curved scissors. Electric clippers should not be used for this procedure. A small amount of ophthalmic ointment may be applied to the scissors, so that trimmed cilia will adhere to the blades and be prevented from falling into the conjunctival fornix. If the surgical site does not include periocular skin and the animal has short hair, it may be possible to avoid or minimize clipping by using an adhesive drape that can be cut to surround the eyelid margins closely.

Disinfection

Povidone–iodine, diluted 1:50 in saline, is the preferred antiseptic. This is easily formulated by adding 20 ml of povidone–iodine solution to 1 litre of sterile saline. It is essential that iodine *solution* is used, since iodine *scrub* contains detergents, and is irritating when applied to the eye. Povidone–iodine has viricidal, bactericidal and fungicidal activity at this concentration, but is minimally toxic to corneal and conjunctival epithelium, and to inflammatory cells.

Chlorhexidine gluconate (0.05%), with 4% isopropyl alcohol, is also safe and effective for ocular surface disinfection. Chlorhexidine diacetate, detergents and surgical alcohol or spirit are toxic to ocular tissues, and should not be used (Fowler and Schuh, 1992).

The conjunctival fornix should be liberally flushed with antiseptic solution, using a small syringe. Cotton-tipped applicators provide an excellent means of gently removing mucus, trimmed hairs and debris from the conjunctival fornix, but should not be permitted to touch the cornea. More concentrated povidone–iodine solution (10%) may be applied to the eyelid skin, but this solution should not be allowed to contact the cornea or conjunctiva. Some dogs may develop blepharoedema or wheals in reaction to this agent. Preoperative treatment with ophthalmic ointments should be avoided, since these will create a greasy operating surface, and because the vehicle can lead to granulomatous inflammation if it contacts subcutaneous, subconjunctival or intraocular tissues.

Relevant anatomy and physiology

The orbit, adnexa and globe are composed of a diverse range of tissues, each with different anatomy and physiology. The ophthalmic surgeon is, therefore, confronted by tissues that demonstrate diverse inflammatory responses to surgical trauma, heal at very different rates, and require different handling skills, surgical techniques and instrumentation. One feature that is consistent among all ocular tissues is their exquisite sensitivity. This necessitates an adequate plane of anaesthesia and, sometimes, postoperative analgesia. An Elizabethan collar is usually provided postoperatively.

Orbit

The orbit is the most anatomically complex region that the ophthalmic surgeon faces. Intimate knowledge of orbital structures is essential when considering specialist procedures, such as orbitotomy or orbitectomy. However, there are a number of anatomical and physiological considerations pertinent to more commonly performed procedures, such as enucleation and exenteration.

First, the orbit communicates with the central nervous system, via a number of foramina. Following enucleation or exenteration, there are also potential communications with nasal sinuses (via the nasolacrimal duct), and the skin surface (via the surgical wound). Careful attention to asepsis is, therefore, critical, particularly if an orbital prosthesis is used. Secondly, care must be taken not to exert excessive traction on the optic nerve during orbital procedures, because this may cause damage to the contralateral nerve, via the optic chiasm, particularly in the cat, or may be associated with cardiac bradyarrhythmias, via the oculocardiac reflex. Finally, the orbit contains a number of large vascular structures that may require special care and, sometimes, surgical ligation.

Eyelids

The primary functions of the eyelids are to protect the cornea, and to retain and disperse the tear film. Therefore, normal blinking motions and eyelid position must be preserved following any surgical procedure involving the lids. In practice, this requires that the facial nerve is protected from trauma as it traverses the lateral aspect of the face, and that special attention is given to preserving eyelid margin anatomy.

There are two landmarks that are useful for eyelid surgery (Figure 2.20). The first is the meibomian gland orifices. This line of small whitish-tan circles demarcates the eyelid margin and provides an important landmark for its realignment following surgical procedures. Sutures that are placed in the eyelid margin should always emerge just anterior to the meibomian gland orifices, so that they are unlikely to rub the cornea.

The second important landmark is the border between periocular skin bearing hairs and hairless eyelid margin tissues. Incisions parallel to the eyelid margin, such as those employed for entropion procedures, should be placed at this site.

The eyelids are highly vascular and, therefore, demonstrate rapid and marked inflammatory responses (e.g. oedema, hyperaemia). They must be handled minimally and extremely gently. The eyelids also heal more rapidly than less vascular sites, and sutures may be removed relatively early postoperatively.

44   Ophthalmic surgery: basic principles

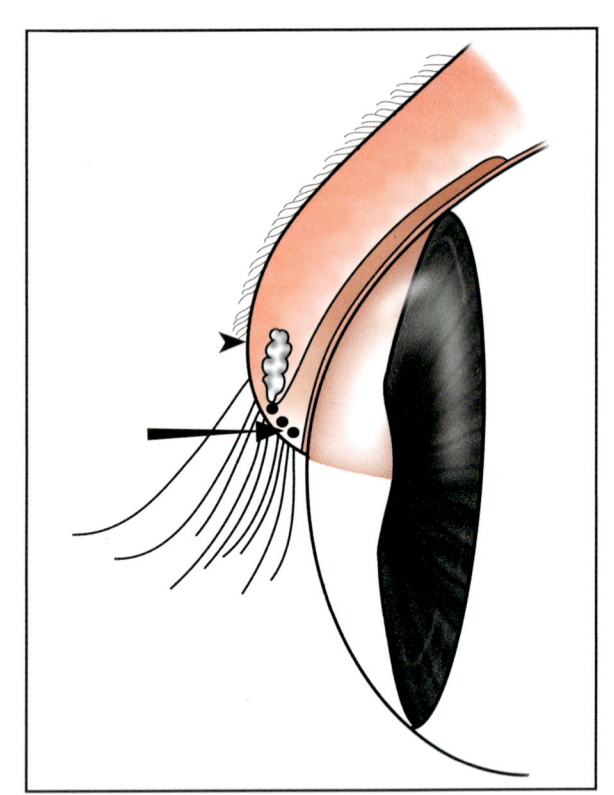

Figure 2.20 Important landmarks for eyelid surgery. The meibomian gland orifices (arrowed) demarcate the eyelid margin. Sutures at the eyelid margin should emerge just anterior to the meibomian gland orifices (to the left of the arrow) so that they are unlikely to rub the cornea. The border (arrowhead) between periocular skin bearing hairs and the hairless eyelid margin tissues is the preferred site for incisions parallel to the margin, such as those employed for entropion procedures.

Conjunctiva

The conjunctiva is divided into four confluent regions: bulbar, palpebral, forniceal and nictitans conjunctivae. The bulbar and forniceal conjunctivae are highly mobile but in close proximity to the globe and, therefore, should be incised and undermined only with blunt-tipped scissors. By contrast, a blade may be used for incising the more firmly adherent palpebral and nictitans conjunctivae.

Tenon's capsule is an important surgical landmark for conjunctival surgery. This fibrous connective tissue attaches the conjunctiva to the underlying sclera. Identification and separation of this layer is an important step in transconjunctival enucleation, and the harvesting of conjunctival grafts. Because conjunctiva heals rapidly and is exposed to minimal forces, smaller conjunctival wounds do not always need to be closed.

Third eyelid and nasolacrimal system

The third eyelid plays a critical role in tear production, retention and dispersion. It is, therefore, important that the gland and free margin of the third eyelid are preserved during surgery. Ideally, mobility of the third eyelid should also be preserved by surgical procedures; however, this is not always possible.

The lacrimal puncta (and canaliculi) should always be located, and sometimes cannulated, prior to eyelid or conjunctival surgery that may endanger them. Inadvertent damage to the lacrimal puncta or canaliculi may lead to chronic epiphora. This is most notable with damage to the ventral punctum or canaliculus.

Cornea

The cornea presents a number of technical challenges to the ophthalmic surgeon:

- The canine or feline cornea is only 0.6–0.7 mm thick. Controlled dissection is, therefore, critical to avoid ocular perforation
- In its normal state, the cornea is avascular, and virtually free of immunologically active cells. This renders it relatively susceptible to microbial invasion as soon as the epithelium is ulcerated and means that corneal repair is slow, compared with that of more vascular structures
- Corneal stromal keratocytes are relatively sparse and inactive. Repair of stromal deficits requires keratocyte activation and subsequent fibroplasia, which occurs slowly. Fibroplasia may be augmented by vascular ingrowth.

The practical significance of these features of corneal anatomy and physiology is that corneal disease may be rapidly progressive and surgical intervention, usually in the form of a conjunctival graft, may be necessary to provide a more rapid supply of blood vessels, fibroblasts, serum and inflammatory cells.

Intraocular structures

Intraocular surgery requires an intimate understanding of relevant anatomy and physiology, specialized surgical training and instrumentation, and an operating microscope. For these reasons, the majority of intraocular surgery is performed by specialists. Discussion of these techniques is beyond the scope of this chapter.

Principles of ophthalmic surgery

Although ocular tissues require special techniques, some general techniques and principles apply to many, or most, ophthalmic procedures. The basic requirements are as follows:

- Adequate restraint – usually general anaesthesia (see Chapter 2a)
- Fine, light surgical instruments (see Chapter 2b)
- Adequate magnification
- Delicate surgical technique.

Surgical techniques can be divided into those intended to separate (incise) tissues and those designed to reunite (suture) them. Tissue stabilization techniques (grasping) are common to both procedures. In all cases, the prevailing principle is to exert fine, three-dimensional control over tissues and instruments, while minimizing tissue trauma.

Tissue stabilization (grasping)

Basic principles

Tissues are grasped during surgical procedures to provide immobilization or mobilization. Adequate *immobilization* is particularly important for surgery of highly mobile tissues, such as the eyelids, the conjunctiva and the globe. On the other hand, tissue *mobilization* may be required to afford better visualization, or to improve the angle of approach for another instrument. All grasping instruments (principally forceps) rely on creating enough friction (grasping pressure) to resist opposing forces applied by the tissue and the surgeon. The ophthalmic surgeon should aim to provide adequate fixation, without damaging delicate ocular tissues. A common error is to apply insufficient force, so that tissues are damaged by the forceps slipping across and abrading their surfaces, and due to frequent re-grasping. Correct instrument choice, close attention and experience will ultimately ensure that the correct force is applied.

Practical applications
The eyelids are not attached to underlying tissue over much of their area; therefore, ensuring that there is adequate eyelid stability, prior to surgical incisions or suture placement is essential. Grasping of the eyelid margin, especially with toothed instruments, should be avoided. Instead, the lids can be tensed by placing firm lateral pressure on skin outside the lateral canthus. If this is performed by an assistant, then the surgeon may further regulate the position and tension of the eyelid in other planes (Figure 2.21). The placement of a Jaeger eyelid plate into the conjunctival fornix and gentle elevation of the lid will also provide adequate support and protect the underlying globe (Figure 2.22).

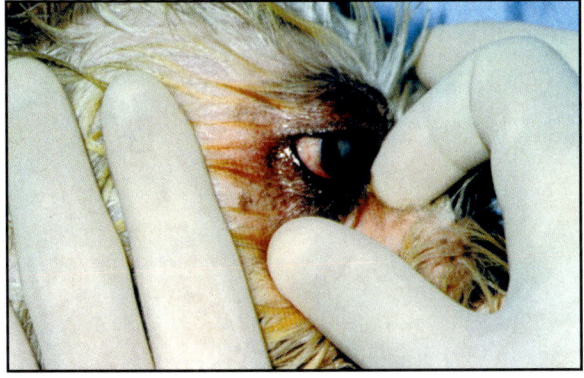

Figure 2.21 The eyelids may be stabilized by an assistant (left) placing firm lateral pressure on skin outside the lateral canthus. The surgeon (right) may further regulate eyelid position and tension in other planes.

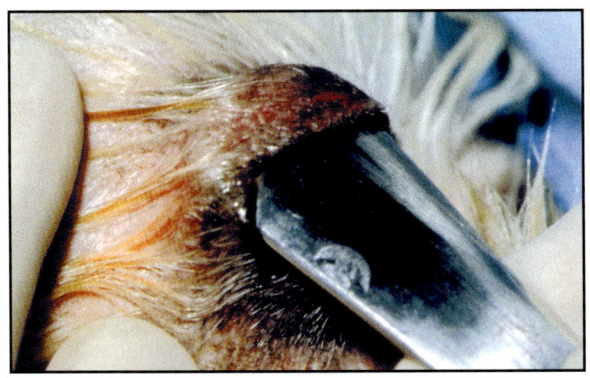

Figure 2.22 Placement of a Jaeger eyelid plate into the conjunctival fornix. Gentle elevation of the lid will provide adequate eyelid support and protection for the globe.

Conjunctiva must be grasped with delicate-toothed forceps (see Chapter 2b). Minimal re-grasping is particularly important, as chemosis, ulceration, hyperaemia and haemorrhage are induced very readily. Due to the extreme mobility of this tissue, incisions should always be made relatively close to the site of fixation. Fixation of the globe itself, for corneal surgery or transconjunctival enucleation, is best achieved by grasping conjunctiva and some underlying Tenon's capsule at a point close to the limbus. For this reason, the perilimbal incision for transconjunctival enucleation should be made a few millimetres from the limbus, thereby leaving a 'handle' of conjunctiva and Tenon's capsule for manipulation of the globe.

The cornea can be grasped only when a free edge is created by an incision, ulcer or laceration. In these cases, the cornea should be grasped with Colibri or Castroviejo forceps.

Tissue separation (incision)

Basic principles
Two common methods of separating tissues are utilized in general and ophthalmic surgery. Sharp dissection relies on the cutting of tissue fibres and requires sharp scissors or scalpel blades. By contrast, blunt dissection relies on the overstretching and rupture of tissue fibres and requires scissors with blunt tips that will stay within a chosen tissue plane. Sharp dissection is preferred in ocular surgery because it tends to cause less inflammation in highly vascular structures. The major roles for blunt dissection are in: the separation of Tenon's capsule for harvesting conjunctival grafts; and dissection within a given corneal tissue plane (lamellar keratectomy).

Whether the surgical goal is a good cosmetic result following an eyelid procedure, or avoidance of globe penetration during corneal surgery, accurately guiding the blade along the desired incision path at the desired depth is of paramount importance. The major determinant of incision path is tissue sectility. *Sectility* is the tendency for tissue fibres to be separated, rather than to be displaced, by a cutting motion. Tissues of high sectility, such as the cornea, are readily incised, with minimal displacement. By contrast, tissues of low sectility, such as conjunctiva, are readily displaced by blade motion. A good general rule is that tissues of lower sectility should be incised with scissors, while those of higher sectility are better incised with a sharp blade. Sectility can vary, due to the amount of tissue stabilization. For example, perilimbal conjunctiva is more firmly attached and, therefore, has greater sectility than other bulbar conjunctiva. Similarly, traction on conjunctiva with grasping forceps will increase the tissue tension and, therefore, its sectility, on the side of the incision on which it is grasped (Figure 2.23). In these cases, the incision will tend to deviate in the direction of lower sectility unless this is corrected for by the surgeon.

46 Ophthalmic surgery: basic principles

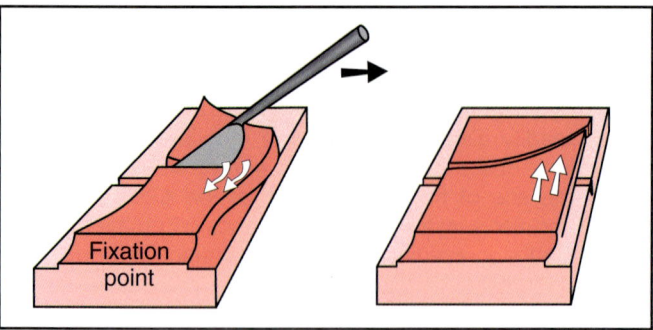

Figure 2.23 Asymmetrical sectility. Fixation of conjunctiva (i.e. at the limbus or where it is grasped by forceps) will create asymmetrical tissue tension. This causes the tissue to shift toward the fixation point (curved arrows) and the incision to deviate away from the point of fixation (straight arrows) unless the surgeon corrects for this. (Redrawn after Eisner (1990) with permission.)

Practical applications

Incisions in the eyelid skin should be made in one fluid movement, following adequate stabilization of the lids. Due to the tendency for scissors, even sharp ones, to exert crushing forces, a number 15 Bard–Parker blade is preferred. If the scalpel is held like a pencil, the surgeon can 'draw' the incision with the wrist rested on the patient (Figure 2.24). The underlying globe should be protected by cutting against a Jaeger eyelid plate, or by displacing the eyelid until it overlies the orbital rim. Undermining the skin should be performed with scissors. Sharp dissection is preferred to blunt dissection, due to the tendency for eyelids to become swollen and contused. The eyelid margin may be incised if necessary; however, incisions should be made with a sharp blade against a lid plate, or with sharp scissors, and should be perpendicular to the margin. This ensures that the margin may be accurately realigned during closure. Eyelids are extremely vascular; however, adequate haemostasis can usually be achieved with firm direct pressure. Cautery should be used in moderation, if at all, to minimize scarring.

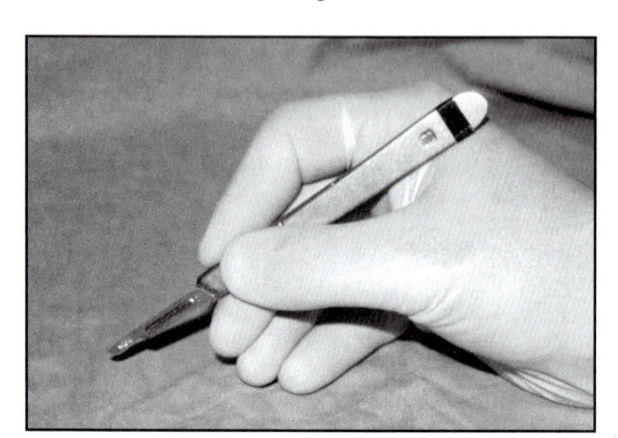

Figure 2.24 Excellent control of the scalpel's path through the tissue is obtained by holding it like a pencil and 'drawing' the incision.

Conjunctival incisions are commonly made, either to harvest a conjunctival graft or during transconjunctival enucleation. In both cases, sharp dissection is used to reach the desired tissue plane (episcleral for enucleation and just subconjunctival for grafts), followed by blunt dissection, until the desired extent of undermining is achieved. Blunt and sharp dissection of conjunctiva is best achieved using Stevens or Westcott tenotomy scissors.

The most common corneal surgery is keratectomy, which is described in full elsewhere. Corneal incisions must be made with a sharp blade, due to the high sectility of this tissue. A number 64 Beaver blade is commonly used and, with experience, allows excellent control of both the incision path and its depth. In many instances, better control of the path of the incision can be achieved if the blade is pushed towards the grasping point (usually a pair of Colibri forceps at the limbus), rather than being drawn away from it. Judgement of the depth of the corneal incision is dependent upon a number of tactile and visual clues; this goes beyond the scope of this chapter. Once the desired dissection plane is achieved, lamellar dissection may be continued with the Beaver blade or a Martinez corneal dissector.

Tissue uniting (suturing)

Basic principles

The aims, when suturing ophthalmic tissues, are to re-establish function and achieve a good cosmetic appearance. This requires attention to the wound alignment and compression.

Wound alignment relies upon:

- Placing the sutures perpendicular to the wound margin. (Oblique sutures tend to cause lateral movement of wound margins)
- Adequately apposing all tissue layers (not just the most superficial layer)
- Using multiple, closely spaced sutures
- Applying the 'rule of bisection' (discussed below).

Wound compression may be increased by:

- Placing the sutures closer together
- Taking larger bites of tissue in each suture (not recommended)
- Tying the sutures more tightly (not recommended).

These two lists highlight the critical role that closely placed sutures play in both wound compression and alignment.

Fine suture material and delicate needles are also essential to the achievement of a good cosmetic result. These must be handled using special instruments (see Chapter 2b) and techniques. Delicate needles must be grasped gently, so as not to bend them, but firmly enough that they can be directed

Ophthalmic surgery: basic principles **47**

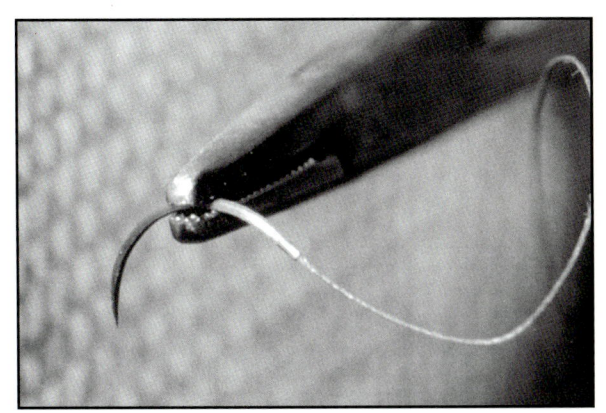

Figure 2.25 Fine suture needles should be grasped in the middle third of their arc, using just the tips of small-tipped needle holders.

accurately through tissues. This is best achieved by using small-tipped needle holders, and by grasping the needle in the middle third of its arc, using just the instrument tips (Figure 2.25).

The 'dangle manoeuvre' is used to aid in grasping small needles (Troutman, 1974). This is technically challenging at first, but can be learnt with practice. The suture material is grasped using a non-toothed instrument, such as tying forceps, and used to dangle or suspend the needle on a tissue surface. The needle is then grasped while stabilized on the tissue surface. Very small needles can be suspended in the tear film, without any risk of corneal injury.

Great care should be taken to avoid bending delicate ophthalmic needles as they are passed through tissue. The best method is to permit the needle to follow a path through the tissue that is determined by its curvature. This is achieved by directing the needle with a rolling motion of the needle holders, and is facilitated by 'palming' larger needle holders, so that the fingers are not restrained by the ring handles (Figure 2.26). Smaller microsurgical needle holders can be rolled in the fingers, using the rounded handles. The rolling technique is illustrated in Figure 2.27.

Standard square knots are used in ophthalmic surgery, but excess tension should be avoided, to prevent suture breakage. Fine suture material should not be grasped with toothed or serrated instruments, such as tissue forceps or standard needle holders.

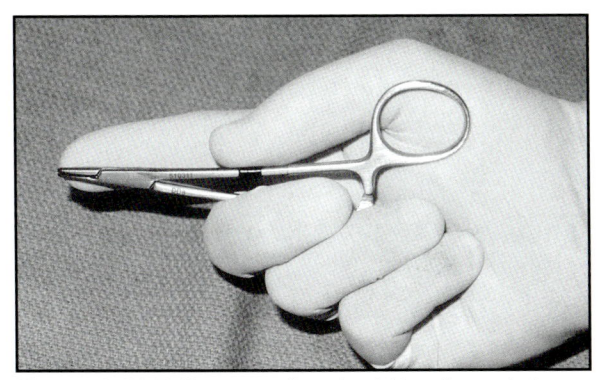

Figure 2.26 Delicate needles should be directed along a curvilinear path with a rolling hand motion. This is facilitated by 'palming' larger needle holders.

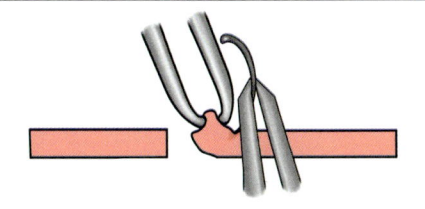

1. The tissue is entered with the needle perpendicular to the tissue surface.

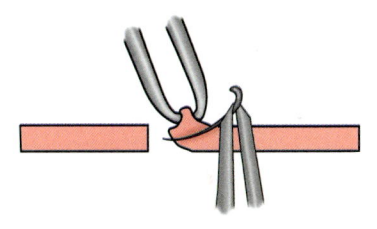

2. The needle is then directed through the tissue using a rolling motion, so that the needle emerges at 90 degrees to the cut tissue surface. The needle may be removed and re-grasped before placement of the next bite, if necessary.

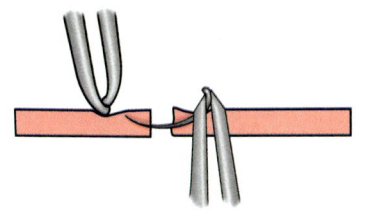

3. The opposite tissue surface is entered exactly opposite the point where the needle emerged, and again at 90 degrees to the cut surface. The needle is rolled up through the tissue to emerge at a point opposite the initial entry point. Forceps can be used to grasp the distal wound edge, or they can be used in a closed position to place gentle pressure at a point just distal to the intended needle emergence site so as to shorten the arc of the needle's tissue path.

Figure 2.27 Minimal tissue trauma and maximal wound alignment are achieved by directing the suture needle along a curvilinear path. This is achieved in a number of steps.

Suture material that is finer than 5-0 should be grasped with tying forceps, and tightened carefully, ensuring that it is not drawn around acute angles of the instruments (Figure 2.28). In all cases, care must be taken to ensure that the suture ends are cut short, and do not abrade the eye or ulcerate the cornea.

Practical applications

Eyelid incisions are, usually, under little tension due to normal muscle actions; however, the cosmetic appearance, and correct alignment of the eyelid margin, are major concerns. Incisions should be closed in one or two layers, with a simple interrupted pattern in the skin, and sometimes with a simple continuous suture pattern in the subcutaneous layer. Care must be taken to ensure that suture material does not penetrate through the conjunctival surface, where it could abrade the cornea. Skin edges should be apposed using multiple closely spaced simple interrupted sutures, placed using a cutting or reverse cutting needle. Eyelid in-

48 Ophthalmic surgery: basic principles

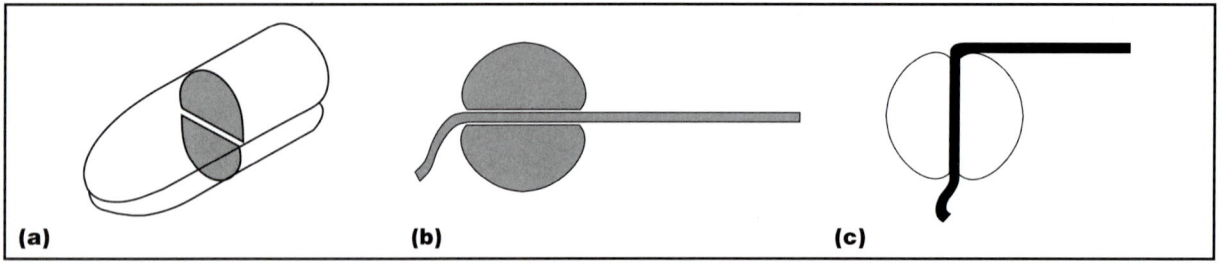

Figure 2.28 (a) Cross-sectional view of the tips of tying forceps. (b) Fine suture material should be grasped with tying forceps and tightened so that it does not pass over sharp edges of the instrument. (c) Suture breakage is likely if it is passed over sharper angles. (Redrawn after Eisner (1990) with permission.)

cisions may be closed using absorbable sutures, such as 4-0 to 6-0 polyglactin 910, both subcutaneously and in the skin. A non-absorbable suture such as 4-0 to 6-0 silk or braided nylon may be used in the skin in a compliant animal, when suture removal is expected to be straightforward. Suture ends should be cut so that they cannot abrade the cornea, but are long enough to be grasped for suture removal, if necessary. In some instances, this is best achieved by cutting the suture end directed towards the cornea relatively short, but by leaving the other end longer. Early removal of eyelid sutures may minimize suture granuloma formation, and is usually possible in this highly vascular site.

Two special techniques are useful for closing eyelid wounds or incisions:

- The 'rule of bisection'. When suturing wound margins of unequal length, such as those that are created with a Hotz–Celsus procedure, sutures should be placed so that each bisects the distance between two previously placed sutures (Figure 2.29). This helps with the wound alignment and minimizes tissue redundancy at the far end of the wound.
- The 'figure-of-eight' closure. This ensures excellent alignment of the eyelid margin, without leaving sutures that may abrade the cornea. The technique is described in Figure 2.30.

Small conjunctival incisions may be left open, because conjunctiva heals so rapidly, and because sutures may be irritating or cause corneal ulceration. Larger conjunctival lacerations should be closed, to

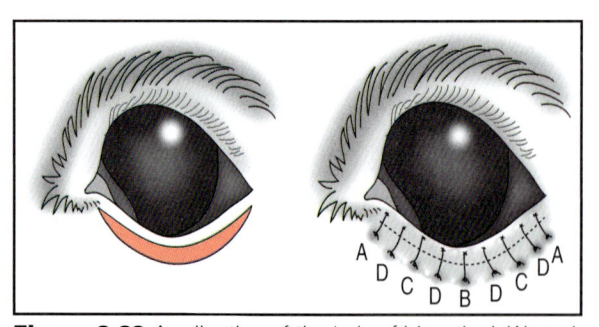

Figure 2.29 Application of the 'rule of bisection'. Wound margins of unequal length, such as those created in a Hotz–Celsus procedure, are sutured so that each suture bisects the distance between two previously placed sutures. In this example, the order of suture placement would be A–B–C–D.

1. A buried horizontal mattress suture is placed as close to the eyelid margin as possible, without penetrating it or the conjunctival surface. The knot should be away from the eyelid margin. This suture is critical for perfect closure of the margin, and should be removed and replaced if the surgeon is not happy with the margin alignment at this point.

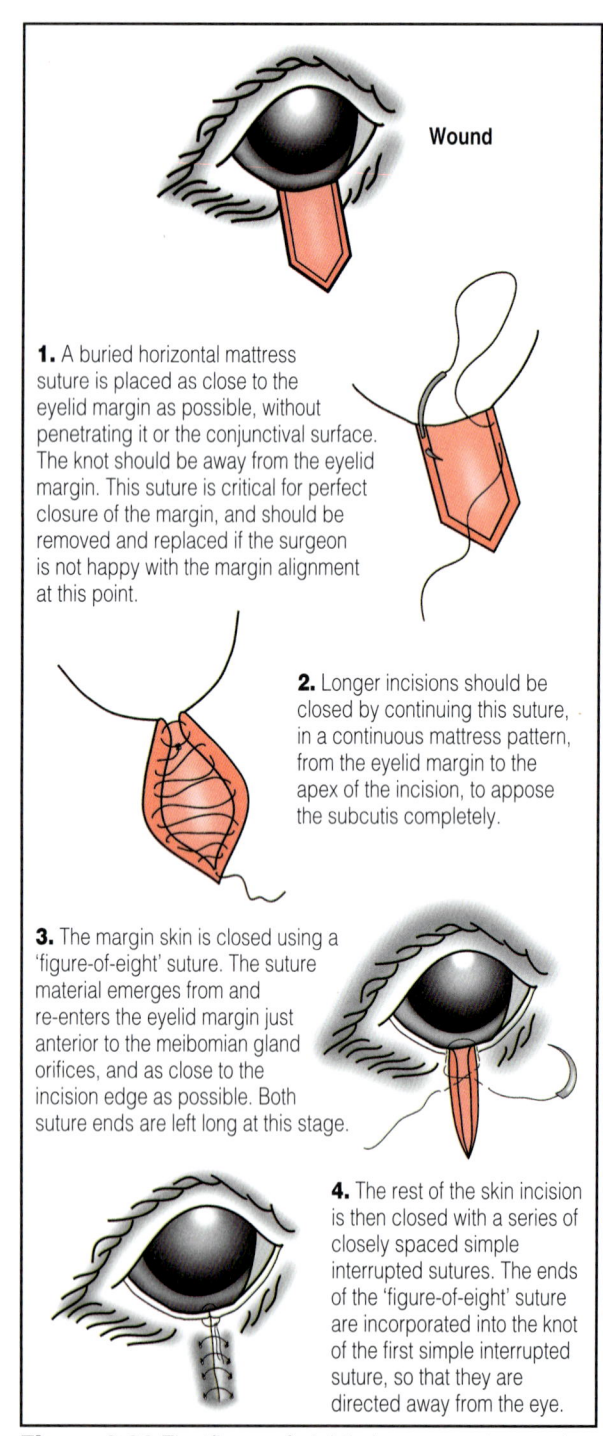

2. Longer incisions should be closed by continuing this suture, in a continuous mattress pattern, from the eyelid margin to the apex of the incision, to appose the subcutis completely.

3. The margin skin is closed using a 'figure-of-eight' suture. The suture material emerges from and re-enters the eyelid margin just anterior to the meibomian gland orifices, and as close to the incision edge as possible. Both suture ends are left long at this stage.

4. The rest of the skin incision is then closed with a series of closely spaced simple interrupted sutures. The ends of the 'figure-of-eight' suture are incorporated into the knot of the first simple interrupted suture, so that they are directed away from the eye.

Figure 2.30 The 'figure-of-eight' closure may be used for any wounds or incisions involving the eyelid margin.

minimize pain and the risk of orbital or subconjunctival infection. A simple continuous pattern with buried knots, using 6-0 to 8-0 absorbable suture, should be used, and suture ends cut short to minimize ocular irritation and risk of corneal ulceration.

Corneal suturing requires magnification, special instrumentation and suture material and some experience. The most commonly used suture material is 8-0 polyglactin 910, with a swaged-on, spatula-tipped needle. Sutures should be placed to approximately three quarters of the corneal depth, or more, but without penetration of the anterior chamber. Careful attention must be given to the apposition of the surgical margins to ensure a 'water-tight' wound. Specific techniques for closing corneal lacerations and suturing conjunctival grafts are described in Chapter 8.

Although descriptions of specific techniques for corneal suturing are beyond the scope of this chapter, the rolling technique of suture placement (see Figure 2.27) is particularly useful.

References and further reading

Eisner G (1990) *Eye Surgery. An Introduction to Operative Technique.* Springer-Verlag, Berlin

Fowler JD and Schuh JCL (1992) Preoperative chemical preparation of the eye: a comparison of chlorhexidine diacetate, chlorhexidine gluconate, and povidone iodine. *Journal of the American Animal Hospital Association* **28**, 451–457

Nasisse MP (ed.) (1997) Surgical management of ocular disease. *Veterinary Clinics of North America – Small Animal Practice* **27**, 963–1271

Troutman RC. (1974) *Microsurgery of the Anterior Segment of the Eye. Vol. 1. Introduction and basic techniques.* CV Mosby, London

3

Ophthalmic drugs

David Gould

Introduction

Both local and systemic routes are used to administer drugs to the eye. Local administration maximizes exposure of drugs to the anterior segment while minimizing systemic exposure and most commonly involves topical application or subconjunctival injection. However, administration of drugs by these routes does not achieve therapeutic levels within the posterior segment and so systemic (or occasionally intravitreal) administration is indicated for conditions of the posterior segment.

Topical therapy allows the clinician to vary the frequency of application of drugs depending on the response to treatment. Frequent application achieves high local concentrations, which can be quickly reduced if necessary. The major disadvantage of topical treatment is variable owner compliance.

Subconjunctival injection should be reserved for cases where topical therapy is not possible, such as in fractious animals or if owner compliance is poor. A small amount of the drug (typically 0.25–0.5 ml) is injected beneath the bulbar conjunctiva after application of a topical anaesthetic. Injection of drug into the palpebral conjunctiva is not recommended, since most will be absorbed into the eyelid and rapidly enter the systemic circulation rather than be absorbed across the eye. Iatrogenic globe injury and subconjunctival granuloma formation are potential risks of subconjunctival injection.

Intravitreal injection is uncommonly used in veterinary practice, since it requires general anaesthesia and carries a risk of iatrogenic damage to the intraocular structures. It is the treatment route of choice for endophthalmitis, since it provides therapeutic concentrations of drugs within the vitreous. Intravitreal injection of gentamicin, which is cyclodestructive (i.e. destroys the ciliary body) in high concentrations, has been used to treat end-stage glaucoma. Since this treatment induces significant intraocular inflammation it generally is not recommended.

The ability of systemically administered drugs to reach therapeutic concentrations within the eye depends on their ability to cross the blood–ocular barrier (BOB). Lipophilic drugs are most efficient at this, but other drugs may cross if the BOB is disrupted by uveitis. Systemic administration is indicated for conditions of the posterior segment but is also suitable for conditions of the anterior segment, usually in combination with topical therapy.

Topical drug preparations

Topically applied drugs may be in ointment or drop formulation.

Ointments have a prolonged corneal contact time, which allows a lower frequency of application. They are used to deliver lipophilic drugs or to act as long-acting ocular lubricants. In humans they cause blurring of vision, but this is less of a problem in the veterinary species.

Drop preparations (solutions, suspensions and emulsions) are easier to apply and cause less blurring of vision. Solutions are used for water-soluble drugs, suspensions for poorly water-soluble drugs and emulsions for lipid-soluble drugs. The delivery volume of a topical eye drop is typically 50 µl, of which only around 20 µl is retained on the eye, with the rest draining down the canaliculi or spilling over the eyelid margin (Mathis et al., 1999). Therefore, from a practical point of view, it is pointless applying more than 1 drop to the surface of the eye at a time. If applying more than one topical drug, it is advisable to wait 5 minutes between applications.

Drop preparations are rapidly washed away in the tear film. Therapeutic levels of topically applied drugs can be increased by improving the drug retention time (by the use of corneal adherents or viscous agents; see Tear substitutes, below), increasing the frequency of application, reducing the washout time (by manual occlusion of canaliculi immediately after application) or by increasing the concentration of the drug (e.g. by the use of fortified drug preparations).

Intraocular penetration of topical drugs

Topically applied drugs vary in their ability to penetrate the cornea and enter the eye. This is of utmost importance when selecting drugs to treat intraocular disease. To enter the anterior chamber, drugs must cross the lipophilic corneal epithelium and then the hydrophilic corneal stroma. Therefore, they should have both lipophilic and hydrophilic properties.

Stabilizers and preservatives

Most topical drug formulations contain stabilizers such as ethylenediamine tetra-acetic acid (EDTA), α-tocopherol or sodium bisulphate, and preservatives such as benzalkonium chloride or alcohol. These can be irritant, and some are epitheliotoxic. Single-use formulations bypass the need for such additives, but are more expensive.

Antibacterials

Systemic antibacterials are indicated for bacterial infections of the eyelids, posterior segment and retrobulbar space. Topical antibacterials are used for bacterial conjunctivitis, keratitis, anterior uveitis and, prophylactically, in cases of ulcerative keratitis.

β-Lactam antibiotics

Penicillins and cephalosporins are bactericidal drugs that block bacterial cell wall synthesis. They are not metabolized by the body and are excreted rapidly via the kidneys. Tissue distribution following systemic administration varies between drugs, and intraocular penetration may be poor unless the BOB is inflamed. Topically applied penicillins and cephalosporins will penetrate to the anterior chamber when the corneal epithelium is disrupted.

The penicillins are mostly active against Gram-positive organisms. An increased Gram-negative range of activity is seen in the aminopenicillins (e.g. ampicillin, amoxicillin) and the carboxypenicillins (e.g. carbenicillin, ticarcillin). Penicillins may be combined with clavulanic acid, a β-lactamase inhibitor, to overcome bacterial resistance.

Cephalosporins are closely related to the penicillins. However, unlike the penicillins, they can be used safely in rabbits and rodents. First-generation cephalosporins (e.g. cephalexin, cephazolin, cefadroxil) are active against Gram-positive and Gram-negative organisms, but not against *Proteus* or *Pseudomonas* spp. Second-, third-, and fourth-generation cephalosporins (e.g. cefuroxime, ceftiofur and cefquinome, respectively) have increasing anti-Gram-negative activity and reducing anti-Gram-positive activity. The cephalosporins have a useful synergistic action with aminoglycosides (which are mostly active against Gram-negative organisms).

Cephalexin and amoxicillin/clavulanic acid are commonly used systemic preparations.

Topical preparations are uncommonly used in small animal practice but include cloxacillin and cephalonium.

Sulphonamides

These are broad-spectrum bacteriostatic agents that block bacterial folic acid synthesis. Systemic administration gives good tissue and ocular penetration. Potential side-effects with long-term use include keratoconjunctivitis sicca and, in Dobermann Pinschers, immune-mediated polyarthritis. Because of these potential side-effects and because of increasing bacterial resistance, sulphonamides are now used less frequently in veterinary ophthalmic practice.

Tetracyclines

The tetracyclines are broad-spectrum bacteriostatic drugs that bind the 30S subunit of bacterial ribosomes and block amino acid attachment. Tetracyclines are excreted in the gastrointestinal tract, via the biliary system, and in the urinary system. Systemically administered tetracycline, oxytetracycline and chlortetracycline penetrate the BOB poorly, but the more lipophilic doxycycline has good ocular penetration. Topically applied tetracyclines may achieve therapeutic concentrations within the anterior chamber.

Tetracyclines are active against intracellular bacteria including *Chlamydophila*, *Mycoplasma* and *Rickettsia*, plus a range of Gram-positive and Gram-negative bacteria. However, resistance is common and they are generally ineffective against *Escherichia coli*, *Salmonella*, *Proteus* and *Pseudomonas*.

Systemic doxycycline is used to treat chlamydial conjunctivitis in cats. It generally is not recommended in young animals since it can discolour the enamel of the permanent teeth.

The only topical preparation available in the UK is chlortetracycline. It can be used to treat chlamydial and mycoplasmal conjunctivitis in cats. However, it may be an irritant and the frequency and duration of application (up to six times daily for 6 weeks in chlamydial conjunctivitis) may limit owner compliance.

Aminoglycosides

These are bactericidal agents that bind the 30S subunit of bacterial ribosomes and inhibit protein synthesis by causing misreading of mRNA. They are excreted via the kidneys. Systemically administered aminoglycosides do not penetrate the BOB effectively and are not used in veterinary ophthalmic practice. Topically applied aminoglycosides have poor corneal penetration, but subconjunctival injection leads to therapeutic concentrations within the anterior chamber. Intravitreal injection of aminoglycosides may be retinotoxic.

Aminoglycosides are effective against Gram-negative and some aerobic Gram-positive organisms (e.g. staphylococci). Aminoglycosides are ineffective against streptococci and against anaerobes. They are synergistic with β-lactam antibacterials.

Gentamicin is indicated for *Pseudomonas aeruginosa* conjunctivitis or keratitis. Tobramycin has broad-spectrum activity including activity against gentamicin-resistant *Pseudomonas aeruginosa*. Neomycin is a broad-spectrum topical antibiotic with poor corneal penetration, used for superficial infections.

Macrolides and lincosamides

These related drugs bind the 50S subunit of bacterial ribosomes and block protein translocation. Erythromycin, tylosin, lincomycin and clindamycin are bacteriostatic and predominantly have a Gram-positive range of activity. Newer macrolide antibiotics, such as azithromycin, are bactericidal and have a wider spectrum of activity. They are metabolized in the liver. Systemic administration leads to good tissue penetration.

Clindamycin is effective against anaerobic bacteria and *Toxoplasma gondii*. Azithromycin is an effective treatment for chlamydial disease in humans and shows promise in the treatment of feline chlamydiosis (Ramsey, 2000). It is also effective against *Pseudomonas* spp., *Branhamella* spp., *Pasteurella multocida* and streptococci (Chu, 1999).

Fluoroquinolones

Fluoroquinolones have broad-spectrum bactericidal activity; they act by inhibiting bacterial DNA gyrase, an enzyme which is essential for folding of bacterial DNA. Most fluoroquinolones are partly metabolized in the liver before being eliminated, although some (e.g.

enrofloxacin) are excreted unchanged. Excretion is mainly via the renal system, and clearance is significantly impaired in the presence of renal failure. Tissue distribution after systemic administration is good and topical application achieves high anterior chamber concentrations.

Fluoroquinolones are effective against most Gram-negative organisms including *Pseudomonas* spp. They have some activity against Gram-positive organisms, but some staphylococci and streptococci may be resistant (Miller *et al.*, 1996). They have poor activity against anaerobes and, therefore, they are a poor choice of treatment for orbital infections.

Enrofloxacin, difloxacin and marbofloxacin are systemic preparations. Enrofloxacin appears to have a narrow therapeutic index in cats, with reports of blindness due to a rapidly developing generalized retinal degeneration resulting when the drug has been given at doses greater than the manufacturer's recommendation. Care should be taken to keep to the manufacturer's recommended dose rate. Ciprofloxacin is available in topical formulation, but is not licensed for veterinary use.

Other antibacterials

Fusidic acid blocks binding of transfer RNA to the bacterial ribosome, inhibiting protein synthesis. It has good anti-Gram-positive and some anti-Gram-negative activity. It is poorly effective against *Chlamydophila* and *Pseudomonas*. It has good corneal penetration.

Chloramphenicol is a broad-spectrum bacteriostatic agent that binds the 50S subunit of bacterial ribosomes to block protein synthesis. If used systemically it also may bind to mitochondrial ribosomes of bone marrow cells to cause reversible, dose-related bone marrow suppression and, very rarely, aplastic anaemia. Topical use is not associated with such side-effects. Chloramphenicol is active against *Pasteurella* spp., *Chlamydophila* spp., most anaerobes and most Gram-positive aerobes. It is unreliable against *Mycoplasma* spp., *Proteus* spp. and enterobacteria. Although theoretically effective against *Pseudomonas aeruginosa*, resistance is high.

Topically applied chloramphenicol is an excellent choice for superficial eye infections in the dog; it also has good corneal penetration and is used prophylactically following intraocular surgery. It is not as effective against *Chlamydophila* spp. as the tetracycline group, and so is not the first choice antibiotic for superficial eye infections in the cat.

Bacitracin, gramicidin and polymixin B are polypeptide antibiotics that are bactericidal in action by inhibiting cell wall or cell membrane synthesis. They are toxic if given systemically. They do not penetrate the cornea and are used to treat superficial bacterial infections. Since bacitracin has a Gram-positive range of activity and polymixin B a Gram-negative range, they may be combined as part of a broad-spectrum double or triple antibiotic preparation (e.g. polymixin B/ zinc bacitracin or neomycin/ polymixin B/ zinc bacitracin).

Metronidazole is a bactericidal nitroimidazole antibiotic that is effective against anaerobic bacteria. It has good tissue penetration when given systemically. It may be used to treat anaerobic orbital infections. In mixed infections it can be combined with a drug active against aerobes, such as a cephalosporin.

Fortified antibacterial solutions

Use of a fortified antibiotic solution rapidly achieves a high therapeutic drug concentration and is indicated for rapidly progressive conditions such as liquefactive corneal necrosis ('melting' ulcer). For Gram-positive bacterial infections, 15 ml artificial tear solution added to one 500 mg vial of cephazolin makes 33 mg/ml fortified cephazolin solution for topical use, stable for 48 hours. For Gram-negative infections, 100 mg gentamicin solution added to a 5 ml vial of topical makes 14.3 mg/ml fortified gentamicin solution for topical use, stable for 30 days.

Since cephalosporins and aminoglycosides are synergistic, the above fortified solutions can be used in combination for mixed infections, or when the causal organism is unknown.

Commonly used systemic and topical antibacterials are summarized in Figures 3.1 and 3.2, respectively.

Antibacterial agent	Tissue distribution	Range of activity	Main indications
Cephalexin	Good	Broad-spectrum. Ineffective against anaerobes or *Pseudomonas* spp.	Aerobic infections of orbit, eyelids or globe
Amoxycillin/clavulanic acid	Good	Broad-spectrum. Ineffective against anaerobes or *Pseudomonas* spp.	Aerobic infections of orbit, eyelids or globe
Doxycycline	Good	Broad-spectrum but most effective against intracellular bacteria	Chlamydial, mycoplasmal and rickettsial infections
Azithromycin	Good	Intracellular bacteria, *Pasteurella* spp., *Pseudomonas* spp. Gram-positive bacteria may be resistant	Promising for treatment of chlamydial, mycoplasmal and rickettsial infections
Enrofloxacin	Good	Broad-spectrum but some staphylococci and streptococci are resistant. Ineffective against anaerobic bacteria	Gram-negative infections including *Pseudomonas aeruginosa*
Clindamycin	Good	Gram-positive bacteria, anaerobic bacteria, protozoa	Toxoplasmosis, anaerobic orbital infections
Metronidazole	Good	Anaerobic bacteria	Anaerobic orbital infections

Figure 3.1 Selected antibacterials for systemic use.

Antibacterial agent	Corneal penetration	Range of activity	Main indications
Fusidic acid	Good	Broad-spectrum, but ineffective against *Pseudomonas aeruginosa*	Gram-positive ocular surface infections, in particular canine bacterial conjunctivitis
Gentamicin	Poor	Broad-spectrum, but streptococci usually resistant	Gram-negative ocular surface infections, in particular *Pseudomonas aeruginosa*
Chloramphenicol	Good	Broad-spectrum, but *Pseudomonas* spp. may be resistant. Also effective against anaerobes	Superficial eye infections, intraocular infections, prophylaxis following intraocular surgery or penetrating corneal injury
Ciprofloxacin	Good	Broad-spectrum, but some staphylococci and streptococci are resistant	Gentamicin-resistant *Pseudomonas aeruginosa* infections
Chlortetracycline	Reasonable	Broad-spectrum, but resistance is common	Feline chlamydial conjunctivitis
Neomycin	Poor	Broad-spectrum	Mixed ocular surface infections
Polymixin B	Poor	Gram-negative bacteria, including *Pseudomonas* spp.	Often used in combination for mixed ocular surface infections
Bacitracin	Poor	Gram-positive bacteria, in particular streptococci	

Figure 3.2 Selected antibacterials for topical use.

Antivirals

Antiviral medications are used to treat feline herpetic keratitis. They are most commonly used for acute ulcerative disease; the efficacy of these agents in the treatment of chronic stromal keratitis is unknown.

Trifluorothymidine, idoxuridine, vidarabine, bromovinyldeoxuridine and acyclovir have decreasing *in vitro* efficacy against feline herpesvirus (FHV-1), with trifluorothymidine being the most effective. The only one of these currently available in the UK is acyclovir. It has low effectiveness against FHV-1 *in vitro* but may have some effect if used in conjunction with human interferon-α_2 (IFN-α_2). Trifluorothymidine can be imported into the UK but is expensive and requires frequent application: four to six times daily for a maximum of 3 weeks (Stiles, 2000).

Human IFN-α_2 has been used to treat FHV-1 infections but controlled studies have not been published. Systemically administered IFN-α_2 is unlikely to be effective since it is degraded by gastric secretions. Very low dose topically applied IFN-α_2 (25–50 IU/ml) has been used but reports are anecdotal. Since the drug is supplied in high concentrations (5 million IU/ml), serial dilutions are required to obtain such low concentrations. Controlled studies in human viral dendritic keratitis comparing the effects of trifluorothymidine alone with those of trifluorothymidine plus high-dose IFN-α_2 (30×10^6 IU/ml) showed that combination therapy reduced healing time from 6 days to 3 days (Sundmacher *et al.*, 1978).

Oral L-lysine (250 mg to 500 mg daily) has been used in the treatment of chronic FHV-1 infection, based on the *in vitro* observation that it inhibits viral replication in the presence of low arginine levels. Uncontrolled clinical trials indicated a beneficial effect in human herpes simplex infections (Griffith *et al.*, 1978) but controlled studies have not been published. Clinical trials are under way to determine the validity of using this amino acid for FHV-1 infections. L-Lysine can be obtained from health food shops, but preparations containing propylene glycol should be avoided since they may be toxic to cats.

Antifungals

Fungal infections are rarely encountered in small animals in the UK but may occur in immunocompromised animals or in animals imported from tropical climates. Antifungal agents may be used topically (for mycotic keratitis) or systemically (for mycotic chorioretinitis). However, there are no antifungal preparations licensed for topical use in small animals in the UK. Intravenous preparations may be diluted and used topically (e.g. amphotericin B 0.2% in aqueous solution) or unlicensed topical preparations may be supplied by hospital pharmacies (e.g. clotrimazole 1% solution in peanut oil). The antiseptic agent chlorhexidine (0.2% in aqueous solution) has been reported to be effective against human keratomycoses (Martin *et al.*, 1996).

For systemic mycoses, combination therapy using amphotericin B and ketoconazole is often used. Newer drugs that show promise include itraconazole and fluconazole, both of which have good intraocular and CSF penetration.

Anti-inflammatories

Anti-inflammatory drugs are indicated for extra- and intraocular immune-mediated diseases, including keratoconjunctivitis sicca (KCS), chronic superficial keratoconjunctivitis, allergic conjunctivitis, eosinophilic keratoconjunctivitis and uveitis.

Corticosteroids

The corticosteroids used in ophthalmic practice are glucocorticoids, which have minimal mineralocorticoid activity and powerful anti-inflammatory activity. Their anti-inflammatory activity is mediated in a number of ways but their primary action is to induce lipocortin, an intracellular protein which inhibits phospholipase A_2 (PLA_2). PLA_2 is an endogenous enzyme that catalyses the breakdown of cell membrane phospholipids to arachidonic acid, the precursor to proinflammatory leucotrienes and prostaglandins (Figure 3.3). Since

54 Ophthalmic drugs

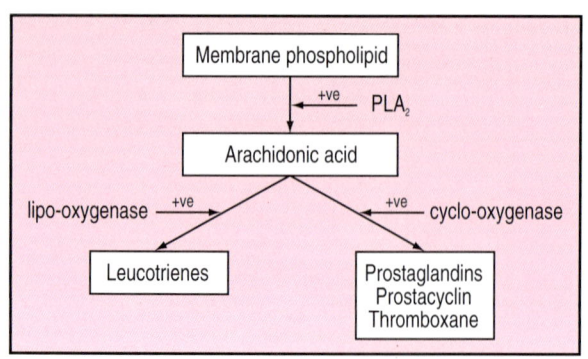

Figure 3.3 Inflammatory pathway. Phospholipase A_2 (PLA_2) catalyses the breakdown of membrane phospholipids into arachidonic acid, the precursor of the proinflammatory leucotrienes and prostaglandins. Glucocorticoids block PLA_2. NSAIDs block cyclo-oxygenase.

Generic name	Primary indication
Betamethasone sodium phosphate 0.1%	Superficial ocular inflammation
Dexamethasone acetate 0.1% in hypromellose	Anterior uveitis
Fluorometholone acetate 1.4% in polyvinyl alcohol	Superficial ocular inflammation and anterior uveitis
Prednisolone acetate 1%	Anterior uveitis
Prednisolone sodium phosphate 0.5%	Superficial ocular inflammation

Figure 3.4 Topical glucocorticoid preparations.

Glucocorticoid	Relative anti-inflammatory potency
Hydrocortisone	1
Prednisolone	4
Fluorometholone	>20
Dexamethasone	40
Betamethasone	50

Figure 3.5 Relative potency of glucocorticoids.

glucocorticoids act upstream of both lipo-oxygenase and cyclo-oxygenase pathways of inflammation, they are potent anti-inflammatory agents. At higher concentrations they are immunosuppressive.

The major ophthalmic contraindication for the use of glucocorticoids is corneal ulceration. Glucocorticoids can exacerbate acute stromal collagenolysis ('melting' corneal ulcer) which can lead to globe perforation.

Long-term topical glucocorticoid use in humans may cause cataract and glaucoma. Neither complication has been reported in veterinary clinical practice, but in experimental cats medium-term topical glucocorticoid administration (three times daily application for 2–3 weeks) has been reported to cause a reversible increase in intraocular pressure (IOP), while longer treatment (more than 7 weeks) caused subcapsular cataract formation (Zhan et al., 1992). Topical treatment also causes a reversible increase in IOP in experimental Beagles (Gelatt and Brooks, 1999).

Topical glucocorticoids
Several topical glucocorticoid preparations are available (Figure 3.4). They vary in their relative anti-inflammatory activities and in their ability to cross the cornea and reach therapeutic concentrations within the anterior chamber. It is important that these differences are appreciated, since they influence the choice of topical preparation for different inflammatory conditions. Dexamethasone and betamethasone have the greatest anti-inflammatory potency of all the glucocorticoids (Figure 3.5). However, to be effective inside the eye, glucocorticoids must be able to cross the cornea and reach therapeutic concentrations within the anterior chamber. The ability of a glucocorticoid preparation to cross the cornea depends on its lipid solubility, since a major barrier to intraocular penetration is the lipophilic epithelium. Lipid solubility is a feature of the ester base to which the glucocorticoid is bound. Phosphate bases are water-soluble and penetrate poorly, so are suitable for superficial inflammatory conditions (e.g. chronic superficial keratoconjunctivitis, eosinophilic keratoconjunctivitis). Acetate, diacetate and alcohol bases are lipophilic and penetrate well, so are suitable for the treatment of anterior uveitis.

For superficial inflammatory conditions a suitable first-choice preparation is fluoromethalone, which combines good anti-inflammatory activity with minimal systemic side-effects.

The first choice preparation for treatment of anterior uveitis is prednisolone acetate, since it has excellent corneal penetration.

Topical antibacterial and glucocorticoid combinations are probably over-used in clinical practice, but they are indicated when both inflammation and bacterial infection are present.

Non-steroidal anti-inflammatory agents
NSAIDs inhibit the cyclo-oxygenase pathway of inflammation (see Figure 3.3) but have a number of additional actions too, including effects at the spinal level which may account for some of their analgesic properties. At least two isoforms of cyclo-oxygenase (COX) exist. COX-1 is constitutively expressed and is thought to have physiological functions. Its inhibition may lead to the side-effects occasionally seen with NSAIDs, such as gastrointestinal bleeding. COX-2 is induced at sites of inflammation and is the main anti-inflammatory mediator. Thus, NSAIDs that specifically target COX-2 should have effective anti-inflammatory and analgesic properties with fewer side-effects.

NSAIDs are used for post-operative pain relief and for the treatment of uveitis. Studies have shown that topical flurbiprofen is as effective as prednisolone acetate in reducing aqueous flare (Ward et al., 1991). Topical NSAIDs can be used in addition to topical glucocorticoids and appear to be additive in effect. They are contraindicated if anterior segment bleeding is present.

A variety of topical preparations is available (Figure 3.6). Many are supplied in single-use vials and are used perioperatively during cataract surgery. Ketorolac is supplied as a 5 ml multi-use formulation and is useful for treatment of anterior uveitis when corneal ulceration is present; although topical NSAIDs delay corneal

Generic name	Indication and frequency of use
Diclofenac sodium 0.1%	Cataract surgery; every 30 minutes for 2 hours preoperatively
Flurbiprofen sodium 0.03%	Cataract surgery; every 30 minutes for 2 hours preoperatively
Ketorolac trometamol 0.5%	Anterior uveitis; four times daily

Figure 3.6 Topical NSAID preparations.

re-epithelialization (and so should be used with care in such cases) they do not potentiate collagenolysis as do topical corticosteroids.

Systemic NSAIDs should not be used concurrently with systemic corticosteroids, or in cases of gastrointestinal bleeding. Carprofen and meloxicam are commonly used in small animal practice. They have some preferential COX-2 inhibition and should therefore have fewer side-effects than some of the other NSAIDs available, such as ketoprofen, aspirin, phenylbutazone and flunixin.

Cyclosporin

Cyclosporin is a chemotherapeutic agent that is used topically for a variety of superficial immune-mediated and autoimmune conditions. It has multiple mechanisms of action. It acts as a T cell suppressor by inhibiting the interleukin 2 expression required for clonal expansion of T cells during the immune response (Figure 3.7). More recent work shows that it also induces production of transforming growth factor-β (TGF-β), a potent endogenous immunosupressant (Nabel, 1999).

In addition (and relevant to its ophthalmic use), cyclosporin increases tear production in normal dogs, possibly via effects on a prolactin receptor (Kaswan et al., 1989).

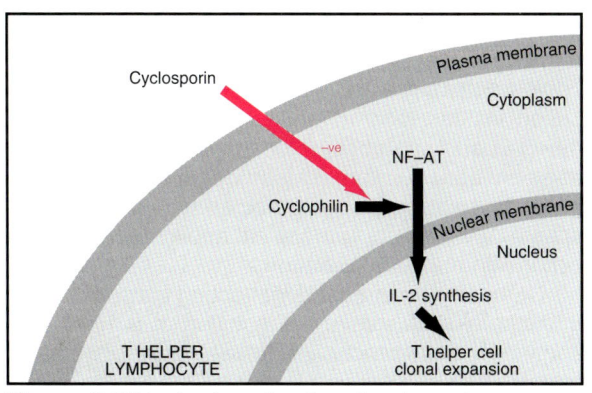

Figure 3.7 Mechanism of action of cyclosporin. Cyclosporin binds and inhibits cyclophilin, preventing it from activating (by dephosphorylation) NF-AT (nuclear factor of activated T lymphocytes). NF-AT activation leads to upregulation of IL-2 expression. IL-2 induces clonal expansion of T helper cells.

Cyclosporin is used to treat canine autoimmune KCS. In view of its direct neurogenic action, it may also potentially be of benefit in the treatment of non-autoimmune (e.g. neurogenic) KCS.

Cyclosporin is also an effective treatment for other canine immune-mediated diseases such as chronic superficial keratoconjunctivitis, plasmacytic conjunctivitis and episcleritis. In cats it has been reported as a treatment for proliferative eosinophilic keratoconjunctivitis.

Topically applied cyclosporin does not penetrate the intact cornea well and therefore has no therapeutic value in the treatment of anterior uveitis.

Azathioprine

Azathioprine is a systemic cytotoxic agent with powerful immunosuppressive effect via its action on helper T lymphocytes. In veterinary ophthalmological practice it is used to treat autoimmune diseases such as uveodermatological syndrome and nodular granulomatous episclerokeratitis. A typical dose protocol would be 2 mg/kg daily until remission is achieved, followed by a slowly tapering course. Routine haematological examination is required throughout the course of treatment, since azathioprine can induce bone marrow suppression. Other side-effects include vomiting, diarrhoea and acute hepatic necrosis.

Megoestrol acetate

Megoestrol acetate is a progestogen with immunosuppressive activity, which has been used to treat eosinophilic keratoconjunctivitis in cats. A typical dosage regimen is 5 mg orally for 5 days, then 5 mg every other day for one week, then 5 mg weekly as maintenance. Serious adverse effects include behavioural changes, adrenocortical suppression and diabetes mellitus; therefore, treatment is generally reserved for patients that do not respond to topical or subconjunctival corticosteroid therapy.

Antiallergic agents

Antihistamines competitively inhibit histamine binding to cellular receptors. Sodium cromoglycate inhibits mast cell degranulation. These agents are used in the treatment of allergic conjunctivitis in humans. There are anecdotal reports of their use in allergic conjunctivitis in small animals but their efficacy is unknown (Mathis et al., 1999).

Anti-glaucoma drugs

Anti-glaucoma drugs work by reducing aqueous humour formation or by increasing its outflow. One should bear in mind that many of these drugs have been developed for treatment of human open-angle glaucoma and are poorly effective as a treatment for canine or feline glaucoma, which is usually closed-angle. For this reason, many veterinary ophthalmologists consider glaucoma primarily a surgical problem rather than a medical one.

Of the anti-glaucoma drug classes available, amongst the most effective are the osmotic diuretics and the carbonic anhydrase inhibitors. The recently introduced prostaglandin analogues also show promise, although their use in veterinary ophthalmic practice is not yet well evaluated. Beta-blockers may be of some use in selected cases. Parasympathomimetics (miotics) and adrenergics are of limited use in canine and feline glaucoma.

Osmotic diuretics

Osmotic diuretics are the first-line emergency treatment for acute glaucoma. They are hyperosmotic agents that promote water retention within the kidney tubules, leading to dilution of tubular sodium and a reduction in sodium and water reabsorption. Their administration leads to a rapid reduction in intraocular pressure (IOP), as water is drawn out of the aqueous and vitreous to compensate for the increase in blood osmolarity. IOP is reduced within 30 minutes and the effect lasts for at least 5 hours. Since their effect is short-lived, alternative medical or surgical treatment is needed after osmotic diuretics have been used to reduce the IOP in the acute stage of disease.

The BOB must be intact for these drugs to be effective, as uveitis will reduce their efficacy. Excessive administration of osmotic diuretics can cause acute hypovolaemia; in patients with compromised renal function this could lead to pre-renal azotaemia or renal failure.

Mannitol is supplied in 10% (100 mg/ml) and 20% (200 mg/ml) concentrations for intravenous administration. It is used at a dose rate of 1 g/kg in dogs (10 ml/kg of 10% solution) usually given rapidly over 30 minutes, then as a slow drip.

Glycerol is given orally at a dose rate of 1–2 g/kg (2–4 ml/kg of 50% solution), but is unpalatable to dogs and may cause vomiting.

Carbonic anhydrase inhibitors

Carbonic anhydrase promotes aqueous humour production within the non-pigmented epithelium of the ciliary processes by catalysing the reaction:

$$CO_2 + H_2O \rightleftharpoons HCO_3^- + H^+$$

Bicarbonate neutralizes sodium ions, which are actively pumped into the posterior chamber from the ciliary epithelium, and water follows by osmosis. By reducing bicarbonate levels, carbonic anhydrase inhibitors thus reduce aqueous humour formation. IOP is lowered by up to 50% and, unlike the osmotic diuretics, these agents can be used long term.

Systemic carbonic anhydrase inhibitors have been largely superseded by topical carbonic anhydrase inhibitors, which appear to be just as effective but have minimal adverse effects. Side-effects of systemic carbonic anhydrase inhibitors are relatively common and include depression, anorexia, vomiting, diarrhoea, polyuria/polydipsia and increased respiratory rate. These are related to alterations in metabolic state including metabolic acidosis (due to increased urinary bicarbonate) and hypokalaemia. The side-effects can be so severe as to necessitate discontinuation of these drugs. Acetazolamide is the only systemic preparation currently available in the UK. It is associated with more severe side-effects than dichlorphenamide and methazolamide.

Dorzolamide is a topical preparation used three or four times daily. It can be used in combination with other drugs such at topical beta-blockers.

Prostaglandin analogues

Low concentrations of certain prostaglandins (notably $PGF_{2\alpha}$) lower IOP by increasing uveoscleral outflow and so are of use as anti-glaucoma drugs. Since topically applied prostaglandins do not readily penetrate the cornea, prostaglandin analogues have been developed. These combine a prostaglandin with a lipid-soluble ester, which allows ocular penetration. An analogue of $PGF_{2\alpha}$, latanoprost, has been developed and is less irritating than its parent molecule.

Latanoprost 0.005% applied once daily causes effective and long-lasting reduction in IOP in glaucomatous human patients. Potential side-effects include miosis and mild conjunctival irritation. Increased iris pigmentation, reported in primate and human studies, has not been documented in dogs or cats. Latanoprost shows promise as a treatment for canine and feline glaucoma and can be used in conjunction with other agents such as dorzolamide.

Parasympathomimetics

Parasympathomimetics increase the outflow of aqueous humour by causing ciliary muscle contraction and miosis, which widens the filtration angle. In severe cases of glaucoma where the filtration angle is obliterated, these drugs may be ineffective.

Direct acting parasympathomimetics

These directly stimulate the muscarinic acetylcholine (Ach) receptors of the iris and ciliary body.

Pilocarpine hydrochloride is available as 0.5%, 1% or 2% solutions. Topical application will induce miosis within 10 minutes in a normal eye. Other local parasympathomimetic effects include conjunctival vasodilation and increased lacrimation. Its lacrimomimetic property is used in the treatment of neurogenic keratoconjunctivitis sicca (KCS). Side-effects of topical application include local irritation (due to the low pH of 4.5–5.5) and salivation. Pilocarpine may also induce transient aqueous flare. Systemic side-effects (gastrointestinal tract irritation, cardiac arrhythmia, bronchospasm) are unlikely with topical application, but may occur with oral administration.

Carbachol is another direct-acting parasympathomimetic, available as a 3% solution. It is used less commonly than pilocarpine in veterinary ophthalmic practice.

Indirect acting parasympathomimetics

Indirect acting parasympathomimetics inhibit acetylcholinesterase and so prolong the action of endogenously released acetylcholine. These rarely used agents are classed as reversible carbamate inhibitors (such as demecarium bromide) and irreversible organophosphates (such as echothiophate). They are more potent and longer acting than direct acting parasympathomimetics, but cause more severe local side-effects (ocular irritation, ciliary spasm) and carry a higher risk of systemic toxicity.

Adrenergic agents

α- and β-adrenoreceptors are found in smooth muscle of the arterioles and within the iris and ciliary body musculature. Alpha stimulation lowers IOP via an $α_1$-mediated vasoconstriction of ciliary processes causing reduced aqueous production and an $α_2$-mediated increase in aqueous outflow via the trabecular meshwork. Beta-stimulation increases IOP by inducing cAMP which increases aqueous production. Therefore alpha-stimulation or beta-blockade should lower IOP. In practice, however, α-agonists (adrenaline, phenylephrine, apraclonidine) are poorly effective in canine and feline closed-angle glaucoma and, paradoxically, may even reduce aqueous outflow further via their mydriatic action. For this reason they are not recommended.

Beta-blockers are commonly used in human open-angle glaucoma, but again their efficacy in canine and feline closed-angle glaucoma is poorly documented and likely to be limited. Timolol maleate 0.5% is most commonly used, usually in combination with other agents such as dorzolamide. Other beta-blockers include carteolol, metipranolol and levobunolol. Side-effects of topical beta-blockers include local irritation, miosis, and bradycardia.

Mydriatics and cycloplegics

Mydriatics are used to dilate the pupil for both diagnostic and therapeutic purposes. Pupil dilation is necessary for examination of the peripheral lens and fundus, for cataract surgery and to reduce the incidence of synechiae in anterior uveitis. Cycloplegics relax the ciliary body musculature and are used to relieve the painful ciliary spasm associated with anterior uveitis.

Mydriatics are either sympathomimetic or parasympatholytic in their mechanism of action. Sympathomimetic drugs (phenylephrine, adrenaline) bind and stimulate adrenoreceptors of the pupillary dilator muscle to cause pupil dilation. There are few adrenoreceptors within the ciliary body, however, so these drugs have no effective cycloplegic action. Parasympatholytic drugs (atropine, tropicamide, cyclopentolate) bind and block acetylcholine receptors within the iris sphincter and ciliary body musculature to cause mydriasis and cycloplegia. This dual action makes parasympatholytics useful drugs in the treatment of anterior uveitis.

Topical sympathomimetics can be used to localize the site of a nerve lesion during the investigation of Horner's syndrome (Bistner et al., 1970). Topical application of 10% phenylephrine will resolve the signs of a post-ganglionic (third-order) lesion within 5–10 minutes, while pre-ganglionic lesions respond more slowly.

Phenylephrine also causes rapid vasoconstriction of conjunctival blood vessels and a slower vasoconstriction of episcleral blood vessels, so can be used to distinguish conjunctival from episcleral hyperaemia. It may also be used as an adjunct to parasympatholytics to induce optimal mydriasis, but is too short acting to be effective as a sole agent. The mydriatic action of phenylephrine is more variable in cats than in dogs.

Topical adrenaline is ineffective as a mydriatic agent, as it has poor corneal penetration. An adrenaline prodrug, dipivefrin, has been developed; this penetrates the cornea and is converted to adrenaline once in the anterior chamber, but this is not yet available in the UK. Adrenaline may be added to intraocular irrigating solutions to maintain mydriasis during phacoemulsification cataract surgery.

Atropine (atropine sulphate 1%) has mydriatic and cycloplegic effects. Its relatively slow onset and long duration of action limit its use as a diagnostic agent, but it is ideal for the treatment of ciliary spasm due to anterior uveitis. In the normal canine and feline eye, maximal dilation is achieved within one hour and lasts 60–120 hours. Its effect is more variable in the inflamed eye, and it is usually applied four to six times daily until mydriasis is achieved and then used to effect. Atropine will reduce tear secretion, and so tear production should be monitored with long-term use. Side-effects include hypersalivation due to its bitter taste and, less commonly, systemic parasympatholytic effects such as bradycardia and constipation. Atropine is contraindicated in canine and feline glaucoma, since it increases IOP.

Tropicamide (0.5%, 1%) has a more rapid onset and shorter duration of action than atropine, so its primary use is to cause mydriasis for diagnostic purposes or prior to cataract surgery. Maximal mydriasis occurs 30 minutes after application of 1% solution and lasts for 8–12 hours.

Cyclopentolate (1%) has a range of activity intermediate to atropine and tropicamide. Maximal mydriasis is achieved within 30–45 minutes and lasts around 60 hours. It is used commonly in human ophthalmology as a cycloplegic, but is not commonly used in small animals.

Tear substitutes

Tear substitutes (lacrimomimetics) are important in the treatment of KCS. Their major disadvantage is the frequency of application necessary to maintain adequate ocular lubrication, and they are usually used in conjunction with a lacrimostimulant such as cyclosporine or pilocarpine. Mimicking the three layers of the tear film, the main classes of tear substitutes are aqueous drops, mucinomimetics and lipid-based ointments, or combinations of these.

Aqueous tear substitutes

Aqueous preparations drain so quickly from the corneal surface that additives are required to prolong their action and give them therapeutic benefit. Many preparations contain methylcellulose or its derivatives. Methylcellulose is a soluble and non-irritant colloid that increases viscosity and prolongs corneal retention. Polyvinyl alcohol is a synthetic resin that has corneal adhesive properties but is less viscous than methylcellulose. Methylcellulose and polyvinyl alcohol are common components of human artificial tear preparations, but the severity of canine KCS is such that these are usually inadequate as a tear replacement in this disease.

Mucinomimetics

Linear polymers such as dextran, polyvinylpyrrolidone and polyacrylic acid (carbomer 980) have mucinomimetic properties and longer corneal contact times than aqueous tear substitutes. For this reason they are more suitable for the treatment of canine KCS.

Carbomer 980 is used four to six times daily and appears to be one of the most effective artificial tear preparations in dogs.

Some artificial tear preparations combine linear polymers with methylcellulose-based preparations to combat both aqueous and mucin tear deficits.

Viscoelastics such as hyaluronic acid and chondroitin sulphate also have mucinomimetic properties and a hyaluron derivative has been used as a tear replacement, although current reports are anecdotal.

Lipid-based tear substitutes

Lanolin, petrolatum and mineral oil are ointments that mimic the lipid portion of the tear film and prevent evaporation of existing tears. They have good corneal retention and so are useful when frequency of application is a problem. They are used three or four times daily. However, they may be more difficult to apply than less viscous preparations and are likely to cause blurring of vision. They are also useful as ocular protectants during anaesthesia or if eyelid paresis is present.

Local anaesthetics

Local anaesthetics are weak bases that reversibly block afferent and efferent nerve impulses by interfering with sodium ion influx into the neuron. Topical local anaesthetics are used as analgesics for diagnostic and minor surgical procedures. Injectable local anaesthetics are used for periorbital nerve blocks or for orbital anaesthesia following enucleation surgery.

Topical local anaesthetics

Proxymetacaine (proparacaine) acts rapidly and its effect lasts for 10–20 minutes. Amethocaine (tetracaine) has a similar effect but appears to be more irritant when applied and is more toxic to epithelial cells. Optimum analgesia is achieved by applying 4 or 5 drops over 2–3 minutes. Topical anaesthetics must not be used therapeutically to alleviate pain associated with corneal ulcers since they are epitheliotoxic. Since they block reflex tear production, they must not be applied prior to Schirmer I Tear Test measurements.

Injectable local anaesthetics

Lignocaine (lidocaine) (1–2%) has a rapid onset of action (10 minutes) and is relatively short-acting (60 minutes). Bupivacaine (0.25–0.75%) has a slower onset of action (45 minutes) and is long-acting (6 hours). Mepivacaine (1–2%) has an intermediate duration of action (2 hours). Lignocaine is commonly used for periorbital nerve blocks, while bupivacaine is useful for postoperative analgesia. An orbital injection of lignocaine and bupivacaine gives good peri- and postoperative pain relief during enucleation surgery. Typically, 1–3 ml of a 1:4 mix of lignocaine 1%: bupivacaine 0.25% is given.

Ocular irrigating solutions

Surface irrigants

Ocular surface irrigants are used to remove debris and bacteria from the cornea and conjunctival sac. Sterile physiological saline (normal saline 0.9%) is commonly used. Balanced salt solution (BSS) is supplied in sterile 15 ml dropper bottles. Sterile distilled water is hypotonic and therefore is not ideal. Many commercially available eyewashes contain preservatives which may be irritant to canine and feline eyes, so their use generally is discouraged.

The addition of an antiseptic agent to reduce bacterial load is strongly advised prior to extraocular and intraocular surgical procedures. Povidone–iodine is most commonly used. It is important to use aqueous solution (rather than alcoholic solution or surgical scrub) to avoid damage to the corneal epithelium. It is also vital to dilute the solution adequately to prevent tissue toxicity. A 10% commercial solution of povidone–iodine should be diluted 1:50 to 1:20 in normal saline to give a final concentration of 0.2–0.5%, which can be safely used to rinse the corneal surface.

Dilute chlorhexidine solution is also an effective antiseptic. Dilute solutions (0.05%) are non-toxic to the cornea, although high concentrations are irritant. As with povidone–iodine, it is important that aqueous solution is used. Since chlorhexidine is unstable in saline solution, it should be diluted with water.

Intraocular irrigants

Intraocular irrigation is required during intraocular surgery, in particular during phacoemulsification cataract surgery. Irrigating fluids must be isotonic and non-irritant and should have a physiological pH to prevent damage to the corneal endothelium. Intraocular use of normal saline or BSS caused corneal oedema in experimental rabbits and although no such problems were found in a canine study (Nasisse et al., 1986), many ophthalmic surgeons avoid their use during prolonged intraocular surgery. Either BSS or sodium lactate solution (Lactated Ringers' or Hartmann's solution) is satisfactory for short-term intraocular irrigation and is commonly used during phacoemulsification surgery. BSS Plus contains glutathione, which is protective to the corneal endothelium and is more suitable for prolonged intraocular irrigation.

Anticollagenases

Matric metalloproteases (MMPs) and serine proteases are collagenases that may cause acute corneal stromal lysis ('melting' corneal ulcer). Collagenases may be released from bacteria (particularly Pseudomonas and Streptococcus), neutrophils or keratocytes. Topical corticosteroids predispose to release of collagenases by neutrophils and therefore are contraindicated when corneal ulceration is present.

A wide variety of anti-collagenase agents have been proposed, but clinical studies are limited and the efficacy of these drugs in a clinical setting is uncertain.

MMPs require zinc and calcium, therefore metal chelating agents such as sodium or potassium EDTA, acetylcysteine, citrate and tetracycline have been recommended as anti-collagenase drugs (Mathis et al., 1999). Acetylcysteine 5% is applied hourly in an attempt to inhibit collagenolysis due to MMPs. It should be noted, however, that metal-chelating agents do not inhibit serine proteases. Autologous serum contains both serine protease inhibitors and MMP inhibitors so should be an effective 'broad-spectrum' anti-collagenase. It is probably the treatment of choice for medical treatment of collagenolysis. One drop of autologous serum (collected from a recently centrifuged blood sample) is applied hourly during the acute stage of the melt. Alternatively, the placement of a conjunctival pedicle graft allows a constant supply of serum to the ulcer in addition to providing physical support.

Antifibrotic agents

Mitomycin C and 5-fluorouracil are drugs that inhibit fibroplasia. Their main use in ophthalmic surgery is to prevent fibrosis around glaucoma drainage implant sites and thus prolong their lifespan. Although seemingly effective in humans, controlled clinical trials have not been reported in dogs, so their benefit in canine glaucoma surgery is unknown. They are not commonly used.

Mitomycin C is applied to the scleral drainage site at the time of surgery, using a cellulose sponge. One application is effective in prolonging drainage implant life in humans but its efficacy in dogs is unknown. Side-effects include breakdown of overlying conjunctival tissue and ocular hypotony.

5-Fluorouracil is less commonly used, since it requires repeated subconjunctival injections and is associated with more severe side-effects.

Fibrinolytics

Tissue-type plasminogen activator (tPA) may be injected intracamerally (i.e. into the anterior chamber) to lyse blood clots within the anterior chamber. tPA for intraocular injection is usually reconstituted from 20 mg powder to a 1 mg/ml solution, which is further diluted to a final concentration of 0.25 mg/ml. Aliquots of 100 μl (containing 25 μg tPA) can be stored at −70°C until ready for use. Injection of the drug across the limbus into the anterior chamber causes rapid clot lysis within hours.

Intracameral injection should only be performed by experienced ophthalmic surgeons, since incorrect injection technique can cause severe intraocular complications including iris haemorrhage, uveitis and lens rupture.

References and further reading

Bistner S, Rubin L, Cox TA and Condon WE (1970) Pharmacological diagnosis of Horner's syndrome in the dog. Journal of the American Veterinary Medical Association **157**, 1220–1224

Chu DT (1999) Recent progress in novel macrolides, quinolones, and 2-pyridones to overcome bacterial resistance. Medicinal Research Reviews **19**, 497–520

Gelatt KN and Brooks DE (1999) The canine glaucomas. In: Veterinary Ophthalmology, 3rd edn, ed. KN Gelatt, pp.701–754. Lippincott, Williams and Wilkins, Philadelphia

Griffith RS, Norins AL and Kagan CK (1978) A multicentered study of lysine therapy in herpes simplex infection. Dermatologica **156**, 257–267

Kaswan RL, Salisbury MA and Ward DA (1989) Spontaneous keratoconjuctivitis sicca. A useful model for human keratoconjunctivitis sicca: treatment with cyclosporine eye drops. Archives of Ophthalmology **107(8)**, 1210–1216.

Martin MJ, Rahman MR, Johnson GJ, Srinivasan and Clayton YM (1996) Mycotic keratitis: susceptibility to antiseptic agents. International Ophthalmology **19**, 299–302

Mathis GA, Reigner A and Ward DA (1999) Clinical ophthalmic pharmacology and therapeutics. In: Veterinary Ophthalmology, 3rd edn, ed. KN Gelatt, pp.291–354. Lippincott, Williams and Wilkins, Philadelphia

Miller CW, Prescott JF, Mathews KA, Betschel SD, Yager JA, Guru V, DeWinter L and Low DE (1996). Streptococcal toxic shock syndrome in dogs. Journal of the American Veterinary Medicine Association **209**, 1421–1426

Moore CP (1995) Ophthalmic pharmacology. In: Veterinary Pharmacology and Therapeutics, 7th edn, ed. HR Adams, pp.1105–1129. Iowa University Press, Ames

Nabel GJ (1999) A transformed view of cyclosporine. Nature **397**, 471–472

Nasisse MP, Cook CS and Harling DE (1986) Response of the canine corneal endothelium to intraocular irrigation with saline solution, balanced salt solution, and balanced salt solution with glutathione. American Journal of Veterinary Research **47**, 2261–2265

Papich MG (1998) Antibacterial drug therapy. Focus on new drugs. Veterinary Clinics of North America: Small Animal Practice **28**, 215–231

Ramsey DT (2000) Feline chlamydia and calicivirus infections. Veterinary Clinics of North America: Small Animal Practice **30**, 1015–1028

Stiles J (2000) Feline herpesvirus. Veterinary Clinics of North America: Small Animal Practice **30**, 1001–1014

Sundmacher R, Cantell K and Neumann-Haefelin D (1978) Combination therapy of dendritic keratitis with trifluorothymidine and interferon. Lancet **II**, 687

Ward DA, Ferguson DC, Ward SL, Green K and Kaswan RL (1991) Comparison of blood–aqueous barrier stabilizing effects of steroidal and nonsteroidal anti-inflammatory agents in the dog. Progress in Veterinary and Comparative Ophthalmology **2**, 117–124

Weiss R (1989) Synergistic antiviral activities of acyclovir and recombinant human leukocyte (alpha) interferon on feline herpesvirus replication. American Journal of Veterinary Research **50**, 1672–1677

Zhan G-L, Miranda OC and Bito LZ (1992) Steroid glaucoma: corticosteroid-induced ocular hypertension in cats. Experimental Eye Research **54**, 211–218

4

The orbit and globe

John R.B. Mould

Introduction

Conditions of the orbit and globe in the dog and the cat are sufficiently similar to justify considering the two species together. Before describing specific conditions, the clinical anatomy of the orbit and the general principles of pathogenesis and investigation of orbital disease will be outlined. An appreciation of these principles helps greatly in understanding orbital disease (McCalla and Moore, 1989).

Clinical anatomy

The orbit is the anatomical region containing the eye, optic nerve, lacrimal gland, extraocular muscles and associated nerves and blood vessels. These structures form a cone, with the base rostrally and the apex caudally. In humans this soft tissue cone is enclosed in a distinct bony cone so that the anatomical concept of the orbit is easy to grasp. In domestic carnivores, however, these structures are only partially enclosed in bone and large areas are bordered by soft tissue. The terms 'orbital' and 'retrobulbar' tend, therefore, to be used less precisely in these species.

A dog's skull is shown in Figure 4.1. The rostral margin of the orbit is bony for about three-quarters of its circumference, the dorsolateral part being completed by the orbital ligament running from the frontal to the zygomatic bone. This is palpable as a strong taut band in the live animal.

Dorsally, the frontal sinus overhangs the globe. Medially, the wall of the orbit is very thin where it overlies the ethmoturbinates; this may be a site for the invasion of nasal tumours into the orbit. Laterally, the orbit is bordered by the zygomatic arch, which is easily palpable, and ventral and medial to this are the masseter and pterygoid muscles. The lacrimal gland is situated deep to the orbital ligament. The zygomatic salivary gland lies in a recess of the maxilla ventral to the eye. The extraocular muscles enclose the optic nerve and form a cone directed caudally, ventrally and medially towards the optic foramen, where the optic nerve enters the cranium.

These anatomical relationships have important clinical consequences:

- The close proximity of masticatory muscles, frontal and maxillary sinuses, caudal molar tooth roots, caudal nasal chamber, pharynx and zygomatic gland means that disease processes in these structures may extend into or distort the orbit and its contents
- The incomplete nature of the bony orbit means that one option in the management of retrobulbar abscess is drainage into the mouth
- The direction taken by the extraocular muscle cone places the structures within it very deep to the surface and surgical access is difficult.

Differential diagnosis and investigation

Clinical signs of orbital disease

Orbital structures lie deep to the surface and so the clinical signs of orbital disease often relate to the effect that the primary lesion has on adjacent structures. Clinical signs may include the following:

- Exophthalmos
- Protrusion of the nictitating membrane
- Strabismus
- Periorbital swelling
- Conjunctival hyperaemia or congestion/chemosis
- Lagophthalmos
- Pain or difficulty in opening the mouth.

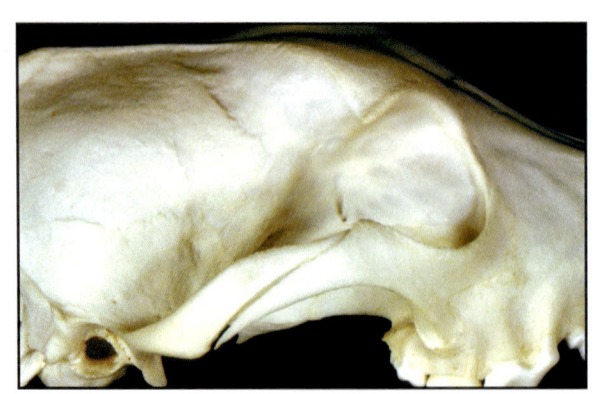

Figure 4.1 Lateral view of a dog's skull, showing the incomplete rostral bony margin to the orbit and the frontal sinus overlying the orbit. The pattern of the ethmoturbinates can just be made out through the thin medial wall of the orbit; this may be a site for the extension of nasal tumours. Note that there is only soft tissue continuity between the soft palate caudal to the last molar and the orbital region.

Some of these signs are not specific for orbital disease: there are, for example, many other causes of prominence of the nictitating membrane and strabismus.

Differential diagnosis of retrobulbar swellings

- Retrobulbar abscess/cellulitis
- Retrobulbar neoplasia
- Extraocular polymyositis (dog only)
- Masticatory myositis (dog only)

and, less commonly,

- Retrobulbar haemorrhage
- Retrobulbar foreign body
- Cysts and tumours of the lacrimal, nictitans and zygomatic glands
- Arteriovenous shunts (congenital)
- Eosinophilic infiltration (cat).

Investigation of orbital disease

History
A sudden onset with pain, malaise and difficulty in opening the mouth strongly suggests abscess/cellulitis (or acute myositis). A gradual onset with slow progression and relatively little pain suggests neoplasia or cyst formation. These are only broad distinctions and must be interpreted in the light of all other findings.

Clinical examination
A full examination of the eyes and adnexa is required, but certain points may be particularly informative here. The eyes should be examined from both in front and above to determine whether prominence is due to buphthalmos or exophthalmos (Figure 4.2).

Chronic glaucoma causes enlargement of the globe (buphthalmos). The enlargement is obvious when viewing the eye from in front, but when the eye is viewed from above, the anterior cornea is only displaced in proportion to the enlargement of the eye. Chronically glaucomatous eyes will also show numerous abnormalities, so it should be relatively easy to establish that the primary problem is ocular.

Exophthalmos (abnormal anterior displacement of the globe) is more striking from above than from in front.

Retropulsion of the globe can be a sensitive test for the presence of an orbital lesion. Pressure should be applied to the globe through the upper lid. There is little resistance in the normal animal or in the presence of an enlarged globe (unless the globe is painful to external pressure) and the eye can be repelled a surprisingly long way. The brachycephalic breeds are an exception, in that they have very shallow orbits and no space for retropulsion of the globe. In most breeds, however, the presence of a retrobulbar mass produces considerable resistance to retropulsion, especially when compared to the normal side. A unilateral problem suggests the presence of an abscess or of neoplasia, but a bilateral symmetrical problem suggests masticatory or extraocular polymyositis.

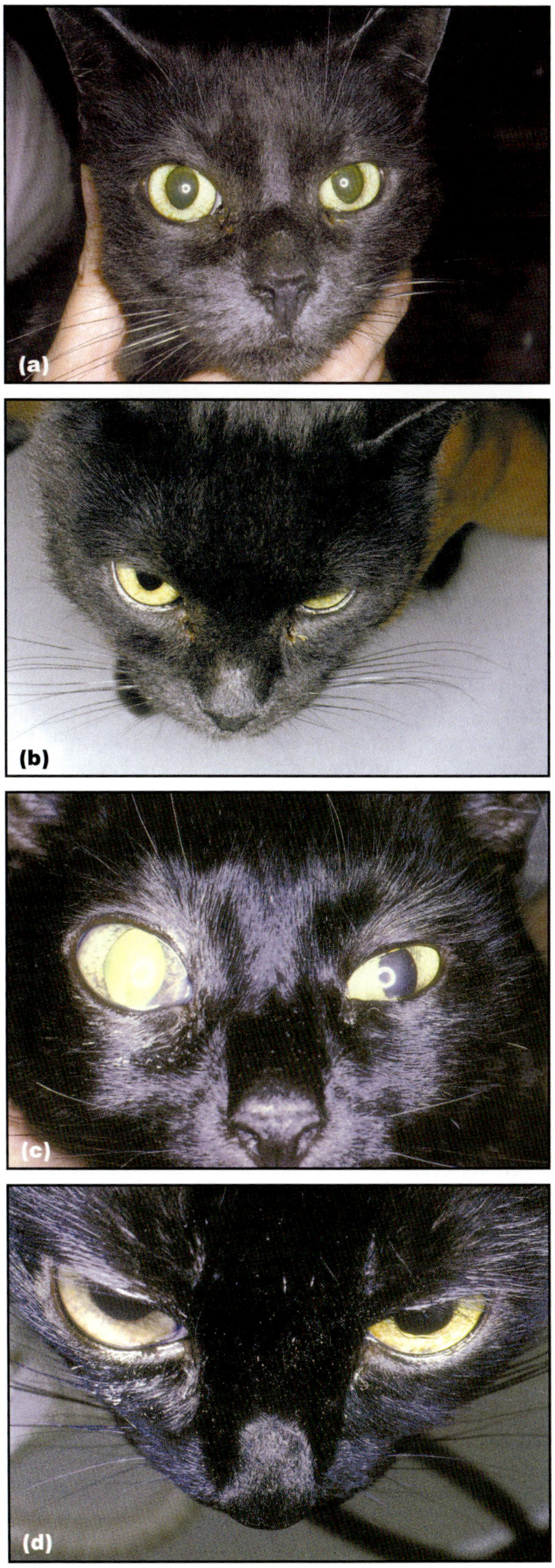

Figure 4.2 Two cats illustrate the value of examination from in front and above. (a) There is a relatively subtle widening of the palpebral fissure as a result of an orbital mass. (b) Viewed from above, the exophthalmos is more obvious. (c) This cat has greatly increased prominence of the right eye, as a result of chronic glaucoma causing globe enlargement. (d) However, there is relatively little difference when viewed from above.

62 The orbit and globe

Some of the above clinical signs are rather non-specific, although exophthalmos with displacement of the globe (strabismus, squint) and a long history without pain suggests the presence of a focal mass such as a tumour. A focal mass displaces the eye away from the mass.

Diffuse retrobulbar swelling (as in abscessation or myositis) usually causes an axial proptosis without deviation, but this is variable. An intra-oral examination should be attempted, but this may not be possible. Severe pain on attempting to open the mouth suggests abscessation/cellulitis or myositis rather than a tumour, unless the vertical ramus of the mandible is involved.

Diagnostic imaging

There are considerable limitations to the use of plain radiography in orbital disease. Most of the structures of interest in the orbit are soft tissue. Problems of superimposition produce poor soft tissue definition. Too often they do not add to the information gained from the clinical examination, with the important exception of the demonstration of bony change.

Radiography: The three most useful views are the dorsoventral, the ventrodorsal (open mouth), and the rostrocaudal (frontal) views (see Chapter 1b). The lateral view is less useful due to superimposition. In all views, it is useful to include both sides for comparison.

The dorsoventral view shows the bony margins of the orbit and the vertical ramus of the mandible well. Although not the ideal view for the nasal cavity, the films should be checked for caudal nasal disease, and an intraoral nasal view taken where indicated.

For the ventrodorsal (open mouth) view, general anaesthesia is required and the jaws must be held as far apart as possible. The maxilla should be as parallel to the table as possible and the beam should be centred on a line joining the upper molar teeth.

For the rostrocaudal (frontal) view, the patient's nose should be pointing directly to the ceiling and the beam should be directed along the long axis of the skull. This is the view normally used for the 'skyline' view of the frontal sinuses, but the beam should be opened out ventrally to include the zygomatic arch and vertical ramus of the mandible.

While the bony structures are well demonstrated in these views, the soft tissues appear homogenous and, in particular, the globes, optic nerves and muscle cones cannot be delineated. The main purpose of plain radiography is to indicate any bony involvement, particularly in the case of suspected orbital tumours, and it is useful for that reason alone.

Several contrast techniques have been described with a view to enhancing the soft tissue information provided by radiographs, but, for various good reasons, are little used and are not described here.

Suturing a metal ring around the limbus is a simple way of locating the globe in radiographs.

Zygomatic sialography may be useful in suspected zygomatic salivary gland disease. The zygomatic papilla is located caudal to the parotid papilla, close to the gum margin. The duct is then cannulated with a fine cannula and contrast medium is injected.

Computed tomography (CT) and magnetic resonance imaging (MRI): Both CT and MRI overcome many of the problems of conventional radiography and give better soft tissue resolution and more precise delineation of orbital lesions (Figure 4.3). Both methods are now much more accessible to veterinary patients than in the past, and their use should be considered in appropriate cases, especially if surgery is contemplated (LeCouteur *et al.*, 1982; Calia *et al.*, 1994).

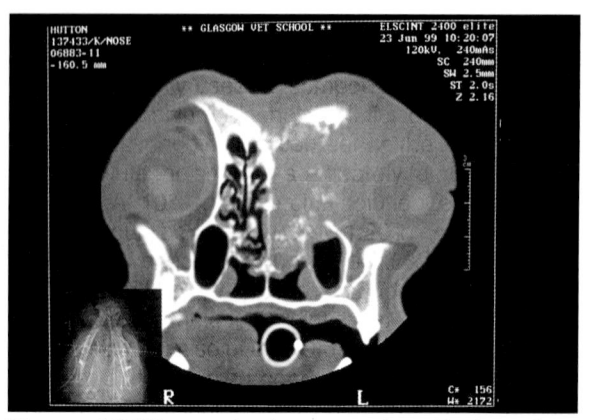

Figure 4.3 CT scan of a dog presenting with signs of an orbital mass. The two globes with the lenses can be made out laterally. A tumour is present in the turbinates, which have been largely destroyed, and in the orbit on the affected side. This illustrates the superior tissue definition provided by CT scanning, though conventional radiography is usually capable of demonstrating nasal tumours and bony involvement.

Ultrasonography: The resolution of ultrasonography is not as good as that of CT or MRI. Most of the structures of interest are a significant distance below the surface and must, therefore, be imaged through the globe itself, or through the lateral periorbital tissues in the region of the orbital ligament (Morgan, 1989). If the lateral oblique view is used, good ultrasonic contact is required, which will involve close clipping of the hairs.

Diseases of the orbit and globe

Conditions causing exophthalmos

Retrobulbar abscessation/cellulitis

Retrobulbar abscessation/cellulitis causes acute pain and dysfunction, and usually requires prompt diagnosis and attention. It is much less common in the cat than the dog. Retrobulbar cellulitis refers to diffuse inflammation of the orbital tissues without localization of pus. The cellulitis phase may precede the formation of a true abscess. The two conditions may be difficult to distinguish and are similar in many respects.

Pathogenesis: A retrobulbar abscess may arise from periorbital skin trauma such as a bite, from extension of sinus, tooth root or zygomatic gland infection, or from foreign body penetration into the pharynx. In many cases, however, the cause remains obscure. Most cases are unilateral.

Clinical signs: The onset is usually fairly rapid. There is painful swelling of the periorbital region and exophthalmos (Figure 4.4), which is generally axial, but there may be some deviation of the globe. There is often congestion of the conjunctiva with a purulent ocular discharge and protrusion of the nictitating membrane. There is severe pain on opening the mouth, because the movement of the vertical ramus of the mandible applies traction and pressure to the orbital tissues. This painful reaction is highly suggestive of the condition. The area behind the last upper molar should be examined for redness and swelling, although this is variable, or the presence of fistulous tracts. This may not be possible without general anaesthesia. There is usually malaise and inappetence (as a result of the pain elicited by eating).

Further investigation: An accurate diagnosis can often be made from the history and clinical examination. There can be quite good symptomatic relief with antibiotics, so the picture may be confused if short courses of antibiotics have been used, followed by recurrences. Radiology usually demonstrates only soft tissue swelling and adds no further information, except in cases of tooth root or sinus infection. Some foreign bodies may be radio-opaque, but the majority are not. Ultrasonography may reveal the presence of a fluid-filled cavity in cases with a discrete abscess. Under anaesthesia, a full examination of the mouth should be made.

Management: The traditional treatment has been to drain the abscess into the mouth. A cuffed endotracheal tube is used and the pharynx is packed with a known number of swabs or a wet gauze bandage (the bandage may be tied to the endotracheal tube). An incision is made with a No.11 scalpel blade approximately 1 cm behind the last molar tooth, but not penetrating deeply. A pair of fine haemostats is inserted and directed dorsally to a greater depth. The blades are gently opened to establish drainage. There may be a free flow of pus, but this is variable. Gentle probing is permitted, as the abscess may be loculated.

Damage to the globe or muscle cone is unlikely unless the probing is very deep (2–3 cm should be adequate in a medium-sized dog) or directed too far medially. Swab samples of the pus should be taken and smears made so that the appropriate antibiotic therapy can begin immediately. If this is not done, it should be assumed that Gram-positive or mixed infections are present. Irrigation of the area has been suggested but is probably unnecessary if adequate drainage is established. Use of indwelling drains has also been advocated, but these are only advisable where there has been unusually extensive orbital involvement. After the procedure, if swabs have been used, they should be removed from the pharynx and counted.

Some clinicians maintain that this drainage procedure is neither necessary nor desirable. A large artery runs across the floor of the orbit, and considerable haemorrhage may be expected if it is ruptured. Instead of drainage, patients are placed on a course of broad-spectrum antibiotics. Medical therapy should produce a noticeable improvement over 24–48 hours and treatment should be maintained for 3–4 weeks, although the length of the course is rather empirical. With this approach, a general anaesthetic is avoided.

Prognosis: With both treatment approaches there is usually prompt improvement and return to normal function within 2–3 days. In the event of recurrence, the antibiotics should be restarted or further investigations considered.

Orbital neoplasia

Pathogenesis: Orbital neoplasia is poorly documented in the literature, but it tends to be serious and difficult to manage when it occurs (Kern, 1985; Gilger *at al.*, 1992; Attali-Sousay *et al.*, 2001). The range of possible tumour types is wide. Obtaining a tissue diagnosis and good imaging of the area are difficult. The prognosis is guarded to poor in many cases.

The most common type of tumour to be found in the orbit of the dog is probably nasal carcinoma invading through the thin medial wall of the orbit and causing exophthalmos and lateral deviation of the globe. The most common primary tumour of the orbit in the dog is meningioma of the optic nerve (Mauldin *et al.*, 2000) (Figure 4.5). The normal orbit contains a variety of tissue types, however, and many of these have been described as giving rise to tumours. Metastatic neoplasia also occurs, and the orbit may be involved in multifocal disease such as lymphoma.

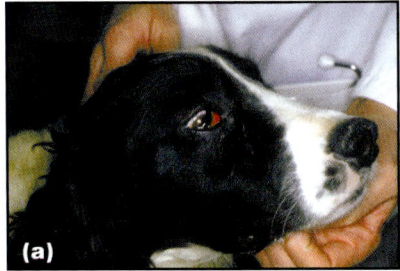

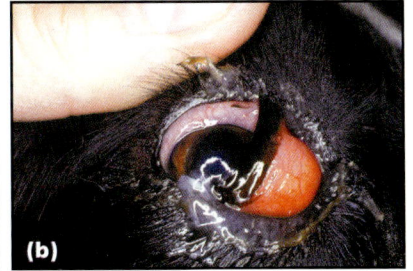

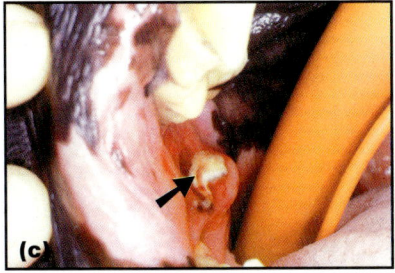

Figure 4.4 An English Springer Spaniel with a retrobulbar abscess. (a) There is painful swelling of the temporal and masseter muscle areas and protrusion of the nictitating membrane. Considerable pain was evinced on opening the mouth. (b) A closer view of the right eye shows chemosis (oedema of the conjunctiva), protrusion of the nictitating membrane and a mucopurulent discharge. Chemosis is uncommon in the dog (unlike the cat) but may occur in orbital disease. (c) The interior of the mouth (under general anaesthesia) shows a fistulous tract (arrowed) caudal to the last molar. Pus was released on enlarging this opening.

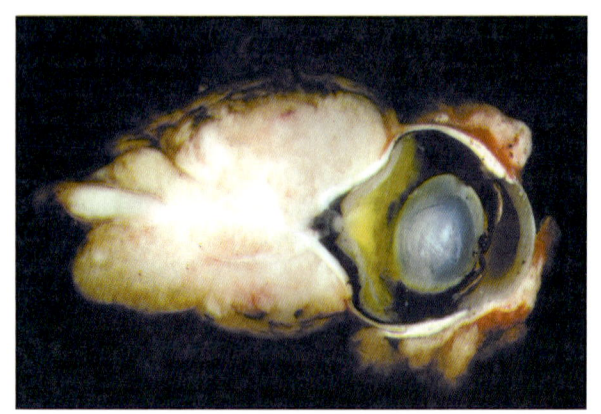

Figure 4.5 Optic nerve meningioma in a dog. The tumour is wrapped around the optic nerve. Local and intracranial recurrence is a risk with optic nerve meningiomas. Histology showed that this example was not fully removed posteriorly.

History and clinical signs: Orbital tumours are seldom directly visible or palpable from the surface, so that the clinical signs are the result of secondary changes in adjacent structures. The onset is typically gradual and tumour growth results in slowly progressive exophthalmos, deviation of the globe and protrusion of the nictitating membrane (Figure 4.6). The degree of nictitating membrane protrusion varies with the site of the tumour. It is likely to be greatest with medial extraconal tumours and less with intraconal tumours. Enophthalmos is sometimes seen where scirrhous tumours retract the globe into the orbit, but these cases are unusual.

Progressive deviation of the globe is suggestive of neoplasia or possibly cyst formation. There may be secondary problems such as keratitis and conjunctivitis resulting from exposure of the ocular surface. The orbital swelling and congestion may be transmitted to the conjunctiva, causing chemosis.

Affected patients usually retain a normal demeanour and continue to eat for a long time and there is usually little pain on opening the mouth, although in some cases there may be mechanical restriction to jaw movement. In ventral tumours there may be convexity behind the last molar tooth. Retropulsion of the globe is usually obviously impaired, and the two sides should be compared. Bilateral involvement is rare, but is occasionally encountered with multifocal and locally invasive tumours. Other accompanying signs which have been described include papilloedema (in tumours applying direct pressure to the optic nerve), indentation of the posterior globe and retinal detachment.

Further investigation: A full clinical examination should be carried out, checking for evidence of lymphoma or primary tumours elsewhere. The possibility of orbital extension of a nasal tumour via the ethmoturbinates or frontal sinus must always be considered, and so evidence of nasal discharge (Figures 4.7 and 4.8), poor airflow or distortion in the frontal sinus region must be sought.

It is rare to be able to make a histopathological diagnosis based on clinical findings alone; the location of the mass may be suggestive, but no more. Radiographs should be taken as described above, recognizing the limitations of standard methods. The radiographs should be examined for any bony involvement attributable to neoplasia and any indications of neoplastic processes within adjacent structures such as nasal chambers, frontal sinuses and zygomatic arch (Figure 4.9). As with any tumour type, bone involvement represents a serious complication.

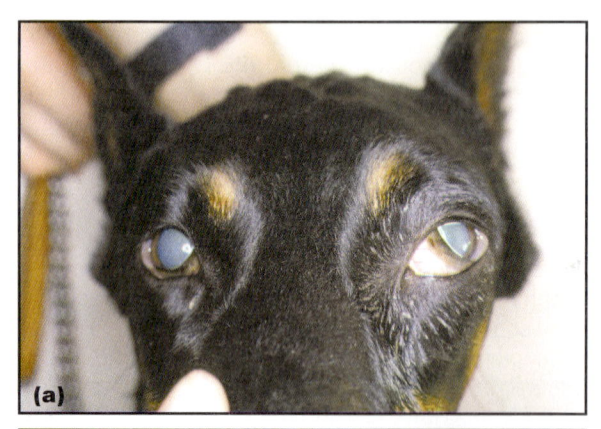

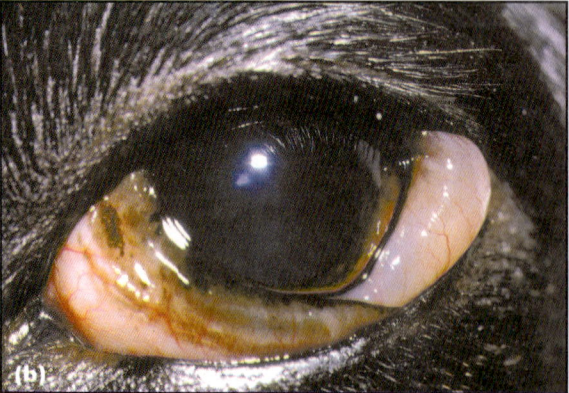

Figure 4.6 (a) Left-sided orbital lymphoma in a Dobermann, which also had cutaneous lesions (visible on the top of the head). (b) There is protrusion of the nictitating membrane and chemosis, both of which may have other causes, but there is also dorsolateral deviation of the globe, which is pathognomonic of an orbital lesion.

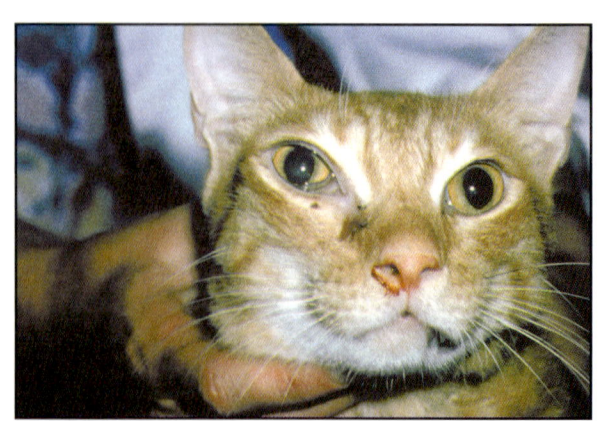

Figure 4.7 Dorsolateral deviation of the globe and protrusion of the nictitating membrane indicate the presence of an orbital lesion in this cat. There is also an ipsilateral nasal discharge, suggesting the orbital lesion may have arisen by extension from a nasal tumour. The tumour was confirmed as a nasal adenocarcinoma at post-mortem examination. (Courtesy of SM Crispin.)

The orbit and globe 65

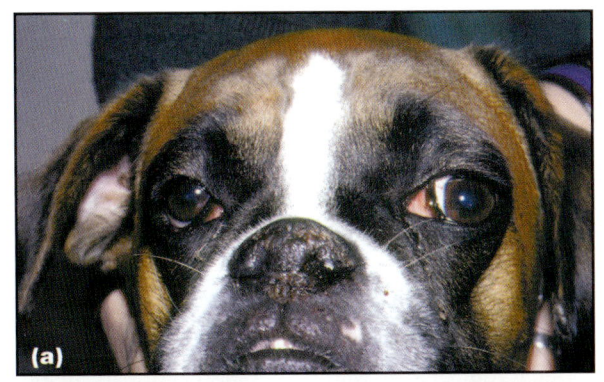

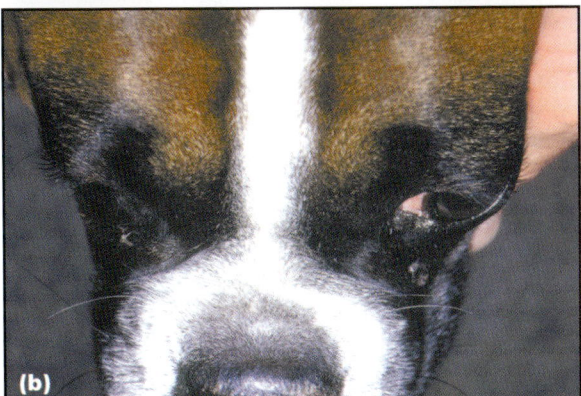

Figure 4.8 (a) Boxer with left-sided protrusion of the nictitating membrane and marked lateral deviation of the globe. The fact that the nictitating membrane is also protruded can mask the degree of displacement of the globe. The degree of anterior displacement, however, is difficult to judge on this view. With lateral deviation of the globe, signs of nasal carcinoma should always be sought and ruled out. Note that the dog has a bloody left-sided nasal discharge. (b) The same dog viewed from above. The exophthalmos is now obvious.

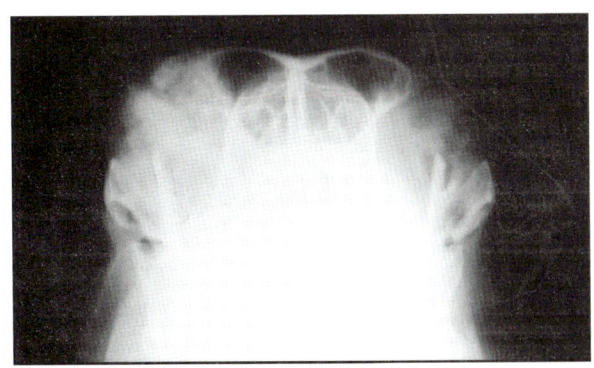

Figure 4.9 'Orbital skyline' view of a canine skull with an orbital tumour on the left side of the radiograph. There is a mineralized mass in the orbit and bony involvement of the frontal sinus wall and possibly the vertical ramus of the mandible and zygomatic arch. These features considerably reduce the feasibility of surgical excision, regardless of the histological type.

Wherever possible and practical, CT or MRI scanning should be seriously considered. Zygomatic sialography should be considered where the clinical signs indicate a mass in the region of the zygomatic gland. Ultrasonography may be carried out if available.

In a few cases, there may be neoplastic tissue that is sufficiently near an accessible surface such as the skin, oral mucosa or conjunctiva to be accessible for biopsy. Fine needle aspiration biopsy is also feasible, but it requires familiarity with the regional anatomy. It does offer, however, the most realistic chance of a histological diagnosis without exploratory orbitotomy, and may avoid major orbital surgery on patients with grave prognoses and those with conditions that are better managed medically, such as lymphoma (Boydell, 1991; Tijl and Koornneef, 1991).

Management: After a tumour has been diagnosed and it has been located, as far as possible, the next decision is whether it is operable (or amenable to chemotherapy) and, if so, whether a functional eye can be preserved. Orbital surgery is difficult, for a number of reasons, and referral should always be considered (Gilger and Whitley, 1994). In many cases, surgery is undertaken with an imprecise knowledge of the relationship of the tumour to other structures and without a histological diagnosis. Ideally, CT or MRI scanning should be undertaken prior to orbital surgery (Figure 4.10).

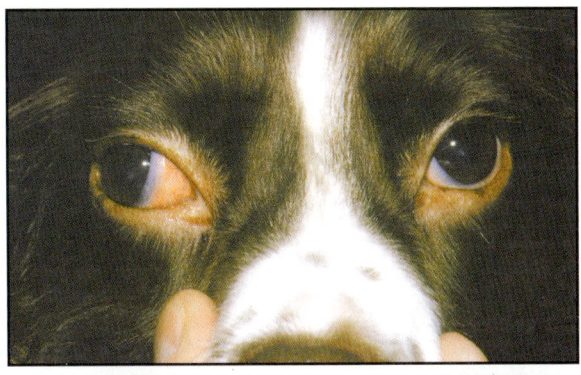

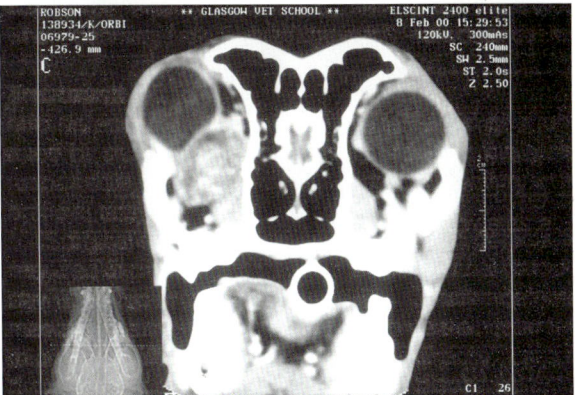

Figure 4.10 English Springer Spaniel with a right-sided orbital mass. Clinical signs and conventional radiography are of limited help in surgical planning. The CT scan clearly shows the tumour. Its position indicates that it is unlikely to be accessible without section of the zygomatic arch.

Problems associated with surgical treatment: It is unusual to be able to remove an orbital tumour and to preserve a functional eye. Most lesions are located relatively deep to the surface, so surgical access is difficult. Access may only be feasible by elevating the temporal muscle (which is very thick and closely applied to the frontal bone) or by sectioning the zygomatic arch. It can also be difficult to avoid damage to small nerves in the orbit, leading to muscle palsies or dry eye,

The orbit and globe

or to extraocular muscles. In most cases, the eye must be removed, and the enucleation technique is extended or modified to include the mass.

The prognosis depends on the histological type, but most orbital tumours are malignant and long-term survival rates are moderate to poor.

Masticatory myositis

Pathogenesis: Masticatory myositis is an immune-mediated condition of the dog in which autoantibodies are formed against type IIM muscle fibres found only in the masticatory muscles. In the acute stage there is infiltration with eosinophils and lymphocytes, hence the alternative name of eosinophilic myositis. The condition occurs in German Shepherd Dogs and Weimaraners, but can be seen in other breeds. The incidence is low.

Clinical signs: In the acute form, there is a sudden onset of pain and swelling of the whole of the masticatory muscle mass, usually symmetrically. The swelling is sufficient to cause exophthalmos and protrusion of the nictitating membrane (Figure 4.11). There is pain on attempting to open the mouth. In time, atrophy and fibrosis of the muscles may occur, resulting in visible wasting of the region, enophthalmos and restricted mobility of the mandible, sometimes resulting in a much reduced range of jaw movement. Alternatively, the onset may be insidious, with the atrophy and fibrosis occurring more slowly and without a prior acute episode (Figure 4.12).

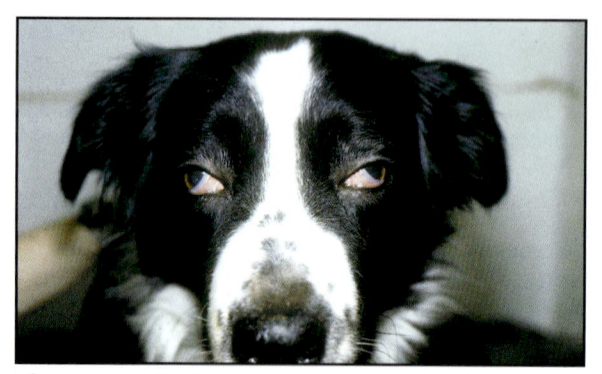

Figure 4.11 Acute masticatory myositis in a Border Collie with symmetrical painful swelling of all the masticatory muscles, leading to protrusion of the nictitating membranes.

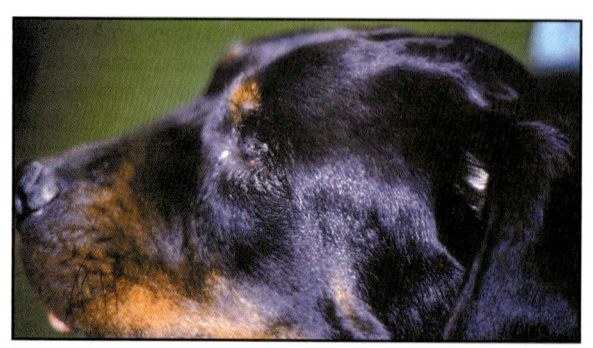

Figure 4.12 Rottweiler with chronic masticatory myositis, leading to secondary atrophy and fibrosis. There is wasting of the masticatory muscles, leading to prominence of the zygomatic arch. The dog was otherwise heavily muscled.

Further investigation: The clinical signs are suggestive, but it is usual to confirm the diagnosis with a biopsy of the temporal muscle, taking care not to sample in error the more mobile subcutaneous muscle overlying it.

Treatment: Dogs are treated with immunosuppressive doses of corticosteroids, the dose being reduced slowly according to clinical response.

Extraocular polymyositis

Extraocular polymyositis is a recently described syndrome affecting young dogs of the larger breeds at about 1 year of age, with the Golden Retriever being over-represented (Carpenter *et al.*, 1989).

Clinical signs: There is inflammation and swelling of the extraocular muscles, producing obvious bilateral exophthalmos that is not accompanied by third eyelid protrusion (Figure 4.13). There may be secondary conjunctival hyperaemia, but there appears to be little pain. The dogs remain well, with no malaise or other systemic signs, although the local appearance may be striking. There is little resistance to retropulsion of the globes, and the globes and vision remain normal. The pathogenesis is unknown.

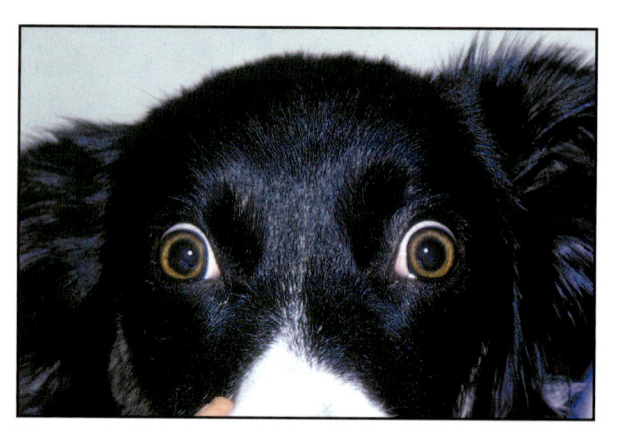

Figure 4.13 A 1-year-old female Border Collie with symmetrical painless exophthalmos due to extraocular polymyositis. There was complete resolution with an extended course of systemic corticosteroids.

Diagnosis: The diagnosis may be confirmed from a biopsy, but this would be a specialist procedure and may not be necessary. Good ultrasound scanning will demonstrate thickening of the extraocular muscles.

Treatment: Systemic corticosteroids are an effective treatment given at immunosuppressive doses initially. Recurrences may occur, though not through life, and the treatment should only be reduced very slowly.

Prognosis: With appropriate early treatment, most dogs respond well, but the prognosis is guarded initially. Some dogs present in the fibrotic stage, with enophthalmos and strabismus, and some may develop these even after early diagnosis and treatment. Contracture may be confirmed by carrying out forced duction tests which will suggest fibrosis of one or more muscles.

To undergo a forced duction test the dog is usually anaesthetized. Forceps are used to grasp the conjunctiva adjacent to the limbus plus the underlying Tenon's capsule, and the mobility of the globe is checked in all directions in which it normally moves. This helps differentiate altered globe position due to extraocular muscle contracture from altered globe position due to an abnormality in the nerve supply to the extraocular muscles (see Chapter 15). in the latter case the globe can be moved freely.

Zygomatic salivary gland mucocoele

Zygomatic gland mucocoele is an uncommon condition in the dog. There is a suggestion that previous trauma may be responsible in some cases. It is important to distinguish this from an orbital tumour, as the prognosis is much better.

The dog is presented with a fluid-filled mass in the ventral orbit but the position is variable. The affected area has a soft fluid feel and this should distinguish it from an orbital tumour (Figure 4.14). There may be prominent convexity in the oropharynx. On aspiration at the most accessible point, usually the oral mucosa, a tenacious fluid typical of stagnant saliva may be found. Zygomatic sialography will demonstrate a fluid-filled cavity, thus distinguishing it from neoplasia of the gland or other tissue. Drainage or fistulation of the mucocoele into the mouth is often sufficient as a means of management, but extirpation of the gland via an oral or lateral approach may be required in recurrent cases.

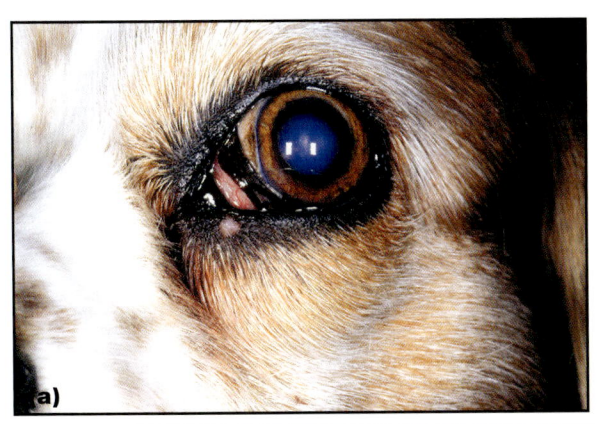

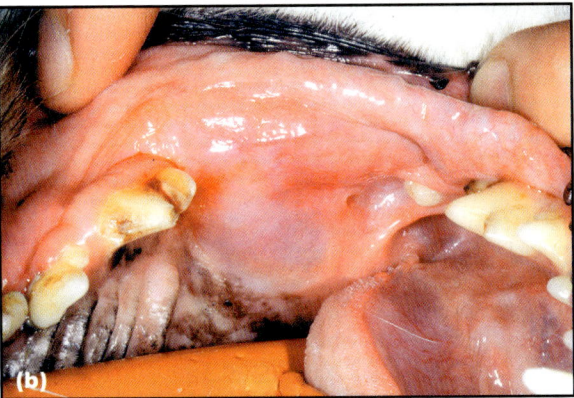

Figure 4.14 Zygomatic mucocoele in a Cavalier King Charles Spaniel. (a) There is a painless soft fluid-filled swelling above and below the zygomatic arch. (b) The area behind the last molar is abnormally convex, again with a soft fluid feel.

Arteriovenous shunts

Arteriovenous shunts are congenital vascular malformations resulting in a large vascular, possibly pulsating, mass in the orbit. They are quite rare but worth noting, as they are the only recognized congenital cause of exophthalmos. Contrast venography or arteriography may confirm the diagnosis. Surgical treatment is difficult, with or without preservation of the eye, as there is a risk of severe haemorrhage. Arteriovenous shunts may also, rarely, result from trauma or invasive neoplasia.

Temporomandibular osteopathy

Periosteal proliferation of new bone may occur on the mandible and temporal bones in juvenile Scottish and West Highland White Terriers. Very occasionally, it may cause exophthalmos, but in most cases the proliferation is ventral and the position of the globe is not affected.

Conditions causing a small or recessed eye

Enophthalmos

Enophthalmos refers to an abnormally deep globe position. It occurs most commonly as a variation of normal in some larger breeds of dog such as Rough Collie, Great Dane, Dobermann and Flat-coated Retriever, all of which are bred for a relatively small eye and deep orbit. The result is a deep set to the eye, often with marked protrusion of the nictitating membrane. These dogs may accumulate large quantities of mucus at the medial canthus (see Figure 7.5) and this should not be confused with a purulent discharge. No treatment is required; the nictitating membranes should not be excised, as this may impair the quantity and distribution of the tear film and will not relieve the enophthalmos. Enophthalmos may also occur as an acquired lesion in a number of conditions.

Horner's syndrome: Horner's syndrome is functional sympathetic denervation of the eye and orbit (see Chapter 15) and results in enophthalmos because of loss of tone in the smooth muscle of the periorbita, which normally acts to maintain the eye in an anterior position. The presence of miosis and nictitating membrane protrusion will support the diagnosis. Care should be taken not to mistake the difference in appearance between the normal and affected eyes as being due to exophthalmos of the normal eye.

Active retraction of a painful eye: Dogs and, to a lesser extent, cats are able to retract the eye in response to pain, by the action of the retractor bulbi muscle. Other signs of pain should also be present.

Atrophy of orbital tissues: Enophthalmos may result from significant loss of orbital tissue mass, giving the eye a hollow, sunken appearance. This may arise in fibrosis and atrophy of the masticatory or extraocular muscles, and in cachexia or severe wasting from any cause (Figure 4.15).

Orbital neoplasia: Enophthalmos occurs in rare cases, but exophthalmos is more common (see above).

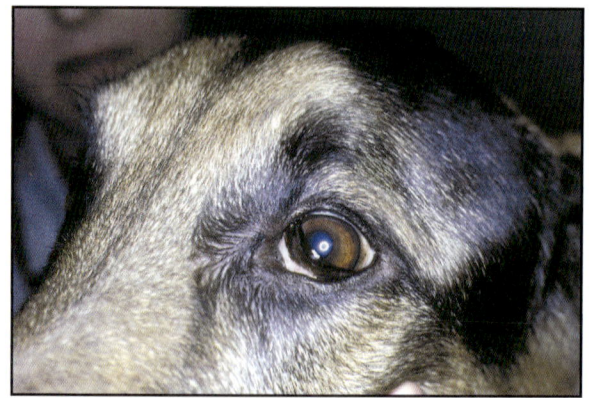

Figure 4.15 German Shepherd Dog with neoplasia at multiple sites. Severe wasting has led to enophthalmos and protrusion of the nictitating membrane.

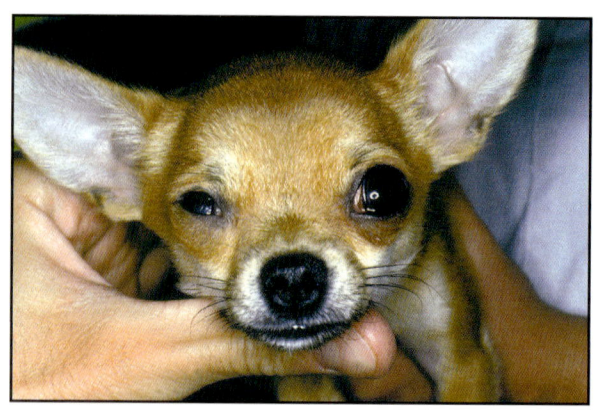

Figure 4.17 A young Chihuahua with right-sided microphthalmos and dry eye.

Microphthalmos

Microphthalmos (or microphthalmia) refers to a congenitally small eye. This may vary from a small but fully functional eye, referred to as *nanophthalmos*, to one with multiple intraocular abnormalities and no visual function. *Cryptophthalmos* refers to an ocular structure that is concealed by other adnexal defects, or is so small as to be difficult to find (Figure 4.16) and *anophthalmos* refers to complete absence of ocular tissue, which is a very rare occurrence.

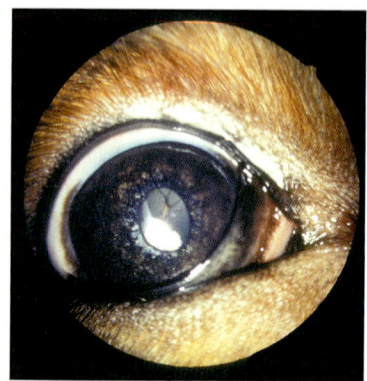

Figure 4.18 Microphthalmic eye in a Cocker Spaniel, in association with cataract and pupillary membrane strands running from the iris to the anterior lens capsule. (Courtesy of SM Crispin.)

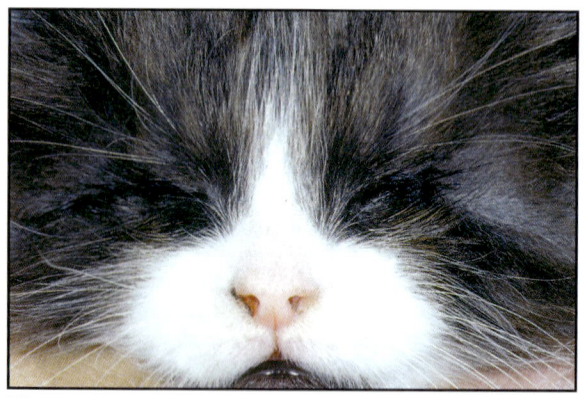

Figure 4.16 An 8-week-old Maine Coon kitten with no detectable ocular tissue, although there are rudimentary lids with slit-like openings.

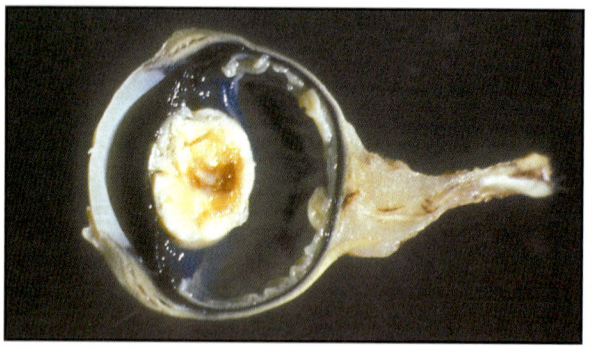

Figure 4.19 Microphthalmic eye from a Cocker Spaniel with extensive cataract and retinal dysplasia, visible as folding of the neuroretina. (Courtesy of SM Crispin.)

Certain breeds, most notably the Rough Collie, have small eyes as a feature of the breed. In other breeds, as a sporadic event, one eye may simply be smaller than the other, but functional, or may have other abnormalities (Figure 4.17). Associated abnormalities may include corneal opacities, persistent pupillary membrane, cataract, detachment or dysplasia of the retina and nystagmus. The cause in these sporadic cases remains obscure.

Microphthalmos is also seen as a proven or suspected hereditary defect in association with cataract or other malformations (Figures 4.18 and 4.19). It may also occur in association with hereditary retinal dysplasia in affected breeds (see Chapter 14). None of these hereditary forms of microphthalmos is common, but they may have implications for breeding when they occur.

Phthisis bulbi: Phthisis bulbi (phthisical eye, phthitic eye) refers to an acquired end-stage eye in which the aqueous production has ceased and the eye has shrunk. Severe intraocular pathology is always implied by the term, although intraocular examination may not be possible due to greyish corneal opacity. Causes include primary or secondary glaucoma, severe intraocular inflammation and severe penetrating wounds or blunt trauma (Figure 4.20).

In those cases which result from chronic glaucoma, the eye is initially enlarged. Glaucoma-induced destruction of the ciliary body may occur in time, resulting in loss of aqueous production and eventual collapse of the globe (Figure 4.21). This may take years, however, or may not occur at all, and so waiting for phthisis is not an acceptable management option

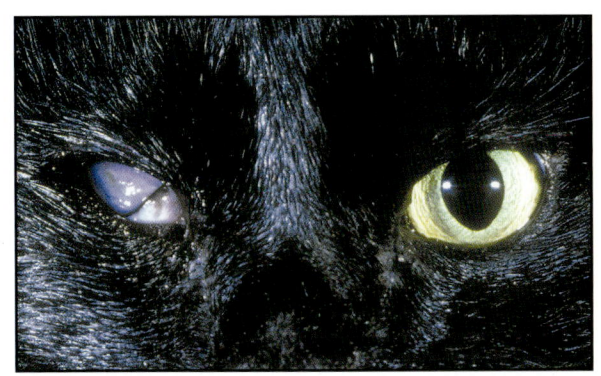

Figure 4.20 Phthisis bulbi in a cat that had sustained ocular trauma in a road traffic accident. Severe blunt trauma to the eye can cause the sclera to split posteriorly, which usually then leads to permanent loss of pressure and phthisis.

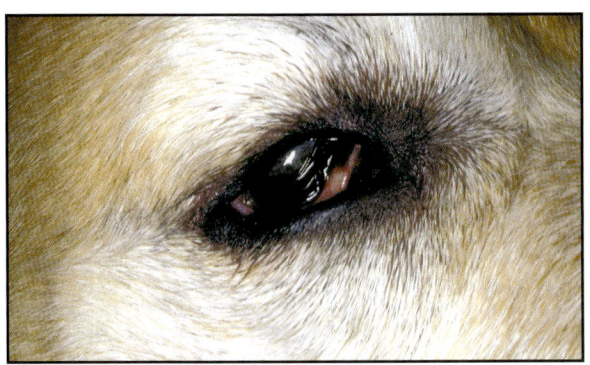

Figure 4.21 Phthisis bulbi in a dog following chronic glaucoma. The small globe is partly concealed behind a permanently protruded nictitating membrane. The cornea is usually diffusely grey and partly pigmented in such cases.

for chronically glaucomatous painful eyes. Phthisical eyes often appear not to be painful, although mild pain may be difficult to detect.

Malignant sarcomas can develop in feline eyes that are phthisical or that have sustained chronic intraocular inflammation. The history may be of several years' duration. The eye may be opaque by the time of examination, preventing a clinical diagnosis of neoplasia. These sarcomas are relatively uncommon, but their malignant nature should be borne in mind when considering the management of such eyes, and enucleation is recommended (Figure 4.22).

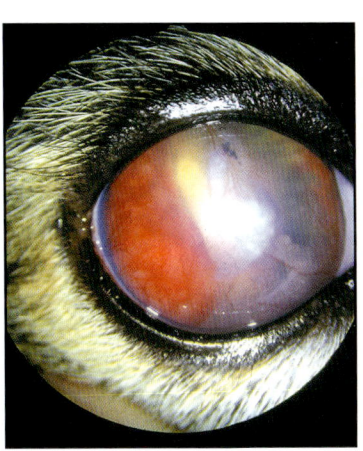

Figure 4.22 There is central corneal scarring in this cat's eye from a penetrating injury years earlier. A sarcoma is now present laterally in the iris, appearing as a red mass. There is said to be an association between these sarcomas and previous trauma in the cat, but the risk cannot be quantified.

Buphthalmos

Buphthalmos means 'ox eye' and tends to be used synonymously with the terms hydrophthalmos and megaloglobus. All refer to a pathologically enlarged eye as a result of glaucoma. Generally, the globe of the dog and cat is unable to withstand sustained high pressure without stretching and enlarging. This process occurs most readily in young animals, and in the cat more than the dog. By the time the globe is visibly enlarged, there will be other pathological changes attributable to the glaucoma and enlargement. These may include corneal changes such as oedema, neovascularization, pigmentation and tears in Descemet's membrane; subluxation of the lens as a result of tearing of zonular fibres; visible retinal atrophy; and cupping and atrophy of the optic disc.

Buphthalmos implies severe irreversible damage and a blind eye, with the possible exceptions of the early stages of chronic open angle glaucoma (which is relatively uncommon), ocular melanosis with secondary glaucoma of Cairn Terriers (which is very breed specific) and some cats with painless enlargement of the globe. It must be emphasized that globe enlargement is a chronic change resulting from prolonged glaucoma and is not a presenting feature of acute angle-closure glaucoma.

The degree of pain in buphthalmic eyes is variable and can be difficult to judge. In many cases, there is little clinical evidence of pain and certainly not of the severe pain and malaise accompanying acute glaucoma. Some owners, however, will volunteer that the patient cries out when it knocks the eye, which may indicate underlying discomfort.

Buphthalmic eyes are frequently unsightly. Options for management of these eyes are discussed fully in Chapter 11, but in view of the severe changes, enucleation is justified in many cases.

Prolapse of the globe and orbital trauma

Prolapse of the globe

Prolapse of the globe is acute dislocation of the globe beyond the plane of the lids and should be distinguished from proptosis or exophthalmos; both of these terms imply only a degree of anterior displacement. The condition occurs as a result of trauma such as road traffic accidents, attacks by larger dogs or non-accidental injury caused by humans. Prolapse is much more common in the exophthalmic breeds and especially the Pekingese, where there is less protection to the eye from the anterior orbital margin. In some cases, the trauma may be apparently minor.

Pathogenesis and clinical signs: With prolapse of the globe, there is traction on the optic and other nerves and on blood vessels. There is also immediate oedema of the conjunctiva and other tissues surrounding the globe. The eyelids go into spasm behind the equator of the globe, making reduction more difficult and adding to the oedema and congestion (Figure 4.23). In addition, the patient is likely to be very distressed. The situation is an emergency.

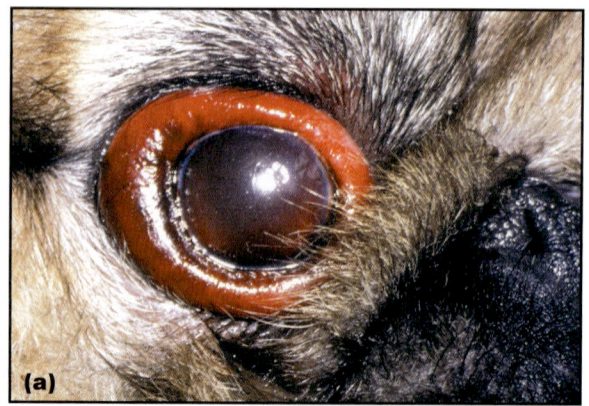

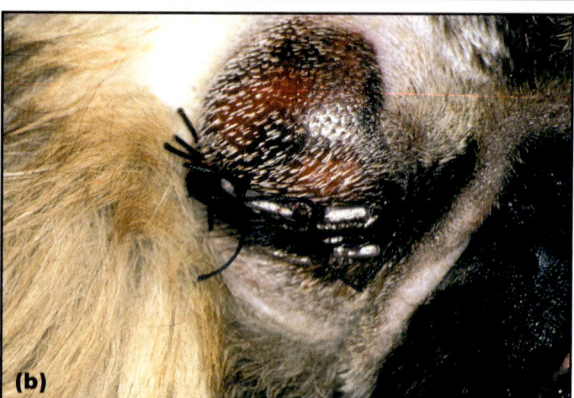

Figure 4.23 Pekingese which sustained prolapse of the globe after being kicked by a man. (a) The lids are in spasm behind the equator of the globe, resulting in extensive chemosis and subconjunctival haemorrhage. There was also a fracture of the zygomatic arch. At this stage, simple reduction of the prolapsed globe is not possible without a lateral canthotomy. (b) Following reduction of the prolapsed globe, the eyelids have been sutured together with horizontal mattress sutures and stents have been used to minimize damage to the lids. There must be no possibility of the sutures abrading the cornea while in place. (Courtesy of SM Crispin.)

Treatment: Attempts should be made to replace the globe immediately before this vicious circle of congestion, pain and lid spasm is established. The simplest way to do this is to apply pressure on the surface of the eye with wet cotton wool as soon as possible, to hold the eye in a more normal position. In many cases, this is not done or it is impossible, and the appearance will be as in Figure 4.23 on presentation. The cornea must be protected with copious lubrication while it is exposed. A general examination should be made and the patient should, if other injuries allow, be anaesthetized without delay. If simple reduction is not feasible, then other steps will be necessary, such as lateral canthotomy or the use of traction sutures or Allis tissue forceps on the lid margin while gently repelling the globe. Once the prolapse is reduced, the lids should be sutured together for 14 days using horizontal mattress sutures positioned so as to prevent contact between the sutures and the globe. Systemic corticosteroids and antibiotics should be administered.

Prognosis: Even with prompt and correct management, the prognosis for restoring a functional eye is very guarded. The objective of the emergency treatment is to prevent the development of severe swelling, corneal desiccation and lid spasm. The prolapse itself, however, may cause tractional damage to the optic nerve, resulting in blindness, to the trigeminal nerve, resulting in a desensitized ocular surface, and to the medial rectus muscle, resulting in avulsion and lateral strabismus, all of which can be permanent and can occur regardless of the initial management. The end result is often the situation in Figure 4.24, and some of these globes will require enucleation at a later date. Where most of the attachments are ruptured at the time of presentation (Figure 4.25), enucleation should be carried out immediately.

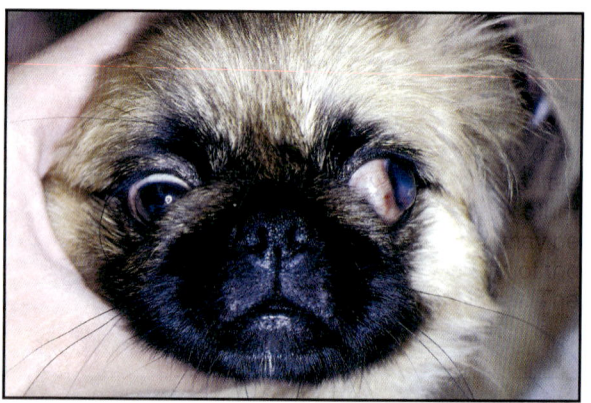

Figure 4.24 This Pekingese had sustained a prolapse of the left globe 3 months previously while in a room on its own. The globe was replaced promptly and correctly at the time, but there is now lateral strabismus, exposure keratopathy, no corneal sensation and no pupillary light response. Such sequelae can occur regardless of the initial management.

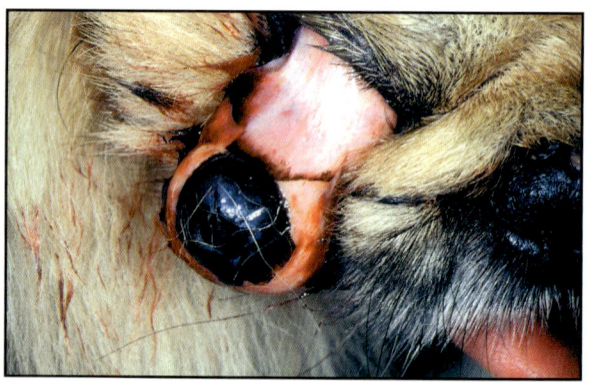

Figure 4.25 This Pekingese was found in this condition in the morning, having been normal the night before. It lived with another dog of the same breed. The eye was attached only by conjunctiva. Repair was not attempted and the eye was removed.

Orbital trauma

Other than prolapse of the globe and trauma to the lids and ocular surface (see Chapters 5 and 8), orbital trauma, as such, is not common. However, there may be traumatic damage to the surrounding structures (see below). The orbital contents are protected by the thick masticatory muscles and the zygomatic arch. Bruising and superficial trauma to the masticatory muscles can be managed conservatively. Orbital haemorrhage is a potentially more serious problem in that it may cause exophthalmos and exposure keratopathy. Where this occurs, the ocular surface should be protected with copious lubrication or by closure of the lids until the problem subsides.

Fractures of the zygomatic arch: Zygomatic arch fractures can occur in, for example, road traffic accidents (Figure 4.26). In general, the fracture is stabilized by the fixed ends of the temporal and zygomatic bones and internal fixation is not often required. Where there is considerable displacement or depression, the fracture ends can be elevated and stabilized with wire sutures.

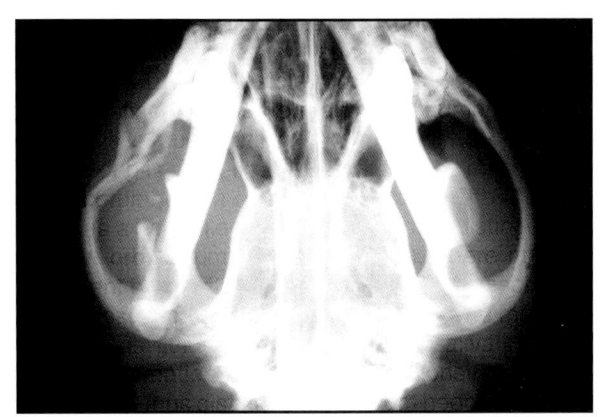

Figure 4.26 Radiograph of a Staffordshire bull terrier that had sustained fractures of the scapula, mandible and zygomatic arch in a road accident. The zygomatic arch fracture is comminuted, but there is minimal displacement, and surgical repair was not required.

Fractures of the frontal sinus: Depression fractures of the frontal sinus can lead to retention mucocoeles, which may erode the sinus wall and cause orbital swelling or a discharging sinus. The fractured wall should be elevated, if possible, and communication with the nasal cavity re-established. Care is required in the interpretation of radiographs, as frontal sinus tumours can also lead to erosion of the frontal sinus wall, the presence of free mucus in the orbit and mucous discharge through the conjunctival surface.

Shotgun pellets: Shotgun pellets may occasionally lodge in the orbit. Any trauma to the globe is likely to have serious implications and should receive priority. Radiographs should be taken: at least two views are necessary to localize foreign bodies in the orbit, and the problems of soft tissue definition and localization of the globe and muscle cone apply as before. The simplest way of localizing the eye is to use metal limbal markers sutured to the conjunctiva (Figure 4.27). The potential value of these procedures should be carefully considered in the case of lead shot because it is relatively inert in tissues and the damage caused by the shot may be less than that caused by orbital exploration (see Chapter 13).

Penetrating trauma to the globe

The intraocular structures are enclosed within the tough fibrous coat of the cornea and sclera, which limit penetrating injury. When penetration does

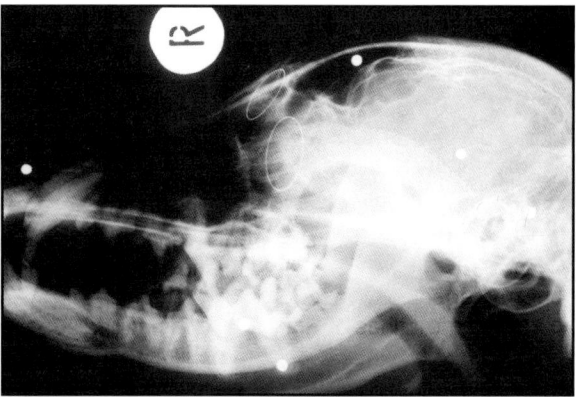

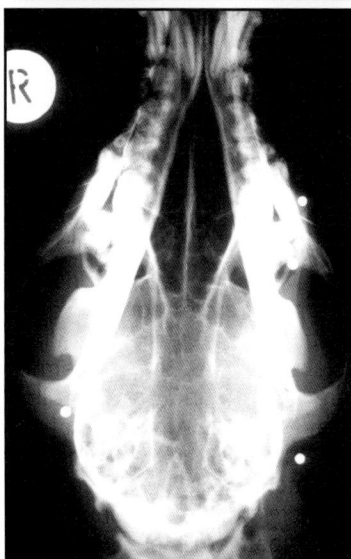

Figure 4.27 Shotgun injury to a 2-year-old Border Collie. Two views are essential in locating foreign bodies. Circular metal rings have been sutured around the limbus in both eyes (more clearly seen in the lateral view) to indicate the positions of the globes.

occur, however, the consequences for the eye are potentially serious.

Most penetrating injuries are anterior, through the cornea or anterior sclera. Initially, the aqueous humour escapes and the iris moves anteriorly, adhering to the underside of a small wound or becoming incorporated within a larger one. This is the eye's natural mechanism for healing a penetration, and it is often successful in doing so, but it may result in considerable disruption of the local anatomy, including drainage angle closure as a result of the anterior displacement of the plane of the iris. If the entry site is not healed and there is prolonged leakage of aqueous, the reduced intraocular pressure, referred to as hypotonia, may also lead to angle closure.

Objects penetrating the anterior coat of the eye may continue onwards to cause direct damage to the iris, or to cause rupture or displacement of the lens, or even to damage posterior structures. Sometimes objects may exit the eye again through the posterior wall.

Clinical signs

A corneal wound should be easy to detect, but a scleral wound less so. Miosis (constriction of the pupil) is likely in all cases, but this may be accompanied by blood or exudate in the anterior chamber, lens and vitreous opacities, retinal detachment, choroidal haemorrhage or any combination of these. Intraocular examination may, therefore, be very difficult and serious intraocular changes may be undetected.

When faced with a traumatized eye, the clinician must never pronounce on the integrity of structures that cannot be examined (Figure 4.28). As full an examination as possible should be made. The pupil should be dilated with mydriatics to assist examination of the lens and posterior structures. Good quality ultrasonography may also provide useful information in the same area.

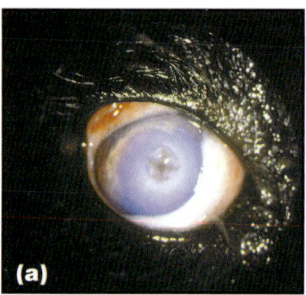

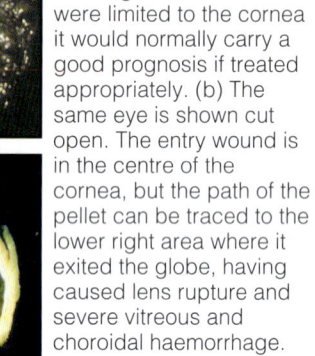

Figure 4.28 (a) A shotgun pellet has caused a small penetrating wound to the cornea with surrounding oedema in this dog. If the wound were limited to the cornea it would normally carry a good prognosis if treated appropriately. (b) The same eye is shown cut open. The entry wound is in the centre of the cornea, but the path of the pellet can be traced to the lower right area where it exited the globe, having caused lens rupture and severe vitreous and choroidal haemorrhage.

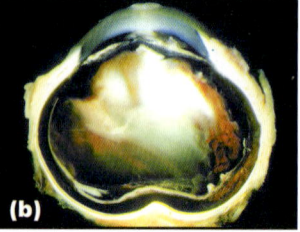

Treatment
Corneal wounds should be sutured, achieving a good seal in order to restore the integrity of the eye (see Chapter 8). Repair of corneal wounds involving the iris should be carried out promptly as adhesions readily develop (Figure 4.29).

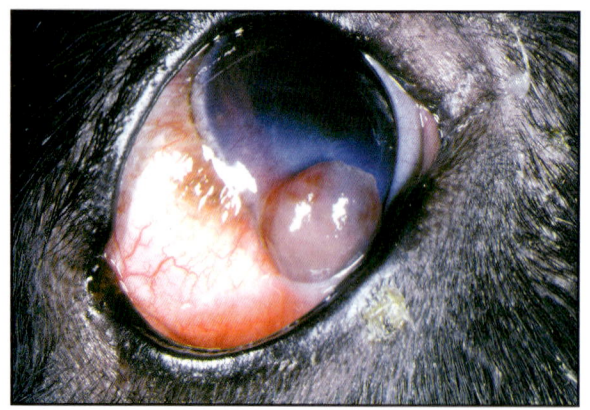

Figure 4.29 This Border Collie had sustained a laceration of the ventrolateral limbus of the right eye 7 days previously. There is iris prolapse; the normal iris appearance is lost as it is now covered by a fibrinous membrane. The cornea and sclera have contracted around the laceration and all the tissues are adherent. The prolapse cannot now be reduced without enlarging the wound and freeing all the structures involved.

A third eyelid flap should not be used for treatment of a penetrating wound or perforated ulcer. If the third eyelid flap has a place, it is in facilitating healing of the corneal surface, but it will not seal a full thickness defect which requires direct surgery for a secure repair.

Topical antibiotics with good intraocular penetration such as gentamicin or chloramphenicol should be applied frequently. Systemic broad-spectrum antibiotics with good effectiveness against Gram-positive bacteria should be given at full doses. Even if the iris itself is not traumatized, there is always likely to be a reflex anterior uveitis with accompanying miosis. Topical steroids should be avoided, however, as they will inhibit healing of the ocular surface. Topical atropine should be used to relieve pain and dilate the pupil; topical and systemic non-steroidal anti-inflammatory preparations may also be used.

Lens rupture
Lens rupture can occur and is a potentially serious complication; it presents problems in both diagnosis and management. The penetration site is easily obscured by constriction of the iris and the iris readily adheres to the site, so that mydriatics may be ineffective.

Possible sequelae of lens rupture include progressive and, ultimately, total cataract, severe lens-induced uveitis and intralenticular infection. Small lens capsule penetrations may heal spontaneously, leaving a focal opacity, but this is exceptional.

Because of the serious consequences of lens rupture, it is often recommended that the lens matter be removed by phacoemulsification as soon as the diagnosis is made (see Chapter 12). Any attempt to repair more posterior lesions is likely to require a specialist, and is probably rarely undertaken.

Blunt trauma to the globe

The consequences of blunt (closed, non-penetrating) trauma to the globe are largely dependent on the force applied at the time of the injury. Changes may be minor and heal uneventfully but, at its worst, blunt trauma can be devastating to the eye, and can do considerably more damage than sharp penetrating injury. When an eye is struck forcefully, there is an instantaneous and potentially considerable rise in intraocular pressure. There are several possible consequences, including iris dialysis (tear), angle recession (posterior displacement of the iris with abnormal opening of the drainage angle), lens rupture and displacement, retinal detachment, massive intraocular haemorrhage and scleral rupture. In the worst cases, there is total intraocular disruption. Since the pressure is exerted evenly over the entire surface of the globe, it ruptures at the weakest point rather than at the point of impact. Dog and cat globes therefore rupture posteriorly, but the intraocular changes are so severe that this cannot be seen clinically.

Clinical signs
Severe blunt trauma is much more common in the cat than in the dog, although the appearances tend to be similar in the two species when it occurs. Most cases result from road traffic accidents. Cats may also have facial and mandibular trauma, such as symphyseal separations, but in many cases the eye suffers massive damage without other injuries (Figure 4.30). The eye usually shows total hyphaema and intraocular examination is not possible. There may also be subconjunctival haemorrhage and poor lid movement, resulting in drying of the ocular surface.

The orbit and globe 73

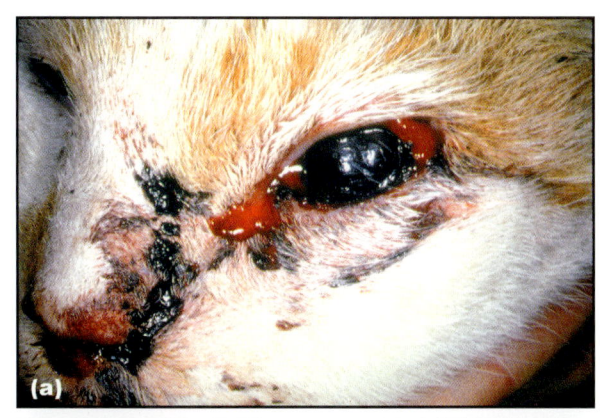

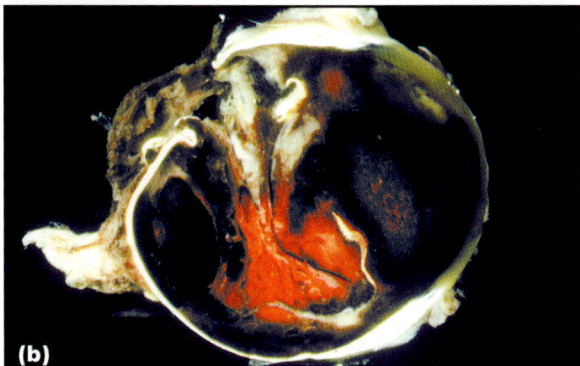

Figure 4.30 This cat had been hit by a car. (a) The eye shows total hyphaema and some drying of the surface. There were no other injuries. (b) The same eye is shown opened. The eye is full of blood. Most of the lens was found free in the orbit, having left the eye through a large posterior scleral wound.

Treatment
Assessment of airway, breathing and circulation take priority, followed by ranking of any other injuries present. Emergency rescuscitation, if indicated, is followed by rehydration and pain relief, provided that intracranial injuries do not dictate otherwise.

Patients may be very distressed, unable to close the mouth and unable or unwilling to eat or drink. The surface of the eye should be treated with lubricants and/or antibiotic ointment, and a guarded prognosis should be given. As with penetrating trauma, no assurances can be given regarding tissues that cannot be examined. If there has been a simple bleed into the anterior chamber, this will resolve well without treatment. If massive intraocular disruption and posterior rupture have occurred, there is no alternative to enucleation, and the eye can safely be maintained on lubricants until this can be carried out. In time, the extraocular tissues become adherent to the site of the rupture, and some limitation to the movement of the globe may be noticed at surgery. If not removed, these eyes readily become phthisical but, although they are presumably pain free by that stage, enucleation is still advisable in the cat in view of the risk of sarcoma in the future.

Intraocular infection
Infection may enter the eye through a penetrating injury (including surgery), via a perforated ulcer or endogenously, as a metastatic process. Systemic infections with ocular involvement are important in some regions of the world and may be due to a variety of organisms. Infections restricted to the eye, however, nearly always enter through penetrating wounds, with or without a retained foreign body. In a perforated ulcer, the defect is usually sealed rapidly. This limits the potential for organisms to enter the eye via the ulcer site and, as a consequence, infection is unusual. It is much more common, however, for organisms to be introduced by thorn injuries, cat claw penetrations, bite injuries, intraocular and glaucoma filtering surgery and migrating foreign bodies.

Prognosis
Established intraocular infection carries a very poor prognosis. There are often large amounts of pus within the eye and there is widespread inflammation. Irreversible changes such as adhesions and angle closure readily occur. Intraocular bacterial infection is also usually very painful.

The index of suspicion for intraocular infection among clinicians is probably low, and this may delay diagnosis. The clinical signs are of chronic uveitis with or without lens rupture or cataract, vitreous opacities, secondary glaucoma and pain. There are probably no pathognomonic signs, and vitreocentesis and culture are required to confirm the diagnosis. Most cases will have a history of trauma (including surgery), but trauma often occurs unobserved in animals and there may simply be a history of a sudden onset of pain.

Bacteria flourish within the vitreous, regardless of the site of entry (which is usually more anterior), and within the lens, if the lens capsule is ruptured and the lens was inoculated with bacteria at the time of the injury (Figure 4.31). In time, both sites may be difficult to evaluate clinically due to opacity. The vitreous may be obscured by aqueous flare, constriction of the pupil and cataract.

In human cases vitreocentesis is regarded as the most effective way of confirming the diagnosis and obtaining material for culture. Anterior chamber infection can occur but is less common, and so aqueous

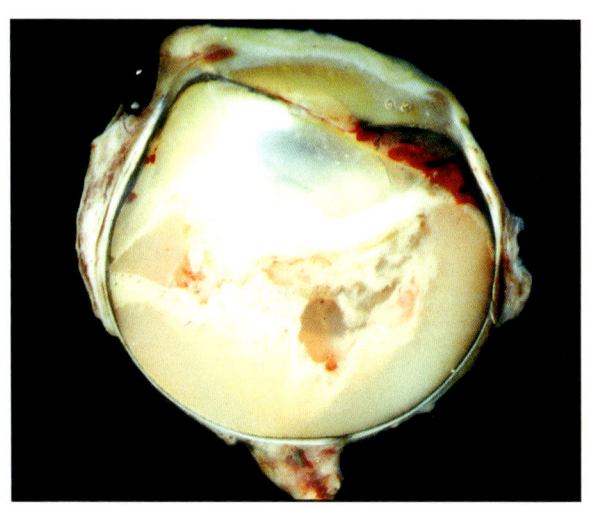

Figure 4.31 This dog's eye had been bitten by another dog one week previously. The lens is ruptured and surrounded by pus and there is further flocculent material in the vitreous. Bacteria were present within the lens matter and the vitreous, but not the aqueous.

centesis alone may give false-negative results. The techniques are described in Chapter 1a. Intralenticular infection is not uncommon but is more difficult to confirm. Gram-positive rods and cocci are the most common organisms found in intraocular infection of the dog and cat.

Prevention

With penetrating injury, every effort should be made to rule in or out a lens penetration by the use of mydriatics and careful examination. Immediate lensectomy may prevent intralenticular infection becoming established; if this is indicated, referral should be considered. All patients that have sustained penetrating injury, perforated corneal ulcers and intraocular surgery should be treated with maximum doses of broad-spectrum antibiotics as soon as possible.

Enucleation

Enucleation is the removal of the globe and is indicated in the following conditions:

- Intractable glaucoma of any cause
- Buphthalmos with pain, poor cosmesis or exposure problems
- Inoperable intraocular tumours
- Some cases of prolapse of the globe
- Unresponsive intraocular infection.

Many of these fall into the category of the 'blind painful eye'. Owners may show a natural resistance to enucleation, and clinicians should take time to explain the usually extensive and irreversible loss of function in the eye and the difficulties of controlling the pain. Chronic glaucoma causes functional transection of the optic nerve at the level of the posterior globe and owners can be reassured that there is no prospect of restoration of sight whatever action is taken. Moreover, human patients with a 'blind painful eye' often request enucleation.

Trans-palpebral enucleation

In this method, the initial incision is made through the lids and the conjunctival sac is not entered at any stage (Figure 4.32). The advantages are that infection and possible tumour cells in the conjunctival tissues are removed with the globe and there is no possibility of conjunctival tissue remaining in the orbit. The disadvantages are the possibility of prolonged haemorrhage from the initial lid incision and difficulty in identifying the reflection of the conjunctiva at the fornices, with the risk

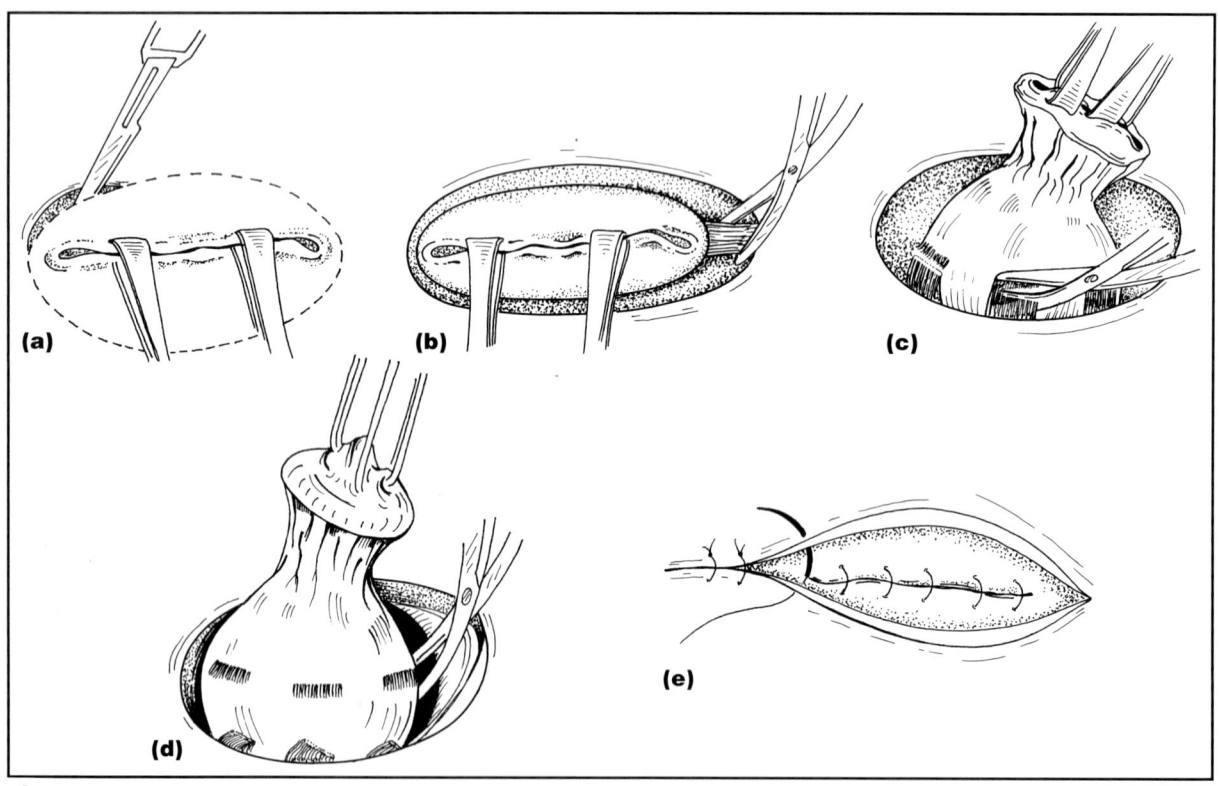

Figure 4.32 Trans-palpebral enucleation in the dog (left eye illustrated): (a) The eyelids are held closed using Allis tissue forceps. An encircling skin incision is made close to the Allis tissue forceps. (b) The underlying tissues are dissected as far as the orbital margin; care should be taken not to penetrate the conjunctival sac. Heavy scissors are used to section the lateral canthal ligament, followed by the shorter medial canthal ligament. (c) The lids are now mobile and can be elevated further. The sheet of tissue attaching the lids to the orbital margin is sectioned around its full circumference. This frees the lids, and only the globe attachments remain. As far as possible, each extraocular muscle is identified in turn and sectioned. In some cases, the attachments are very thin and traction on the lids tends to flatten them against the globe, making them difficult to identify. (d) When all the other visible attachments to the globe have been sectioned, the optic nerve is identified and clamped with curved artery forceps. It is not always possible to visualize the optic nerve, but it may be felt with the tips of the forceps before clamping. Curved scissors are then introduced between the globe and the forceps and the remaining attachments cut. (e) A continuous absorbable suture is placed subcutaneously to provide a tight seal of the orbital cavity, followed by simple interrupted skin sutures.

of inadvertent penetration of the conjunctival sac. Trans-palpebral enucleation tends to be easier in the cat, where the muscles are less fleshy, resulting in less haemorrhage. It is probably the most commonly used method in both dogs and cats.

In most hands, the procedure is conducted in an empirical manner rather than the controlled technique illustrated in textbooks. Practice on cadavers will help, but the procedure on a cadaver is deceptively easy due to lack of haemorrhage. The following suggestions may help the general surgeon:

- An assistant can help the surgeon considerably by manoeuvring the globe as requested, by the use of Allis tissue forceps clamped behind the lid margins. It is absolutely essential that the eye is only positioned and that *no traction is applied*. In the cat, it is certainly possible to damage the contralateral optic nerve by excessive traction in enucleation
- After the initial incision and dissection of the skin away from the conjunctiva, the exposure of the globe is greatly increased by sectioning the lateral and medial canthal ligaments. This should be performed early in the procedure. These ligaments are more easily palpated than seen. The medial ligament is shorter than the lateral one. Both are tough, and delicate instruments should not be used for this. It is important that they are sectioned completely and that there are no strands remaining intact and, again, this is more easily appreciated by touch than by sight
- Once the conjunctival fornix has been passed, the attachments of the globe should be sectioned in a circumferential fashion. It may be difficult to identify each extraocular muscle in turn, but this is not necessary. It is best to insert a fine instrument (or one blade of fine scissors) carefully between the muscle and sclera to separate the two before cutting as closely to the globe as possible. Muscle hooks can be used if available
- There may be diffuse haemorrhage from the lid incision which, in some cases, continues throughout the procedure and is difficult to control. Individual bleeding vessels should be clamped as they are seen during the operation. There may also be haemorrhage from orbital vessels that are obscured by the globe while it is still *in situ*. In general, bleeding is much more likely in the dog than the cat
- It is often not possible to visualize the optic nerve before clamping. The main reason is the presence of the retractor bulbi muscle, the attachments of which are posterior to those of the recti and more difficult to access. The nerve can always be felt with the tip of curved artery forceps and, with care, blind clamping is acceptable
- There is always dead space. The deeper tissues should be closed if possible, but this often achieves little. Sutures hold very poorly in orbital fat and should only engage muscles or connective tissue
- Haemorrhage should be controlled before closure. At least one layer of tight subcutaneous closure should be provided in the orbital fascia. This provides a barrier to haemorrhage escaping from the orbit and extraneous material entering, and also provides a surface for the lids to rest on, thereby preventing sinking of the surface postoperatively. Packing the orbit with foreign material is not recommended.

Enucleation is painful in the short term and a course of postoperative analgesia should always be given. Some clinicians favour the use of retrobulbar or local nerve blocks to reduce postoperative pain (see Chapter 2). Patients usually resume a normal demeanour soon after surgery, probably because the ocular pain has gone. In addition, a course of systemic broad-spectrum antibiotics should always be provided.

Trans-conjunctival enucleation

The lids remain open throughout and the initial incision is made through the conjunctiva close to the limbus. The advantages are that it is easier to remain close to the sclera and to identify and deal with the extraocular muscles. There is less haemorrhage and less extraocular tissue is removed with the globe. The disadvantages are that the conjunctival space is entered and pathogens may enter the orbit. It can be difficult to manoeuvre the globe by the conjunctiva remaining attached at the limbus. Trans-conjunctival enucleation is contraindicated where there is known infection or where there may be tumour cells outside the eye.

After the globe has been removed, the method is completed by removing the entire conjunctival sac and nictitating membrane, followed by the lid margins. Closure is then as described for the trans-palpebral method. Leaving conjunctiva *in situ*, deliberately or inadvertently, may lead to cyst and mucocoele formation and, ultimately, the formation of a draining sinus (Figure 4.33).

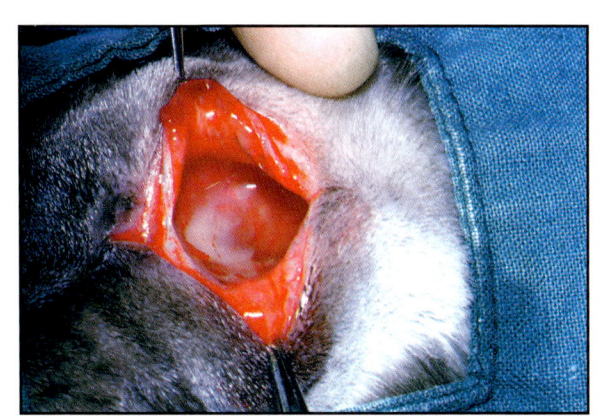

Figure 4.33 Following enucleation this cat suffered recurrent cycles of orbital swelling, followed by discharge of mucoid material through a sinus, leading to temporary resolution. At exploratory surgery, the socket contained mucoid fluid and was partly lined with conjunctiva.

Evisceration and implant

This technique is gaining in popularity. Evisceration refers to the technique of removing the entire ocular contents via a perilimbal incision, leaving a corneoscleral shell. A spherical prosthesis is inserted into the shell and the incision is sutured. A mobile globe and normal adnexa are therefore preserved, but the appearance of the cornea and iris is compromised.

Submission of a globe for pathological examination

The value of pathological examination

There are some clinical situations where gross examination and histology of an enucleated eye may provide useful information, either of historical significance or of relevance to the future management of the patient. Indeed, in medical ophthalmology, it is usually recommended that all enucleated globes be submitted for examination.

However, the submission of an eye for pathology is never a substitute for thorough clinical examination of the affected and the contralateral eyes. For example, in the case of eyes enucleated because of primary glaucoma, the appearance of the drainage angle in the contralateral eye (the 'good eye') may be even more informative than examining the blind eye, except as a rule-out for other diseases.

Fine needle aspiration of cells from within an eye may be useful in some circumstances, e.g. in confirming lymphoma, without an invasive biopsy or enucleation, but the procedure is not often carried out. Best results will be obtained where the clinician and the pathologist are using the technique regularly and that will not often be the case. Aqueous fluid may be aspirated via a limbal approach, or cells may be aspirated from the surface of the iris (see Chapter 1a). Care should be taken not to over-investigate blind painful eyes if the management, i.e. enucleation, is likely to be unaltered by the results.

If the globe is removed for any of the following reasons, surgery should be followed by pathological examination.

The opaque eye

Several disease processes can result in significant opacity due to keratitis or degeneration of the corneal endothelium, which causes corneal oedema. In more extreme cases, the anterior chamber may be full of blood, pus or tumour. The opacity can obscure the signs of the primary disease process.

The blood-filled eye

Intraocular haemorrhage may be minor and resolve rapidly or may be persistent and result in an eye full of blood, usually with secondary glaucoma. Clinical examination of such eyes is very unrewarding (although ultrasonography may be helpful) and the clinician is in the unfortunate position of having to give a poor prognosis without a diagnosis. Possible causes may include bleeding from tumours, collie eye anomaly, retinal detachment, systemic hypertension and trauma, some of which may have a bearing on the future management of the patient.

Non-pigmented tumours

Lymphoma, amelanotic melanoma, ciliary body epithelial tumours and metastatic tumours can all appear as pale masses or thickening within an eye, as may inflammatory thickening of the iris. A tentative clinical diagnosis may be made based on known patterns of behaviour for tumours, but there is no substitute for histopathological confirmation.

Intraocular melanoma

Most intraocular melanomas are pigmented on clinical appearance, but the prognostic factors are mainly histological, and the histological nature of the tumour is not easily inferred from the naked eye appearance. Most eyes with primary tumours, notably canine melanoma, either have glaucoma by the time of diagnosis or are not suitable for any surgery other than enucleation. The diagnosis is therefore best made retrospectively in the enucleated eye.

Glaucoma of unknown cause

Many disease processes lead to glaucoma and a blind painful eye if they are not treated correctly. In late stage glaucoma, the primary cause may not be apparent and the list of possibilities is wide. The findings may be relevant to the management of the patient or of the contralateral eye.

Possible systemic disease

Intraocular haemorrhage, retinal detachment, iris thickening and uveitis may all be indicators of systemic disease. Even where one eye is showing obvious signs, the contralateral eye should be carefully examined, since a systemic disease may not have affected both eyes symmetrically. Systemic diseases that may manifest first or most obviously in the eye include lymphoma, some infections and hypertension. There is no substitute for full clinical investigation in these cases, especially if it will save the patient from the loss of an eye. If it is decided, however, that enucleation is necessary, then the eye should be examined after surgery, as the ocular pathology may elucidate the underlying systemic problem.

Submission of the specimen

The globe should be trimmed of all tissue except the optic nerve. Several fixatives are suitable for eyes, but the best are those that penetrate rapidly through the wall. In the non-specialist situation, formalin is likely to be the only one available. All fixatives are dangerous and should be labelled, stored and handled according to health and safety regulations. Unless instructed otherwise by the laboratory, the eye should not be injected, punctured or cut, but should be trimmed and then immersed whole into the fixative.

The clinician should include details of:

- Breed, age and sex
- History, including medical and surgical treatment
- The location of any focal lesions
- Findings in the contralateral eye.

A fixed eye is always more opaque than a living eye, and a focal lesion may not be visible in the laboratory. This could result in the pathologist opening the eye in an inappropriate plane. Similarly, retinal and fundic lesions are much harder to interpret in a fixed eye and without the magnification provided by ophthalmoscopy, so details must be provided if sections are to be cut through the area of interest.

Laboratory method

In the examination of an enucleated eye, it is important to follow a set protocol; this will ensure that as much information as possible is extracted from the specimen. In the enclosed environment of an eye, the tissues undergo considerable interaction in many diseases. The pathologist will aim to establish what is primary, what is secondary and what is incidental.

Probably the single most useful step in maximizing the information gained from an eye is in choosing the optimum plane of section. This applies to the gross examination, too, as an essential precursor to obtaining histological sections in the right plane. It is not desirable to cut the eye into multiple blocks, but to retain the relationships between the tissues in a single section passing through the pupil, the optic nerve and the area of interest.

References and further reading

Attali-Sousay K, Jegou J-P and Clerc B (2001) Retrobulbar tumours in dogs and cats. *Veterinary Ophthalmology* 4, 19–27

Boydell P (1991) Fine needle aspiration biopsy in the diagnosis of exophthalmos. *Journal of Small Animal Practice* 32, 542–546

Calia CM, Kirschner SE, Baer KE and Steffanacci JD (1994) The use of computed tomography scan for the evaluation of orbital disease in cats and dogs *Veterinary and Comparative Ophthalmology* 4, 24–30

Carpenter JL, Schmidt GM, Moore FM, Albert DM, Abrams KL and Elner VM (1989) Canine bilateral extraocular polymyositis. *Veterinary Pathology* 26, 510–512

Gilger BC, McLaughlin SA, Whitley RD and Wright JC (1992) Orbital neoplasms in cats: 21 cases (1974–1990). *Journal of the American Veterinary Medical Association* 201, 1083–1086

Gilger BC and Whitley RD (1994) Modified lateral orbitotomy for removal of orbital neoplasms in two dogs. *Veterinary Surgery* 23, 53–58

Kern TJ (1985) Orbital neoplasia in 23 dogs. *Journal of the American Veterinary Medical Association* 186, 489–491

LeCouteur RA, Fike JR, Scagliotti RH and Cann CE (1982) Computed tomography of orbital tumors in the dog. *Journal of the American Veterinary Medical Association* 180, 910–913

Mauldin EA, Deehr AJ, Hertzke D and Dubielzig RR (2000) Canine orbital meningiomas: a review of 22 cases. *Veterinary Ophthalmology* 3, 11–16

McCalla TL and Moore CP (1989) Exophthalmos in dogs and cats. *Compendium on Continuing Education for the Practicing Veterinarian* 11, 784–793, 911–927

Morgan RV (1989) Ultrasonography of retrobulbar diseases of the dog and cat. *Journal of the American Animal Hospital Association* 25, 393–399

Tijl JWM and Koornneef L (1991) Fine needle aspiration biopsy in orbital tumours. *British Journal of Ophthalmology* 75, 491–492

Acknowledgements

The author is grateful to Dr SM Crispin for the use of photographic material.

5

The eyelids and nictitating membrane

Simon Petersen-Jones

Embryology, anatomy and physiology

Outer eyelids

The outer eyelids (Figure 5.1) develop as folds from the surface ectoderm, which meet and fuse along the presumptive eyelid opening. Ectoderm gives rise to the epidermis, the lining conjunctiva and the cilia and glands of the eyelid, which develop as an ingrowth of the ectoderm. Neural crest mesenchyme gives rise to the deeper structures of the eyelid, including the dermis and tarsal plate. Striated muscles of the eyelid develop from condensations of mesoderm. The third eyelid, or nictitating membrane, develops as an ectodermal budding with a mesenchymal core. The outer eyelids remain fused at the region of contact between the upper and lower eyelid folds until 10 to 14 days after birth in both cats and dogs.

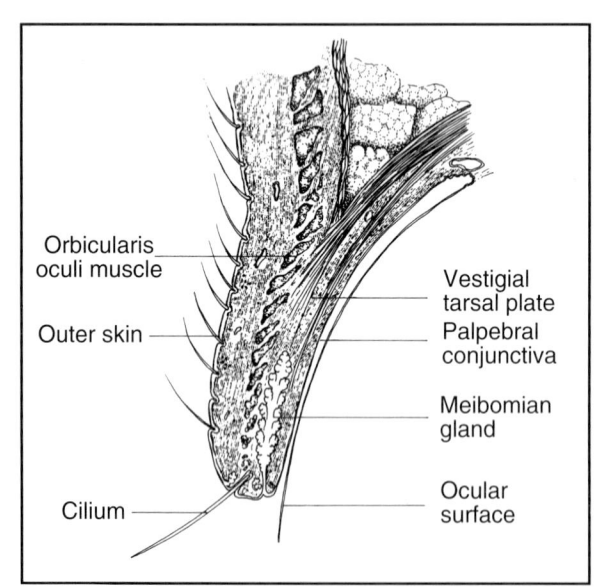

Figure 5.1 Cross-section through an eyelid.

The mature outer eyelids (upper and lower) are tissue flaps which consist of an outer layer of hairy skin; a tarsal plate for support, which is poorly developed in the dog and somewhat better developed in the cat; both striated and smooth muscle; lipid-secreting (meibomian) glands within the tarsal plate and an inner conjunctival lining. There is an excellent blood supply to the eyelids.

The eyelid skin is thin and contains many mast cells. This accounts for the ease with which it becomes inflamed and oedematous. The upper eyelid bears two or more rows of cilia in the dog while, in the cat, the first row of skin hairs are often well developed and act as cilia. Associated with the cilia are two types of gland (glands of Zeis and of Moll); infection of these glands may lead to the formation of a stye. Neither cat nor dog has cilia on the lower lids.

In animals with normal lid–globe conformation, the eyelids rest against the ocular surface and slide across it during the process of blinking. However, in many breeds of dog, and a few breeds of cat, eyelid conformation is far from optimal. This is a common contributory factor in the development of ocular surface disease. The length of the palpebral fissure varies between breeds and it is reported that in breeds that commonly have lid conformational abnormalities, such as entropion and ectropion, the palpebral fissures tend to be longer than average (Stades et al., 1992).

In addition to having an overlong palpebral fissure, there are often loose lateral and, in some cases, medial palpebral ligaments. In some breeds the lid defects are exacerbated by a less than optimal globe position (a relative exophthalmos in some breeds and enophthalmos in others). Conformational lid abnormalities will be discussed further later in this chapter.

Eyelid margin
The eyelid margin is normally free of hairs and is often pigmented. It is a very important region: the zone of transition between skin and palpebral conjunctiva. Lesions of the eyelid margin can result in serious ocular surface pathology, since this region slides across the cornea during blinking and helps spread the tear film. Meibomian gland orifices can be seen with the naked eye, opening along the eyelid margin in a slight longitudinal groove. Meibomian lipid secretion is an important component of the pre-ocular tear film (see Chapter 6). In many animals, it is possible to see the outline of the meibomian glands through the palpebral conjunctiva when the eyelid is everted.

Palpebral conjunctiva
The palpebral conjunctiva lines the inner aspect of the eyelids and is firmly attached where it overlies the meibomian glands.

Nasolacrimal system

The punctal openings into the canaliculi of the nasolacrimal drainage system can be seen at the medial canthal region of upper and lower eyelids, just within the eyelid margin.

Palpebral ligaments

The eyelid opening is known as the palpebral fissure. Musculo-fibrous bands, the medial and lateral palpebral ligaments, serve to anchor the medial and lateral canthal regions and maintain the slit shape of the palpebral fissure during blinking. The medial palpebral ligament is a short fibrous ligament that attaches the medial canthus firmly to the periosteum of the frontal bone. The lateral palpebral ligament is a thickened fibrous band than runs from a position adjacent to the palpebral conjunctiva at the lateral canthus to the craniomedial face of the orbital ligament (Robertson and Roberts, 1995a).

Eyelid musculature and movement

Closure of the fissure (blinking) is achieved by the action of the orbicularis oculi muscle, with most movement involving the upper eyelid. The orbicularis oculi muscle in the upper lid has a high percentage of fast twitch fibres to allow for rapid lid closure (Miller and Braund, 1991). The blink reflex is an important protective reflex. Normal complete blinking is essential for the distribution of the pre-ocular tear film and the maintenance of a healthy ocular surface. Protrusion of the third eyelid across the cornea during blinking also aids in the protection of the ocular surface and the distribution of tears. Portions of the orbicularis oculi muscle surround the lacrimal canaliculi and, during blinking, squeeze the canaliculi and help propel tears through the nasolacrimal drainage system. Other muscles, both striated and smooth, are also involved in maintaining eyelid shape and position. The striated muscles include the retractor anguli oculi medialis and lateralis, which act to lift and widen the medial and lateral portions of the palpebral fissure respectively, and the main elevator of the upper eyelid, the levator palpebrae superioris. Smooth muscle (Müller's muscle) within the eyelid acts to widen the palpebral fissure.

The striated eyelid musculature is innervated by the facial (VII) nerve, with the exception of the levator palpebrae superioris. This is the major elevator of the upper eyelid, and is innervated by the oculomotor (III) nerve. The smooth muscle is innervated by postganglionic sympathetic nerves.

Sensation

Sensation to the eyelids is provided by the trigeminal (V) nerve. The ophthalmic branch supplies the medial and middle portions of the upper eyelid and, along with the maxillary branch, the lateral portion of the upper lid and the medial portion of the lower lid. The rest of the lower eyelid is supplied by the maxillary branch alone.

Third eyelid (nictitating membrane)

The third eyelid (Figure 5.2) occupies the ventromedial portion of the conjunctival sac at the medial canthus. It consists of a T-shaped cartilage skeleton covered by conjunctiva. Flaps of conjunctiva continuous with the leading edge of the third eyelid extend into the upper and lower fornices, thereby partly encircling the globe. Pigment is often present in these flaps of conjunctiva, as a continuation of the pigmentation of the free border of the third eyelid. A lack of pigmentation of the border of the third eyelid can make it more noticeable, and owners may mistakenly think that such an appearance is due to inflammation or partial prolapse of the third eyelid, particularly if the border of the fellow third eyelid is pigmented.

The nictitans gland, or gland of the third eyelid, is situated at the base of the third eyelid. This gland surrounds the base of the upright portion of the

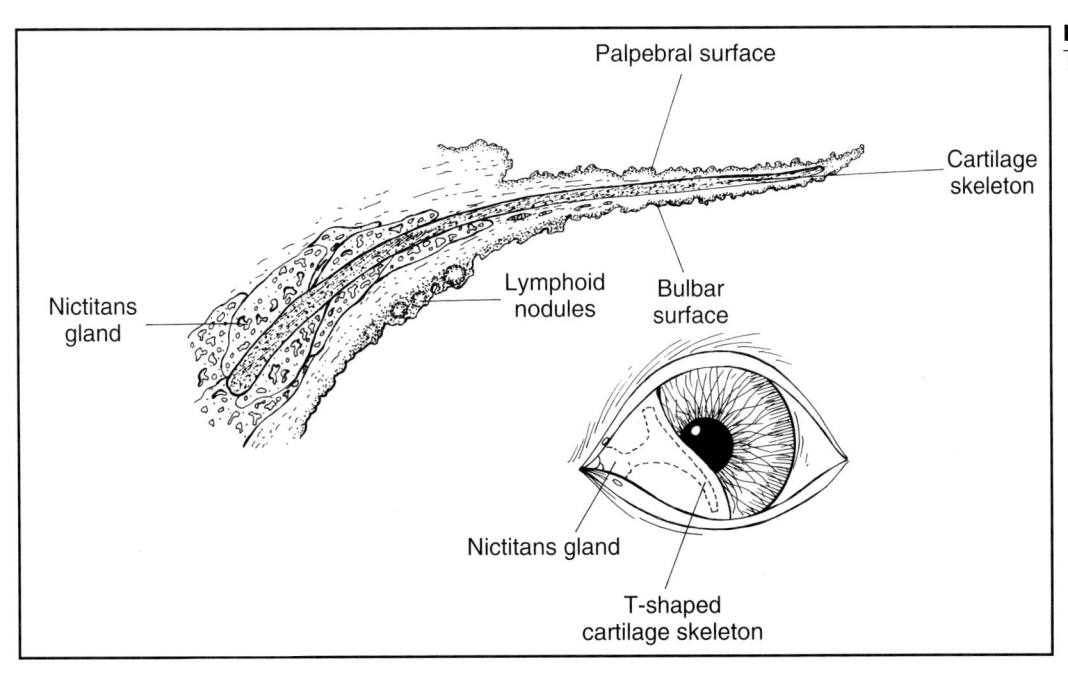

Figure 5.2 The third eyelid.

T-shaped skeleton. It produces a significant proportion of the tears, and its removal can predispose to dry eye problems. The tears from the gland gain access to the conjunctival sac via several small openings on the inner aspect of the third eyelid between an accumulation of lymphoid follicles; these give the bulbar aspect of the third eyelid a roughened and almost hyperaemic appearance.

The third eyelid sweeps passively across the corneal surface when the globe is retracted. This occurs every time the animal blinks. Cats have some striated muscle attachments on the third eyelid which enable active protrusion. There are also smooth muscle attachments with sympathetic innervation which help to keep the third eyelid retracted.

The third eyelid plays an important role in ocular surface protection and tear production. Additionally, it affords some support to the lower eyelid. For these reasons, it is imperative that it is preserved in a functional condition whenever possible.

Congenital conditions of the eyelids of dogs

Coloboma
Colobomas (where part of the eyelid is congenitally absent) are uncommon in the dog. When they do occur, reconstruction to establish complete eyelid closure during blinking is necessary. The technique selected will depend on the extent of the defect; some suitable surgical techniques are described under conditions of the eyelids of the cat.

Epibulbar dermoid
Epibulbar dermoids are congenital lesions in which a piece of histologically normal skin is abnormally located, most commonly on the cornea and/or the conjunctiva (more details are included in Chapters 7 and 8). In some individual animals, the adjacent eyelid may also be involved (Figure 5.3). The skin of the affected portion of eyelid is raised and bears longer hairs than the adjacent normal skin. Surgical excision of the affected portion of eyelid with direct closure of the resulting wound is usually feasible.

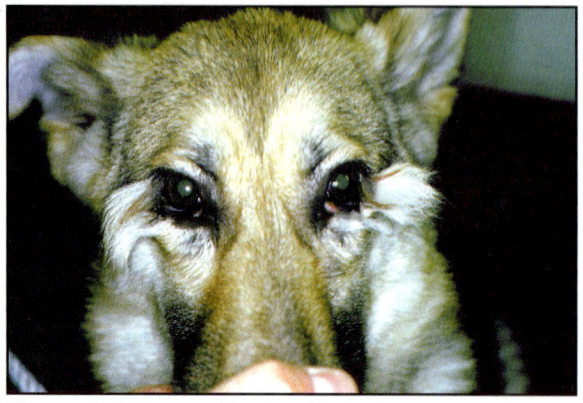

Figure 5.3 German Shepherd Dog with bilateral dermoids affecting both eyelid and conjunctiva. (Courtesy of JRB Mould.)

Ophthalmia neonatorum
The development of an infection within the conjunctival sac before the eyelids open is known as ophthalmia neonatorum, or neonatal conjunctivitis. Often more than one member of a litter is affected.

The first sign is swelling of the still fused eyelids and sometimes the escape of a small amount of purulent discharge at the medial canthus. Ulceration of the ocular surface that is severe enough to result in corneal perforation can develop if the condition is not recognized and treated promptly. Treatment requires opening the lids along their line of fusion using fine, blunt-ended scissors inserted medially. Purulent material is collected for culture and direct smears are taken for Gram staining for rapid assessment of bacterial involvement. The conjunctival sac is then thoroughly irrigated with sterile saline. Broad-spectrum ophthalmic antibiotic ointment is applied, and the corneal surface is kept moist until the infection has resolved and normal tear production has been established.

Ankyloblepharon
The eyelids are normally fused (physiological ankyloblepharon) at birth. Sometimes this continues beyond the normal 10–14 days, in which case the eyelids may be surgically opened by cutting along the presumptive opening with fine blunt-ended scissors.

Macropalpebral fissure
A longer than average palpebral fissure may be associated with eyelid conformational abnormality. When pronounced, it is termed macropalpebral fissure. Breeds such as Bloodhounds, St Bernards and Clumber Spaniels have an overlong palpebral fissure associated with a 'diamond eye' conformation. 'Diamond eye' deformities are always associated with ectropion and sometimes with entropion too, and are discussed later in this chapter. Brachycephalic breeds typically have a macropalpebral fissure which, coupled with a prominent globe, results in exposure of more sclera than is seen in other breeds. Additionally, they may show incomplete eyelid closure during blinking (lagophthalmos) and often incomplete eyelid closure while sleeping. This can lead to corneal dry spot formation and development of an exposure keratopathy (see Chapter 8). Application of tear substitutes may help to halt corneal changes, but if corneal lesions do progress, surgical shortening of the eyelids is required.

Shortening of the palpebral fissure to prevent superficial keratitis in brachycephalic dogs
Shortening the eyelids may be performed at the medial or lateral canthus.

Shortening at the medial canthus: Shortening of the palpebral fissure at the medial canthus is achieved by a medial canthoplasty. This is especially useful in breeds where medial lower lid entropion and medial canthal trichiasis are a problem, resulting in an overflow of tears and development of a medial keratitis. The medial canthoplasty procedure is illustrated in Figure 5.27.

The eyelids and nictitating membrane

Shortening at the lateral canthus: There are a number of methods described for shortening the palpebral fissure at the lateral canthus, and two will be described here. The first technique has the advantage of simplicity, while the second results in a stronger repair that is less likely to break down under the tension of the eyelids.

- Method 1: Simple shortening of the palpebral fissure
  A strip of eyelid margin from both upper and lower eyelids is excised, starting at the lateral canthus, and continuing medially for a length equal to that by which the eyelids need to be shortened. The cut edges are then directly sutured using a two-layer repair (Figure 5.4).
- Method 2: Modified Fuchs' lateral canthoplasty
  Method 1 results in a repair that is usually under some tension due to the prominence of the globe in affected brachycephalic dogs; there is therefore a risk of wound breakdown. The alternative method, illustrated in Figure 5.5, results in a stronger repair, but is more time consuming to perform.

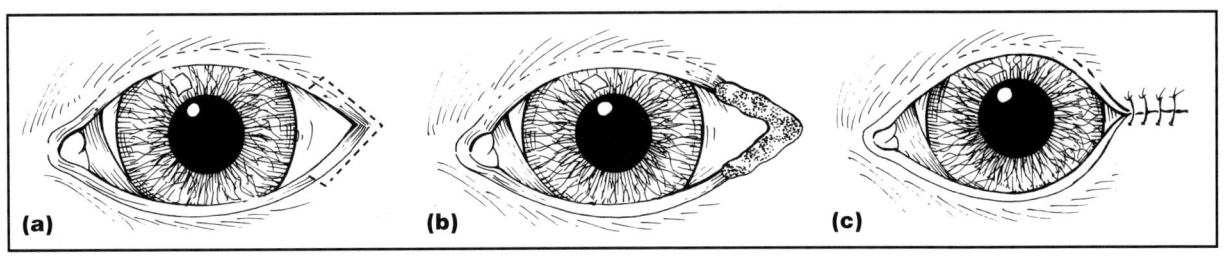

Figure 5.4 Shortening of the eyelids at the lateral canthus by trimming the edges of the eyelids and directly suturing them. (a) A macropalpebral fissure. (b) Skin is excised from corresponding areas of both upper and lower eyelid margins at the lateral canthus. (c) The freshened-up areas of upper and lower lids are sutured directly together; a two-layer repair is recommended for additional strength.

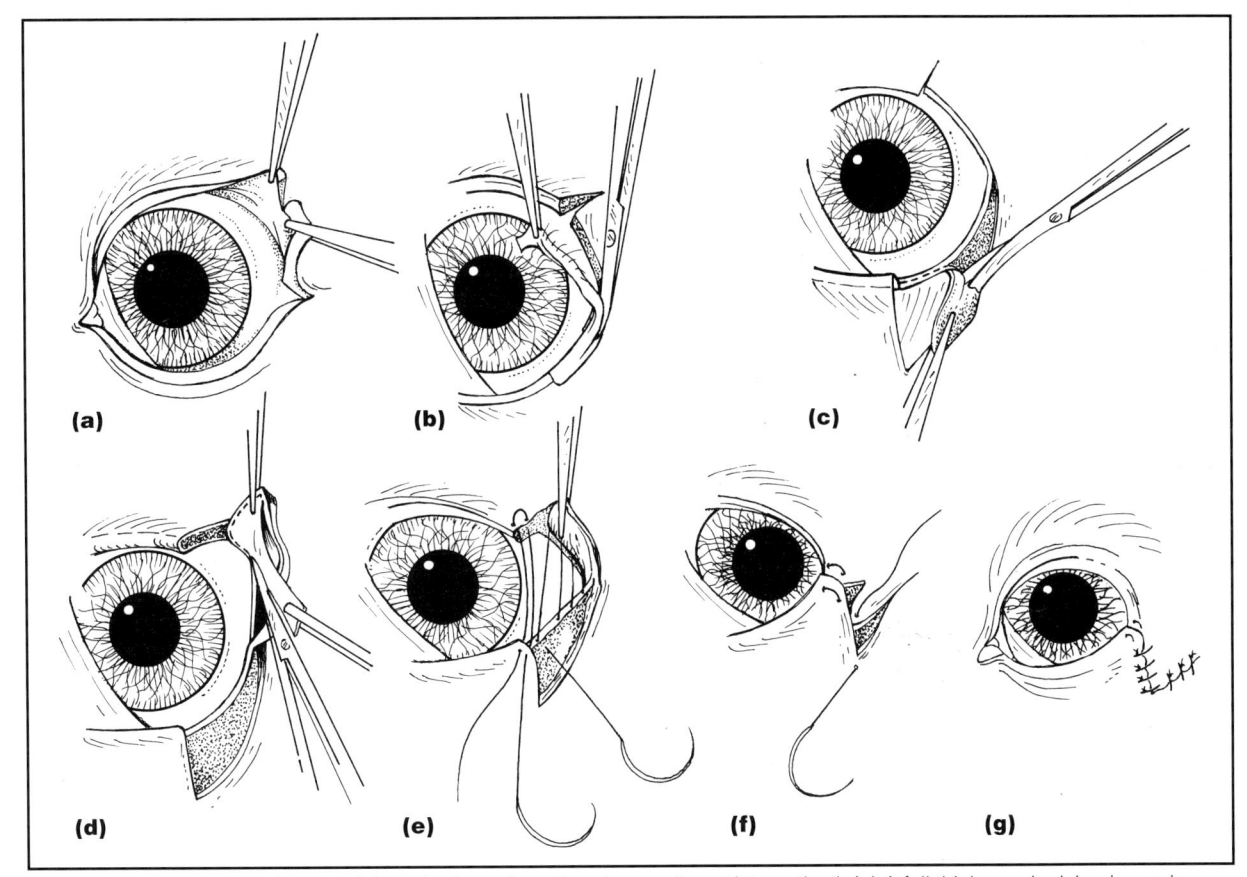

Figure 5.5 Shortening of the eyelids at the lateral canthus by an alternative method. (a) A full thickness incision is made through the upper eyelid at 90 degrees to the eyelid margin at a distance from the lateral canthus equal to the length by which the eyelid needs to be shortened. (b) The eyelid margin is excised from the incision in (a) to the lateral canthus and for an equal distance along the lower eyelid. (c) A triangle of skin is excised from the lower eyelid leaving the tarsoconjunctiva *in situ*. This triangle is equal in size to the upper triangle delineated by a line between the lateral canthus and the end of the initial incision made in the upper eyelid. (d) The conjunctiva of the upper triangle is excised. (e) Sutures are placed to create a new lateral canthus: the cut edge of the upper palpebral conjunctiva is sutured to the edge of the tarsoconjunctiva of the lateral lower lid. (f) The triangle of upper eyelid skin from which the conjunctiva has been excised is pulled down into the triangular skin defect in the lower eyelid. (g) The skin edges are sutured. This results in a very strong repair.

Micropalpebral fissure

An abnormally small palpebral fissure is common in certain breeds of dog, such as the Rough Collie. Surgical lengthening of the palpebral fissure is not usually indicated.

Abnormalities of eyelid position

Entropion

Entropion, which is an inversion or inturning of the eyelids, is a common condition in dogs and frequently results from, or is associated with, poor eyelid conformation.

The following forms of entropion are recognized:

- Breed-related primary entropion (usually juvenile)
- Spastic entropion
- Cicatricial entropion
- Entropion associated with ectropion in dogs with a diamond eye conformation
- Senile entropion
- Medial canthal entropion.

The first five forms of entropion listed above cause discomfort, manifested as increased lacrimation and blepharospasm. Retraction of the globe and blepharospasm can lead to further inturning of the lid and a worsening of the discomfort. This is termed the spastic component of the entropion. In some cases, keratitis or corneal ulceration may develop. As discussed below, dogs with medial canthal entropion usually present with epiphora or medial keratitis rather than ocular discomfort and blepharospasm.

Breed-related primary entropion

The age of onset differs between breeds. Some, such as the Shar Pei, may develop entropion shortly after the lids open. This often involves both upper and lower lids. As the affected puppies grow, however, the tendency for the lids to turn in decreases (sometimes completely), and a temporary eversion of the eyelids using 'tacking sutures' (Figure 5.6) may be the only treatment that is required in this breed (Johnson et al., 1988).

Other breeds, such as Retrievers and Chow Chows, typically develop entropion at a few months of age (Figure 5.7). These animals will usually require a permanent surgical correction rather than a 'tacking' procedure. The commonest portion of the eyelid to be involved is the lateral third to half of the lower lid.

Entropion in the broad-headed breeds (Rottweilers, Mastiffs etc.) may extend around the lateral canthus and involve the lateral portion of the upper lid.

It has been suggested that a tight lateral canthal ligament may contribute to this form of entropion and that sectioning this ligament can play a role in the management of the entropion (Robertson and Roberts 1995 a and b).

Chow Chows, like Shar Peis, commonly suffer from upper as well as lower eyelid entropion.

Most of these forms of entropion can be readily managed using the modified Hotz–Celsus procedure.

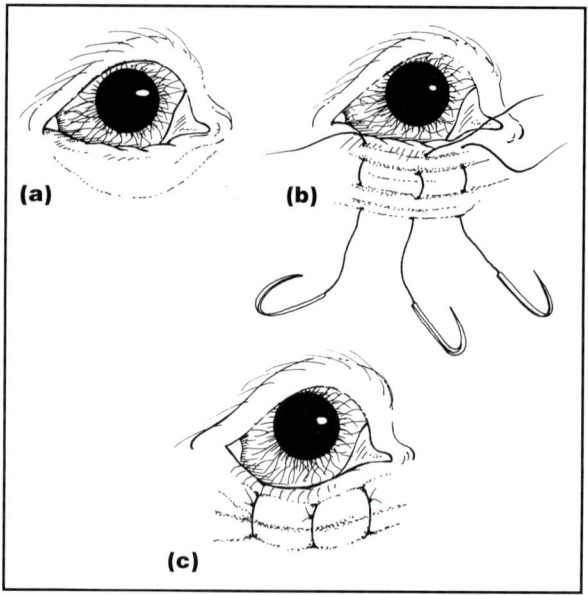

Figure 5.6 Temporary eversion of the eyelid to treat lower eyelid entropion. (a) The lower lid is exhibiting entropion. (b, c) Two or three temporary everting sutures of an interrupted Lembert pattern (Halsted's) are placed and tightened sufficiently to correct the eyelid deformity.

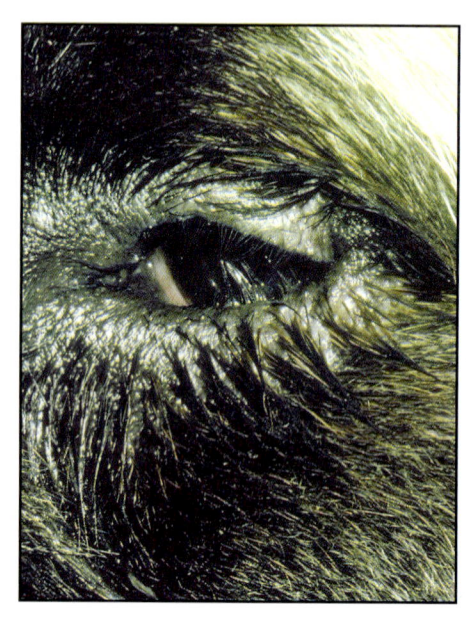

Figure 5.7 Lower eyelid entropion in a dog.

Some breeders are of the opinion that correction should be delayed until the dog is several months of age, as the conformation of the head will alter as the animal matures. It is a mistake to leave the entropion unrelieved, as the dog will be in discomfort or pain, and permanent corneal changes may well develop. Permanent surgical correction is likely to be necessary except in puppies under a few months of age. At the very least, a temporary eversion 'tacking' procedure (Figure 5.6) should be performed to break the cycle of irritation, blepharospasm and further inturning of the eyelid.

Occasionally, in some breeds, such as the Chow Chow, breed-related entropion may develop in middle-aged animals, typically males. This appears to be associated with increased subcutaneous fat deposits. Most commonly, these lead to upper eyelid entropion.

Spastic entropion

Spastic entropion is a secondary entropion that develops as a result of blepharospasm associated with a painful ocular lesion. In some secondary cases of spastic entropion, successful treatment of the painful ocular lesion that causes the blepharospasm may be all that is required. However, once entropion develops, the irritation it causes leads to a worsening of the blepharospasm, thus exacerbating the entropion. A procedure to evert the eyelid, at least temporarily, and break the cycle of entropion and blepharospasm is often required in such cases. For dogs to develop secondary entropion, they must have a lid conformation that allows the lid to turn in if blepharospasm is present. In view of this, permanent slight eversion of the inturning lid may be required. A similar secondary entropion is occasionally seen in dogs with very severe keratoconjunctivitis sicca, where the eyelids turn in as a result of friction between them and the cornea during blinking.

Cicatricial entropion

This results from lid distortion and contracture following injury or severe conjunctival disease.

Entropion associated with ectropion in dogs with a diamond eye conformation

Entropion may be present in some more complicated lid conformational abnormalities. For example, some breeds with long palpebral fissures and redundant facial skin, such as the St Bernard and the Clumber Spaniel, can have a diamond-shaped eyelid opening, with both entropion and ectropion. The correction of this defect is a little more complicated than that required for simple entropion, and is described later in the chapter.

Senile entropion

Elderly English Cocker Spaniels tend to lose elasticity in their facial skin and, when this is coupled with excess facial skin, this can result in a 'slipped facial mask'. This leads to entropion/trichiasis of the upper eyelid and ectropion of the lower lid. Although the upper lid defect can be corrected by a conventional modified Hotz–Celsus procedure, it may recur; other procedures, such as the Stades' correction, give better long-term results (see below).

Medial canthal entropion

Medial canthal entropion of the lower lid (Figure 5.8) is rather different from entropion involving other portions of the eyelid. It results in less irritation, as the firm attachments of the medial canthal region tend to limit the degree of inturning. It is usually associated with epiphora, possibly due to the lower punctum being in a suboptimal position. It may be accompanied by the presence of excessive hairs on the caruncle in the medial canthus. This may lead to the development of a chronic medial keratitis. Some breeds, such as the Miniature Poodle and the Maltese Terrier, tend to have a simple medial lower lid entropion. However, in other breeds, such as the Bichon Frisé and the Shih Tzu, a hairy caruncle is also present.

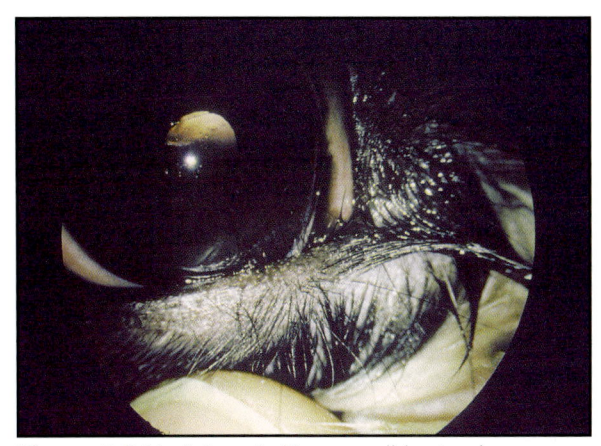

Figure 5.8 Medial canthal lower eyelid entropion.

The medial lower eyelid entropion may need correcting when causing keratitis or epiphora. This can be achieved by a modified Hotz–Celsus procedure or, where there is also a hairy caruncle, a medial canthoplasty can be utilized to deal with both problems (see Figure 5.27).

Management of entropion

The management required depends on the type of entropion present. The following list shows the management commonly used for the various forms of entropion:

- Breed-related primary entropion (usually juvenile)
  - Temporary tacking
  - Permanent eversion (e.g. modified Hotz–Celsus procedure)
- Spastic entropion
  - Treat the underlying cause
  - Temporary tacking
  - Some cases require permanent lid eversion
- Cicatricial entropion
  - Blepharoplastic procedure to correct lid deformity
- Associated with ectropion in dogs with a diamond eye conformation
  - Procedure to shorten eyelids and tighten lateral canthus
- Senile entropion
  - Stades' procedure
- Medial canthal entropion
  - Modified Hotz–Celsus eversion
  - Medial canthoplasty.

Initial assessment: The initial assessment of the required degree of correction must be performed carefully prior to sedation and application of topical anaesthetic. The animal should not be physically restrained (or only minimally restrained), because an assistant pulling on the animal's skin in an effort to restrain it will result in alteration of the eyelid to globe relationship. Good lighting and close examination are required, but not to such a degree that any blepharospasm is worsened. The first thing to ascertain is that the clinical signs are the result of entropion. Once that has been confirmed, the length of lid involved and the degree of inversion should be assessed. To relieve the spastic component of the entropion and to allow the assessment of the anatomical component that must be corrected, a topical anaesthetic is applied and the eyelid conformation reassessed.

Surgical correction of entropion: Liquid paraffin should never be injected into the eyelids as a treatment for entropion because serious granulomas may result. Several procedures of varying complexity are described in the literature for treating entropion. Perhaps the simplest and most effective eversion is the modified Hotz–Celsus procedure.

Modified Hotz–Celsus procedure: This involves the removal of a strip of skin and some of the underlying musculature parallel to and approximately 2 mm from the eyelid margin (Figures 5.9 and 5.10). The length and width of the required correction is estimated, prior to sedation. A Jaeger lid plate (see Chapter 2b), which is shaped rather like a shoe horn, can be used to stabilize the lid and a number 15 blade can be used to make skin incisions demarcating the extent of the required excision. The strip of skin can then be excised using scissors, such as tenotomy scissors. Some experienced surgeons will simply use sharp straight scissors to directly resect the strip of skin. Those unused to performing the entire excision with scissors may find it helpful to 'tent up' the strip of skin to be resected by gently pinching it with forceps. This makes it easier to ensure that only the desired width of tissue is removed. It should be remembered that it is better to under-correct an entropion and have to repeat the procedure, rather than to over-correct entropion and have to perform the more complicated surgery required to restore normal lid conformation in dogs with iatrogenic ectropion.

Upper eyelid entropion/trichiasis

Upper eyelid entropion/trichiasis, often coupled with lower eyelid ectropion, is a common problem in middle-aged to older English Cocker Spaniels. Affected dogs have excessive facial skin that tends to stretch and droop more with age. The resulting deformity varies in severity from a simple upper eyelid entropion/trichiasis (Figure 5.11) to a 'slipped facial mask', where the palpebral fissures are ventral to their normal position; the upper lid may partially obscure vision and the lower lid has a marked ectropion. In dogs with milder deformity, the upper lashes tend to contact the lower conjunctival sac as the eyelids are closed, resulting in conjunctivitis. As this becomes chronic, there is a reduction in tear production. As the condition worsens, the lashes contact the cornea, resulting in keratitis and often ulceration.

The correction employed depends on the severity of the condition at presentation:

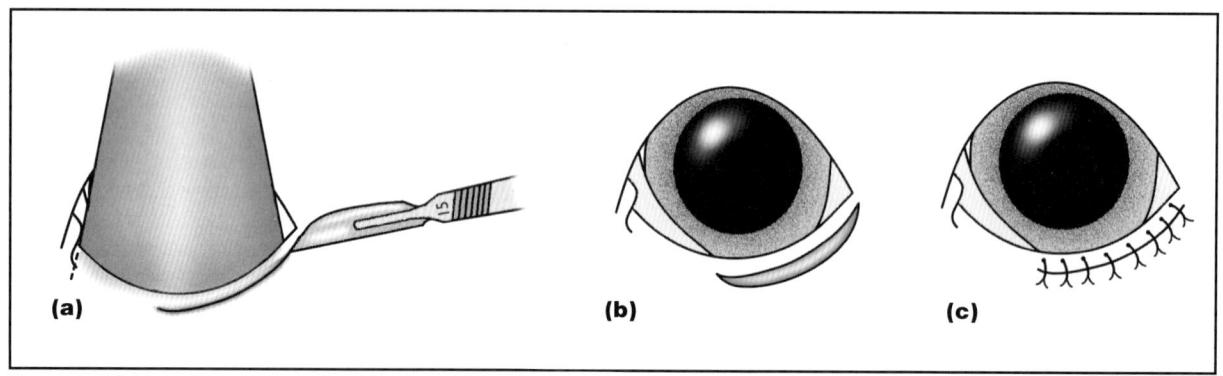

Figure 5.9 Hotz–Celsus correction for lower eyelid entropion. (a) The degree of correction has been assessed in the conscious and unsedated animal. A Jaeger lid plate has been positioned in the conjunctival sac to support the lower eyelid and a No.15 blade is used to incise the strip of skin to be removed. The first incision is parallel to, and 2–3 mm from, the eyelid margin. (b) The required width and length strip of skin and some underlying orbicularis oculi muscle have been excised. (c) 6-0 simple interrupted polyglactin sutures are used to repair the skin defect. The knots are positioned away from the eyelid margin.

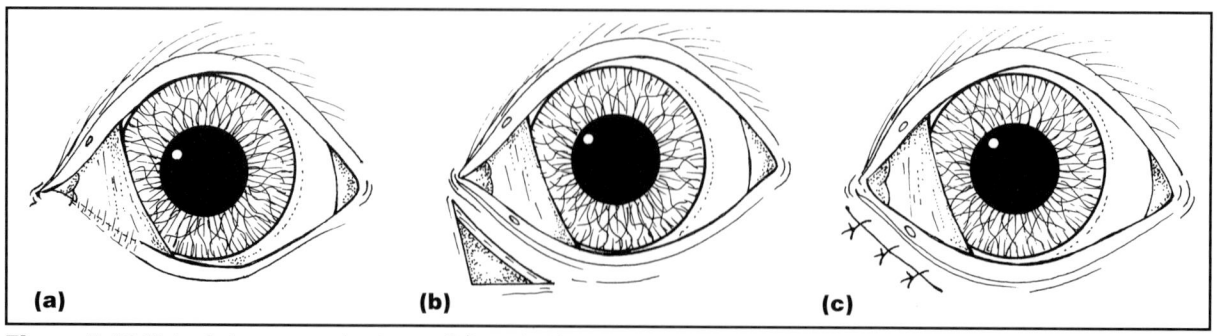

Figure 5.10 Hotz–Celsus correction for medial canthal lower eyelid entropion. (a) Medial canthal entropion is present. (b) A triangular piece of skin is excised. (c) The wound is closed with 6-0 polyglactin.

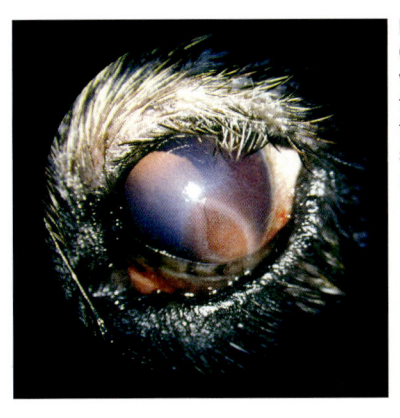

Figure 5.11 A Cocker Spaniel with upper eyelid trichiasis/entropion that has caused superficial ulcerative keratitis.

- Local eversion of the upper lid by a modified Hotz–Celsus procedure is sufficient in milder cases, although recurrence of the problem often occurs several months later
- A Stades' procedure, which everts the lid and creates a band of hairless skin adjacent to the eyelid margin (Figure 5.12) can prevent this recurrence (Stades, 1987). This technique involves removing a strip of skin 15–20 mm wide from the upper eyelid and leaving the resulting defect partly open to granulate, thereby creating a hairless strip of scar tissue adjacent to the eyelid margin that prevents recurrence of the trichiasis
- When there is a marked lower lid ectropion and a drooping upper eyelid that is obscuring vision (a 'slipped facial mask'), a facelift procedure can be utilized (Spreull, 1982; Bedford, 1990). The technique described by Bedford involves removing a strip of skin from the top of the head starting as a narrow strip just dorsal to the level of the medial canthi, widening over the top of the head and extending to the occiput. Spreull recommended removal of a transverse strip of skin from the back of the head, followed by anchoring of the skin to the periosteum to prevent it sliding forward.

Once the eyelids are returned to a normal anatomical relationship to the globe, secondary complications, such as keratitis, corneal ulceration and chronic conjunctivitis, will usually resolve with appropriate topical medication. Tear production will usually increase significantly once the chronic conjunctivitis resolves.

Excessive facial folds/brow ptosis

Some breeds of dog, such as the Shar Pei, that have excessive wrinkling of the skin, may have problems of drooping upper eyelids. In some cases, this is also associated with entropion. Simple surgical excision of the fold dorsal to the eye may be required.

Ectropion

An outward turning of the lower eyelid (ectropion) is quite common in dogs (Figure 5.13). It occurs most commonly as a breed-related problem associated with an overlong palpebral fissure, although cicatricial ectropion and iatrogenic ectropion do occur. Breed-related ectropion tends to worsen with fatigue. More severe cases of

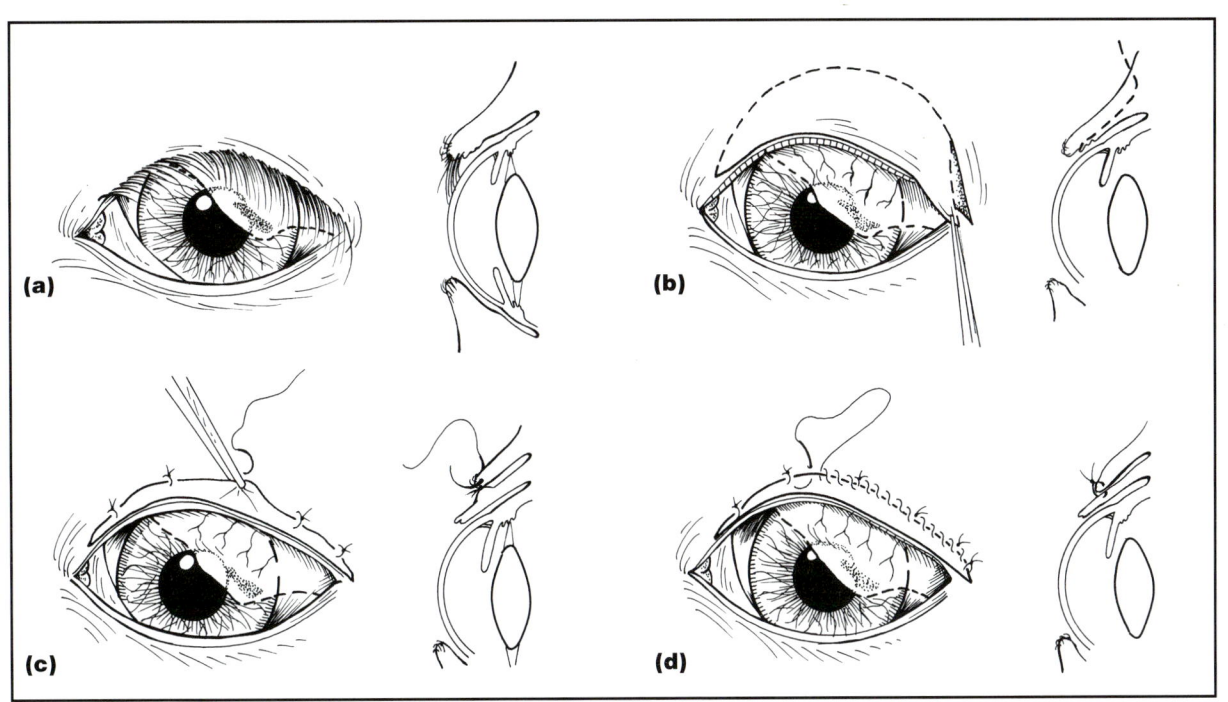

Figure 5.12 Correction of upper eyelid entropion/trichiasis using a Stades' procedure (adapted from Stades, 1987). (a) Upper eyelid entropion/trichiasis is present, resulting in a superficial keratitis. (b) A skin incision is made 1 mm dorsal to the meibomian gland openings so as to remove all the cilia from the upper lid. This strip of skin stretches from 3–4 mm from the medial canthus to 5–10 mm past the lateral canthus and is 15–20 mm wide. (c) Any hair follicles remaining in this area need to be excised. The upper skin edge is then mobilized and sutured down halfway across the wound (to the area of the bases of the meibomian glands), initially using simple interrupted sutures. (d) A continuous suture pattern is finally used to suture the leading skin edge in position. The uncovered portion of the wound is left open to heal by second intention – granulation, epithelialization and contraction – thus creating a hairless strip of scar tissue adjacent to the eyelid margin, preventing recurrence of the trichiasis.

86 The eyelids and nictitating membrane

ectropion have exposure of conjunctiva and accumulation of contaminating debris in the lower conjunctival sac. This results in inflammation, chronic conjunctival changes and an increase in conjunctival mucin production. Dogs with a 'diamond eye' conformation (Figure 5.14) can suffer from entropion in addition to ectropion. This is associated with a macropalpebral fissure and often a weak lateral canthal ligament.

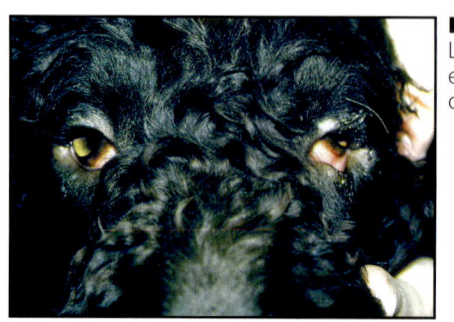

Figure 5.13 Lower eyelid ectropion in a dog.

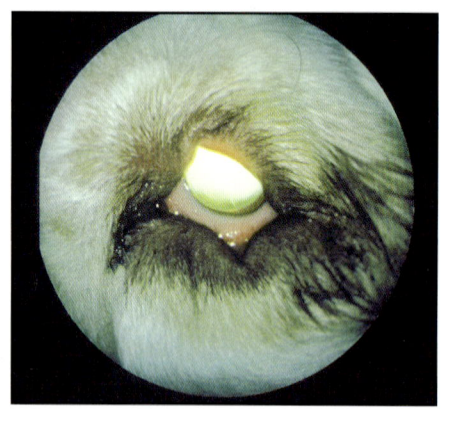

Figure 5.14 Diamond eye in a Clumber Spaniel.

Treatment
Surgical treatment of ectropion is required only when conjunctival (or corneal) pathology results from the deformity. Several techniques have been described, the simplest of which consists of removal of a wedge of affected eyelid at the lateral canthal region. Wedge resection can also be useful for correcting iatrogenic (such as that in Figure 5.15) or cicatricial ectropion. More complicated procedures to correct ectropion include various modifications of the Khunt–Szymanowski procedure. One such method was described by Munger and Carter (1984), and is illustrated in Fig. 5.16.

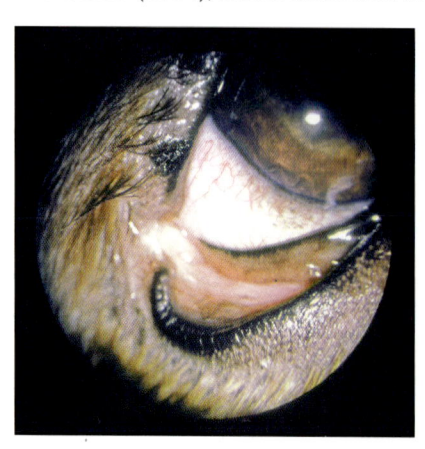

Figure 5.15 Lower eyelid ectropion in a dog due to over-correction of entropion.

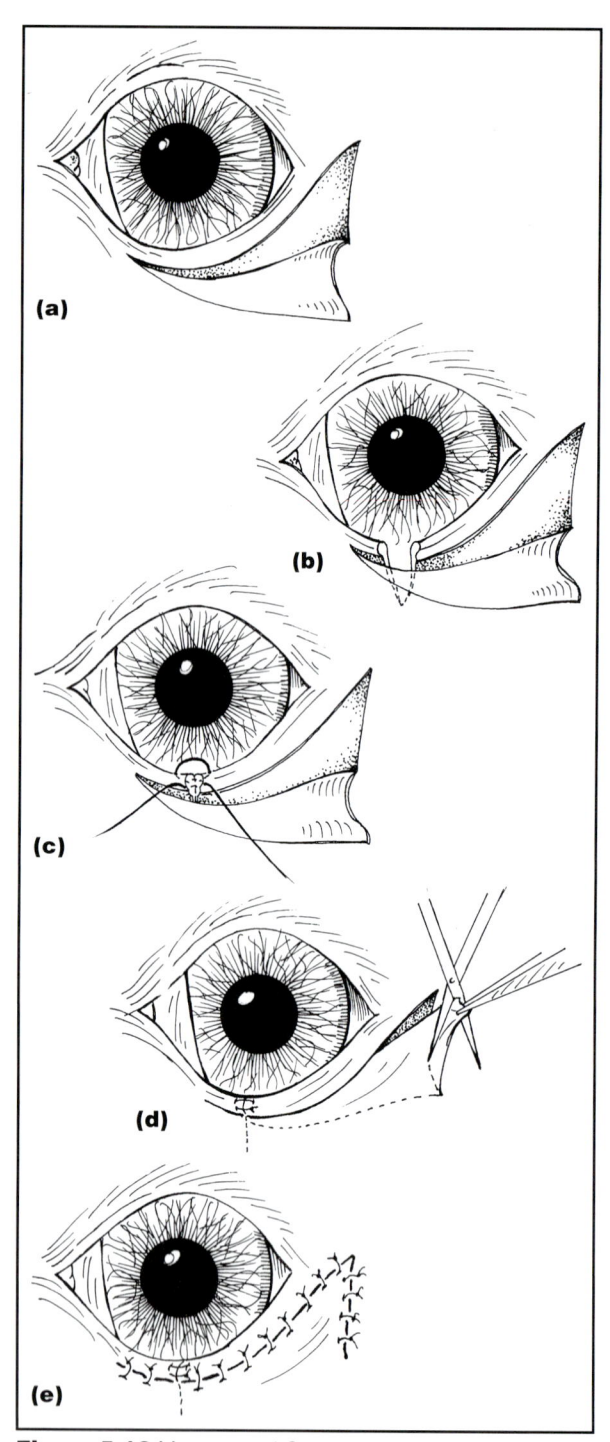

Figure 5.16 Munger and Carter's (1984) modification of the Khunt–Szymanowski procedure for the correction of lower eyelid ectropion. (a) A skin incision is made 3 mm from and parallel to the lower eyelid margin. This is extended dorsolaterally to 1cm beyond the lateral canthus. A second incision is made ventrally from the lateral end of the first incision and the resulting skin flap is undermined and mobilized. (b) A triangular-shaped wedge of tarsoconjunctiva is resected. The width of the triangle base is equal to the length by which the eyelid is to be shortened. (c) The defect created in the tarsoconjuntival half of the lower eyelid is sutured using 6-0 polyglactin, burying the knots. (d) The skin–orbicularis oculi muscle flap is slid laterally and a triangle of it is removed from the lateral end. This is a similar size to the triangle removed from the tarsoconjunctiva. (e) The skin–muscle flap is sutured into its transposed position.

V–Y plasty: Cicatricial ectropion can sometimes be corrected by releasing tension on the lid margin with a V–Y plasty. After making a V-shaped incision, the surrounding skin is undermined with tenotomy scissors and excessive scar tissue is excised, and the wound repaired in a Y shape. The degree of ectropion correction resulting from use of this procedure in dogs is often disappointing, possibly due to the poorly developed tarsal plate in this species. As mentioned previously, a wedge resection of the deformed portion of the lid can produce an effective correction.

Diamond eye correction: When entropion or excessive ectropion accompanies the diamond eye conformation, surgical correction is indicated. A Wyman's lateral canthoplasty (Wyman, 1971) can be performed to create a tighter lateral canthal ligament. The original procedure described by Wyman does not address the problem of overlong eyelids that contribute to the diamond eye conformation. One of the simplest procedures for correcting the diamond eye conformation and shortening the palpebral fissure is a modification of Wyman's lateral canthoplasty. This is utilized by the author, and involves combining the Wyman lateral canthoplasty with the inclusion of wedge resections of upper and lower lids (Figure 5.17).

Ptosis

Ptosis, or drooping of the upper eyelid, may occur as a result of a slipped facial mask (as described above), from denervation of the levator palpebrae superioris muscle (innervated by the oculomotor (III) nerve) or, more commonly, as part of Horner's syndrome. Horner's syndrome is due to interruption of the sympathetic nerve supply to the head. This includes the supply to Müller's muscle within the eyelid. This muscle normally acts to keep the palpebral fissure widened. Horner's syndrome is discussed in more detail in Chapter 15.

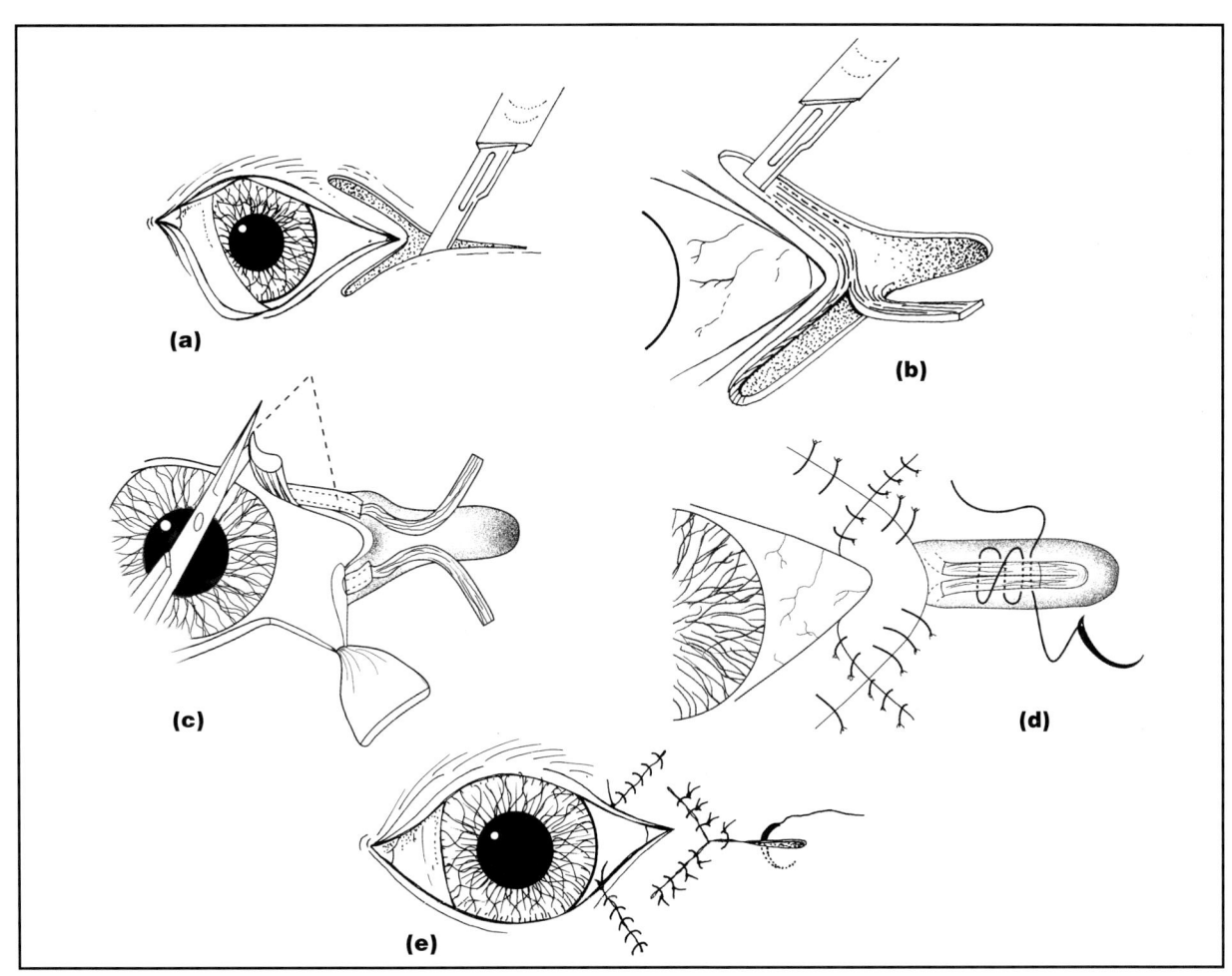

Figure 5.17 Wyman canthoplasty coupled with eyelid shortening for the treatment of diamond eye. (a) A Y-shaped skin incision is made at the lateral canthus with the arms of the Y extending along the upper and lower lids about 5 mm from the margins. (b) The surrounding skin is undermined and strips of orbicularis oculi muscle are dissected out from the upper and lower lids. These muscle strips are finger-shaped and remain attached at the lateral canthal region. (c) Wedges of full thickness eyelid tissue can be resected to shorten the eyelids prior to suturing the muscle flaps to the zygomatic arch. Most dogs with this shape of eyelid have overlong eyelids (especially St Bernards), and eyelid conformation can be improved by shortening the eyelids. The wedge resections are repaired using a two-layer repair. A secure repair is required, as the lids will be under tension following anchoring of the two strips of muscle to the zygomatic arch. (d) The zygomatic arch is exposed by blunt dissection and the strips of orbicularis oculi muscle are reflected laterally and firmly sutured to the periosteum of the zygomatic arch using PDS or monofilament nylon. (e) The skin incisions are closed. If the eyelids still need pulling laterally, the Y-shaped skin incision can be closed as a V. Postoperatively, the eyelid will be under quite a bit of lateral tension, giving a slit-eye appearance. This will tend to loosen over the following few weeks.

Retraction of the upper eyelid
The upper eyelid may be retracted in dogs suffering from the acute phase of extraocular polymyositis. The levator palpebrae superioris muscle originates within the orbit adjacent to the extraocular muscles and can be inflamed and contracted in dogs suffering with this condition (see Chapter 4).

Conditions involving cilia

Distichiasis
Distichiasis is a common condition in dogs. Distichia are abnormally positioned cilia that emerge along the eyelid margin either through or adjacent to the meibomian gland orifices (Figures 5.18 and 5.19). When more than one distichium emerges at one site, the condition is known as distichiasis. Distichia can usually be seen reasonably easily, although magnification is helpful. Distichia that contact the ocular surface often collect a covering of mucus. This can highlight their presence. Distichiasis occurs very commonly in certain breeds of dog, such as the American and English Cocker Spaniel, the Bulldog, the Miniature Long-Haired Dachshund, the Pekingese, the Rough Collie, the Shetland Sheepdog, the Weimeraner and the Welsh Springer Spaniel.

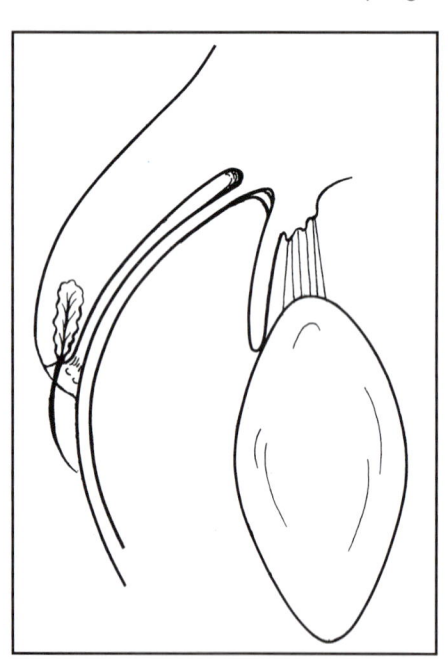

Figure 5.18 Cross-section of the eyelid, showing a distichium.

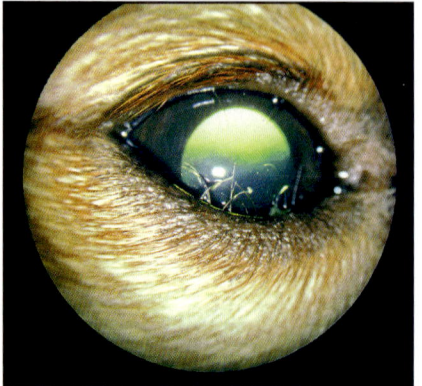

Figure 5.19 Shetland Sheepdog with several long distichia.

Distichia typically emerge when the dog is a few months of age, so if they are going to cause clinical signs, these have usually developed by the time the dog is a young adult. Therefore, if a middle-aged dog that has distichiasis is presented suffering from ocular irritation that has developed for the first time, it is likely that the distichia are not the primary cause of irritation (see below).

Clinical signs
The majority of dogs with distichiasis show few clinical signs, but, in some cases, the distichia do cause irritation or even pain and corneal ulceration. The stiffness, length, number and direction of the cilia are factors that determine how much irritation and corneal damage they cause. It is important not to assume that the presence of distichia always means that they are the cause of any signs of ocular surface disease that may be present. If the dog presents with a simple tear overflow, it is important to differentiate between a straightforward poor drainage of tears and an overflow of tears due to increased lacrimation. Other causes of irritation and ocular surface disease, such as conjunctivitis, ectopic cilia and keratoconjunctivitis sicca, should be ruled out before assuming that the distichia are the cause of the ocular irritation.

Always examine the lid with magnification in the minimally restrained dog and try to identify distichia that are contacting the corneal surface and could thus be significant. In middle-aged and older dogs, distichia that have previously been of no clinical significance can start to cause irritation as predisposing factors develop. Examples of such factors are age-related alterations in lid position leading to more direct corneal contact with the distichia and a reduction in tear production (e.g. development of keratoconjunctivitis sicca) that means that the passage of the distichia over the corneal surface is not so well lubricated.

Treatment
When distichia are causing clinical problems, a surgical procedure to destroy or remove the follicles which bear the distichia is usually indicated (see below).

Simple plucking can be utilized if only one or two troublesome distichia are present. A good pair of epilation forceps are required. The owners should be warned that the cilia will probably grow back. They may cause more severe problems while they are still rather short and therefore less flexible. When managing distichiasis, it should be remembered and explained to owners that, as with hairs elsewhere, the growth of distichia is cyclical. It is only possible to treat the hairs that are there at the time of presentation and, in the future, hairs may emerge at fresh sites on the eyelids. Gently squeezing the eyelid at the time of surgery may reveal distichia which were about to emerge from the eyelid margin. It is sensible to make accurate drawings of the position of the distichia and make a note of those that are contacting the cornea and those that are treated.

Permanent destruction of distichia may be achieved by electrolysis, cryosurgery or surgical excision. All methods should be performed with the aid of adequate magnification to facilitate accurate surgery. Each method has its own advantages and most also have significant disadvantages:

- Electrolysis is performed using a commercial electroepilation unit. Older units have a lead ground plate that may be wrapped around the tongue of larger patients, thus gaining good electrical contact. The needle electrode is slid into the eyelid alongside the cilium shaft to a depth of several millimetres and the current is turned on for 5 to 10 seconds until the cilium extrudes, along with meibomian secretion and hydrogen bubbles, when it may be easily plucked. A setting of 2 to 5 milliamps is recommended. Diathermy or electrocautery should not be used, as excessive tissue damage may result. Electrolysis can be time consuming and occasionally needs to be repeated
- Cryosurgery is performed using a small closed nitrous oxide or liquid nitrogen probe (such as those designed for glaucoma treatment or intracapsular cataract extraction). The probe is pressed on to the palpebral conjunctiva over the suspected site of the offending distichium's follicle. The eyelid is then frozen for several seconds until the ice ball reaches the eyelid margin. A slow thaw is allowed; then the procedure is repeated for all the regions of the lids with distichia that are considered to be clinically significant. The treated eyelids swell initially, although the use of systemic non-steroidal anti-inflammatory drugs helps to limit the swelling, which soon subsides. Depigmentation of eyelid skin and hair is common and in some instances may be permanent.

Several surgical techniques have been developed to excise the follicles from which the distichia originate. These should be left to those familiar with the techniques. It is possible to induce significant scarring and distortion of the eyelid and cause significant tear film instability, and thus end up with more serious clinical problems than resulted from the distichia. Magnification is required to ensure that the surgery is performed accurately and does not result in any distortion of the eyelids. Techniques include partial tarsal plate excision (Bedford, 1973) and excision of a strip of tarsoconjunctiva (Spreull, 1982). A final surgical option is to perform a Hotz–Celsus procedure to evert the eyelid and direct the hairs away from the cornea.

Ectopic cilia

Ectopic cilia (Figures 5.20, 5.21 and 5.22), like distichia, arise from follicles within or adjacent to the meibomian glands. However, unlike distichia, they emerge through the palpebral conjunctiva several millimetres from the eyelid margin. They are usually positioned midway along the upper eyelid; there is most commonly a single cilium here, although they can appear in other sites, and also as groups of ectopic cilia. They are not as common as distichia and are usually unilateral. There appears to be a breed predilection in Flat-Coated Retrievers, but ectopic cilia may be seen in any breed that suffers from distichiasis.

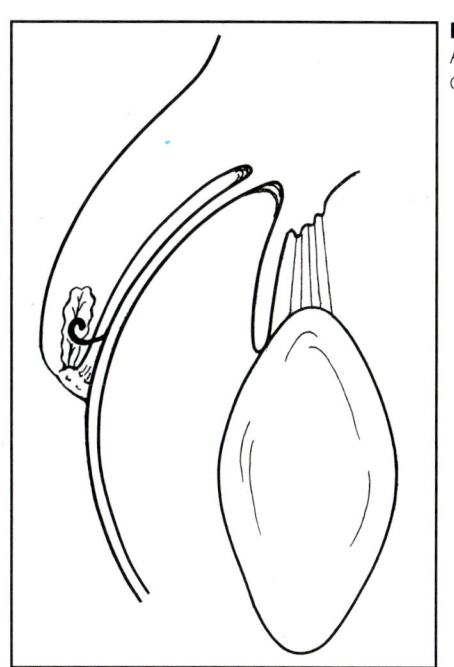

Figure 5.20 An ectopic cilium.

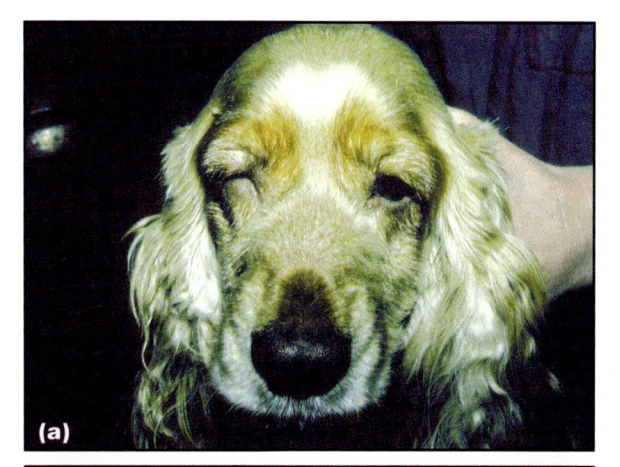

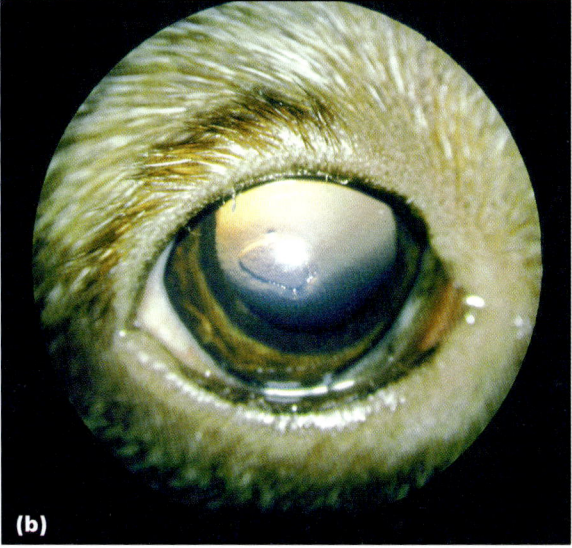

Figure 5.21 English Cocker Spaniel with an ectopic cilium protruding through the palpebral conjunctiva midway along the upper eyelid. (a) The dog presented with blepharospasm and lacrimation. (b) There is a central superficial corneal ulcer. (Note that the dog also has distichia).

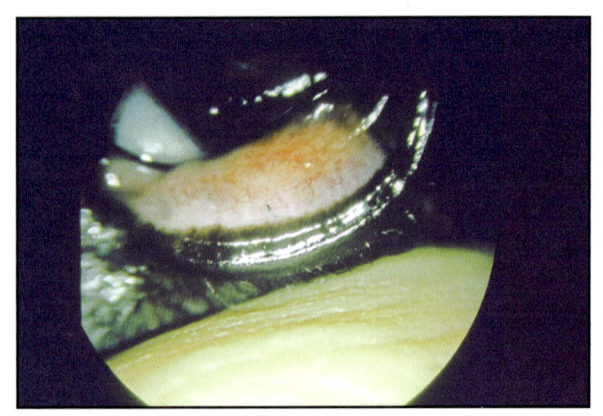

Figure 5.22 Poodle with ectopic cilia emerging through the palpebral conjunctiva of the lower eyelid.

Clinical signs

Young adults are most commonly affected. The offending hair invariably abrades the cornea, causing a superficial keratitis and even ulceration. Although the clinical signs of unilateral blepharospasm accompanied by corneal changes in a young adult dog may lead the examiner to suspect the presence of an ectopic cilium, visualization of the offending hair is difficult without magnification. The cilium sometimes emerges from a pigmented spot, though both may be non-pigmented. Many affected dogs also have distichia, and this may lead the veterinary surgeon to assume, wrongly, that the distichia are responsible for the clinical signs. However, it is uncommon for distichiasis to cause the same degree of discomfort and corneal change as ectopic cilia. Surgical excision of the follicle of the offending cilium with the aid of magnification is the simplest procedure for permanent removal of the ectopic cilium (Figure 5.23).

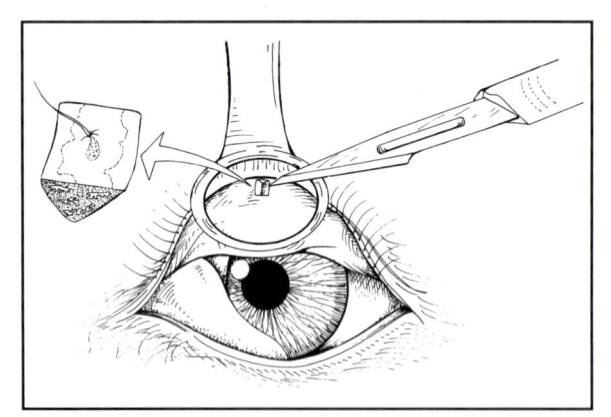

Figure 5.23 Excision of ectopic cilium. A chalazion clamp is applied to the affected eyelid to immobilize it and to prevent any haemorrhage which would obscure the operative field. A small square of tissue surrounding the cilia and including its follicle is excised.

Trichiasis

This is a condition in which facial hair contacts the ocular surface. Upper eyelid trichiasis/entropion in English Cocker Spaniels has already been discussed in the section on entropion.

The nasal folds of some brachycephalic dogs may contact the cornea, causing a superficial pigmentary keratitis (Figure 5.24). Surgical resection of the nasal folds may be required (Carter, 1973) (Figure 5.25).

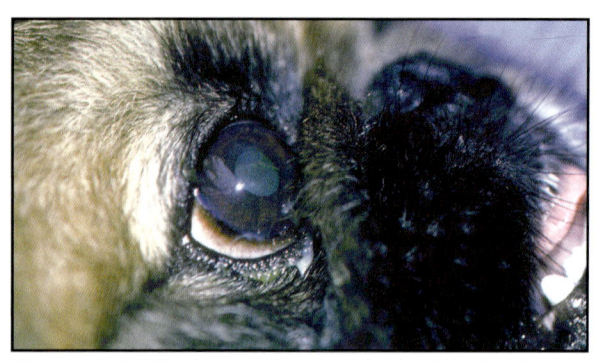

Figure 5.24 The hair on the nasal folds of this Pekingese were in contact with the corneas, and medial pigmentary keratitis had resulted.

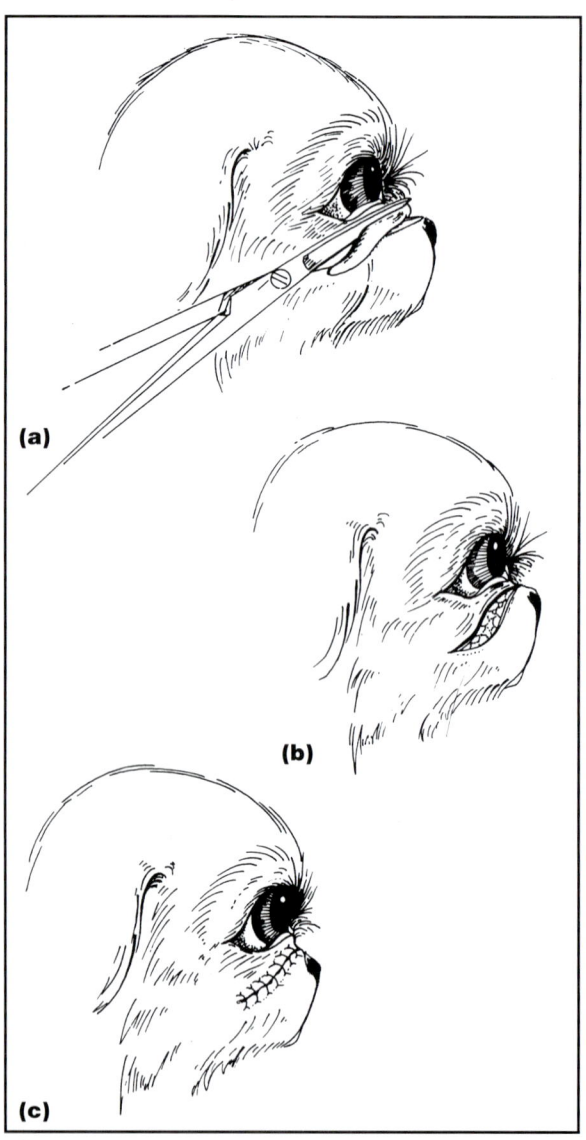

Figure 5.25 Excision of nasal folds. (a) Once the facial hair has been clipped, it is very obvious where to incise in order to resect the nasal fold. Strong sharp scissors are used to excise the offending fold. (b, c) The resulting skin defect is sutured.

The eyelids and nictitating membrane

The presence of hairs emerging from the caruncle at the medial canthus (hairy caruncles) is common in some breeds, such as the Tibetan Spaniel, the Shih Tzu and the Lhasa Apso, and this can be associated with problems (Figure 5.26). They can contribute to tear overflow by wicking tears onto the medial canthal skin as the dog blinks, or, if excessively long, can cause a medial superficial keratitis. Hairy caruncles can be managed by excision of the dermal tissue (taking care to avoid the nasolacrimal drainage system), cryosurgery to destroy the hair follicles or a medial canthoplasty (Figure 5.27).

Trichiasis can also result from lid distortion caused by scarring. Lid lacerations should be carefully repaired to restore accurate anatomical alignment and prevent this problem.

Infections and inflammations of the eyelids (blepharitis)

Blepharitis is a common condition in the dog (Figure 5.28). The various causes of blepharitis and appropriate diagnostic tests are shown in Figure 5.29.

Blepharitis may be associated with a more widespread dermatitis or may accompany ocular surface disease (blepharoconjunctivitis).

Stye (hordeolum)

Abscessation of an individual meibomian gland results in an internal stye (internal hordeolum) (Figure 5.30). An external stye results from infection and abscessation of the glands of Zeis or Moll. Styes are

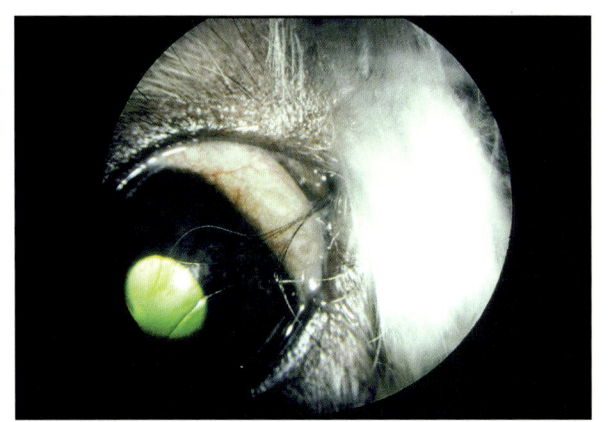

Figure 5.26 A hairy caruncle resulting in medial keratitis and contributing to a tear overflow in this Shih Tzu.

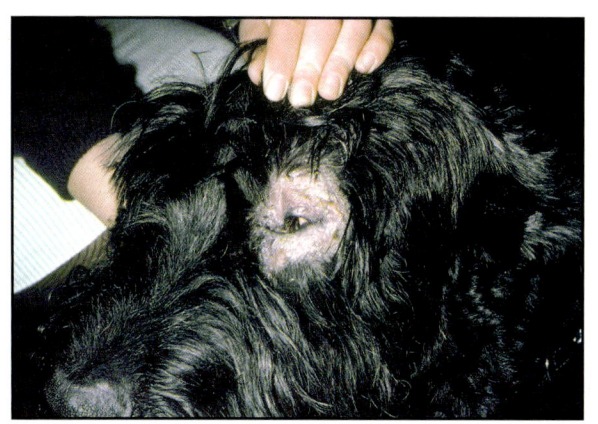

Figure 5.28 Chronic blepharitis in a dog, resulting in periocular alopecia and thickening of the eyelid skin.

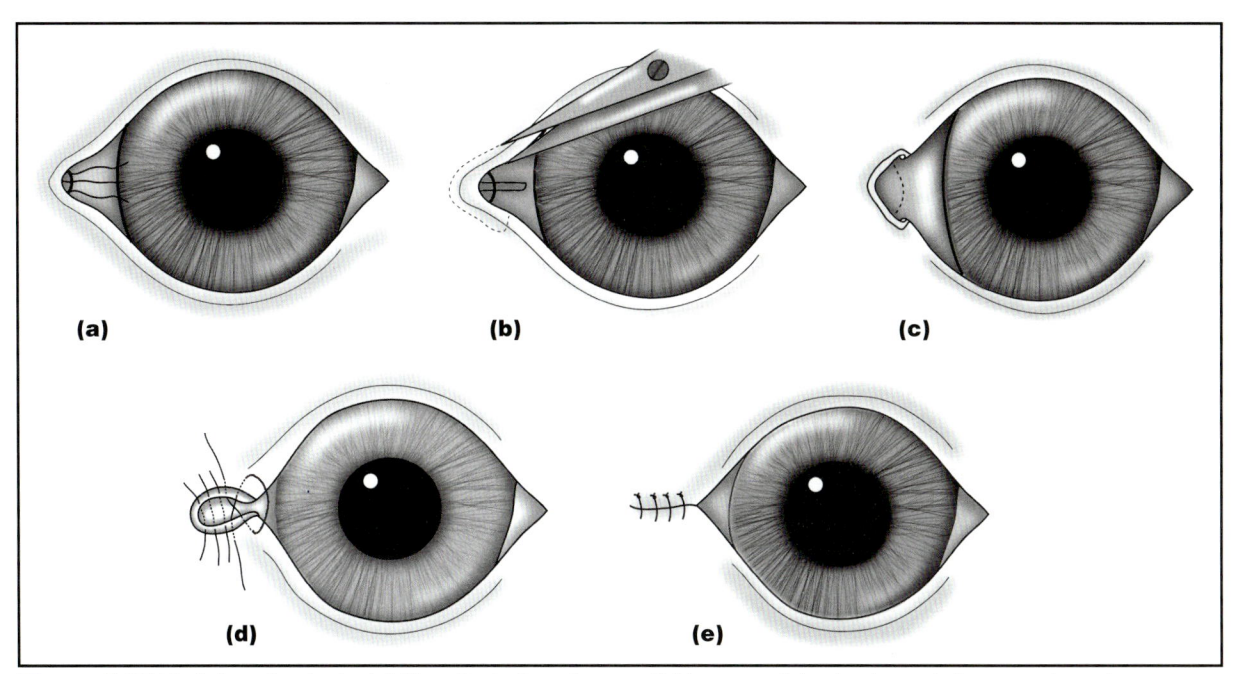

Figure 5.27 Medial canthoplasty. (a) The affected eye has medial lower eyelid entropion, a hairy caruncle and a macropalpebral fissure. This combination can result in tear overflow and the development of medial keratitis. This procedure will remove the source of corneal irritation and shorten the eyelid opening. (b) Strips of eyelid margin are removed from upper and lower eyelids, continuing around the medial canthus to remove all the hair-bearing mucosa of the caruncle. The incisions start just medial to the lacrimal puncta and care is taken to preserve the puncta and canaliculi. (c) The tissue has been removed. (d) A two-layer repair is performed and the medial canthus of the shortened eyelid opening is reformed using a figure-of-eight suture. This repair needs to be secure, since the incision is under tension as these dogs tend to have tight eyelids. (e) The procedure is completed and the eyelid opening has been shortened.

The eyelids and nictitating membrane

Aetiology	Features	Diagnostic tests	Treatment

Parasitic:
  Sarcoptes
  Demodex
	Does not usually occur as an isolated blepharitis	Skin scrapings	Appropriate antiparasitic treatment

Bacterial infection:
  Juvenile pyoderma
  Blepharitis
  External stye
  Meibomianitis and chalazion
		Swabs for bacteriology: drain abscess or express meibomian secretion for culture (staphylococci often isolated)	Hot compresses. Surgical drainage of chalazia or abscesses. Expression of infected meibomian secretions. Appropriate systemic antibiotics

Fungal infection: Ringworm		Wood's lamp examination. Skin scrape. Fungal culture	Griseofulvin

Immune-mediated:
  Pemphigus
  Medial canthal erosion
  Uveodermatological syndrome
	Eyelid poliosis and vitiligo as well as panuveitis (see Chapter 10)	Biopsy. Histopathology and immunopathology. Clinical signs	Appropriate anti-inflammatory medication

Allergic:
  Food
  Contact
  Drugs
  Atopy
		Clinical signs (other skin areas affected). Hypoallergenic diets. Intradermal skin testing	Avoid allergen (hypoallergenic diet). Hyposensitization

Post-parotid duct transposition	Associated with overflow of saliva from the eye	Swab for bacteriology: many conjunctival sacs yield large numbers of bacteria	Regular flushing of conjunctival sac and cleaning of periocular area. Dry the face after feeding. Appropriate topical antibiotics
Secondary to ocular irritation (due to self-inflicted trauma)		Demonstrate primary source of irritation	Correct primary cause
Seborrhoeic	Other areas of skin also affected	Clinical signs	Treat as for seborrhoeic dermatitis elsewhere

Endocrine-related:
  Hyperadrenocorticism (Cushing's syndrome)
  Hypothyroidism
		Clinical signs, endocrine assessment	Treat underlying endocrine disease

Figure 5.29 Causes of blepharitis in the dog.

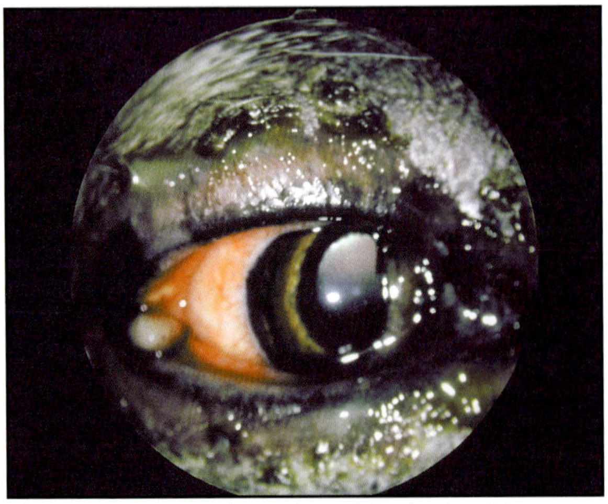

Figure 5.30 Internal stye due to infection involving a meibomian gland in a dog suffering from blepharoconjunctivitis.

painful on manipulation, which can help to distinguish them from chalazia (see below). Styes should be treated like abscesses elsewhere in the body, by drainage, application of warm compresses and, if required, systemic antibiotics.

Meibomianitis

Meibomianitis may result from staphylococcal infection, usually associated with generalized dermatoses. The affected meibomian glands exude a yellow, purulent material instead of the normal clear oily secretion, or, in some cases, no secretion can be expressed. They can be seen through the palpebral conjunctiva as linear yellow-white inflammatory infiltrates perpendicular to the eyelid margin. Treatment should include the expression of material for culture, the use of topical and systemic antibiotics and the application of warm compresses.

Chalazia

Chalazia result from the retention of meibomian secretions, causing rupture of the involved gland and a granulomatous reaction around a core of inspissated meibomian secretion. They appear as a firm nodular painless yellow-grey mass that can be seen through the conjunctival surface of the eyelid. The commonest cause of a chalazion is blockage of meibomian gland secretion by the formation of a meibomian adenoma (Figure 5.31). Multiple chalazia may be present on occasion; this seems to be most common in the Labrador Retriever in the UK.

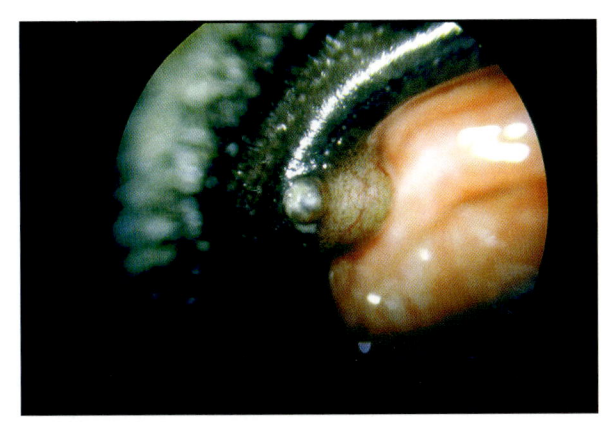

Figure 5.31 Chalazion in a dog as a result of blockage of the meibomian gland orifice by a sebaceous adenoma. (Courtesy of DT Ramsey.)

Treatment is by surgical curettage through the conjunctiva followed by the application of a topical antibiotic–steroid preparation for 5–7 days. When the chalazion is secondary to adenoma formation, surgery to excise both the adenoma and the chalazion is performed.

Juvenile pyoderma

Juvenile pyoderma results from a staphylococcal infection with a marked inflammatory reaction to staphylococcal toxins. It may initially involve the eyelids alone, but other parts of the integument of the head soon become involved. Enlargement and even abscessation of the draining lymph nodes may also occur. Recommended medication includes broad-spectrum antibiotics and oral prednisolone to control the inflammatory response.

Chronic bacterial blepharitis

Chronic bacterial blepharitis can develop in adult dogs (Figure 5.32). Staphylococcal species are often implicated and an allergic response to bacterial toxins may exacerbate the condition. The eyelids can become grossly thickened, with abscessation of glands within the eyelid skin (external styes – see above), which, if recurrent, can lead to cicatricial ectropion (Figure 5.33). The meibomian glands may also become inflamed (meibomianitis – see above).

Treatment consists of surgical drainage of any abscesses or chalazia and applications of hot compresses. The appropriate antibiotics should be given and an Elizabethan collar applied to prevent self-trauma.

Immune-mediated blepharitis

The eyelid has a mucocutaneous junction and, therefore, may be involved in pemphigus conditions.

The uveodermatological syndrome is assumed to have an immune basis. Depigmentation of the eyelids (Figure 5.34), planum nasale and muzzle are accompanied by panuveitis (see Chapter 10).

A medial canthal erosion involving both upper and lower eyelids is seen occasionally in dogs, most commonly German Shepherd Dogs (Figure 5.35); an immune-mediated aetiology is suspected. Affected

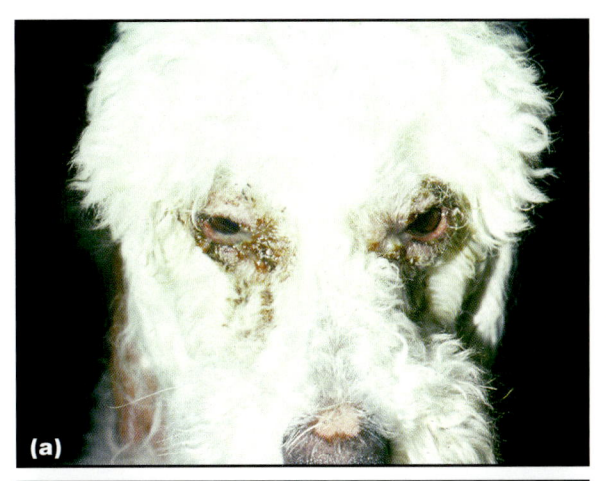

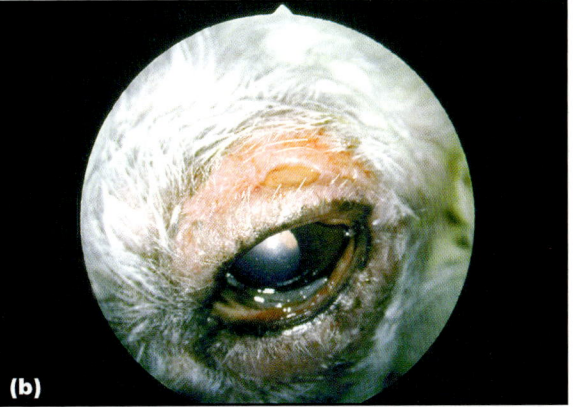

Figure 5.32 Poodle with chronic blepharitis. (a) External view. (b) Close-up after exudate was cleaned away, showing splits in the eyelid skin resulting from rupture of the external styes. Coagulase-positive staphylococci were isolated. The condition resolved after treatment with an appropriate systemic antibiotic and the fitting of an Elizabethan collar. Hot compresses were applied to the eyelids twice daily.

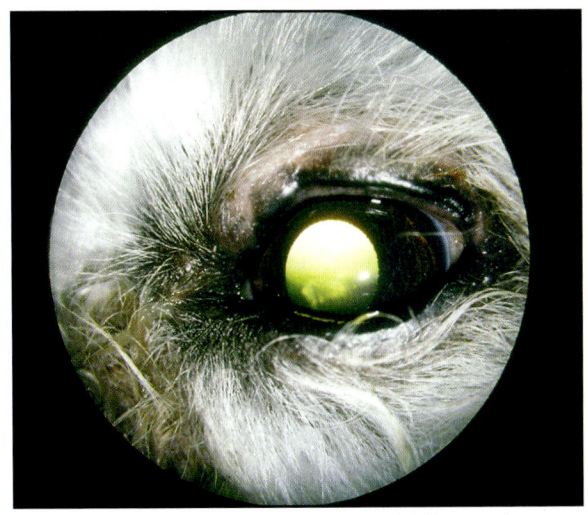

Figure 5.33 Slight upper eyelid cicatricial ectropion resulting from a chronic bacterial blepharitis.

dogs may also suffer from pannus (chronic superficial keratitis/keratoconjunctivitis) and plasma cell infiltration of the third eyelid (see Chapter 8). In some instances, the lateral canthal region will also be ulcerated.

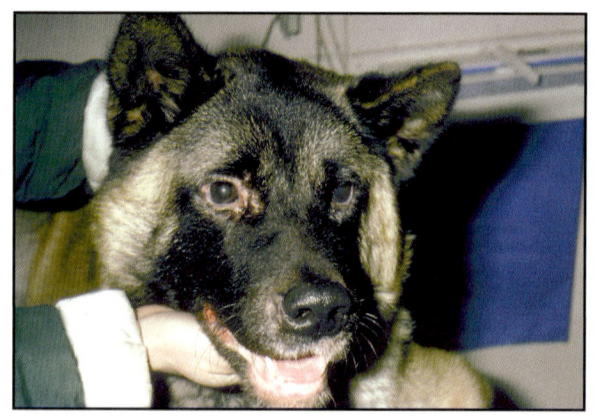

Figure 5.34 Depigmentation of the eyelid margins and muzzle in a dog suffering from the uveodermatological syndrome.

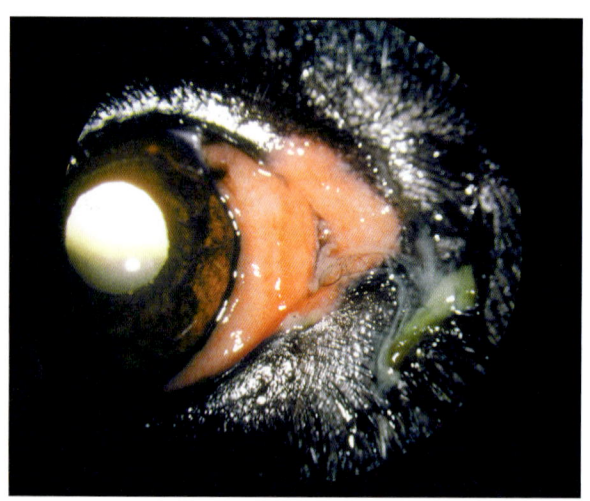

Figure 5.35 Medial canthal ulceration and plasma cell infiltration of the third eyelid in a German Shepherd Dog.

Seborrhoeic blepharitis

Older English Cocker Spaniels with upper eyelid entropion/trichiasis often have an accompanying periocular seborrhoea, otitis externa and labial fold dermatitis. Bacterial infection of the labia and external ear canal may act as reservoirs of infection for the periocular area and conjunctival sac.

Blepharitis following parotid duct transposition

Periocular dermatitis is a complication of transposition of the parotid duct for the management of severe keratoconjunctivitis sicca. Dogs that have undergone this surgery often have a saliva overflow from the eye, particularly at meal times. Additionally, the bacterial flora of the conjunctival sac is markedly changed following parotid duct transposition, with the presence of increased numbers of bacteria (Petersen-Jones, 1997). Constant moistening of the periocular skin with saliva containing many bacteria results in dermatitis. Good nursing helps to control the condition; regular cleaning and drying of the face should be advised (especially after meal times). Topical antibiotics may also be indicated.

Eyelid injuries

Traumatic eyelid injuries are common. They are most frequently the result of bite wounds, cat scratches or road traffic accidents. Immediate first-aid should include application of cold compresses to minimize swelling. The dog should be examined for systemic injury in the case of traumatic injuries and the globe should be carefully examined for involvement. When the nasal regions of the eyelids are involved, a careful examination for damage to the nasolacrimal duct system should be undertaken.

Reconstructive surgery, if necessary, should be performed promptly, paying particular attention to restoring a normal lid–cornea relationship. Cicatrix formation resulting from poor anatomical repair can cause ectropion or trichiasis. The eyelid skin has a good blood supply and it is unusual to see wounds that cause ischaemia and devitalization. Wounds should be thoroughly, but gently, irrigated with saline, cleaned with dilute povidone–iodine and a primary repair performed, preserving as much tissue as possible. Repair using 5-0 or 6-0 suture material should be performed, paying particular attention to accurate restoration of the eyelid margin. A figure-of-eight suture is useful to repair the eyelid margin (see below), followed by the use of 6-0 polyglactin sutures to repair the tarsoconjunctiva, taking care to bury the knots so they do not abrade the corneal surface.

If the nasolacrimal system is involved, it should be cannulated prior to surgery to ensure that patency can be maintained; an indwelling cannula should be left in place for 7 to 10 days postoperatively. Administration of prophylactic topical and systemic antibiotics is recommended and, in acute cases, systemic non-steroidal anti-inflammatory drugs can be beneficial in reducing swelling.

Eyelid neoplasia

Eyelid neoplasia is common in older dogs, but the majority of canine eyelid tumours are benign. Types of tumour include sebaceous adenoma, papilloma, benign melanoma, sebaceous adenocarcinoma, histiocytoma, mast cell tumour, basal cell carcinoma and squamous cell carcinoma (Krehbiel and Langham, 1975; Roberts et al., 1986).

Sebaceous adenoma

The sebaceous adenoma is the commonest eyelid tumour in the dog. It is a benign tumour that arises from the meibomian gland (Figure 5.36). Often only a small portion of the tumour shows at the eyelid margin and eversion of the eyelid reveals the true extent of the tumour on the inner aspect of the eyelid. Treatment can be by sharp excision, or by cryosurgery following surgical debulking, if the tumour is large.

Papilloma

These are usually superficial. They should be removed if they are rapidly increasing in size or irritating the cornea; they are cryosensitive. However, papillomas may spontaneously regress in young dogs.

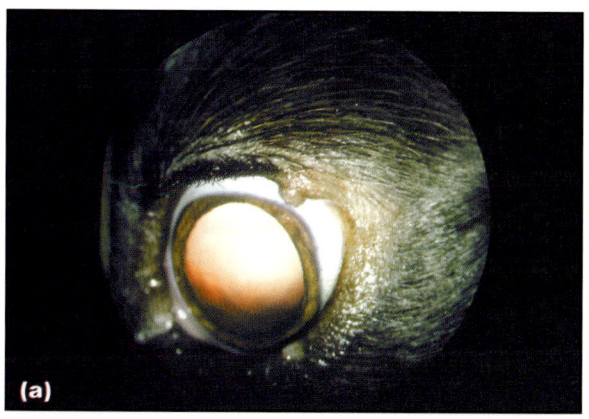

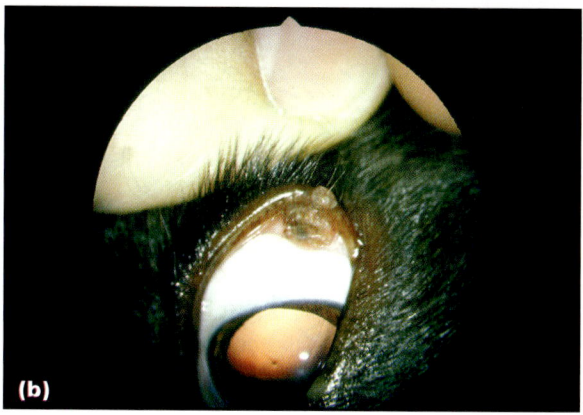

Figure 5.36 Meibomian gland adenoma in a dog. (a) The tip of the tumour shows at the eyelid margin. (b) Eversion of the eyelid reveals the full extent of the tumour.

Melanoma

Canine eyelid melanomas are usually superficial and benign. They occur most frequently in older heavily pigmented breeds of dog. They are usually slow growing and may be multiple. They, too, are cryosensitive.

Sebaceous adenocarcinoma

Clinically, these have the same appearance as meibomian gland adenomas. Although histologically they have features that suggest malignancy, they do not appear to metastasize.

Histiocytoma

Histiocytomas are primarily tumours of young growing dogs and typically develop rapidly. They are raised, usually less than 1 cm in diameter, pink and hairless. Often, they regress spontaneously over a few weeks.

Treatment of eyelid tumours

Complete surgical excision or cryosurgery are the treatments of choice. The advantage of sharp excision is that it is generally easy to ensure that all of the tumour is removed and that regrowth is unlikely. The choice of which eyelid reconstruction is required after removal of a tumour will depend on the position and size of the tumour and the width of free margin required around that particular tumour.

Full thickness excision and direct closure of wound

Many tumours can be removed using a full thickness V-shaped ('cake slice') excision or four-sided ('house-shaped') excision followed by direct closure (Figure 5.37). In most dogs, up to one third of the length of an eyelid can be removed and repaired by direct closure.

The positioning of the first suture is critical: it should accurately reform the eyelid margin. A simple interrupted suture or a figure-of-eight suture can be used for this purpose (Figure 5.37). The advantages of the figure-of-eight suture pattern are that it results in a strong, accurate repair and has the knot positioned well away from the eyelid margin (and hence the corneal surface). Once the eyelid margin is accurately reformed, the rest of the wound is repaired by a one or two layer procedure using simple interrupted sutures. It is important that the sutures do not abrade the cornea, so it is probably best to leave the palpebral conjunctiva unsutured. A suture material such as 6-0 polyglactin is suitable, and avoids the need to remove small sutures from around the eye.

Larger tumours requiring excision of more than one third of the eyelid

Surgical mobilization of adjacent tissues is required to create a functional and fully mobile eyelid. The reconstructed eyelid should be mobile, allowing complete

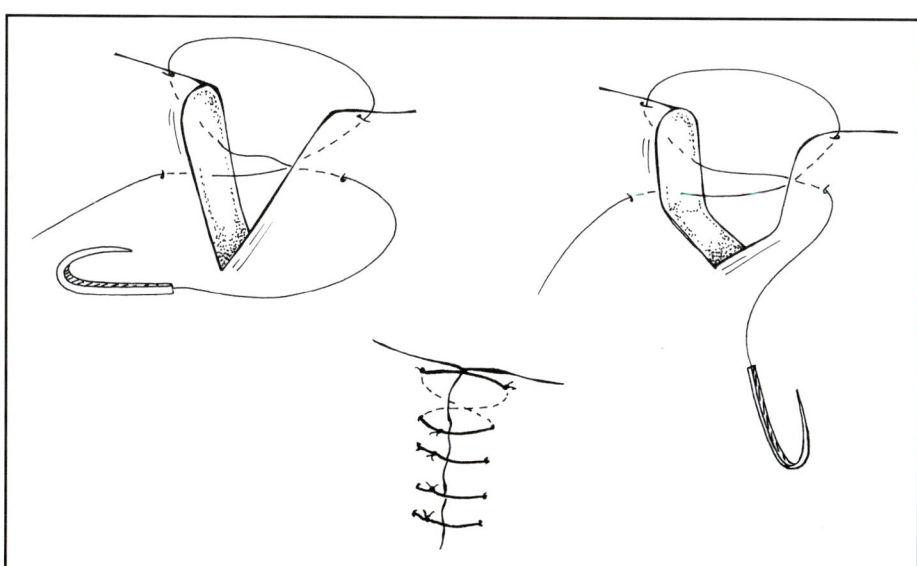

Figure 5.37 V-shaped resection and a four-sided resection to remove an eyelid tumour. A figure-of-eight suture is used to reform the eyelid margin. This suture pattern results in a strong repair, with the knot well away from the ocular surface.

98   The eyelids and nictitating membrane

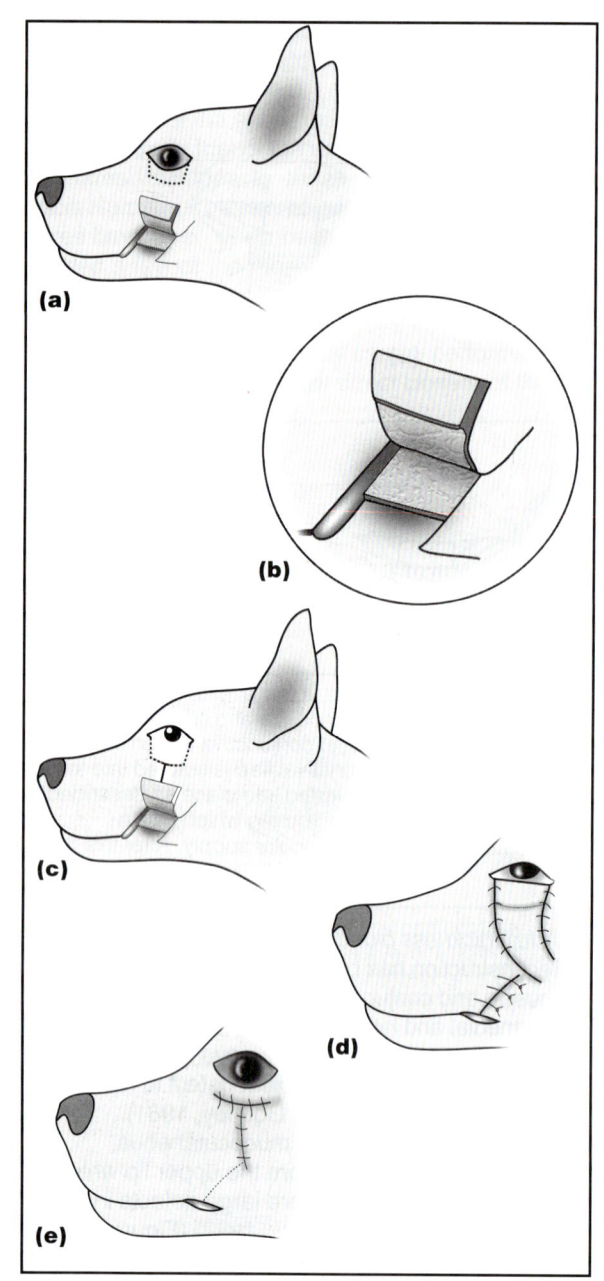

Figure 5.42 Lip to lid graft (mucocutaneous subdermal plexus flap). Rotation of a graft fashioned from the upper lip can be used to replace the lower eyelid. A portion of oral mucosa is included with the flap to replace the lower palpebral conjunctiva, and the oral mucocutaneous junction mimics the eyelid margin. (a) There is a large defect in the lower eyelid. A dissection of full thickness lip has been started. (b) The lip flap only includes oral mucosa for sufficient depth to mimic the depth of the lid itself. The dissection is then continued to separate the skin and subdermal plexus from deeper structures over sufficient length to allow the flap to be rotated to reach the eyelid defect. The skin ventral to the eyelid defect is incised and the edges are separated sufficiently to accommodate the rotated flap. (c) The oral mucosa of the lip flap is sutured to the conjunctiva in the fornix and the lip skin is sutured to the edges of the eyelid defect and the separated edges of the skin incision ventral to the lid defect. The defect in the oral mucosa and the lip skin is closed. (d) 4 to 6 weeks after the surgery, the connecting skin from the lip to the lid may be excised and the edges of the original incision ventral to the lid defect may be reunited. This improves the cosmetic result.

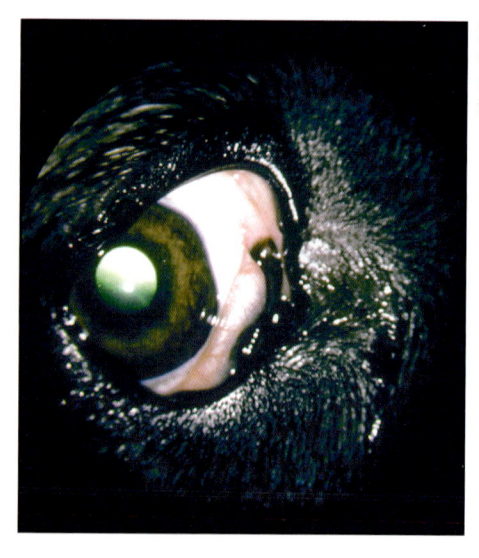

Figure 5.43 A scrolled third eyelid.

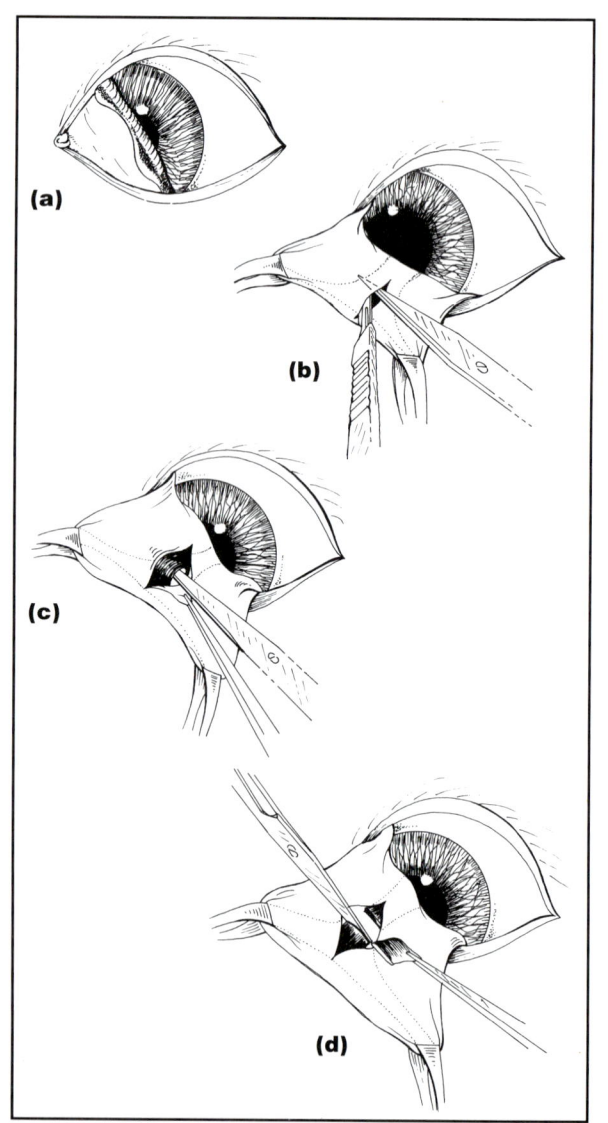

Figure 5.44 Surgical correction of scrolling of the third eyelid. (a, b) The third eyelid is everted and an incision is made through the conjunctiva overlying the horizontal arm of the T skeleton in the region of the deformity. (c) Blunt dissection is performed to isolate the scrolled portion of cartilage, taking care not to 'button-hole' the third eyelid. (d) The abnormal portion of cartilage is excised.

have rather loose third eyelids. If this happens, tightening of the third eyelid can be performed by removing a full-thickness wedge of the third eyelid at the far edge of the free border (so as to avoid the remaining cartilage). The defect is repaired using 6-0 polyglactin.

Prolapse of the gland of the third eyelid

Prolapse of the gland of the third eyelid results in the appearance of a pink swelling at the medial canthus ('cherry eye') (Figure 5.45).

The third eyelid gland produces a significant proportion of the pre-ocular tear film and should, therefore, be preserved. Sometimes it can be manipulated back into position, but it usually prolapses again.

Several procedures to permanently replace the gland have been described. One of the simplest and most effective is the imbrication or pocketing technique (Morgan *et al.*, 1993), illustrated in Figure 5.46; this is the current technique of choice in general practice. An alternative technique favoured by some veterinary ophthalmologists is to suture the prolapsed gland to the orbital rim, as shown in Figure 5.47 (Kaswan and Martin, 1985; Petersen-Jones, 1991; Stanley and Kaswan, 1994). This procedure limits the passage of the third eyelid across the cornea and, therefore, interferes with its function of protecting the eye and spreading the tear film.

Inflammation of the third eyelid

A plasma cell infiltration (plasma cell conjunctivitis) of the free border of the third eyelid resulting in depigmentation and a pink or purple thickening occurs in some breeds, notably the German Shepherd Dog (see Figure 5.35). It may accompany chronic superficial keratitis/keratoconjunctivitis (pannus). Topical corticosteroids and/or cyclosporin are moderately effective in controlling the condition (Bromberg, 1980; Read, 1995).

The third eyelid may also be involved in dogs with inflammatory granulomatous ocular diseases, such as nodular granulomatous episclerokeratitis or ocular nodular fasciitis.

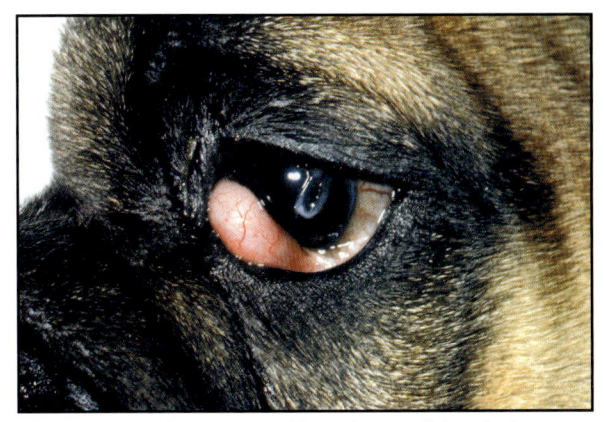

Figure 5.45 Young dog with prolapse of the nictitans gland ('cherry eye').

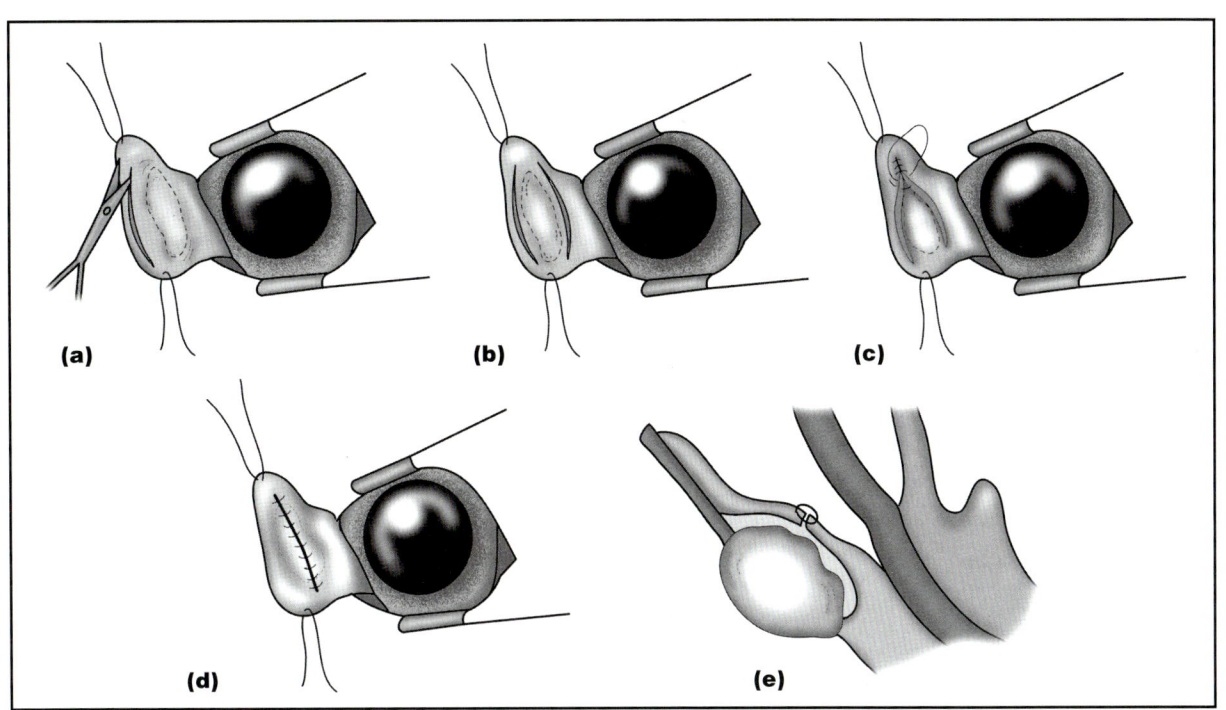

Figure 5.46 Pocketing procedure for repositioning a prolapsed third eyelid gland. (a) The third eyelid is manipulated by stay sutures at either end of the free border. Using these sutures, the third eyelid is held in a protruded and everted position, and a curved incision parallel to the free border of the third eyelid is made proximal to the prolapsed gland.
(b) A second incision is made distal to the prolapsed gland in the smooth-surfaced conjunctiva just distal to the roughened conjunctiva, which marks the presence of lymphoid tissue overlying the gland. (c) Conjunctiva from a position proximal to the first incision and distal to the second incision is sutured together to pull the conjunctiva over the prolapsed gland, creating a pocket to hold it in position. A continuous suture pattern is used, starting with a buried knot. 6-0 polyglactin is suitable for most dogs. Care is taken to not completely close either end of the pocket over the gland. Small spaces left at either end allow the glandular secretions to escape from the pocket and reach the conjunctival sac. (d) The suture line is completed. (e) Cross-section through the third eyelid to show the pocketed and buried gland.

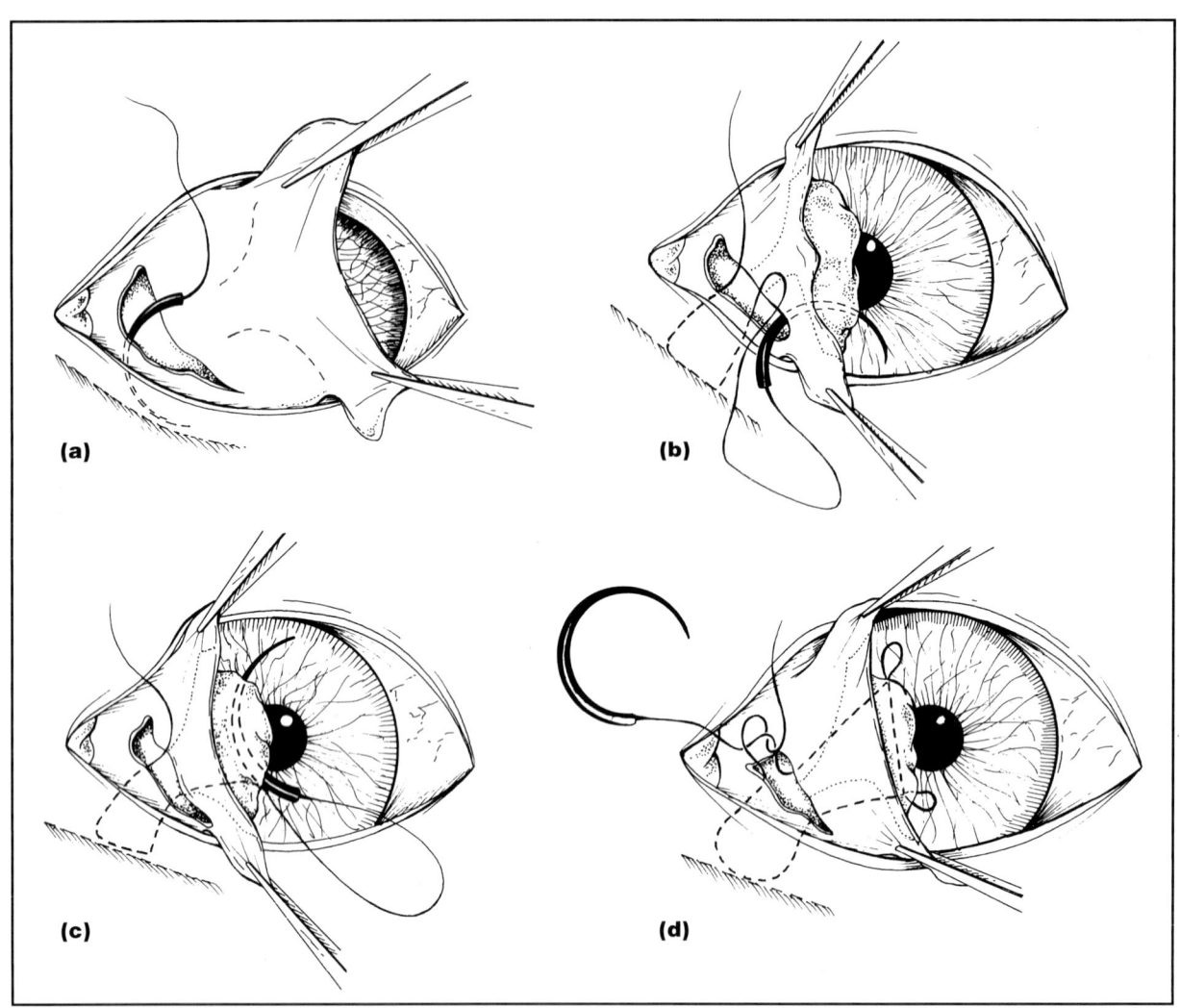

Figure 5.47 The suturing of the gland of the nictitating membrane to the orbital rim as a treatment for prolapse of the gland. (a) Forceps grasp the periphery of the free margin of the third eyelid and pull it across the eye (stay sutures may be used). An incision is made in the medioventral conjunctival fornix (at the base of the third eyelid) using scissors. Blunt dissection allows access to the periosteum of the medioventral orbital rim. A firm bite of periosteum along the orbital rim is taken using 3-0 polydioxanone or monofilament nylon: the suture material (with a swaged-on needle) is introduced through the previously made incision. It can be a little difficult to obtain a bite of periosteum and bring the needle out through the incision, because access to the area is limited. (b) After taking a bite of orbital periosteum, the needle is then passed through the original incision dorsally to the prolapsed gland to emerge from the gland at its most prominent point of prolapse. (c) With the third eyelid everted, the needle is passed back through the exit hole in the gland to take a horizontal bite from the most prominent part of the gland. (d) Finally, the needle is passed back through the last exit hole to emerge through the original incision in the conjunctival fornix, thus encircling a large portion of the gland. The suture ends are then tied. This creates a suture loop through the gland which anchors it to the periosteum of the orbital rim, preventing it from re-prolapsing. The conjunctival incision can now be repaired using 6-0 polyglactin, or it may be left unsutured. Postoperatively, topical antibiotic cover is given.

Trauma to the third eyelid

Lacerations most commonly occur as the result of a cat scratch injury. The underlying globe should always be carefully examined for injury. Full thickness lacerations or avulsion injuries usually require suturing, and care should be taken to reconstruct the free border, while ensuring that the sutures do not abrade the cornea. Lacerations just involving the conjunctiva of the third eyelid do not usually require suturing as, like other conjunctival injuries, they heal rapidly.

Foreign bodies behind the third eyelid

Foreign bodies, such as grass seeds, sometimes lodge between the third eyelid and the globe. This site should always be checked if a conjunctival foreign body is suspected. Signs of the presence of a foreign body include blepharospasm, conjunctivitis, and excessive lacrimation which is followed by a profuse mucopurulent ocular discharge within hours.

Neoplasia of the third eyelid

Neoplasia of the third eyelid is uncommon; it has recently been reviewed by Ward (1999). Reported tumours include adenomas and adenocarcinomas of the third eyelid gland, and squamous cell carcinomas and haemangiomas of the third eyelid conjunctiva. Adenomas and adenocarcinomas may invade the adjacent orbit and cause signs of a space-occupying lesion (Figure 5.48). Surgical removal of the third eyelid as well as the tumour is usually required for adenomas and adenocarcinomas. Local excision is usually possible for conjunctival haemangiomas.

Protrusion of the third eyelid

Protrusion of the third eyelid is a common sign with a variety of causes (Figure 5.49). The underlying aetiology should be identified and treated whenever possible.

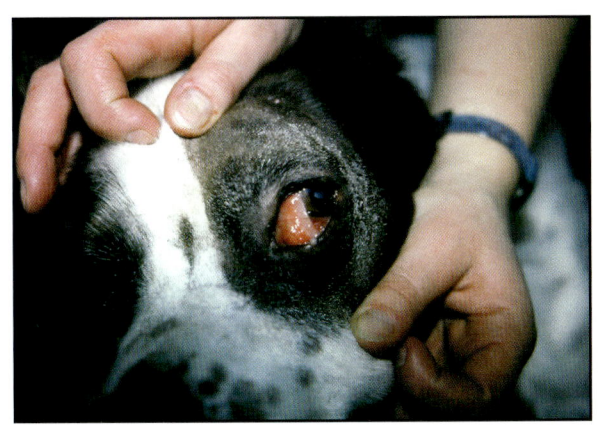

Figure 5.48 Adenocarcinoma of the nictitans gland in an English Springer Spaniel. Note the lateral displacement of the globe.

Cause	Features
Reduced globe size (see Chapter 4)	May be due to microphthalmos or phthisis bulbi
'Haws' syndrome (cats only)	Cats with mild diarrhoea may present with bilateral third eyelid protrusion (viral aetiology suggested)
Enophthalmos (see Chapter 4)	May be due to reduced orbital contents e.g. cachexia, dehydration, masseter and temporal muscle atrophy, contracture of extraocular muscles following extraocular polymyositis
Active globe retraction	Painful ocular lesion – other signs of pain will be present
Orbital space-occupying lesion (see Chapter 4)	Prominent globe
Horner's syndrome (see Chapter 15)	Miosis, ptosis, enophthalmos and possibly conjunctival hyperaemia

Figure 5.49 Causes of third eyelid protrusion in dogs and cats.

Conditions of the eyelids of cats

Ankyloblepharon

The eyelids of kittens usually open by the 12th day after birth. Ophthalmia neonatorum is occasionally encountered. Feline herpesvirus infection may be responsible for the condition and secondary bacterial infection is common. Treatment is as discussed for the dog. Occasionally, ankyloblepharon persists after the age at which the eyelids normally open, in which case the lids can be opened surgically.

Coloboma

Eyelid colobomas occur sporadically in cats (Figure 5.50). The upper lateral portion of the eyelid is most commonly affected, usually bilaterally. There is a range of severity from an abnormally thin portion of lid, to a large defect where the majority of the lid is absent. Inadequate eyelid closure can result in an exposure keratopathy/keratitis. Additionally, facial hair may be directed onto the cornea (trichiasis), leading to an exacerbation of the keratopathy/keratitis.

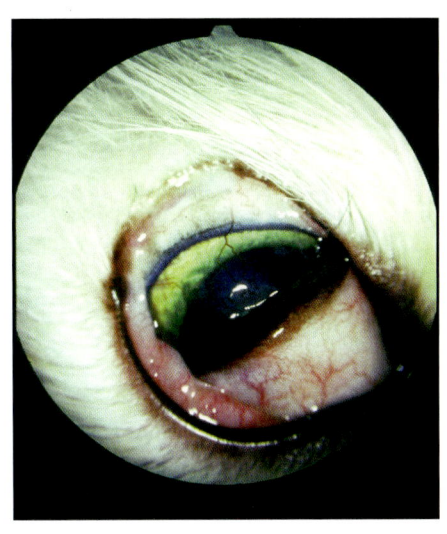

Figure 5.50 A coloboma of the lateral portion of the upper eyelid in a cat.

The extent of corneal coverage during blinking and the degree of trichiasis, as well as any corneal changes that have already developed, should be assessed when deciding how to manage each individual case.

Treatment

Mild defects with little corneal exposure can be managed by performing cryosurgery to remove the hairs responsible for any trichiasis and by treating with artificial tear ointments.

Surgical reconstruction of larger eyelid defects is required to prevent progression of the corneal pathology (Dziezyc and Millichamp, 1989). Smaller defects may be repaired by converting them into triangular full thickness defects and closing them directly. Larger defects require a more complicated blepharoplastic reconstruction. A procedure involving transposing a pedicle of skin from the lower eyelid to reform the upper eyelid and lining it with a pedicle of conjunctiva transposed from the lower conjunctival sac can be used (Dziezyc and Millichamp, 1989). This procedure has disadvantages: the recreated eyelid may not have normal mobility; the eyelid margin is abnormal (this is most important for the upper eyelid as it has greater movement over the cornea than the lower eyelid); and hairs from the new eyelid grow in the direction of the cornea and may result in trichiasis. A more complicated two-stage procedure was developed for reconstruction of the upper lid in humans by Mustardé (1980) (Figure

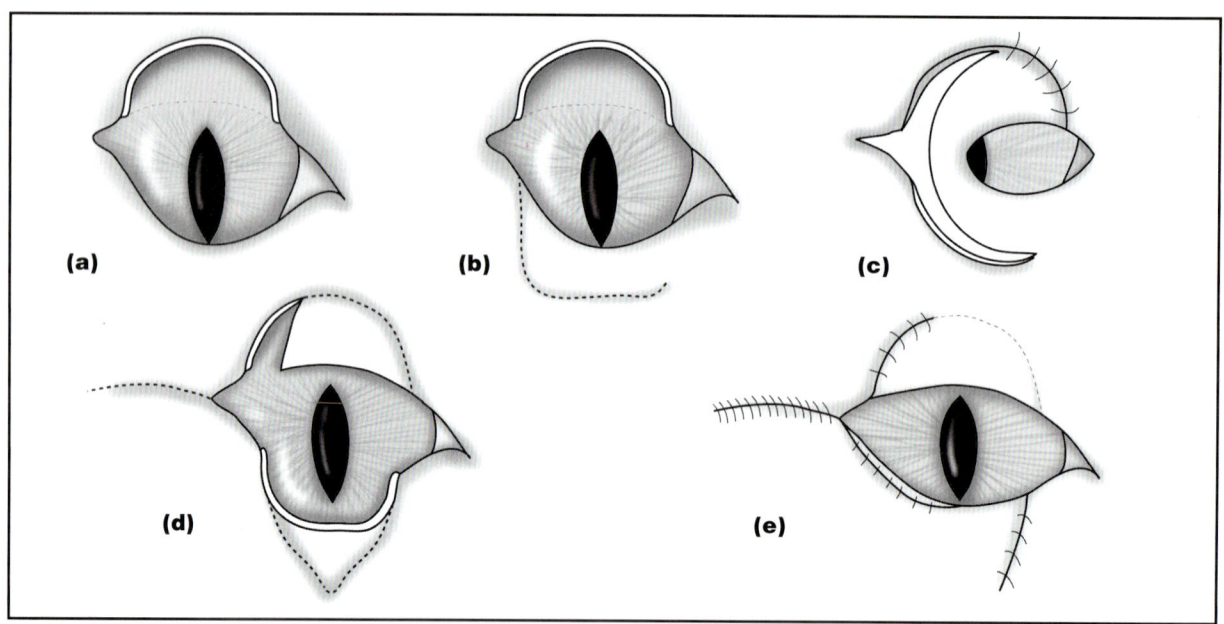

Figure 5.51 The repair of a coloboma of the right upper eyelid using a two-staged Mustardé technique. (a) The upper eyelid has a colobomatous defect affecting the lateral three-quarters of the eyelid, leading to exposure keratopathy/keratitis and trichiasis. (b) The edge of the defect is freshened up medially to received a rotated portion of the lower eyelid and any conjunctiva in the fornix is mobilized. (c) A full-thickness portion of lower eyelid is fashioned and left attached to the remaining lower eyelid medially. This is rotated into the defect of the upper eyelid and partially sutured into place using a two-layer repair. (d) After waiting for two weeks for the transposed lower lid to heal into place in the defect of the upper eyelid, its connection to the medial remaining lower eyelid is sectioned and the lower lid completely swung into position in the upper lid defect. The edges of the remaining defect in the upper eyelid must be freshened to receive the transposed full-thickness eyelid. This leaves a large full-thickness defect in the lower eyelid. (e) The lower eyelid defect is closed by using a cheek rotation flap and lining it with mobilized remaining conjunctiva and an oral mucosal graft.

5.51). This offers the important benefit of a functional eyelid with a normal eyelid margin, lined with conjunctiva. The reconstructions require experience and the correct instrumentation and are best left to those practised in such techniques.

Dermoid
Dermoids are occasionally encountered in cats. They show a familial tendency in the Birman (Hendy-Ibbs, 1985). When the eyelids are involved, a simple surgical excision can usually be performed.

Entropion
Entropion, typically secondary to painful ocular surface lesions, occasionally occurs in cats (Figure 5.52). Surgical correction is usually required. A simple skin–muscle resection (Hotz–Celsus correction) is suitable. Medial lower eyelid entropion is not uncommon in the Persian cat (for correction, see that already described for the dog).

Ectropion
Cicatricial ectropion may result from periocular injuries, such as abscesses or burns. If an isolated portion of eyelid is affected, a V resection of the affected area may correct the abnormality adequately. Following extensive contracture due to burns, reconstructive surgery utilizing techniques such as pedicle advancement flaps may be required to allow restoration of an adequate blink (Figure 5.53).

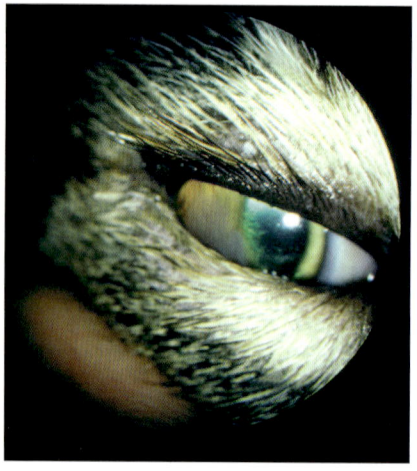

Figure 5.52 Entropion in a cat.

Distortion due to symblepharon
Extensive conjunctival adhesions (symblepharon) resulting from severe conjunctivitis, such as that caused by feline herpesvirus infection, may distort the eyelid margins. Treatment to break down the adhesions does not carry a good success rate and should probably only be attempted if exposure keratopathy has developed (see Chapter 7).

Conditions associated with cilia
Distichiasis and ectopic cilia are rare in cats, but may occasionally be encountered, especially in cats with developmental eyelid defects. Electrolysis or

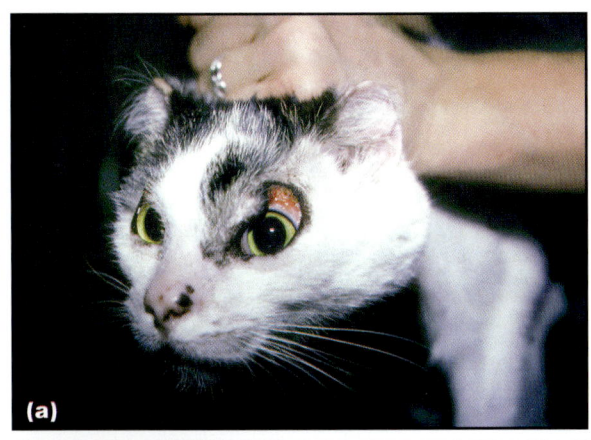

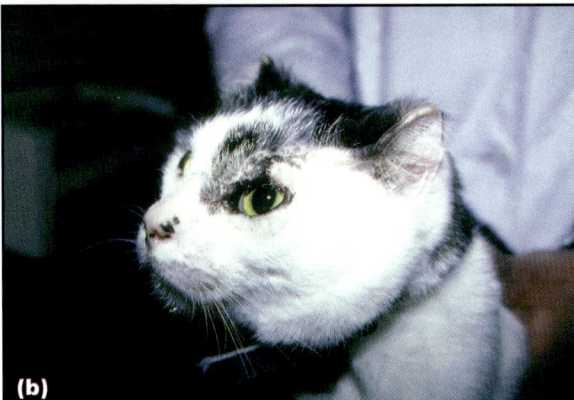

Figure 5.53 This cat was involved in a house fire. (a) There is severe contracture of the skin of the head, resulting in distortion of both upper eyelids. This has resulted in the exposure of the lateral cornea when the eyelids are closed. (b) The left upper eyelid has been reconstructed using a horizontally directed advancement flap developed from skin lateral to the upper eyelid. Following surgery, the cat was able to close its eyelids completely.

cryosurgery can be used to manage distichiasis, and surgical excision performed for removal of ectopic cilia.

Blepharitis

Blepharitis is less common in cats than dogs.

Parasitic blepharitis

Parasitic blepharitis may be caused by *Demodex cati* or *Notoedres cati*, and occurs rarely.

Superficial fungal blepharitis

Superficial fungal infection, most commonly caused by *Microsporum canis*, can involve the eyelids, but it is unlikely to be confined to them.

Bacterial blepharitis

Bacterial blepharitis is rare in cats. Localized abscessation may result from cat fight injuries. Meibomianitis is uncommon, but occasionally retention of meibomian secretion is encountered. Sometimes, the granulomas that result can be extensive and involve a considerable length of the eyelid. Treatment is by conjunctival incision and curettage, as described for the dog.

Eosinophilic eyelid plaques

Eosinophilic plaques involving the eyelids are sometimes encountered. They appear as yellowish plaques involving the palpebral conjunctiva. They may be a manifestation of eosinophilic keratoconjunctivitis and respond to megoestrol acetate therapy, although the systemic side-effects of this drug may make topical corticosteroids a preferred choice of treatment.

Neoplasia

Feline eyelid tumours are usually locally invasive and often appear as raised or ulcerative lesions.

Squamous cell carcinoma is the commonest eyelid neoplasm of the cat; exposure to sunlight is a contributory factor. It is most common in white cats. This tumour appears as a slightly raised or depressed ulcerative lesion, the margins of which can be difficult to identify (Figure 5.54). Treatment may be by surgical excision, cryotherapy or radiotherapy (Nasisse, 1991).

Basal cell carcinoma, fibrosarcoma and mast cell tumours may also affect the eyelids.

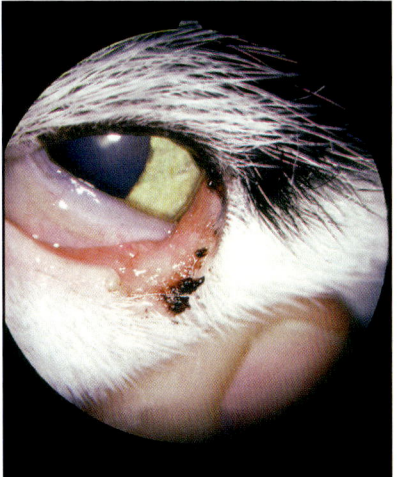

Figure 5.54 Eyelid squamous cell carcinoma in a cat.

Conditions of the third eyelid of cats

The feline third eyelid fulfils an important role in maintaining the health of the ocular surface. Its loss is not tolerated well and so removal is indicated only for primary neoplasia. Removal is not an option when neoplasia is secondary (e.g. multicentric lymphoma).

Scrolling of the third eyelid

Scrolling of the third eyelid (as described above for the dog) occurs rarely in the cat. A similar correction to that employed in the dog can be used.

Prolapse of the nictitans gland

Prolapse of the nictitans gland is occasionally encountered in the cat.

Protrusion of the third eyelid

Protrusion of the third eyelid is a common occurrence in the cat. The causes are listed in Figure 5.49.

Neoplasia of the third eyelid

Neoplasia of the third eyelid is rare in cats. Fibrosarcoma and adenocarcinoma have been reported.

References and further reading

Bedford PGC (1973) Distichiasis and its treatment by method of partial tarsal plate excision. *Journal of Small Animal Practice* **14**, 1–7

Bedford PGC (1990) Surgical correction of facial droop in the English cocker spaniel. *Journal of Small Animal Practice* **31**, 255–258

Bedford PGC (1998) Technique of lateral canthoplasty for correction of macropalpebral fissure in the dog. *Journal of Small Animal Practice* **39**, 117–121

Bedford PGC (1999) Diseases and surgery of the canine eyelid. In: *Veterinary Ophthalmology*, 3rd edn, ed. KN Gelatt, pp. 535–568. Lippincott, Williams and Wilkins, Philadelphia

Blanchard AL and Keller WF (1976) The rhomboid graft-flap for the repair of extensive ocular adnexal defects. *Journal of the American Animal Hospital Association* **12**, 576–580

Bromberg N (1980) The nictitating membrane. *Compendium of Continuing Education for the Practicing Veterinarian* **2**, 627–632

Carter JD (1973) Surgery of congenital eyelid defects. *Veterinary Clinics of North America: Small Animal Practice* **3**, 423–432

Dziezyc J and Millichamp NJ (1989) Surgical correction of eyelid agenesis in a cat. *Journal of the American Animal Hospital Association* **25**, 513–516

Gelatt KN (1972) Surgical correction of everted nictitating membrane in the dog. *Veterinary Medicine / Small Animal Clinician* **67**, 291–292

Gelatt KN (1991) The canine eyelids. In: *Veterinary Ophthalmology*, 2nd edn, ed. KN Gelatt, pp. 256–275. Lea and Febiger, Philadelphia

Gelatt KN and Blogg JP (1994) *Handbook of Small Animal Ophthalmic Surgery. Vol 1: Extraocular Procedures*. Pergamon Press, Oxford

Hendy-Ibbs PM (1985) Familial feline epibulbar dermoids. *Veterinary Record* **116**, 13–14

Johnson BW, Gerding PA, McLaughlan SA, Helper LC, Szajerski ME and Cormany KA (1988) Nonsurgical correction of entropion in shar pei puppies. *Veterinary Medicine / Small Animal Clinician* **83**, 482–483

Kaswan RL and Martin CL (1985) Surgical correction of third eyelid prolapse in dogs. *Journal of the American Veterinary Medical Association* **186**, 83

Krehbiel JD and Langham RF (1975) Eyelid neoplasms of dogs. *American Journal of Veterinary Research* **36**, 115–119

Miller WW and Braund KG (1991) Morphological and histochemical features of the normal canine orbicularis oculi muscle. *Progress in Veterinary and Comparative Ophthalmology* **1**, 150–154

Moore CP and Constantinescu GM (1997) Surgery of the adnexa. *Veterinary Clinics of North America: Small Animal Practice* **27**, 1011–1066

Morgan RV, Duddy JM and McClurg K (1993) Prolapse of the gland of the third eyelid in dogs: a retrospective study of 89 cases (1980 to 1990). *Journal of the American Animal Hospital Association* **29**, 56–60

Munger RJ and Carter JD (1984) A further modification of the Khunt–Szymanowski procedure for correction of atonic ectropion in dogs. *Journal of the American Animal Hospital Association* **20**, 651–656

Munger RJ and Gourley IM (1981) Cross lid flap for repair of larger eyelid defects. *Journal of the American Veterinary Medical Association* **178**, 45–48

Mustardé JC (1980) Reconstruction of the upper lid. In: *Repair and Reconstruction in the Orbital Region. A Practical Guide*. 2nd edn, pp. 130–151. Churchill Livingstone, Edinburgh

Nasisse MP (1991) Feline ophthalmology. In: *Veterinary Ophthalmology*, 2nd edn, ed. KN Gelatt, pp. 529–575. Lea and Febiger, Philadelphia

Pavletic MM, Nafe LA and Confer AW (1982) Mucocutaneous subdermal plexus flap from the lip for lower eyelid restoration in the dog. *Journal of the American Veterinary Medical Association* **180**, 921–926

Petersen-Jones SM (1991) Repositioning prolapsed third eyelid glands while preserving secretory function. *In Practice* **13**, 202–203

Petersen-Jones SM (1997) Quantification of the conjunctival sac bacteria in normal dogs and those suffering from keratoconjunctivitis sicca. *Veterinary and Comparative Ophthalmology* **7**, 29–35

Read RA (1995) Treatment of canine nictitans plasmacytic conjunctivitis with 0.2% cyclosporin ointment. *Journal of Small Animal Practice* **36**, 50–56

Roberts SM, Severin GA and Lavach JD (1986) Prevalence and treatment of palpebral neoplasms in the dog: 200 cases (1975–1983). *Journal of the American Veterinary Medical Association* **189**, 1355–1359

Robertson BF and Roberts SM (1995a) Lateral canthus entropion in the dog, Part 1: Comparative anatomic studies. *Veterinary and Comparative Ophthalmology* **5**, 151–156

Robertson BF and Roberts SM (1995b) Lateral canthus entropion in the dog, Part 2: Surgical correction. Results and follow-up from 21 cases (1991–1994). *Veterinary and Comparative Ophthalmology* **5**, 162–169

Spreull JSA (1982) Surgery of the eyelids in small animals. *Veterinary Annual* **22**, 279–297

Stades FC (1987) A new method for surgical correction of upper eyelid trichiasis-entropion: operation method. *Journal of the American Animal Hospital Association* **23**, 603–610

Stades FC, Boevé MH and van der Woerdt A (1992) Palpebral fissure length in the dog and cat. *Progress in Veterinary and Comparative Ophthalmology* **2**, 155–161

Stanley RG and Kaswan RL (1994) Modification of the orbital rim anchorage method for surgical replacement of the gland of the third eyelid in dogs. *Journal of the American Veterinary Medical Association* **205**, 1412–1414

Ward DA (1999) Diseases and surgery of the canine nictitating membrane. In: *Veterinary Ophthalmology*, 3rd edn, ed. KN Gelatt, pp. 609–618. Lippincott, Williams and Wilkins, Philadelphia

Wyman M (1971) Lateral canthoplasty. *Journal of the American Animal Hospital Association* **7**, 196–201

Wyman M (1979) Ophthalmic surgery for the practioner. *Veterinary Clinics of North America: Small Animal Practice* **9**, 311–348

6

The lacrimal system

Sheila Crispin

Introduction

The lacrimal system or lacrimal apparatus consists of two components: a secretory component; and an excretory component (Figure 6.1). The eyelids in this context are concerned with tear film distribution; defective spreading of the tear film is summarized briefly in this chapter, and further details are given in Chapter 5.

The secretory component produces the pre-ocular tear film, which covers the ocular surface. The ocular surface is the term used to describe the continuous epithelium that begins at the lid margin, extends on to the back of the upper and lower eyelids, both surfaces of the third eyelid, into the fornices and on to the globe. It includes the conjunctival, limbal and corneal epithelium. The close relationship of the tear film with the cornea and conjunctiva means that it is intimately concerned with both of these tissues in health and disease. It is, therefore, important to evaluate the tear film whenever there is ocular surface disease.

The excretory component consists of the upper and lower puncta and their respective canaliculi, which join at the rudimentary lacrimal sac and continue as the nasolacrimal duct.

Anatomy and physiology

The pre-ocular tear film

The pre-ocular tear film ('tear film' or ptf) covers the corneal and conjunctival epithelium. The tear film consists of an outer oily (lipid) layer; a middle aqueous layer and an inner mucin layer however, this classic trilaminar description oversimplifies what is a complex integrated structure (Figure 6.2). Normal canine ptf has a pH of 6.8–8.0, with a mean around 7.5. Normal feline tears are also slightly alkaline, with a pH of 7.2–7.8.

Secretion

The oily layer: This is largely supplied by the modified sebaceous glands known as meibomian or tarsal glands (see Chapter 5). The openings of the glands are clearly visible just anterior to the mucocutaneous junction on the eyelid margin, and the glands themselves are often visible through the semitransparent palpebral conjunctiva. The functions of this tear film component include reducing evaporative loss, enhancing tear film stability and providing an oily barrier at the eyelid margin.

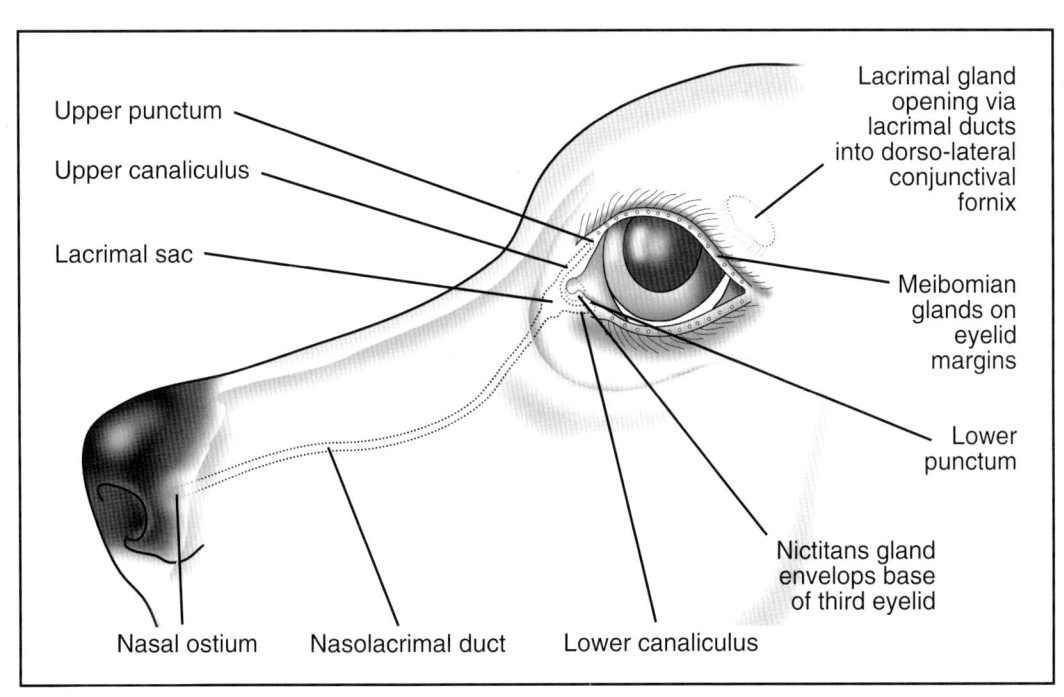

Figure 6.1 Components of the canine lacrimal system.

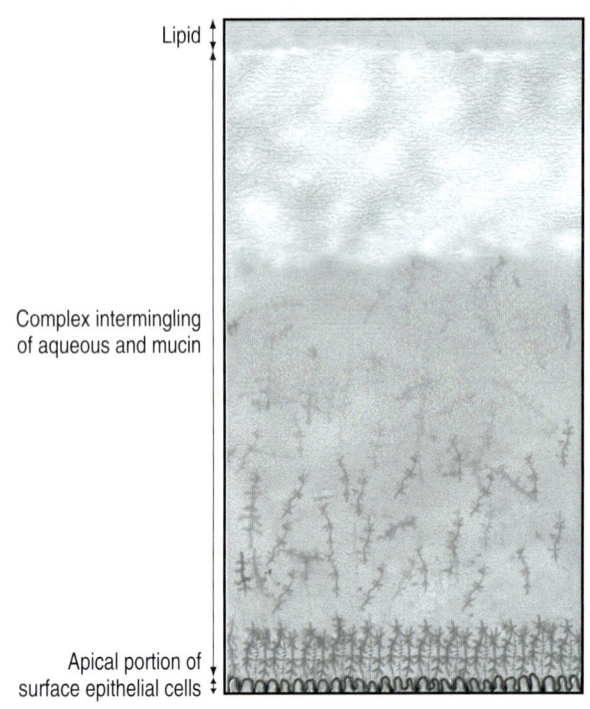

Figure 6.2 Diagrammatic representation of the pre-ocular tear film.

The aqueous layer: This is produced by the lacrimal and accessory lacrimal glands and the nictitans gland. The lacrimal gland lies under the periorbita on the dorsolateral aspect of the globe. It is responsible for most of the basal aqueous tear production. The aqueous tear component leaves the lacrimal gland via 15 to 20 microscopic ducts that open into the dorsal conjunctival sac at the dorsolateral conjunctival fornix. The nictitans gland (membrana nictitans gland) envelops the base of the T-shaped piece of hyaline cartilage that supports the third eyelid. Numerous microscopic ducts open on to the bulbar (inner) surface of the third eyelid and empty their secretion into the ventral conjunctival fornix. The nictitans gland and the lacrimal gland are histologically similar, being mixed tubulo-alveolar and tubulo-acinar secretory units. Acinar cells primarily secrete protein and mucin, while the cells of the tubules and ductules secrete serum.

Neurological control of lacrimal gland secretion is thought to involve an interaction of both cholinergic and adrenergic divisions of the autonomic nervous system. The lacrimal nerve, a branch of the ophthalmic division of the trigeminal nerve (cranial nerve V), carries both post-ganglionic parasympathetic and sympathetic efferent nerve fibres to the lacrimal gland. Pre-ganglionic parasympathetic fibres are derived from the facial (VII) nerve, and synapse with the post-ganglionic fibres at the pterygopalatine ganglion. Cholinergic and adrenergic nerve terminals are distributed in a similar fashion throughout the lacrimal and nictititans glands (Powell and Martin, 1989).

The functions of the aqueous portion of the tear film include corneal lubrication, nutrition and protection. In tear-deficient dry eye, it is the aqueous component that is most commonly inadequate.

The mucin layer: This portion is less well understood; separate goblet cell (secretive) and glycocalyx (membrane-bound) pathways have been demonstrated in the dog (Hicks *et al.*, 1997). The transmembrane mucin derived from surface epithelial cells probably has a crucial role to play in maintaining the structural integrity of the tear film.

Distribution

Normal blinking and third eyelid movement help spread the tear film and aid tear drainage (see Chapter 5).

Excretion

While a portion of the ptf is lost by evaporation, most of the tears drain via the nasolacrimal system.

The lacrimal puncta: The upper and lower lacrimal puncta are located in the upper and lower eyelids, approximately 3–4 mm from the medial canthus at the medial limit of the meibomian glands (Figure 6.3). The puncta are usually situated 1–2 mm to the conjunctival aspect of the eyelid margin. Arising from the lacrimal puncta are the upper and lower lacrimal canaliculi, which course away from the eyelid margin for a short distance and then head medially through the periorbita, where they join to form the lacrimal sac.

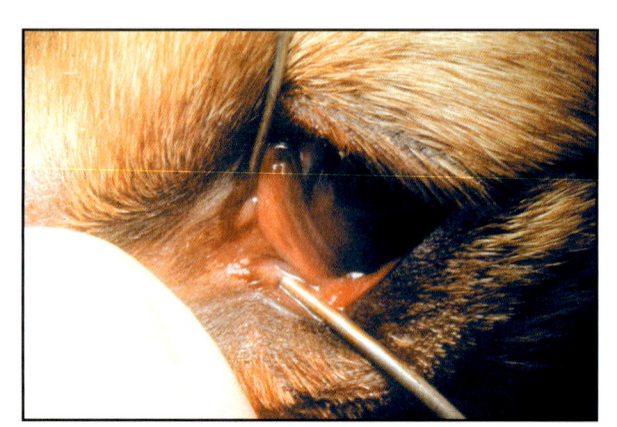

Figure 6.3 Lacrimal probes placed in the upper and lower lacrimal puncta.

The lacrimal sac: The lacrimal sac lies in a funnel-shaped depression within the lacrimal bone, known as the lacrimal fossa. The sac is poorly developed in the dog and cat, being no more than a slight dilation at the meeting of the two lacrimal canaliculi, just beneath the medial canthal ligament.

The nasolacrimal duct: This arises from the lacrimal sac and forms a dorsally concave arch. In non-brachycephalic breeds, it passes rostrally from the lacrimal sac through the lacrimal canal of the lacrimal bone and maxilla and then, no longer covered by bone, on the medial aspect of the maxilla, under the nasal mucosa. It ends by opening on to the ventrolateral floor of the nasal vestibule below the alar fold, approximately 1 cm caudal to the external nares. The rostral opening is known as the nasal ostium or nasal punctum, and cannot be visualized without a speculum or fibreoptic light source. The diameter of the nasolacrimal duct is at its smallest within the lacrimal canal immediately distal to the lacrimal sac. In approximately 50% of dogs there is communication with the nasal cavity via an accessory opening in the medial wall of the nasolacrimal duct, at the level of the root of the upper canine tooth. The nasolacrimal duct distal to the accessory opening remains patent in these individuals.

The nasolacrimal duct is longer and narrower in non-brachycephalic (dolichocephalic and mesocephalic) breeds of dog. In contrast, the brachycephalic breeds have a shorter, wider and more tortuous nasolacrimal duct, and the location of the nasal ostium is more variable.

Tear drainage: Tear drainage mechanisms have not been fully investigated in the dog and cat, most accounts being extrapolated from human studies. The action of blinking propels tears medially into the lacrimal lake, which is the collection of tears at the medial canthus, situated between the nictitating membrane and the lower palpebral conjunctiva. During blinking, contraction of the orbicularis oculi muscle causes the occlusion of the lacrimal puncta and compression of the lacrimal canaliculi, thus forcing tears into the lacrimal sac and the nasolacrimal duct. A valve mechanism within the lacrimal sac prevents reflux. Tear drainage is further aided by the dilation of the lacrimal sac during blinking, due to the insertion of orbicularis oculi muscle fibres on its lateral wall. The subsequent generation of a negative pressure draws tears into the lacrimal sac from the canaliculi. Thus, the canaliculi are primed for a subsequent blink.

Investigation of dysfunction and disease

Investigation of lacrimal dysfunction and ocular surface disease requires careful inspection of the external eye and adnexa. Particular attention should be paid to:

- The animal's conformation
- The presence, position and size of the lacrimal puncta
- The position of normal and extraneous hairs
- The nature and position of any ocular discharge
- The site and extent of any inflammation.

Assessment of tear film distribution is made by observing the rate and adequacy of normal blinks, and also by ensuring that the third eyelid is present and that its mobility is normal (see Chapter 5).

Clinical problems are broadly classified into those associated with tear production and evaporation, and those associated with tear drainage. Dry eye problems are common in veterinary practice and may be developmental or acquired and a consequence of tear deficiency (tear-deficient dry eye – TDDE) or excessive evaporation (evaporative dry eye – EDE), but the categories are not mutually exclusive. Drainage problems are also common, and may be developmental or acquired.

Samples for analysis may be required on occasions: irrigating fluid from a nasolacrimal flush can be collected into a sterile container, and swabs, impression smears and scrapes can be taken from the eyelid margins or conjunctiva for culture and sensitivity. Biopsy material can be obtained by excision or aspiration, but it must be noted that aspiration cytology is often difficult to interpret, and, therefore, not as accurate as histopathology.

Assessing surface damage

Fluorescein

A single drop of sterile saline is placed on a fluorescein-impregnated paper strip which is then applied lightly to the dorsal palpebral conjunctiva. Alternatively, a single drop of fluorescein can be applied to the ocular surface. The ocular surface is best viewed with a slit lamp using the standard blue exciter filter.

Rose bengal

When applied in liquid form, rose bengal causes pain, particularly in patients with dry eye, where the dye is taken up into the surface cells. In the USA, rose bengal is available as an impregnated paper strip, which is well tolerated when released with a drop of sterile saline. Rose bengal is not used routinely, but can be applied after fluorescein, if staining with that is negative. The ocular surface is viewed in white light. Any ocular surface staining is best seen over the white of the sclera where there is good contrast. It is less easily observed where contrast is less, such as when the cornea is viewed over a dark brown iris. Staining is apparently associated with loss of a mucin-like material, which could be glycocalyx, at the apical surface of the epithelial cells (Watanabe and Tanaka, 1996).

Testing tear production

Schirmer tear test (STT)

Tear production is most commonly assessed using the Schirmer I tear test (see Chapter 1a). There are significant differences between the values obtained in the unanaesthetized eye (Schirmer I) and the anaesthetized eye (Schirmer II). In the majority of normal adult dogs and cats, a reading of 20 ± 5 mm/min is obtained. The range is large: in one canine study the values ranged from 13.3–27.2 mm/min (Wyman *et al*, 1995). In another study in the adult cat (Brown *et al.*, 1997), the range was 12.5–31.0 mm/min. Readings of less than 10 mm/min are significant, when taken in conjunction with other signs of ocular surface disease. However, STT readings in young animals can be low in apparently normal eyes.

There is also variation between eyes, individuals and breeds. Furthermore, Håkanson and Arnesson (1997) demonstrated quite wide variation on different days in young normal Beagles, and suggested that serial measurements over several days would provide a more accurate assessment of tear production in individual animals.

Phenol red thread (PRT) test

This provides an indirect measurement of tear production that is subject to less variation than the STT and is better tolerated by the patient. It has been evaluated in both the dog (Brown et al., 1996) and cat (Brown et al, 1997). In 20 dogs (mean age 5.08 years), the mean length of absorption for the PRT test without anaesthesia was 34.15 ± 4.45 mm per 15 seconds, with a range of 20–41 mm/15 s. In 10 dogs of mean age 6.81 years, the mean length of absorption was 32.9 ± 4.89 mm/15 s without topical anaesthesia, and 30.6 ± 7.62 mm/15 s after topical anaesthesia. In a study of 28 normal adult cats (Brown et al., 1997), the mean length of absorption for the PRT test without anaesthesia was 23.04 ± 2.23 mm per 15 seconds, with a range of 18.5–28.0 mm/15 s. After topical anaesthesia, it was 23.89 ± 2.17 mm/15 sec, with a range of 18.5–28.0 mm/15 s. There were, therefore, no significant differences between the means of the PRT test with or without topical anaesthesia in either species.

Testing tear stability

Fluorescein break-up test (FBUT)

Premature break-up of the tear film is a feature of any form of dry eye and may be demonstrated by this test. It is a provocative test, in so far as fluorescein shortens the normal break-up time.

A drop of fluorescein is applied to the eye and the animal is allowed to blink. The eyelids are then held open and the cornea is observed with a slit lamp biomicroscope with blue exciter filter in place. In the dog, the normal average time between the first blink and observation of the first dry spot is approximately 20 ± 5 seconds (Moore et al., 1987). Values of <10 s are indicative of tear film instability.

Testing tear drainage

Dysfunction of the excretory component of the lacrimal apparatus usually gives rise to inadequate drainage of tears with subsequent epiphora (Figure 6.4). Assessment of the patency of the nasolacrimal apparatus is crucial in the investigation of epiphora.

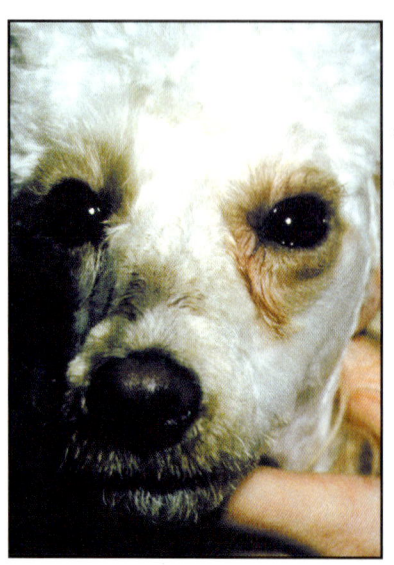

Figure 6.4 Bilateral epiphora in a Miniature Poodle. The tear staining is unsightly in light-coated dogs.

Direct examination

The presence, size and position of the upper and lower lacrimal puncta should be noted as part of any ophthalmological examination. The openings can be examined by slightly everting the eyelid margins in this region. The tissue in their immediate vicinity is usually unpigmented. The eyelid margin in the punctal region will kink slightly when the eyelid is manipulated. Examination of the lacrimal puncta is facilitated by both magnification and illumination with either a slit-lamp biomicroscope, a direct ophthalmoscope, an examination loupe and transilluminator, or an otoscope with the speculum removed.

Fluorescein drainage test

This assesses the entire mechanism of tear drainage by determining both anatomical and physiological patency. It involves installing fluorescein into the conjunctival sac and noting the time taken for dye to emerge from the ipsilateral nostril (Figure 6.5). If the dye is applied to both eyes simultaneously, it is important to observe fluorescein as it emerges from the ventrolateral surface of the external nares before licking spreads the dye over both sides of the nose. It is often less confusing to test each side separately. In normal mesocephalic and dolichocephalic dogs, fluorescein should be visible at the ipsilateral nostril within 4 minutes. There is little value in continuing observation if fluorescein is not apparent 10 minutes after its administration.

The test is most useful when there is a unilateral obstruction to tear passage, in which case the difference in transit time between the two eyes is readily apparent. A standard blue exciter filter and dark conditions will facilitate the detection of fluorescein, which fluoresces green. The limitation of this test lies in the number of false negative results it gives. Tear drainage into the caudal nasal cavity and thence into the nasopharynx is common in the brachycephalic breeds of dog, and in cats. Such individuals are negative for a fluorescein drainage test, although the excretory component of the nasolacrimal system is patent. Sometimes the caudal drainage of tears can be determined by the observation of fluorescein in the oropharynx or on the tongue.

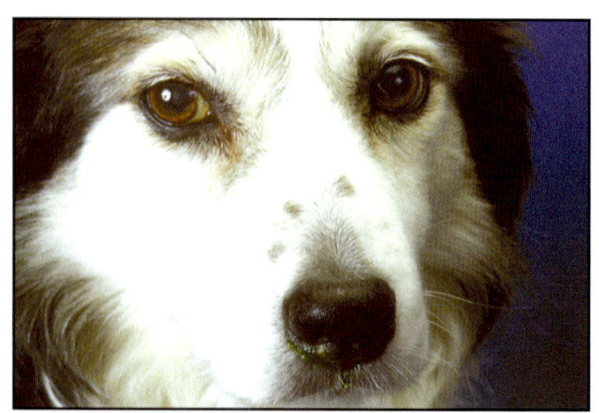

Figure 6.5 Normal passage of fluorescein, which appeared at the ipsilateral nostril within 30 seconds of application to the conjunctival sac.

Fibreoptic illumination

Bright illumination from a narrow fibreoptic light source cannulating the proximal part of the drainage system is a useful device in the investigation of lacrimal drainage problems involving the canaliculi or lacrimal sac. Alternatively, the puncta and canaliculi can be probed very gently using an appropriately sized lacrimal probe (e.g. Bowman).

Cannulation and irrigation

This is essentially a test of the anatomical patency of the nasolacrimal system. In many dogs it is possible to perform it under topical anaesthesia, but general anaesthesia should always be used in small dogs and cats to avoid causing inadvertent damage. When performed under general anaesthesia, the head should be tilted downwards and the pharynx packed with moistened gauze bandage or swabs, to prevent aspiration. Different types of metal and plastic cannulae are available, but the design and properties (e.g. malleability coupled with rigidity) of silver lacrimal cannulae make them the best choice; they are also readily sterilized for repeated use (Figure 6.6). Disposable plastic cannulae are also available (Figure 6.6). Plastic lacrimal cannulae can be rendered more rigid by cutting them shorter, but the sharp-edged tip should be blunted by flaming prior to use. Both plastic and metal cannulae should be used with care to avoid damaging the puncta and canaliculi.

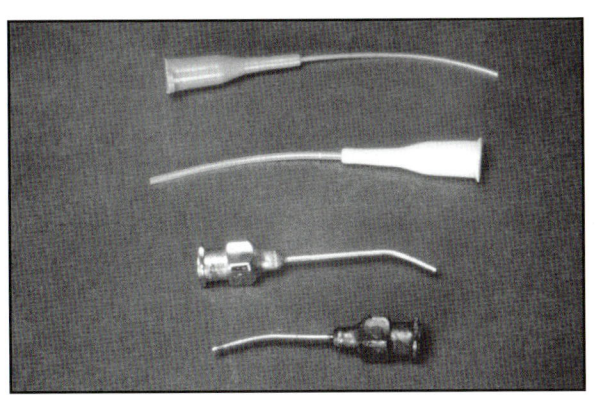

Figure 6.6 Plastic and metal lacrimal cannulae.

1. Cannulate the dorsal punctum with a sterile lacrimal cannula, which is then attached to a syringe of sterile saline or sterile water (Figure 6.7).
2. Establish patency of the lower punctum and canaliculus by applying digital pressure to the lacrimal sac region while slowly injecting the irrigating fluid. If fluid emerges from the lower punctum, it confirms the anatomical patency of the upper and lower lacrimal puncta and canaliculi and the lacrimal sac.
3. Occlude the lower punctum by applying direct digital pressure, so that patency of the nasolacrimal duct can be demonstrated when the head is lowered. When the tears drain caudally, as in brachycephalic dogs and cats, the saline passes into the nasopharynx and elicits an obvious swallowing response in the conscious animal.
4. If the irrigant is required for culture and sensitivity testing, it is usually collected from the nostrils.

Gentle sustained pressure should be all that is required to irrigate the lacrimal drainage apparatus. If resistance is met, then the cannula should be repositioned before assuming the presence of an obstruction.

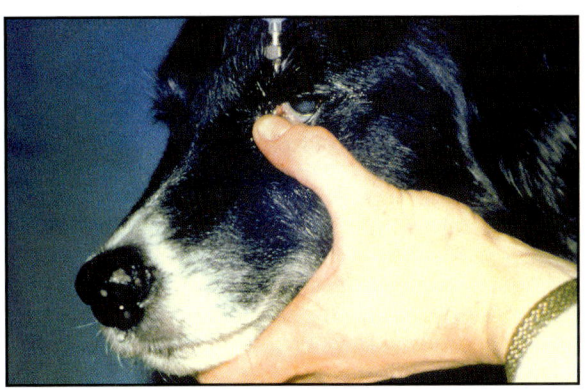

Figure 6.7 Irrigation of the nasolacrimal drainage system with sterile water via the upper punctum in a conscious, non-sedated dog; note the water dripping from the nose. A lacrimal cannula has been passed into the upper punctum and canaliculus after applying a drop of local anaesthetic to the upper punctum.

It is better to use a urinary catheter rather than a cannula if the whole of the excretory component of the lacrimal system is to be explored, albeit indirectly. The upper punctum is the entry point of choice:

1. Introduce a suitably sized sterile urinary catheter into the upper punctum.
2. Pass the catheter without any force via the upper canaliculus and lacrimal sac into the nasolacrimal duct.
3. Advance the catheter until it exits at the external nares via the nasal ostium (Crispin, 1987).

Minor difficulties in manipulating the catheter may be encountered in the region of the lacrimal foramen and nasal ostium; if so, the catheter should be withdrawn slightly before the manoeuvre is repeated.

Less commonly, the system is catheterized in retrograde fashion via the nasal ostium, after placing a nasal speculum to spread the exteral nares and using a fine fibre optic light source to improve visibility.

Dacryocystorhinography

This radiographic technique (see also Chapter 1) can be used to delineate the nasolacrimal system. It is indicated in some cases of persistent or recurrent epiphora, in order to evaluate anatomical patency of the nasolacrimal system. The site, extent and degree of nasolacrimal obstruction can be visualized. In addition, developmental defects, dilations, deviations and stenosis of the nasolacrimal system may also be seen.

Under general anaesthesia, the upper punctum is cannulated, and 1–2 ml of contrast agent (meglumine iothalamate 60% w/v) is injected, after occluding the lower punctum by applying tissue forceps. Lateral and dorsoventral radiographic views should be taken as the radiopaque medium is injected, or immediately afterwards. Delineation of the nasolacrimal duct in brachycephalic breeds is often obscured by the rapid appearance of contrast medium in the nasal cavity and nasopharynx.

Canine lacrimal apparatus – secretory problems

The wet eye
Epiphora is defined as tear overflow because of impaired tear drainage, and must be distinguished from increased lacrimation due to painful or irritating ocular conditions (reflex tear secretion), as well as disease of the paranasal sinuses and mechanical or olfactory stimulation of the nasal mucosa. Increased lacrimation and inadequate tear drainage can exist concurrently.

The dry eye
Dry eye is a consequence of tear deficiency (TDDE) or increased evaporative loss (EDE), or a combination of the two. EDE is often related to meibomian gland disease, but may also be caused by abnormal eyelid structure or function (e.g. overlong palpebral aperture, poor eyelid/globe congruity, inadequate blink). A standard protocol should be adopted for investigation (Figure 6.8).

1. Find out the age, breed, sex, history (including previous and present treatment) and clinical signs
2. Observe the normal blink and protective blink
3. Perform a detailed examination, with magnification, of all three eyelids and the ocular surface
4. Perform a Schirmer I tear test
5. Perform a phenol red thread test
6. Perform a fluorescein break-up test (FBUT)
7. Apply rose bengal

Figure 6.8 Protocol for the investigation of dry eye problems. Investigations 5–7 are not a routine part of the assessment.

Lipid abnormalities
Meibomian gland dysfunction is an important cause of evaporative dry eye. Developmental eyelid defects may affect the number and distribution of the meibomian glands. Both qualitative and quantitative alterations in meibomian gland secretion may be of significance.

Acquired lipid abnormalities involving the meibomian glands include marginal blepharitis (inflammation of the eyelid margins), which is commonly caused by bacteria (staphylococci and streptococci) or, less commonly, by parasites, yeasts and fungi (see Chapter 5). In addition to meibomian gland involvement as part of eyelid inflammation, the glands can themselves become inflamed (meibomianitis) or infected. Meibomian gland secretions become inspissated because of obstruction of the gland duct, resulting in a sterile lipogranulomatous response (chalazion). Rupture of the affected glands will result in a more diffuse granulomatous response, and secondary infection will also result in extensive eyelid swelling.

While meibomian gland dysfunction is usually a feature of local eyelid disease, more generalized involvement of the skin and mucous membranes should alert the clinician to less common disorders, such as erythema multiforme (Figure 6.9), that are apparently connected with acute hypersensitivity reactions which result in immune complex-mediated vasculitis.

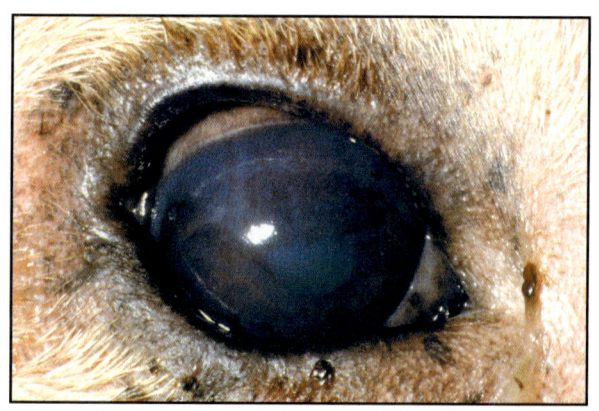

Figure 6.9 Complex tear film abnormalities in a Labrador Retriever with erythema multiforme.

Surgical techniques that remove the meibomian glands, for example, partial tarsal plate excision as a treatment for distichiasis, may be complicated subsequently by evaporative dry eye.

Clinical problems, most seriously corneal ulceration, can occur in breeds susceptible to exposure keratopathy, such as the Pekingese (Figure 6.10).

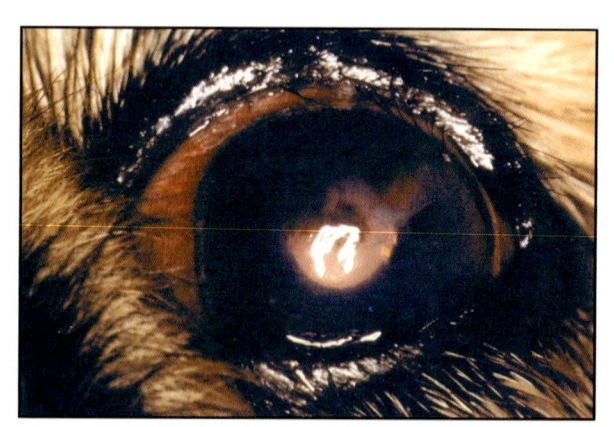

Figure 6.10 Dysfunctional tear film and ulcerative keratitis in a Pekingese. Distichiasis had been treated by partial tarsal plate excision. The tear film was unstable, with a fluorescein break-up time of <8 seconds. The eyelids were scarred, some facial hairs were contacting the cornea and the dog still had distichiasis.

Clinical features: In developmental disease, the number and distribution of the glands may be abnormal; for example, no glands are apparent in regions with colobomatous eyelid defects, and the number and distribution of the glands may be irregular in dogs which develop distichiasis.

In acquired disease, there are a great many potential alterations: the eyelids may be thickened, their margin distorted, or the meibomian gland openings may be prominent, inflamed or obliterated. Excessive secretion or secretions of abnormal appearance may be present; alternatively, there may be no obvious secretion. Gentle pressure may fail to express meibomian oil from the orifices, or the secretion which emerges is of abnormal appearance.

The consequences of abnormal meibomian gland function are to increase evaporative loss, with premature break-up of the tear film; the latter phenomenon is common to all forms of dry eye. Swabs, impression smears and scrapes can be taken from the eyelid margins for microscopy; culture and sensitivity may also be performed when infection is suspected. Biopsy material can be obtained by total or partial excision of the affected portion of the eyelids or gland incision.

Diagnosis: The diagnosis of meibomian lipid abnormalities is largely subjective, based on history and clinical appearance; tests of increased evaporative loss, such as tear film break-up time, may be suggestive. Careful observation of blinking and examination of the eyelids is essential, particularly the number and distribution of the openings of the meibomian glands at the eyelid margin, and the glands themselves, beneath the eyelid. The tear film break-up time may be decreased. In severe meibomian gland disease there may be keratoconjunctivitis, with or without punctate epitheliopathy.

Treatment: Local meibomianitis can be treated with an ointment containing an antibiotic and corticosteroid combination applied to the eyelid margin. Warm compresses may also be useful if the condition has not been present for long and involvement is focal. In other respects, treatment is as for blepharitis (see Chapter 5). Treatment of chalazia, either single or multiple, usually requires incision of the overlying palpebral conjunctiva and curettage or surgical excision.

Treatment of eyelid infections consists of careful cleaning using bland isotonic solutions or baby shampoo (diluted 1 in 20 with isotonic solution), combined with the use of appropriate therapeutic agents. Topical application of a suitable antibiotic, antifungal or parasiticide is required and, most importantly, systemic administration of an appropriate drug for a minimum of 3–4 weeks may also be required (see Chapter 5).

Meibomian gland dysfunction associated with systemic disease may be treated symptomatically while the systemic disease is managed.

Aqueous deficiency

Deficiency in the lacrimal and nictitans component of the tear film produces the classic tear-deficient dry eye (Figures 6.11–6.13). Abnormalities of lacrimation associated with neurological dysfunction are described in Chapter 15.

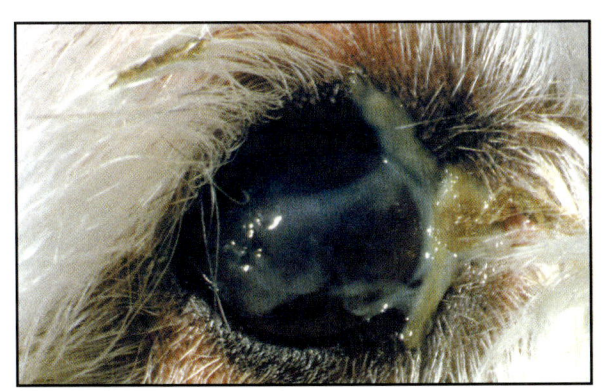

Figure 6.11 Immune-mediated keratoconjunctivitis sicca (KCS) in a West Highland White Terrier. There is an extensive ocular discharge and the cornea has a dull and lacklustre appearance.

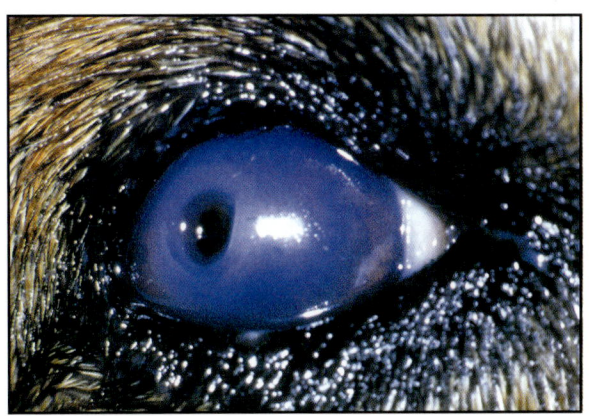

Figure 6.12 Acute KCS and ulcerative keratitis (from which *Pseudomonas aeruginosa* was cultured). The dog, a Jack Russell Terrier, had suffered multiple injuries in a road traffic accident, including urethral rupture, and was uraemic and severely dehydrated on presentation.

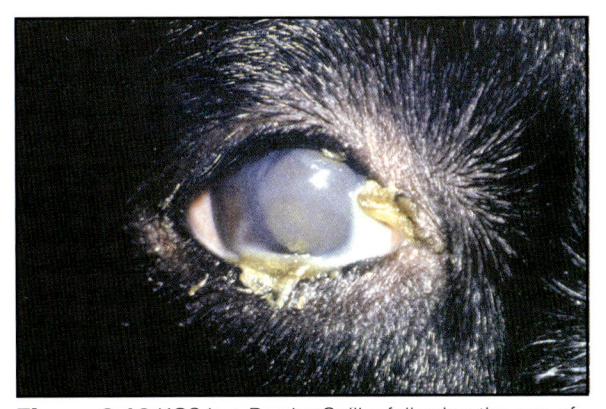

Figure 6.13 KCS in a Border Collie, following the use of the sulphonamide salazopyrin for colitis.

Developmental causes: These may be a consequence of aplasia or hypoplasia of the lacrimal gland and/or the nictitans gland and the associated nerve supply. In affected animals the nose is often dry. Yorkshire Terriers, Pugs and English Springer Spaniels are most commonly affected.

Acquired causes: These include immune-mediated disease; systemic diseases (e.g. distemper); surgery (e.g. removal of the nictitans gland); direct trauma (bite wounds, blows to the head, chemical injury, irradiation); afferent and efferent arm lesions, including facial (VII) nerve damage (neurogenic origin); lacrimotoxic drugs (e.g. sulphonamides); ageing; and metabolic disease (e.g. hypothyroidism). The disease may also be idiopathic. Immune-mediated disease is probably the commonest of the possible acquired causes. Neutered animals, irrespective of their gender, are predisposed to age-related keratoconjunctivitis sicca (KCS) (Kaswan *et al.*, 1991).

A number of sedatives and general anaesthetics will produce transient reductions in tear production; some combinations, e.g. xylazine and butorphanol (Dodam *et al.*, 1998), cause a profound decrease. Topically or parenterally administered atropine will also reduce tear production. The results of Schirmer tear testing should not form the basis of diagnosis and future management of KCS under these circumstances.

Keratoconjunctivitis sicca

KCS is primarily a result of aqueous deficiency, but the problem is chronically exacerbated by abnormalities of mucin production. Certain breeds appear to be particularly at risk of developing KCS; these include the English Bulldog, West Highland White Terrier, Cavalier King Charles Spaniel, Lhasa Apso and Shih Tsu.

Clinical signs: The appearance is variable: disruption of the corneal reflex, a lacklustre appearance of the cornea, superficial keratitis and diffuse conjunctivitis are common. Pain, blepharospasm and sometimes corneal ulceration are more likely in acute-onset KCS. Chronic KCS, however, is uncomfortable rather than painful, and affected animals present with conjunctival thickening, corneal vascularization, pigmentation and, eventually, xerosis. Xerosis is the extreme dryness associated with keratinization of the ocular surface in chronic disease. In all cases, there is an ocular discharge but this is of variable appearance and quantity. The discharge is most commonly yellow or green in colour and of a tenacious consistency; it is particularly obvious where it is adherent to the cornea. Secondary opportunist bacterial conjunctivitis is frequently associated with KCS and is a common reason for failure to diagnose the underlying primary problem.

Diagnosis: The diagnosis is made on the basis of clinical signs and Schirmer tear tests; the Schirmer I tear test (STT I) is employed routinely (see Chapter 1a and above). It is important to test both eyes and to recheck regularly as part of the management regime.

Drug treatment: This depends on investigating the primary cause and treating it if possible. While thyroid hormone replacement therapy will be effective as treatment for KCS in hypothyroid animals, sulphonamide-induced KCS is rarely completely reversible. As clinical signs of KCS have been reported within 30 days of starting sulphonamide therapy in susceptible dogs (Diehl and Roberts, 1991), systemic use of sulphonamides should be avoided in these cases if possible. Failing this, tear production should be monitored during their use. Animals with immune-mediated KCS invariably require treatment for life.

KCS is usually managed medically with a variety of drug combinations after, most importantly, cleaning the eyes carefully with tepid boiled water to remove the tenacious discharge. Drugs used include lacrimostimulants, lacrimomimetics, mucolytics, antibiotics and anti-inflammmatories. Medical management is also discussed in Chapter 3.

- Lacrostimulants:
  - Topical cyclosporin is the drug of choice for management of most types of canine KCS (Kaswan and Salisbury, 1990; Gilger and Allen, 1998). It is most commonly applied twice daily and, as the maximal response to treatment may take many weeks, it is important not to discontinue treatment without a trial of at least 6–8 weeks, monitoring any changes in STT levels. However, as cyclosporin helps to reduce the ocular surface changes seen in chronic disease, it could be argued that it is indicated even without an increase in STT values. Responsive cases (improved appearance and comfort, with or without increased STT values) usually require treatment for life with once- or twice-daily maintenance therapy.
  - Pilocarpine has been used much less frequently since the introduction of cyclosporin. KCS of neurogenic origin may respond well to treatment with oral pilocarpine 1%, although its use is not devoid of potential side-effects; Moore (1999) sets out the guidelines which should be followed.
- Lacrimomimetics/mucinomimetics: There are many commercially available preparations, but those of particular value are a hyaluron derivative (available in North America), carbomer 940 and polyacrylic acid (both available in Europe). These preparations are an important aspect of long-term medical management
- Mucolytics: Mucolytics such as acetylcysteine are rather expensive for extended use, but may be useful in the initial stages to remove excessive mucin.
- Antibiotics: A course of broad-spectrum topical antibiotic may be required if bacterial overgrowth exacerbates the clinical presentation. The antibiotic should be selected on the basis of bacterial culture and sensitivity testing, and may be discontinued once the infection is brought under control.
- Anti-inflammatories: Topical corticosteroids are useful when immune-mediated KCS is suspected and in those cases in which there is a vascular non-ulcerative keratitis. Prednisolone acetate, although a potent topical anti-inflammatory agent, should be reserved for the treatment of intraocular inflammation. Preparations such as betamethasone sodium phosphate, prednisolone sodium phosphate, dexamethasone with hypromellose, and fluorometholone are effective anti-inflammatories. Fluorometholone penetrates less well into the eye than the other preparations and this may be of advantage in the treatment of the superficial corneal and conjunctival changes associated with KCS. There are also preparations that contain antibiotics and ocular lubricants as well as corticosteroids, and this is a treatment option when secondary opportunist infection is present. Corticosteroids should not be used if corneal ulceration is present, and owners should be warned that, if ulcers develop, their use should be discontinued and veterinary advice sought.

Surgical management: If the loss of tear production is absolute and permanent, if the owners cannot manage medical therapy or if the clinical signs are not kept under control with medical treatment, then parotid duct transposition (pdt), should be considered. Parotid duct transposition should only be performed after checking that the KCS is permanent and that the parotid salivary gland actually produces saliva, and after discussing the possible postoperative management and appearance with the owners, at some length. Possible immediate complications of parotid duct transposition (pdt) include those associated with poor assessment and surgical mishaps. Postoperative problems include ocular discomfort, blepharitis, excessively wet eyes and face, periorbital hair loss, skin excoriation and corneal deposition (usually calcium salts). Owners should be warned that they may find an over-wet eye as unpleasant as one that is too dry, and advised on how they can best manage long-term complications such as blepharitis (see Chapter 5). Ocular discomfort may be associated with excessively alkaline parotid saliva (pH may be above 8.3); standard pH test papers can be used to test the pH of the parotid saliva before surgery is performed, so that owners can be alerted to this possibility. The bacteria isolated from the conjunctival sac change both qualitatively and quantitatively following pdt and bacterial overgrowth may be a contributory factor in post-pdt blepharitis (Petersen-Jones, 1997). The immunological composition of tears and parotid saliva differs, in that tears are richest in IgA, followed by IgG, and IgM is absent, whereas parotid saliva is richest in IgA, there is less IgG than in tears, and IgM is present (Jiménez et al., 1992).

It is worth being particularly cautious in advising surgery for very greedy dogs, and it is always sensible to divide the feeds up over a 24-hour period to provide optimum lubrication after surgery has been performed. There are many minor variations in the way the surgery can be carried out (Wyman, 1979; Moore, 1999). If patients are selected carefully, the results of surgery are very rewarding (Figure 6.14). On rare occasions, the effects of parotid duct transposition may need to be reversed by repositioning the duct in the mouth, a more reliable procedure than ligation of the parotid duct.

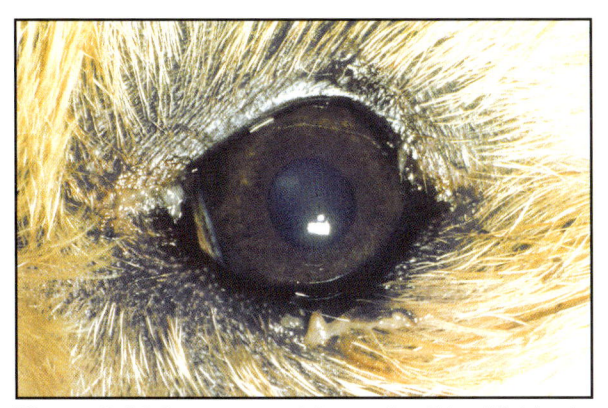

Figure 6.14 Appearance of the eye in a West Highland White Terrier two years after parotid duct transposition.

Mucin abnormality

Mucin deficiency may lead to evaporative dry eye and is seen most commonly as a consequence of chronic conjunctivitis and in association with KCS. Generalized conditions, including burns, immune-mediated disease, infection and chronic inflammation may also be a cause of mucin abnormality. Dry eye syndromes, for example, those associated with erythema multiforme and toxic epidermal necrosis, may be a consequence of goblet cell loss and damage to the lacrimal and meibomian gland orifices.

Clinical signs: The clinical signs are those of EDE, i.e. usually chronic keratoconjunctivitis, often coupled with no ocular discharge and normal aqueous production (Moore, 1990). Punctate epitheliopathy with frank fluorescein-positive erosions may be part of the clinical presentation and typically responds poorly to treatment, or tends to recur once treatment is stopped.

Diagnosis: This is based on the clinical signs, the fluorescein break-up test and conjunctival biopsy. Fluorescein break-up time is approximately 20 seconds in the normal dog, but, in mucin-deficient animals, the tear film usually breaks up in less than 5 seconds (Moore, 1990). Conjunctival biopsy allows epithelial goblet cells to be quantified; samples should be taken from the lower conjunctival fornix (between the third eyelid and lower eyelid), an area with a high density of goblet cells in the normal dog.

Treatment: The mainstay of treatment is the topical application of mucinomimetics or mucin replacers (e.g. polyvinyl alcohol or polyacrylic acid). Topical corticosteroids are also indicated in those cases in which there is marked mononuclear cell infiltration, provided that no ulceration is present.

Canine tear film – distribution problems

Evaporative tear loss leading to exposure keratopathy is the commonest consequence of defective spreading of the tear film (Figure 6.15). There are a great number of possible reasons for defective tear film distribution, including poor congruity between the eyelids and globe, and inadequate blinking. Possible causes are summarized in Figure 6.16.

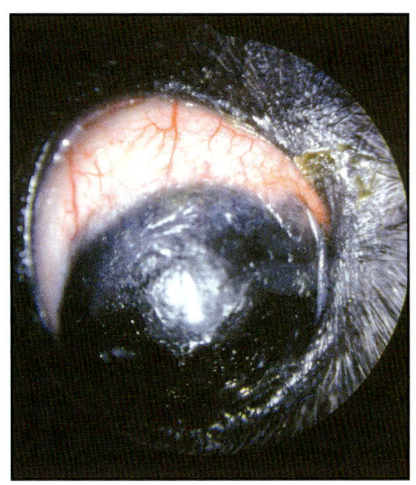

Figure 6.15 Exposure keratopathy and dry eye in a Lhasa Apso from which the third eyelid had been removed some years earlier.

The lacrimal system

Eyelid problems
Developmental defects: e.g. agenesis, coloboma, oversized palpebral aperture (macropalpebral fissure), entropion, ectropion
Breed-related anatomical anomalies: e.g. the deep medial canthus of long-nosed breeds, such as the Dobermann
Breed-related anatomical abnormalities: e.g. the various manifestations of 'diamond' eye in some large breeds
Acquired defects: e.g. absence of the third eyelid; deformities resulting from trauma, surgery, infection and ageing
Eyelid, conjunctival, limbal or corneal masses may also interfere with congruity and the distribution of the ptf
Prominent or enlarged eye
Anatomical/breed-related: e.g Pekingese and Pug
Exophthalmos and proptosis due to retrobulbar or periorbital swelling/infiltration
Buphthalmos or hydrophthalmos as a result of glaucoma
A result of intraocular space-occupying lesions
Globe prolapse
Inadequate blink response
Reduced or absent blinking usually involves defective motor function (cranial nerve VII), deficient corneal sensation (cranial nerve V) or, less commonly, intracranial lesions

Figure 6.16 Causes of defective tear film distribution in dogs.

Canine tear film – excretory problems

Developmental defects

Lacrimal punctal aplasia or imperforate punctum
This is a common developmental abnormality of the nasolacrimal system in the dog. It occurs in all breeds, although the American and English Cocker Spaniel, Bedlington Terrier, Golden Retriever, Miniature and Toy Poodle, Samoyed and Sealyham Terrier appear to be predisposed. Studies in the Golden Retriever and Cocker Spaniel indicated a familial tendency but have not revealed a mode of inheritance (Barnett, 1979).

The cause of the condition has not been fully determined. The nasolacrimal system develops embryologically from a solid cord of ectodermal cells that becomes canalized during development. Incomplete canalization might result in an imperforate lacrimal punctum, micropunctum or aplasia of any part of the nasolacrimal system. The problem is probably present from birth, but the presenting signs of epiphora due to inadequate tear drainage are usually not seen until after 8 weeks of age. The severity of the epiphora is variable, but it generally gives rise to rust-coloured staining of the medial canthal skin and the hair ventral to this region. Epiphora is more obvious in dogs with a pale coat.

This condition can affect the upper or lower punctum, or both, and may be unilateral or bilateral. The lower punctum is more commonly affected than the upper punctum. In unilateral cases, the other eye may be normal or have some other developmental defect, such as micropunctum.

Diagnosis: Veterinary advice is usually sought because the dog has epiphora. A diagnosis of lacrimal punctal aplasia may be made by careful examination using magnification and illumination (Figure 6.17). The position of an imperforate punctum is sometimes marked by the presence of a thin translucent sheet of mucous membrane overlying the canaliculus. Other indications of its position include a small depression in the conjunctiva overlying the canaliculus, or a small pigmented spot. In cases where there are no such indications, the diagnosis of imperforate punctum should be confirmed prior to surgical treatment by cannulating and flushing the nasolacrimal system with sterile saline via the ipsilateral patent punctum (usually the upper punctum). The position of the imperforate punctum is revealed by transient ballooning of the overlying mucous membrane (palpebral conjunctiva) during irrigation. Absence of any changes during irrigation may indicate that the associated canaliculus is also absent. If this is suspected, investigation with fibreoptic endoscopy, a lacrimal probe (e.g. Leibreich), a pigtail probe (e.g. Worst) or dacryocystorhinography is necessary to demonstrate the degree of aplasia of the associated canaliculus (see below).

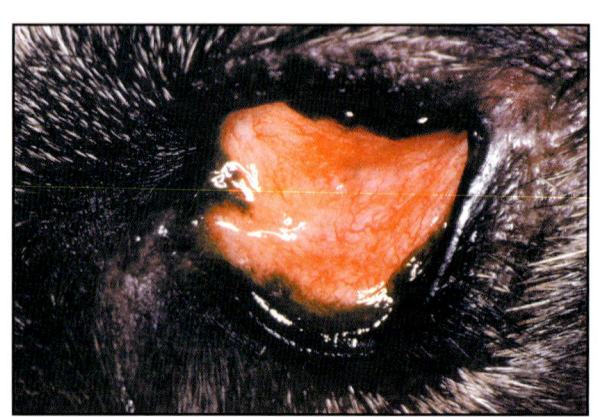

Figure 6.17 Absence of lower lacrimal punctum in a Tibetan Mastiff. The dog had first presented with painless epiphora; tear drainage was not investigated and lower eyelid entropion surgery was performed in error, producing lower eyelid ectropion. The lower punctum was recreated using a one-snip technique and a lid-shortening procedure restored normal eyelid congruity.

Treatment: Under general anaesthesia, the sheet of conjunctiva overlying the canaliculus is grasped with fine forceps and cleanly excised (one-snip technique) with fine, sharp scissors, leaving an obvious round to oval defect beneath (Figure 6.18). The procedure is facilitated by magnification. Patency is confirmed after surgery by irrigation via the ipsilateral punctum. The risk of postoperative fibrosis and subsequent occlusion or stenosis of the canaliculus is small. Postoperative treatment consists of topical ophthalmic antibiotic and corticosteroid solution for approximately 7 days. In the event of postoperative punctal occlusion, the area overlying the canaliculus is once again excised using the three-snip technique, in which three equidistant incisions are made around the punctum and the three conjunc-

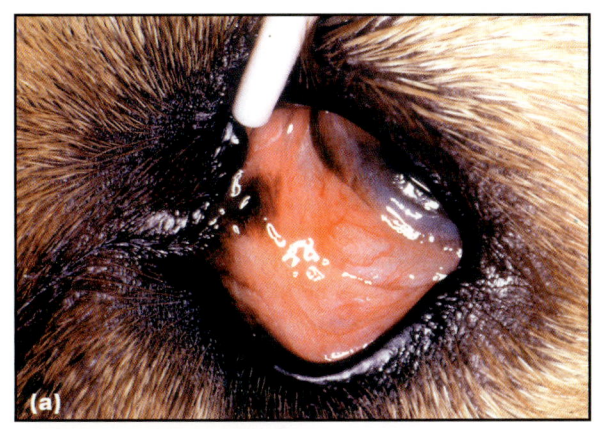

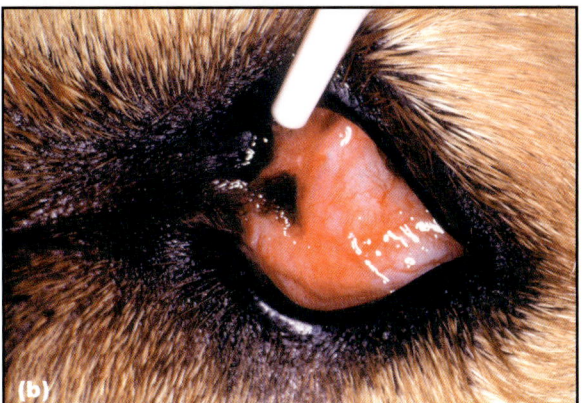

Figure 6.18 Basic lacrimal surgery in a Golden Retriever with lower lacrimal punctal aplasia. The upper punctum and canaliculus have been cannulated. In (a) there is no sign of a lower punctum, but injection of sterile saline via the upper punctum has raised a transient bleb where the punctum should be. A one-snip technique has been used to create a lower punctum (b).

tival flaps that are created are removed. Punctal patency is maintained by catheterizing the entire nasolacrimal system with 0 or 00 monofilament nylon, or with silastic tubing.

Micropunctum

The clinical signs associated with incomplete development of the punctum, or micropunctum, are similar to those exhibited by patients with imperforate lacrimal punctum (Barnett, 1979). Diagnosis is based on a history of epiphora, together with observation of an abnormally small lacrimal punctum by direct examination using magnification and illumination. Fluorescein drainage is delayed on the affected side. Lower micropunctum is more frequently diagnosed than upper.

Treatment: Micropuncta can be enlarged using a punctum/canaliculus dilator (e.g. Nettleship), or using one of two surgical techniques. The first technique involves inserting one blade of a fine pair of straight scissors into the punctum and making two small parallel incisions directed toward the medial canthus, thereby creating a small flap of conjunctiva overlying the canaliculus which is then excised. The second technique is the three-snip technique described above.

Aplasia of other parts of the lacrimal drainage system

Lacrimal canalicular aplasia is a rare condition similar in both aetiology and presentation to imperforate lacrimal puncta. Clinical signs of epiphora are usually only seen in cases of lower canalicular aplasia. The main problem lies in its differentiation from imperforate lacrimal punctum. If there is no evidence of a transient swelling of the conjunctiva over the presumed position of the lacrimal punctum on irrigation via the other punctum, then a malleable lacrimal probe, pigtail probe, or a fibreoptic light source may be inserted via the normal punctum, to gain some idea of the extent of the defect. Dacryocystorhinography may also be required.

Treatment of canalicular aplasia consists of cutting down on the end of a malleable lacrimal probe or pigtail probe if the instrument can be aligned close to the normal punctal position, in order to create a communicating canaliculus and punctum. Canalization is maintained by catheterizing the entire nasolacrimal system with 0 or 00 monofilament nylon, or with silastic or polyethylene tubing.

Alternatively, if there is no obvious canaliculus and punctum, surgical treatment should be considered; this consists of creating an alternative tear drainage pathway into the maxillary sinus (conjunctival maxillary sinosotomy), the nose (conjunctival rhinostomy) or the mouth (conjunctival buccostomy). This type of invasive surgery is not without risk of complications and may not be justifiable if the problem is only cosmetic.

Epiphora in the miniature breeds

Epiphora with obvious tear staining is a common problem in some of the smaller breeds (Figures 6.4 and 6.19), especially in the Bichon Frisé, Maltese Terrier, Miniature and Toy Poodle and Tibetan Spaniel. It is particularly apparent in pale-coated animals. Certain anatomical features of these breeds predispose them to impaired tear drainage, and this results in epiphora. The onset of epiphora is variable, but it is generally observed from 2–3 months of age onwards, as bilateral rust-coloured staining of the medial canthal skin and the hair beneath. Ocular irritation and conjunctival hyperaemia are not features of the condition, although it has been reported that some affected individuals may

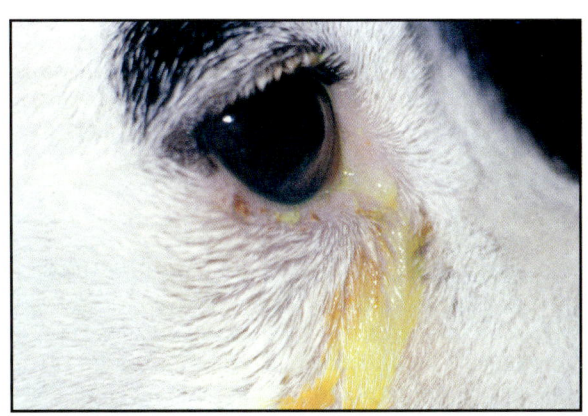

Figure 6.19 Epiphora demonstrated with topical fluorescein. No fluorescein appeared at the nostril after application of one drop to the lower conjunctival sac.

have higher than average Schirmer I tear test readings and that nictitans gland hypertrophy may be present in some dogs with this problem (Read et al., 1996).

Animals with epiphora should be examined meticulously, as there are a great number of possible contributory factors, some of which may interact. Fluorescein passage may be delayed or absent in affected eyes. Nasolacrimal cannulation and flushing should be performed to confirm patency of the nasolacrimal system and to exclude other possible causes of epiphora. Anatomical patency of the nasolacrimal system in such cases suggests that tears do not enter the drainage apparatus at a rate sufficient to allow the complete drainage of tears.

Diagnosis: This is based on the absence of findings suggesting other causes of epiphora, and the presence of certain anatomical features which may interact to predispose the individual to epiphora. These features include:

- A shallow orbit with a prominent globe
- Close apposition of the eyelids to the globe, resulting in a shallow lacrimal lake and close apposition of the lower lacrimal punctum to the prominent cornea, thereby effectively occluding it. Tears tend to be squeezed on to the face on eyelid closure, due to the shallow lacrimal lake
- Medial lower eyelid entropion, causing ventral displacement and functional closure of the lower lacrimal punctum and canaliculus, with subsequent impairment of tear drainage
- Misplacement of the lower punctum without medial lower eyelid entropion
- Hair at the medial canthus, of both the eyelids and the lacrimal caruncle, tends to impinge on the ptf, acting as a wick to entrain tears on to the skin and hair of the medial canthus. These hairs may impinge on to the cornea (trichiasis), causing increased lacrimation, which further compounds the problem
- Distichiasis
- Tight medial canthal ligaments, which displace the medial canthus ventrally.

Treatment: This is not always necessary if the problem is one of cosmetic appearance of no concern. If there is medial lower eyelid entropion, this should be repaired with the Hotz–Celsus technique, or medial canthoplasty can be used to correct the entropion, caruncular trichiasis and tight medial canthal ligaments (see Chapter 5). Surgery to realign the misplaced lower punctum may also be necessary (Grahn, 1999). If distichiasis is contributing to the epiphora, it should be treated (see Chapter 5).

Some reduction in the severity of the tear staining has been reported during treatment with either oral metronidazole or oral oxytetracycline. Treatment is empirical, as the mechanism is not understood, although it may relate to the interaction of the antibiotics with tear porphyrins. As this effect is only seen during treatment, it cannot be used for long-term management.

Other

Congenital or acquired cystic dilation of the lacrimal canaliculus is termed canaliculops; there is a single case report in the dog (Gerding, 1991). The cystic dilation of the lower canaliculus gave rise to a palpable firm painless swelling below the medial lower eyelid margin. Epiphora was due to partial obstruction of the lower canaliculus by the cyst, and patency of the canaliculus was restored by surgical excision. The history and clinical presentation were consistent with a congenital lesion, but an acquired origin could not be excluded.

Two cases of cystic nasolacrimal duct obstruction presumed to be of developmental origin have been reported (White et al., 1984; Grahn and Mason, 1995).

Canine nasolacrimal system – acquired conditions

Traumatic damage

Eyelid surgery in the canalicular region may result in iatrogenic damage and it is always sensible to cannulate both puncta and canaliculi when performing surgery in this region.

Medial eyelid lacerations can involve the lacrimal canaliculi. Those that occur are usually due to bite or scratch wounds. Marked eyelid oedema and inflammation develops following eyelid laceration. Prompt primary repair of the laceration is indicated if canalicular patency is to be maintained, and requires good microsurgical facilities and meticulous surgical technique. The proximal portion of the lacerated canaliculus can generally be cannulated via its punctum, either directly, or via a Worst pigtail probe, through which silastic tubing is passed. The distal portion of the canaliculus is often difficult to locate and the task is made easier if viscous fluid (e.g. tear replacement polymers) and air bubbles are mixed in a syringe and injected via the undamaged punctum. The bubbles that emerge from the distal portion enable the damaged canaliculus to be identified and cannulated with silastic tubing (Loff et al., 1996). Following microsurgical repair of the damaged tissues, the eye is treated with topical antibiotic solution until the cannula is removed some 3 weeks later.

The prognosis for maintaining canalicular patency is poor in cases of long-standing canalicular laceration or where cannulation and catheterization of the lacerated canaliculus is not possible. Subsequent canalicular obstruction usually gives rise to epiphora.

Acquired obstructions

Both external and internal factors may influence the patency of the lacrimal drainage apparatus. Traumatic injury (see earlier), foreign bodies, inflammatory disease and neoplasia are possible causes.

External factors are:

- Eyelid neoplasia in the region of the lacrimal punctum (an uncommon cause of external obstruction)
- Dental disease, which may involve the nasolacrimal duct (e.g. molar abscess)

- Extramural space-occupying lesions from the nasal cavity or maxillary sinus, which can cause nasolacrimal duct compression, deviation or infiltration (Gelatt et al., 1972). Chronic inflammatory nasal conditions can bring about secondary inflammatory changes in the adjacent nasolacrimal duct, and subsequent obstruction. Clinical signs such as chronic nasal discharge, epistaxis and facial swelling may suggest primary nasal cavity pathology. Plain radiographs of the maxillary and nasal regions should be taken. Dacryocystorhinography enables deviation, obstruction and invasion of the nasolacrimal duct by such lesions to be visualized and located (Gelatt et al., 1972).

In addition to the standard investigations of inadequate lacrimal drainage, review of the possible external factors requires careful examination of the head and neck, paying particular attention to the adnexa, oral cavity and nose. Diagnostic imaging techniques, including plain radiographs, will aid diagnosis.

Internal factors are:

- Foreign bodies
- Inflammation
- Neoplasia.

Foreign bodies

These may gain access to the drainage system via either punctum; organic material is a common cause of internal obstruction (Figures 6.20 and 6.21). Clinically, such cases present with discomfort and conjunctivitis. Initial epiphora is superseded by a profuse mucopurulent discharge within a matter of hours and, if the material causes local trauma, there may be bleeding from one or both puncta. Initially, some part of the foreign body may be visible extruding from the lacrimal punctum. Later, it becomes hidden as it migrates via the canaliculus towards the lacrimal sac and, in these cases, fluorescein drainage is delayed or absent on the affected side. If some part of the foreign body is visible, topical local anaesthetic is applied and the foreign body is grasped with fine forceps and removed. The shapes of some foreign bodies (e.g. barley awns) make them difficult to remove in their entirety and, in these cases, it is important to flush any debris out through the unaffected punctum. This is effected by applying digital pressure in the region of the lacrimal sac prior to irrigation, to avoid flushing material into the narrow intraosseous portion of the nasolacrimal duct. A similar approach can be used for foreign bodies that are identified within the canaliculus. Again, the aim of irrigation is to flush the foreign body out and not to force it into the nasolacrimal duct, where it is inaccessible. On occasions, the canaliculus must be surgically explored to effect complete removal of the foreign body. Following removal, the patient is given a 5–7 day course of a topical antibiotic and corticosteroid solution.

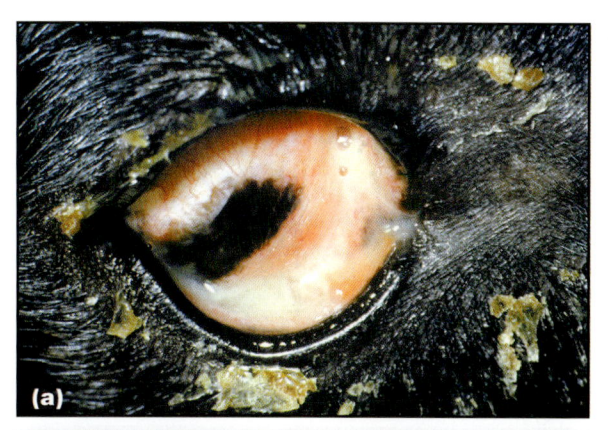

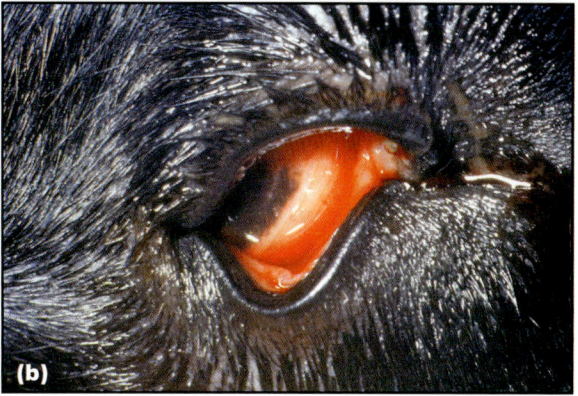

Figure 6.20 Foreign body in the upper punctum. The dog had an acute onset of pain, blepharospasm and lacrimation initially. A mucopurulent discharge soon developed (a) and the owner noticed within a week that there was intermittent bleeding from the corner of the eye. (b) The profuse mucopurulent discharge has been cleaned away and a grass seed is just visible in the upper punctum. The intermittent bleeding was the result of mechanical trauma to the canaliculus.

If the diagnosis is missed, particularly when the foreign body becomes lodged in the intraosseous portion of the nasolacrimal duct, the problem can be exacerbated by intramural inflammatory changes, intraluminal inflammatory debris and fibrosis. Dacryocystorhinography can be useful in confirming the diagnosis (Figure 6.21b). Unless the patency of the system can be restored by catheterization of the entire system via the upper punctum (Figure 6.21c), or, less commonly, via the nasal ostium, permanent obstruction may result.

Canaliculitis and dacryocystitis

Canaliculitis is defined as inflammation of either the canaliculus or canaliculi. Dacryocystitis is defined as inflammation of the lacrimal sac, although the inflammatory processes rarely involve the lacrimal sac in isolation. In practice, therefore, the term dacryocystitis is applied to inflammation of the whole of the excretory system. Acute and chronic forms exist and are usually accompanied by inflammation of the canaliculi and nasolacrimal duct. Most cases result from the presence of a foreign body within the drainage system, and all cases should be investigated with regard to this aetiology. Continuous tear flow plays a role in flushing both bacteria and debris through the nasolacrimal

118 The lacrimal system

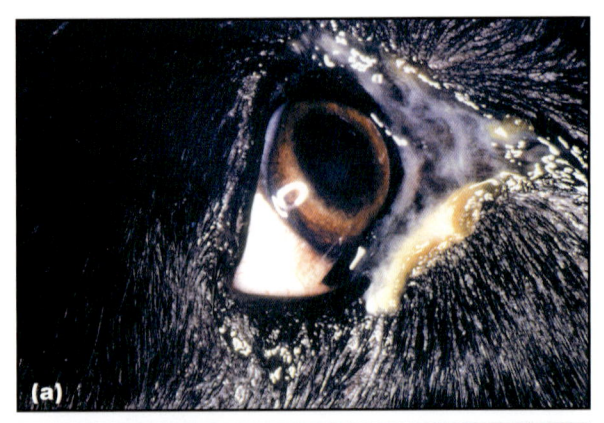

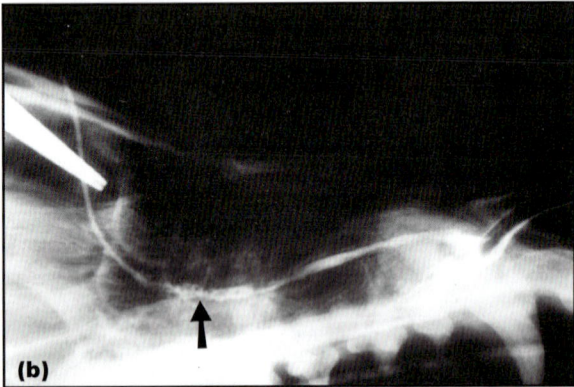

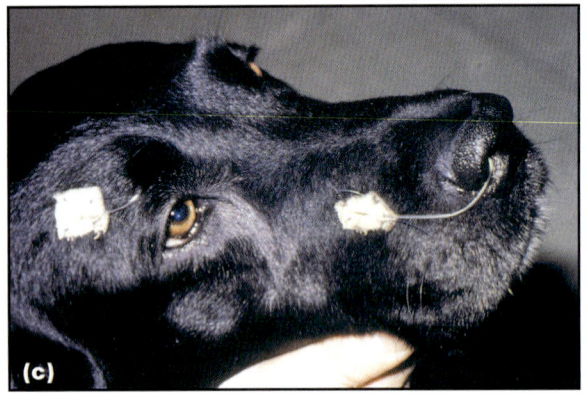

Figure 6.21 (a) Chronic dacryocystitis associated with disintegration of a foreign body in a Labrador Retriever. The foreign body was inadvertently flushed down the nasolacrimal duct and lodged in the intraosseous portion of the nasolacrimal duct. Repeated irrigation failed to restore patency of the duct, and the dog was referred to a specialist. (b) Dacryocystorhinography demonstrated the abnormal region in the narrowest part of the intraosseous portion of the nasolacrimal duct (arrowed). (c) Patency was restored and retained by cannulating the entire system using a feline urinary catheter; the abnormal region of the nasolacrimal duct was apparent when the catheter was passed. The catheter (FG 6) was sutured in place to retain patency. The condition resolved completely within 2 weeks and the catheter was removed.

system, so any obstruction to tear drainage allows debris to accumulate within the system and possible overgrowth of bacteria. The epithelial lining of the nasolacrimal system is a potent barrier to bacterial infection. Foreign body-induced trauma and concurrent nasolacrimal obstruction allow the development of dacryocystitis. A wide number of different bacterial species have been isolated from patients with dacryocystitis and are usually those which form part of the normal conjunctival flora. This suggests that dacryocystitis is an opportunistic infection rather than a primary bacterial infection (Lavach et al., 1984).

Clinical signs
Dacryocystitis is characterized by a profuse mucoid to mucopurulent ocular discharge which is occasionally malodorous, and which is most marked at the medial canthus (see Figure 6.21a). It is usually unilateral; bilateral involvement is more likely to signify nasal disease. Mild secondary conjunctivitis is usually present, but the quantity of discharge is far more profuse than would be expected from mild conjunctivitis. The discharge may be streaked with tears, whereas the discharge in primary conjunctivitis tends to be homogeneous in nature. Medial canthal swelling and pain are occasionally present. The application of digital pressure in the medial canthal area in the region of the lacrimal sac results in the expulsion of mucopurulent material from the puncta, especially the lower punctum. Abscessation and rupture of the lacrimal sac can occur, resulting in a fistula at the medial canthus.

Diagnosis
Diagnosis is based on clinical findings and delayed or absent fluorescein drainage; it is confirmed by cannulation of one of the two lacrimal puncta on the affected side. On flushing the nasolacrimal system in the order described earlier in this chapter, thick purulent material is seen emerging from the other punctum, followed by material emerging from the nostril. If no purulent material or irrigant emerges from the nostril, then complete obstruction of the lacrimal sac and/or nasolacrimal duct is likely. If a fistula is present, irrigating saline will escape from the fistulous tract.

Treatment
Treatment of dacryocystitis is aimed primarily at re-establishing patency of the nasolacrimal system and combating bacterial infection. Bacterial culture, both aerobic and anaerobic, and sensitivity should be performed on debris flushed from the nasolacrimal system. In acute dacryocystitis, repeated daily flushing with sterile saline is performed until normal patency of the system has been re-established and no abnormal material emerges on irrigation. The appropriate topical (aqueous preparations, not ointments) and systemic antibiotics are also administered. The prognosis is good in acute cases where a mucus plug or a foreign body is expelled on flushing.

Catheterization of the nasolacrimal system may be necessary in cases where complete nasolacrimal obstruction prevents flushing, or if the degree of patency achieved by repeated flushing and antibiotics is minimal, or if recrudescence of dacryocystitis follows the cessation of treatment. Chronic dacryocystitis, with or without fistula formation, is best treated in this manner from the outset. Nasolacrimal catheterization is performed under general anaesthesia via the upper lacrimal punctum, and silastic or polyethylene tubing (e.g. a feline urinary catheter) is sutured in place. It is usually possible when placing the catheter to irrigate the system and collect material for culture and sensitivity. Appropriate topical solutions of antibiotic, usually combined with corticosteroid, and systemic antibiotics, are both given until the nasolacrimal catheter is removed after 3 weeks. Most fistulae close following restoration of nasolacrimal patency and control of bacterial infection. The persistence or recurrence of clinical signs, despite the above treatment, is suggestive of a retained foreign body or other outflow obstruction. Surgical exploration of the lacrimal sac via dacryocystotomy has been successful in treating recurrent dacryocystitis associated with retained foreign bodies (Laing et al., 1988). In cases where nasolacrimal catheterization is not possible, due to complete nasolacrimal obstruction, permanent epiphora will result, unless alternative tear drainage pathways are created into the maxillary sinus, oral or nasal cavity.

Neoplasia and cysts

Primary neoplasia of the lacrimal apparatus is rare in all species. In the secretory portion, tumours of the orbital lacrimal gland (Rehbun and Edwards, 1977) or the nictitans gland (see Chapter 5) may occur. There are no reports of primary tumours of the excretory portion in dogs, but glandular tumours of the lacrimal sac in human beings have been reviewed by Pe'er et al., (1996). It is, however, not uncommon for tumours in neighbouring tissues (e.g. nose and sinuses) to impinge upon, or even to invade, the excretory lacrimal apparatus.

Cysts of the excretory portion of the lacrimal apparatus have been described earlier. Cysts of the secretory portion, the orbital lacrimal gland (Playter and Adams, 1977) and nictitans gland (see Chapter 5) are rare. Cystic lesions of the periorbital region have been reviewed by Martin et al. (1987).

Feline lacrimal apparatus – anatomical differences from the dog

The tear film is a trilaminar complex of lipid, aqueous and mucin (Carrington et al., 1987). The excretory component differs slightly from that of the dog: the nasolacrimal duct passes into the lacrimal bone via the lacrimal foramen, then passes along the medial surface of the maxilla, and it exits in the vestibule of the nasal cavity beneath the ventral nasal concha (maxilloturbinate). Tear drainage into the caudal nasal cavity and thence into the nasopharynx is common in cats, so that fluorescein passage to the ipsilateral nostril is seen in only 50% of normal cats.

Dacryoadenitis

Inflammation of the lacrimal gland (dacryoadenitis) is rare. Granulomatous diseases, such as eosinophilic granuloma of the orbit and tuberculosis of the lacrimal gland, are rare causes of dacryoadenitis (Peiffer, 1981).

Feline lacrimal apparatus – secretory problems

The wet eye

The causes are similar to those described for the dog and, additionally, there is a single case report of unilateral paradoxical lacrimation (Hacker, 1990), in which excessive tear production occurred each time the cat ate (gustolacrimal reflex). No cause was established.

The dry eye

Abnormalities of the pre-ocular tear film in cats have received little study. The lower blink rate of cats compared with dogs indicates that the tear film is more stable, and this is usually a function of the constitution of the lipid portion of the tear film.

Lipid abnormalities

Congenital absence of meibomian glands associated with eyelid agenesis and colobomatous eyelid defects is commoner in cats than dogs; blepharoplasty is the treatment of choice for restoration of eyelid congruence (see Chapter 5). Acquired feline meibomianitis is an infrequent condition of unknown cause which is most likely to be diagnosed when there is multiple involvement of the meibomian glands and lipogranuloma formation. The quality and quantity of the ptf is likely to be affected adversely, and secondary corneal pathology is not unusual. Lipogranulomatous masses also have the potential to produce further problems, as their shape and size can be a cause of corneal irritation and even ulceration.

Diagnosis: Diagnosis is based on the clinical appearance of the eyelid margins and the inner aspects of the eyelids. Possible eyelid changes include swelling, pigment loss, prominence of the meibomian gland orifices and of the glands themselves.

Treatment: Treatment of these problems is as already outlined for the dog. The lipogranulomatous masses are best removed surgically by incision and curettage.

Keratoconjunctivitis sicca

Keratoconjunctivitis sicca (KCS) (Figure 6.22) is less common in the cat than in the dog. Feline KCS can be caused by disease, especially that associated with the complications of feline herpesvirus infection; trauma, including surgically induced damage to the facial nerve associated with techniques such as bulla osteotomy (where the effects are often temporary); and systemic disorders, such as dysautonomia. Lacrimotoxic agents, such as sulphonamides, which are an important cause of iatrogenic KCS in the dog, do not appear to be of significance in the cat. Transient reductions in tear production will be seen following the use of sedatives and general anaesthetic agents, as well as parasympatholytics such as atropine.

Clinical features: The clinical presentation largely relates to the severity of the problem and the time for which it has been present, but there are usually fewer corneal changes and less of an ocular discharge in cats

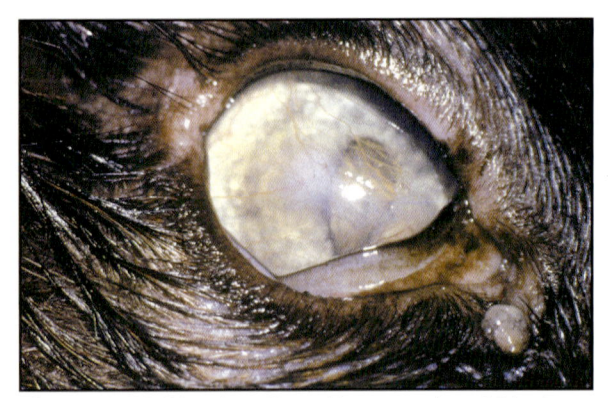

Figure 6.22 Chronic unilateral keratoconjunctivitis sicca of unknown cause in a domestic short hair cat. There is chemosis, a rather dull cornea, disruption of the corneal reflex and a scanty ocular discharge.

than dogs. Both conjunctival hyperaemia and mild diffuse corneal opacification are common; blepharoconjunctivitis may also be present. Corneal ulceration may occur in acute cases and those with underlying herpetic keratitis (see Chapter 8) and can be extensive.

Diagnosis: Diagnosis is based on the history, clinical appearance and on Schirmer tear testing. Confirmation of feline herpesvirus infection should be attempted, because it is a common underlying cause. Pharmacological testing (Guildford *et al.*, 1988) can aid a diagnosis of feline dysautonomia (see Chapter 15).

Treatment: The treatment options are largely as set out for the dog, except that immune-mediated causes of feline KCS have not been identified, so there is no suggestion that cyclosporin is effective, and its use would be contraindicated in FHV-positive animals. Tear substitutes (lacrimomimetics) are most commonly used for palliative treatment, and are reasonably effective in cats. For presumed neurogenic types of KCS, oral pilocarpine would be the treatment of choice, but treatment is difficult, as most cats refuse to eat medicated food. Topical pilocarpine may have some beneficial effect, but has not been clinically evaluated.

Parotid duct transposition is reserved for those cases in which medical therapy is either unsuccessful or impractical, When surgery is anticipated, the technique should be practised first. Parotid duct transposition in cats is sufficiently different from the technique in dogs that it may form a trap for the unwary (Gwin *et al.*, 1977).

If the underlying cause is irreversible (e.g. destruction of the lacrimal ductules by feline herpesvirus), treatment options include palliative medical treatment for life, or surgical parotid duct transposition.

Feline dysautonomia

This is an autonomic gangliopathy that produces widespread effects on organs innervated by parasympathetic nerves. KCS may be one of the presenting signs, although other ocular features, such as prominent third eyelids and dilated, non-responsive pupils (with normal vision), may be more obvious in the acute phase. Tear replacement therapy (e.g. 0.2% polyacrylic acid or 0.2% w/w carbomer 940) will be needed to mitigate the effects of reduced tear production.

Mucin abnormality

Conditions producing mucin abnormality have received little critical evaluation in the cat; their diagnosis is essentially similar to that for the dog. Rapid tear film break-up times were reported in a series of four cases: three cats with indolent corneal ulcers and one with bilateral corneal sequestration (Cullen, 1999). Palpebral conjunctival biopsies revealed a marked decrease or complete absence of goblet cells, conjunctival epithelial dysplasia, squamous metaplasia and submucosal infiltration with polymorphonuclear leucocytes and mononuclear cells. Goblet cell regeneration was confirmed after 5 months of mucinomimetic tear replacement in two cats, but no cause was established.

Feline tear film – distribution problems

The causes of evaporative dry eye are as already set out for the dog. As anatomical eyelid abnormalities are less frequent in cats than dogs, there are fewer tear film distribution problems in most breeds of cat. The exception is any type of flat-faced cat, especially some Persians, with an extended palpebral aperture and lagophthalmos. In such animals, blinking may not close the palpebral aperture effectively, so that low-grade exposure keratopathy ensues. In this breed, a number of anatomical problems combine to complicate the presentation: there is a poorly defined orbit, prominent globe, shallow lacrimal lake, misalignment or maldevelopment of the puncta, kinking of the canaliculus and tight apposition between the eyelid and eye. There may also be medial lower eyelid entropion and a wick effect from hairs at the medial canthus.

Third eyelid removal in cats is accompanied by complications that include a reduction in tear quantity and inadequate tear film distribution, both of which will result in secondary corneal pathology without tear replacement therapy (Figure 6.23). It is important, therefore, to preserve third eyelid function in the cat whenever possible; the only indication for partial or total removal of the third eyelid is primary neoplasia.

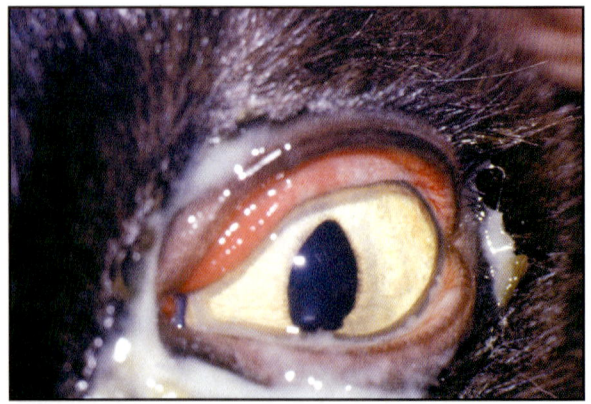

Figure 6.23 Adult domestic shorthair cat from which the third eyelid had been removed about 12 months previously by another veterinary surgeon for reasons unknown. There is a marked ocular discharge and chronic chemosis. The cat had severe ocular discomfort.

Feline tear film – excretory problems

Drainage problems are investigated as described above. The protocol adopted for basic investigation of the lacrimal apparatus is to start with visual inspection, then measure the tear production; finally, samples may be collected, if indicated. The patency of the system can be assessed, somewhat imperfectly in the cat, with fluorescein dye, as outlined previously.

If there is doubt as to the patency of the system, it is logical to proceed next to cannulation of the upper punctum and canaliculus under general anaesthesia, as a means of investigating the entire drainage system. When it is impossible to irrigate the system via the upper or lower punctum, dacryocystorhinography can be performed, or the examiner may decide to try and pass a very fine catheter through the entire system. Either technique will indicate the site of obstruction. Both techniques are usually attempted via the upper punctum and canaliculus, although the lower punctum and canaliculus can be used. It is not possible to carry out any investigations via the nasal ostium.

Developmental defects

Aplasia and hypoplasia

Partial or complete absence of parts of the nasolacrimal drainage system is an unusual developmental problem in cats (Figures 6.24 and 6.25). The upper or lower punctum is absent and, on occasions, the associated canaliculus is also missing. Occasionally, the punctum is misplaced. In cats, the upper punctum and canaliculus are often involved, whereas in dogs it is usually the lower punctum which is imperforate or hypoplastic (micropunctum).

Clinical features: Epiphora is the commonest clinical manifestation, although in chronic cases there may be a mucoid, or even mucopurulent, ocular discharge. The Persian is the breed most commonly affected; in addition to punctal abnormalities, epiphora may be a consequence of the head conformation and of medial lower eyelid entropion (Figure 6.26). Nasolacrimal drainage can become obstructed secondarily, but irrigation of the drainage system will produce only temporary improvement, unless the primary problem is also addressed.

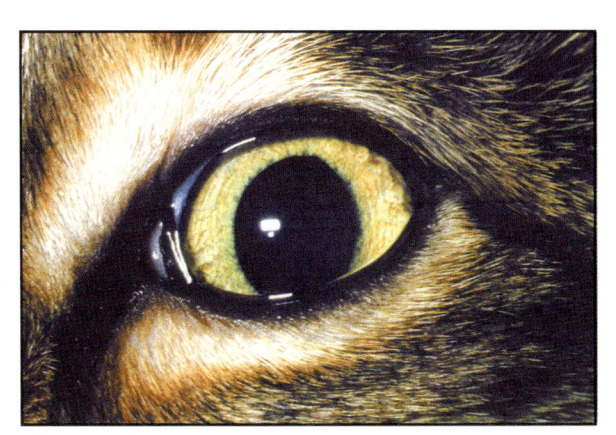

Figure 6.24 The left eye of a 7-month-old Bengal cat with bilateral absence of the lower punctum and canaliculus, and associated epiphora.

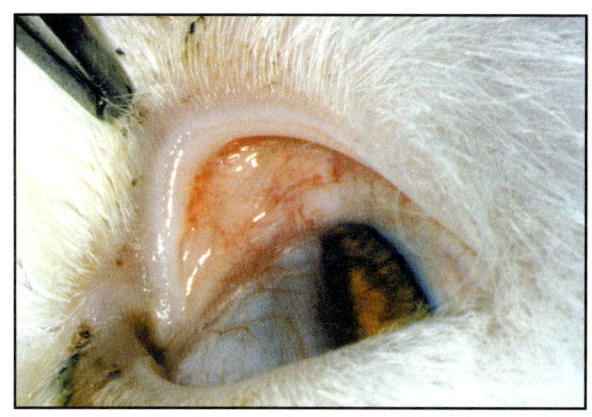

Figure 6.25 The left eye of a 1-year-old Persian cat that presented with mild bilateral epiphora. The upper punctum was absent in both eyes. A depression is apparent where the punctum should be.

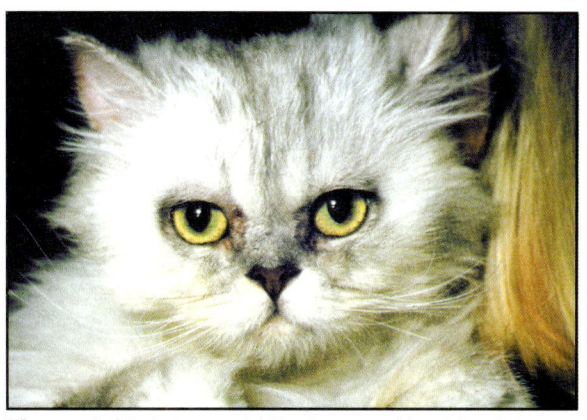

Figure 6.26 A 1-year-old Persian cat with mild epiphora, the right eye being slightly more affected than the left. In addition to the characteristic features of Persian anatomy, this cat had upper punctal aplasia on the right side.

Treatment: When examination reveals that the upper or lower punctum is absent, the other punctum should be cannulated and the system irrigated with the cat under general anaesthesia. If a sheet of mucous membrane covering the punctum is the only defect, a transient bleb may form when the saline is injected, and simple excision of the overlying mucous membrane will be all that is required to establish patency. A topical antibiotic and corticosteroid ophthalmic solution is applied for 5–7 days after surgery to minimize scar formation.

If the defect involves more of the drainage system than the punctum, then dacryocystorhinography may help to establish the extent of the problem. Treatment to produce an alternative drainage route may be required. It is sometimes possible to create patency by feeding a fine, malleable, lacrimal cannula or pigtail probe via the normal punctum, canaliculus and lacrimal sac to the affected area. The conjunctiva over the tip of the cannula or probe is removed to create a punctum, and fine nylon or silastic tubing is then passed through the new punctum and into the nasolacrimal duct. The nylon is retained in place with butterfly sutures and should remain *in situ* for 3–4 weeks to maintain patency. For more extensive defects, it is possible, but more difficult, to create an alternative outflow channel into the nose or mouth, as described earlier for the dog. Surgery should only be contemplated in those cases in which the epiphora is producing serious problems.

Acquired obstructions

Acquired partial or complete obstruction (Figure 6.27) may be a consequence of: active or previous inflammation (e.g. symblepharon); trauma; or abnormalities external to the drainage system (e.g. medial canthus, nose, sinuses and teeth roots) or within it (e.g. foreign bodies, infection).

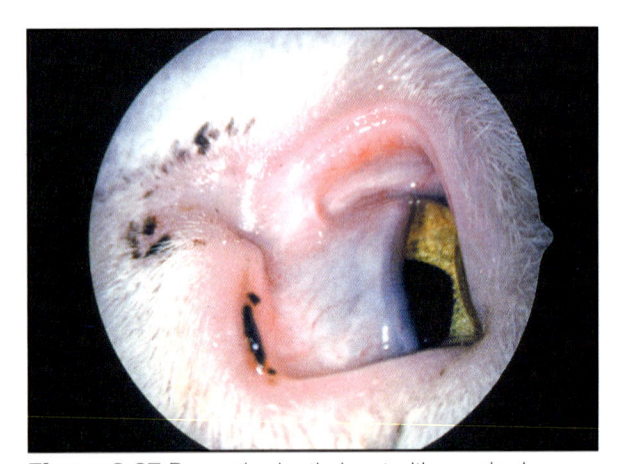

Figure 6.27 Domestic shorthair cat with acquired blockage of the upper and lower puncta as a result of extensive symblepharon formation (feline herpesvirus infection). The ventral fornix had been obliterated by the extensive adhesions and the dorsal fornix was also compromised.

Comprehensive investigation is required to establish the cause and may include visual inspection, nasolacrimal and nasal flushes for cytology and culture, dacryocystorhinography and imaging techniques. Epiphora is the commonest presenting sign, but occasionally a more florid ocular discharge is present, usually when dacryocystitis complicates the presentation.

In differentiating the causes of epiphora, it is important to rule out other causes, such as blepharitis, blepharoconjunctivitis and the idiopathic facial dermatitis syndrome of Persian cats.

The severe ocular surface inflammation provoked by FHV-1 infection in kittens is the commonest cause of acquired stenosis or occlusion, as symblepharon formation obliterates one or both of the punctal openings early in life. Careful examination confirms the punctal obliteration, but surgical treatment to restore patency may be unsuccessful, as adhesions recur.

Other causes of obstruction or partial obstruction include dental disease, especially tooth root problems; nasopharyngeal or nasal problems, such as previous upper respiratory tract infections; chronic rhinitis; nasal polyps; neoplasia and, rarely, inflammatory and neoplastic diseases of the sinuses.

Squamous cell carcinoma is the most likely local tumour to involve the lacrimal drainage system; less commonly, other tumours, such as lymphoma, may infiltrate the region.

The lacrimal drainage system can also be damaged by traumatic injury, usually caused by cat claws; it usually involves the medial canthus. Microsurgical facilities are essential if primary repair is to be performed. Chronic complications of damage to this region include dacryocystitis, abscessation, bone sequestration and formation of a draining sinus below the medial canthus.

Dacryocystitis is a possible sequel to established obstructive disease, whatever the initiating cause, and the clinical signs are typical. A profuse and purulent ocular or periocular discharge may be present in chronic cases (Figure 6.28). Gentle digital pressure at the medial canthus in the region of the lacrimal sac can be used to express purulent material, and there may be slight reddening in the medial canthus area.

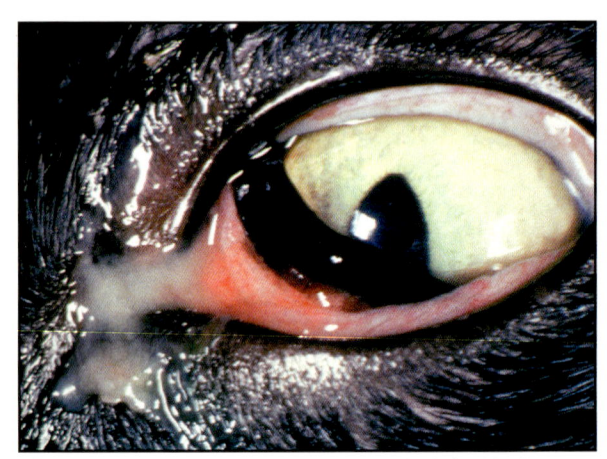

Figure 6.28 Domestic shorthair cat with left-sided dacryocystitis as a complication of chronic rhinitis. Investigation demonstrated that there was communication between the left nasolacrimal duct and nasal cavity and also between the right and left nasal cavities, resulting from chronic destructive changes associated with rhinitis. Initial culture had revealed *Bacteroides* sp.; later culture demonstrated anaerobic Gram-negative cocci. On the basis of culture and sensitivity testing, the cat was given a course of topical and oral tetracycline, to which she responded well. (Courtesy of JRB Mould.)

Identifying the cause of the dacryocystitis may not be easy; initially, it is sensible to establish whether the inflammation is entirely internal (i.e. in the lumen of the drainage apparatus) or if there is an external component (e.g. teeth, nose or sinuses). The discharge should be cultured (both aerobically and anaerobically) and antibiotic sensitivity established. Both systemic antibiotic and topical antibiotic solution should be given for 7–10 days in uncomplicated cases, whereas more complicated cases may require antibiotic treatment for at least a month, combined with cannulation of the entire system. If abscessation or sinus formation is present, surgery (to drain the abscess and extirpate necrotic tissue and fistulous tracts) may be required; surgical bypass may also be required.

References and further reading

Barnett KC (1979) Imperforate and micro-lacrimal puncta in the dog. *Journal of Small Animal Practice* **20**, 481–490

Brown MH, Brightman AH, Butine MD and Moore TL (1997) The phenol red thread test in healthy cats. *Veterinary and Comparative Ophthalmology* **7**, 249–252

Brown MH, Galland JC, Davidson HJ and Brightman AH (1996) The phenol red thread test in dogs. *Veterinary and Comparative Ophthalmology* **6**, 274–277

Carrington, SD, Bedford, PGC, Guillon J-P and Woodward EG (1987) Polarized light biomicroscopic observations on the pre-corneal tear film. 3. The normal tear film of the cat. *Journal of Small Animal Practice* **28**, 821–826

Crispin SM (1987) Nasolacrimal cannulation in the dog. *In Practice* **19**, 205–207

Cullen CL (1999) Ulcerative keratitis associated with qualitative tear film abnormalities in cats. *Veterinary Ophthalmology* **2**, 197–204

Diehl KJ and Roberts SM (1991) Keratoconjunctivitis sicca in dogs associated with sulphonamide therapy: 16 cases (1980–1990). *Progress in Veterinary and Comparative Ophthalmology* **1**, 276–282

Dodam JR, Branson KR and Martin DD (1998) Effects of intramuscular sedative and opioid combinations on tear production in dogs. *Veterinary Ophthalmology* **1**, 57–59

Gelatt KN, Cure TH, Guffy MM and Jessen C (1972) Dacryocystorhinography in the dog and cat. *Journal of Small Animal Practice* **13**, 381–393

Gerding PA (1991) Epiphora associated with canaliculops in a dog. *Journal of the American Animal Hospital Association* **27**, 424–426

Gilger BC and Allen JB (1998) Cyclosporine A in veterinary ophthalmology. *Veterinary Ophthalmology* **1**, 181–187

Grahn BH (1999) Diseases and surgery of the canine nasolacrimal system. In: *Veterinary Ophthalmology, 3rd edn,* ed. K.N. Gelatt, pp. 569–581. Lippincott, Williams and Wilkins, Philadelphia

Grahn BH and Mason RA (1995) Epiphora associated with dacryops in a dog. *Journal of the American Animal Hospital Association* **31**, 15–19

Guildford WG, O'Brien DP, Albert A and Emerling HM (1988) Diagnosis of dysautonomia in a cat by autonomic nervous system function testing. *Journal of the American Veterinary Medical Association* **193**, 823–828

Gwin RM, Gelatt KN and Peiffer RL (1977) Parotid duct transposition in a cat with keratoconjunctivitis sicca. *Journal of the American Animal Hospital Association* **13**, 42–45

Hacker DV (1990) 'Crocodile tears' syndrome in a domestic cat: case report. *Journal of the American Animal Hospital Association* **26**, 245–246

Håkanson NW and Arnesson K (1997) Temporal variation in tear production in normal Beagle dogs as determined by Schirmer Tear Test. *Veterinary and Comparative Ophthalmology* **7**, 196–203

Hicks SJ, Carrington SD, Kaswan RL, Adam SM, Bara J and Corfield AP (1997) Demonstration of discrete secreted and membrane-bound ocular mucins in the dog. *Experimental Eye Research* **64**, 597–607

Jiménez A, Barrera R, Mañé MC, Andrés S, López R and Molleda JM (1992) Immunoglobulins of tears and parotid saliva in the dog. *Progress in Veterinary and Comparative Ophthalmology* **2**, 55–57

Kaswan RL and Salisbury MA (1990) A new perspective on canine keratoconjunctivitis sicca. *Veterinary Clinics of North America* **20**, 583–613

Kaswan RL, Salisbury MA and Lothrop CD (1991) Interaction of age and gender on occurrence of canine keratoconjunctivitis sicca. *Progress in Veterinary and Comparative Ophthalmology* **1**, 93–97

Laing EJ, Speiss B and Binnington AG (1988) Dacryocystotomy: a treatment for chronic dacryocystitis in the dog. *Journal of the American Animal Hospital Association* **24**, 223–226

Lavach JD, Severin GA and Roberts SM (1984) Dacryocystitis in dogs: a review of 22 cases. *Journal of the American Animal Hospital Association* **20**, 463–467

Loff HJ, Wobig JL and Dailey RA (1996) The bubble test: an atraumatic method for canalicular laceration repair. *Ophthalmic Plastic Reconstructive Surgery* **1**, 61–64

Martin CL, Kaswan RI and Doran CC (1987) Cystic lesions of the periorbital region. *Compendium of Continuing Education for the Practicing Veterinarian* **9**, 1022–1029

Moore CP, Wilsman NJ, Nordheim EV et al. (1987) Density and distribution of conjunctival goblet cells. *Investigative Ophthalmology and Visual Science* **28**, 1925–1932

Moore CP (1990) Qualitative tear film disease. *Veterinary Clinics of North America* **20**, 565–581

Moore CP (1999) Diseases and surgery of the lacrimal secretory system. In: *Veterinary Ophthalmology, 3rd edn,* ed. K. N. Gelatt, pp. 583–607. Lippincott, Williams and Wilkins, Philadelphia

Pe'er J, Hidayat AA, Ilsar M, Landou L and Stefanyszyn MA (1996) Glandular tumours of the lacrimal sac. Their histological patterns and possible origins. *Ophthalmology* **103**, 1601–1605

Peiffer RL (1981) Feline ophthalmology. In: *Veterinary Ophthalmology, 1st edn,* ed. K.N. Gelatt, pp. 521–568. Lea and Febiger, Philadelphia

Petersen-Jones SM (1997) Quantification of conjunctival sac bacteria in normal dogs and those suffering from keratoconjunctivitis sicca. *Veterinary and Comparative Ophthalmology* **7**, 29–35

Playter RF and Adams LB (1977) Lacrimal cyst (dacryops) in 2 dogs. *Journal of the American Veterinary Medical Association* **171**, 736–737

Powell CC and Martin CL (1989) Distribution of cholinergic and adrenergic nerve fibres in the lacrimal gland of dogs. *American Journal of Veterinary Research* **30**, 2084–2088

Read RA, Dunn KA, Smith KC and Barnett KC (1996) A histological study of nictitans glands from dogs with tear overflow of unknown cause. *Veterinary and Comparative Ophthalmology* **6**, 195–204

Rehbun WC and Edwards NJ (1977) Two cases of orbital adenocarcinoma of probable lacrimal gland origin. *Journal of the American Animal Hospital Association* **13**, 691–694

Saito A and Kotani T (1999) Tear production in dogs with epiphora and corneal epitheliopathy. *Veterinary Ophthalmology* **2**, 173–178

Watanabe H and Tanaka M (1996) Rose Bengal staining and expression of a mucin-like glycoprotein in corneal epithelium (abstract 1649). *Investigative Ophthalmology and Visual Science (ARVO Supplement)* **37**, S357

White RAS, Herrtage ME and Watkins SB (1984) Endoscopic management of a cystic naso-lacrimal obstruction in a dog. *Journal of Small Animal Practice* **25**, 729–735

Wyman M (1979) Ophthalmic surgery for the practitioner. *Veterinary Clinics of North America* **9**, 311–348

Wyman M, Gilger B, Mueller P and Norris K (1995) Clinical evaluation of a new Schirmer tear test in the dog. *Veterinary and Comparative Ophthalmology* **5**, 211–217

7

The conjunctiva

Sheila Crispin

Embryology, anatomy and physiology

The conjunctiva is derived embryologically from ectoderm and mesenchyme. It is a thin semi-transparent variably pigmented mucous membrane. Figure 7.1 shows the anatomy of the conjunctiva. The *nictitating conjunctiva* covers both the inner and outer surfaces of the third eyelid. The *palpebral conjunctiva* covers the posterior surface of the upper and lower eyelids. The palpebral conjunctiva terminates at the lid margin and is reflected at the dorsal and ventral fornices, to continue on to the globe as the *bulbar conjunctiva*, which covers the anterior surface of the episclera and sclera. The bulbar conjunctiva fuses with Tenon's capsule (vagina bulbi) close to the limbus. The space lined by the conjunctiva beneath the upper and lower eyelids is called the conjunctival sac.

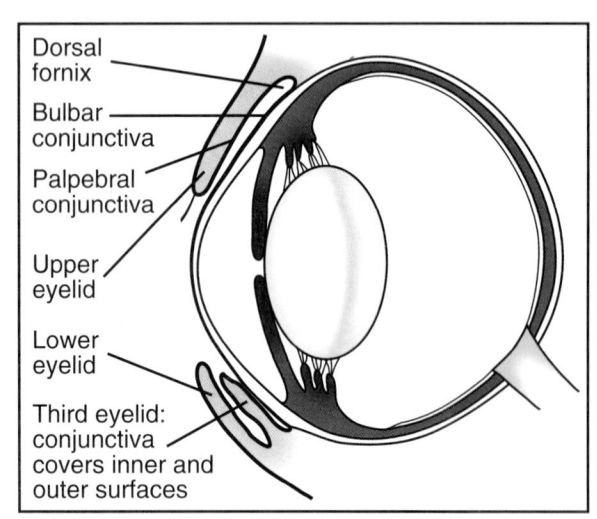

Figure 7.1 Anatomy of the conjunctiva.

The pre-ocular tear film (see Chapter 6) covers the epithelium of both the conjunctiva and cornea, and may be regarded as their outermost 'layer'. Normal conjunctiva consists of: an outer non-keratinized epithelium containing goblet cells; and an underlying conjunctival stroma, which is divided into a superficial (adenoid) layer and a deep (fibrous) layer. The superficial layer contains lymphoid tissue and cells such as lymphocytes and histiocytes; conjunctiva-associated lymphoid tissue (CALT) is an important component of this layer. The deep layer consists mainly of connective tissue, nerves and blood vessels.

The conjunctiva has a rich vascular supply. The bright red, freely branching blood vessels are obvious in non-pigmented areas. In corneal disease, endothelial budding may occur from the terminal arcades of the conjunctival vessels at the limbus, with consequent superficial corneal vascularization. The only lymphatic drainage of the eye is situated in the conjunctiva. Pain fibres are somewhat sparse, and the sensory nerve supply to the conjunctiva is from the ophthalmic division of the fifth cranial nerve.

Pathology

The conjunctiva is freely mobile, except in areas of closer attachment at the limbus, the fornices and towards, and including, the lid margins. Because of the loose arrangement, conjunctival oedema (chemosis) and subconjunctival haemorrhage form readily after insult.

Acute conjunctivitis
Oedema, hyperaemia and cellular infiltrates are characteristic of acute conjunctivitis. The cell types may be helpful in establishing a broad diagnosis (see Chapter 1) but, on many occasions, cytology is non-specific.

Chronic conjunctivitis
In chronic conjunctivitis there may be an increase in the number of epithelial goblet cells. Reduction in the number of goblet cells can also occur, however, possibly as a consequence of diffuse infiltration by chronic inflammatory cells associated with infectious and immune-mediated disorders. The changes are usually permanent.

Follicular hypertrophy
This is basically lymphoid hyperplasia with secondary vascularization; it is usually a non-specific response to chronic inflammation and does not help in reaching a specific diagnosis.

Canine conjunctival problems

Epibulbar dermoid
Epibulbar dermoids are superficial masses (choristomas) of developmental origin that contain many elements of normal skin and frequently sprout hairs. They often involve the cornea and are usually located in the region of the lateral limbus (Figure 7.2). In dogs, they may be unilateral or bilateral, although the former is more common.

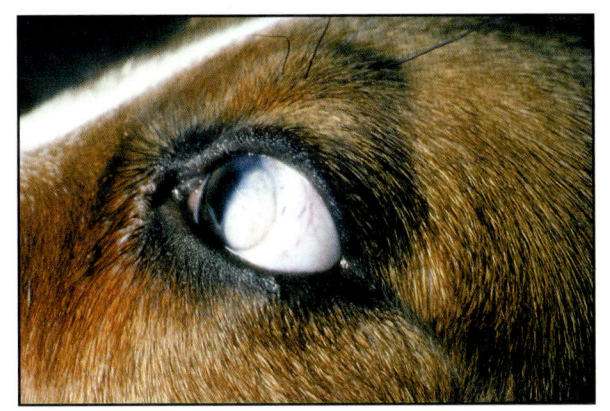

Figure 7.2 Epibulbar dermoid in a crossbred dog.

Treatment

Surgical excision is the treatment of choice. A lateral canthotomy may be required for adequate exposure. The mass is excised by superficial conjunctivectomy and also by keratectomy if there is corneal involvement (Figure 7.3). A bridle suture is passed through the dermoid to make manipulation easier. The initial incision is made in normal tissue on the corneal side of the mass and the mass is undermined and dissected off. No suturing is required. Topical application of surface-active corticosteroids may be necessary to minimize scarring once epithelium has covered the defect. The canthotomy is repaired with absorbable (e.g. 5-0 or 6-0 polyglactin 910) or non-absorbable (e.g. 5-0 or 6-0 silk) material.

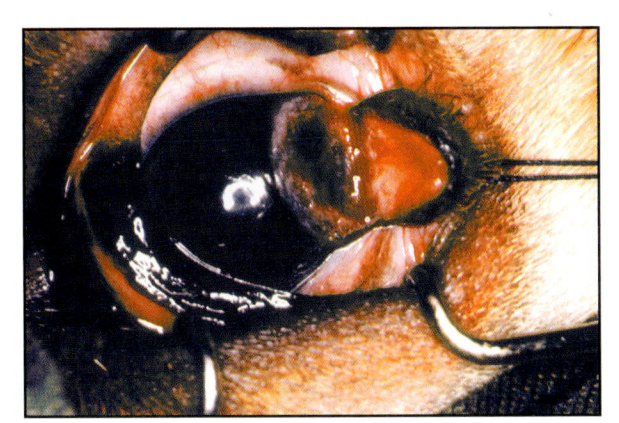

Figure 7.3 Removal of an epibulbar dermoid. A bridle suture through the dermoid makes the surgery easier. Note that a lateral canthotomy has been performed to improve access.

Canine conjunctivitis

Inflammation of the conjunctiva (conjunctivitis) is one of the most common conditions encountered in small animal practice; however, it is important to differentiate conjunctivitis from other problems of similar appearance (see Appendix) and to establish the cause of the inflammation, so that treatment can be both economical and effective.

Conjunctivitis can occur in animals of any age. Canine neonatal conjunctivitis (ophthalmia neonatorum) is described in Chapter 5 and will not be discussed further in this section.

Reports of the conjunctival bacterial flora isolated from clinically normal dogs, dogs with external eye disease and dogs with keratoconjunctivitis sicca have been reviewed (Whitley, 2000). *Staphylococcus* spp. emerged as the commonest isolate in all three situations, particularly S. *intermedius* and S. *epidermidis*.

History

An accurate history is required and should seek to establish:

- The vaccination status, and recent contact with other dogs
- Whether the inflammation is unilateral or bilateral
- Whether other dogs are affected
- Whether there is any apparent environmental or seasonal incidence
- Whether there have been similar episodes in the past
- The dog's general health
- Any treatment the dog has received.

Clinical signs

The clinical signs of conjunctivitis are typical. The condition is usually uncomfortable or irritating, rather than obviously painful.

In acute cases there is an active hyperaemia, which is often more marked towards the fornices, conjunctival chemosis (oedema) and lacrimation or an ocular discharge (Figure 7.4). The nature of the discharge is variable; for example, it may be serous, mucoid, mucopurulent, purulent or haemorrhagic. It is worth noting that a mild mucoid ocular discharge may persist for some time after the other acute signs have resolved. An ocular discharge with no other clinical signs does not constitute a reason for treatment. Furthermore, mucus accumulation at the medial canthus is an almost universal 'normal' feature of certain breeds of long-nosed dogs, such as the Dobermann (Figure 7.5) and Rough Collie, and should not be confused with conjunctivitis.

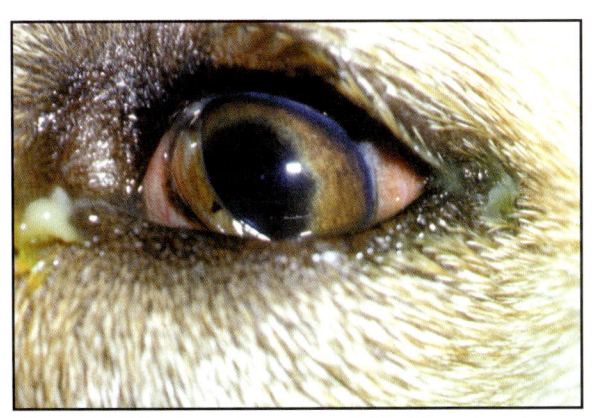

Figure 7.4 Acute canine conjunctivitis. There is active hyperaemia of the conjunctival vessels, chemosis and an ocular discharge, and the eye is uncomfortable. The aetiology was not established, despite intensive investigations, and no treatment was given. The clinical signs of conjunctivitis resolved completely in a week, except for a mild ocular discharge which persisted for about 3 weeks.

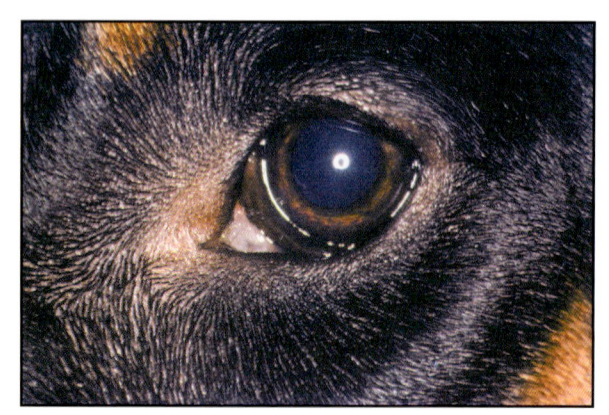

Figure 7.5 Dobermann with mucus accumulation at the medial canthus. This is a feature of breeds with a deep-set medial canthus.

Follicle formation is an indication of non-specific immune stimulation and is more likely to be found in chronic conjunctivitis (Figure 7.6). Other signs of chronic conjunctivitis include thickening of the conjunctiva and an associated dull redness. While many cases of conjunctivitis are self-limiting, a small proportion persist, particularly when the treatment is incorrect. The changes within the conjunctiva can become irreversible, so that treatment is ineffective.

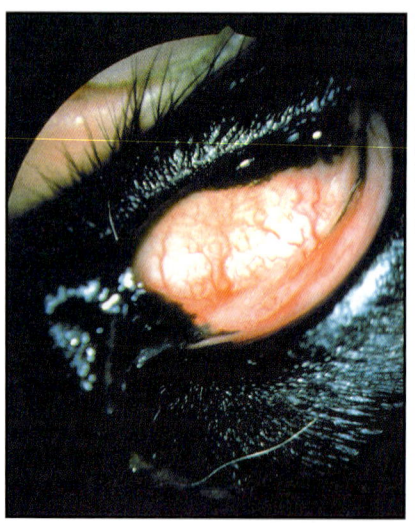

Figure 7.6 Chronic canine conjunctivitis. Note the obvious lymphoid hyperplasia (follicular conjunctivitis).

Aetiology

Conjunctivitis is unsatisfactorily classified unless the aetiology can be determined; it is better to avoid classifications based on duration and appearance.

Primary conjunctivitis:

- Infectious agents include viruses (most notably distemper), which typically produce bilateral involvement. Bacterial conjunctivitis is usually secondary to other underlying dysfunction, such as poor eyelid anatomy or dry eye syndromes (see below)
- Irritants such as chemicals, dust and wind may cause conjunctivitis, as may some topically applied drugs or home remedies, especially if applied for long periods
- Allergic conjunctivitis is common and may be associated with immediate or delayed hypersensitivity reactions. It is usually bilateral. Allergic conjunctivitis is often a feature of the type 1 hypersensitivity that characterizes atopy
- Autoimmune conjunctivitis is less common. It occurs when the conjunctiva of both eyes is involved in the bullous or interface autoimmune skin diseases, such as the pemphigus and pemphigoid group of disorders
- Ligneous conjunctivitis is a rare disorder of unknown cause (Figure 7.7). The Dobermann appears to be more susceptible than other breeds (Ramsey *et al.*, 1996). The conjunctival lesion consists of a bilateral membranous or pseudomembranous conjunctivitis and is invariably part of a multisystemic disease, with similar changes in the oral mucosa or urinary tract mucosa, or upper respiratory tract infection. In humans, ligneous conjunctivitis is sometimes due to plasminogen gene mutations.

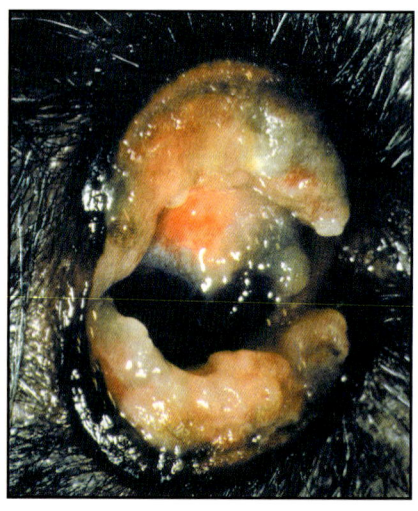

Figure 7.7 Ligneous conjunctivitis in a crossbred dog with multisystemic disease.

Secondary conjunctivitis: This may be associated with:

- Bacterial overgrowth (predominantly staphylococci and streptococci). *Chlamydia* spp. are unproven as a cause of canine conjunctivitis in the UK
- Mechanical irritation from eyelid problems (e.g. agenesis, blepharitis, ectropion, entropion, other types of imperfect anatomy and neoplasia) or from lash and hair abnormalities (e.g. trichiasis, distichiasis, ectopic cilia, hairs from epibulbar dermoids, dermal hairs from nasal folds)
- Pre-ocular tear film problems
- Dacryocystitis
- Orbital and periorbital problems.

It is important to identify and treat the primary problem in order to ensure resolution of the secondary conjunctivitis. For example, in ectropion the ventral conjunctiva is permanently exposed to the environment and debris tends to collect in the ventral conjunctival sac; this is only rectified when normal eyelid congruity is achieved after surgery.

Diagnosis

- Assessment of the pre-ocular tear film and a Schirmer I tear test should be a routine part of the investigation of conjunctivitis, as keratoconjunctivitis sicca (dry eye) is frequently misdiagnosed as conjunctivitis
- Samples for cytology are easy to obtain at the initial consultation (Bauer et al., 1996; Willis et al., 1997) and may help to differentiate bacterial, viral and allergic conjunctivitis
- Bacterial culture and sensitivity testing are less essential initially, but should always be performed in cases of conjunctivitis that persist for more than 10–14 days, ideally at least 48 hours after antibiotic treatment has been stopped
- Conjunctival biopsy can be of value in establishing the extent of any conjunctival changes and in enabling a specific diagnosis of immune-mediated conjunctivitis.

Investigative procedures are set out in Chapter 1.

Treatment

Treatment of primary conjunctivitis depends upon the cause. Thus, for distemper there is no specific therapy, but supportive nursing care and treatment of secondary bacterial infection may be required.

Topical fusidic acid is the treatment of choice for Gram-positive infections, especially those caused by staphylococci. The judicious use of corticosteroids is also valuable in confirmed staphylococcal infection, as hypersensitivity to staphylococcal toxins exacerbates the condition. Topical chloramphenicol has a broad spectrum of activity, and it remains an excellent choice for superficial eye infections, although it should not be selected if *Pseudomonas* spp. are involved. Topical gentamicin should be used for Gram-negative infections, including *P. aeruginosa*. For mixed infections, a combination of antibiotics, such as polymixin B with bacitracin, or gramicidin with polymixin B and neomycin sulphate, is appropriate. Useful topical preparations are summarized in Chapter 3.

Allergic conjunctivitis may be successfully treated if the allergen or allergens (e.g. house dust components, fleas, moulds and vegetation) can be identified (e.g. by intradermal skin testing) and then avoided. Hyposensitization may be effective in more than 50% of cases if undertaken early in the course of disease. Symptomatic treatment (e.g. antihistamines or short courses of topical corticosteroids) is less satisfactory, but may be an option when allergens cannot be avoided and the condition has become chronic. Any secondary infection will require appropriate antibiotic treatment.

Symblepharon

Conjunctival adhesions of the palpebral, bulbar or nictitating conjunctiva, either to each other or to the cornea, may be seen as a distinct entity, or in conjunction with other ocular defects such as microphthalmos. Acquired symblepharon is sometimes seen in dogs as an iatrogenic problem following eyelid surgery; it may also occur after injury, especially chemical.

No treatment is required unless the patient is indisposed by the symblepharon, in which case the adhesions can be freed surgically, utilizing a technique that prevents the adhesions from re-forming (see feline section of this chapter).

Conjunctival trauma

The majority of conjunctival injuries are of traumatic origin. They present with a history of sudden onset and there is usually a change in the appearance of one eye or, rarely, both eyes. The aetiology is varied and includes lacerations from sharp objects, claw and bite wounds, and blunt trauma.

Blunt trauma, usually a result of blunt injury to the head, is a common cause of subconjunctival haemorrhage. It is important to remember that blunt trauma to the globe and orbit, or to the head region itself, can be very damaging to the globe. The possibility that this type of trauma could be non-accidental should be considered if there is not an obvious cause. The degree of intraocular damage must be carefully assessed by examination. Imaging techniques, such as ultrasonography, are especially important when intraocular haemorrhage prevents complete examination.

Clinical signs

These include ocular discomfort, chemosis and reddening. Conjunctival injuries can seal quickly, so there may or may not be signs of local tissue damage. Subconjunctival haemorrhage may be spectacular but can be left to resorb naturally in uncomplicated cases. Fresh haemorrhage is bright red (Figure 7.8).

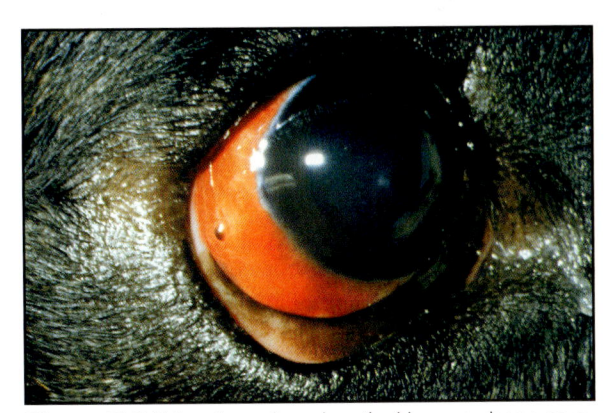

Figure 7.8 Extensive subconjunctival haemorrhage as a result of head trauma.

Treatment

Full-thickness conjunctival injury is common but few cases require direct suturing. Healing is usually rapid and uncomplicated, provided that the damage is limited to the conjunctiva and does not involve deeper structures. On rare occasions, minimal debridement is required, perhaps combined with repair using buried absorbable 7-0 suture material.

Following conjunctival injury, it is usual to give topical antibiotic ointment for 3–5 days; this is particularly important following scratches and bites from other animals. If the conjunctiva is very swollen, a topical preparation with an oily excipient should be used, to prevent conjunctival desiccation.

Differential diagnosis

Haematological disorders (e.g. clotting defects, platelet disorders) can underlie cases of spontaneous subconjunctival haemorrhage not associated with trauma; both eyes are usually affected. Sudden or sustained increases in venous pressure, as in crush injuries and asphyxia, may result in diffuse haemorrhage or petechial haemorrhage.

Foreign bodies

Foreign bodies are a relatively common source of conjunctival injury. They frequently consist of organic matter such as seeds or wood. The conjunctival sac can accommodate surprisingly large foreign bodies. Less spectacular, but usually more traumatic, are foreign bodies located beneath the third eyelid. Most foreign bodies are superficial, but on occasions they may penetrate more deeply.

Clinical signs and diagnosis

There is an acute onset of discomfort or pain, with chemosis and inflammation. There may also be profuse lacrimation initially, and an ocular discharge within hours (Figures 7.9 and 7.10). The foreign body is usually visible once topical local anaesthetic has been applied and the eye and its adnexa have been examined carefully. Occasionally, examination under general anaesthesia and ancillary aids, such as diagnostic imaging, will be needed. If the foreign body is not identified initially, it may erode through the conjunctiva and migrate, usually in the orbital and paraorbital regions, rarely into the globe itself. Single or multiple discharging tracts may develop in such cases.

Differential diagnosis

The ocular discharge associated with a conjunctival foreign body should be differentiated from that of orbital infections and inflammations (which may include orbital foreign bodies), cysts and mucocoeles.

Treatment

Most conjunctival foreign bodies can be removed under direct vision, following the application of topical local anaesthetic. General anaesthesia is needed if surgical exploration is required.

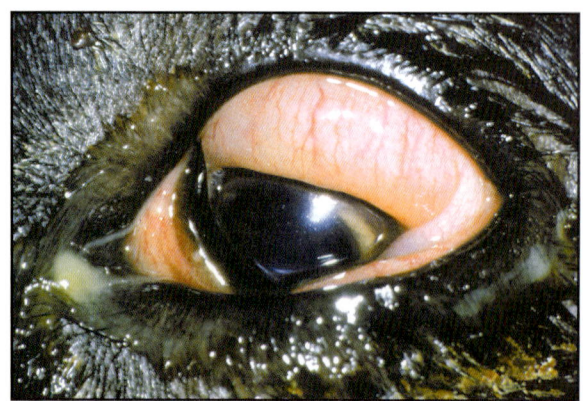

Figure 7.9 Conjunctival foreign body in the upper conjunctival fornix. The foreign body (a piece of wood) is not visible because of the extensive chemosis.

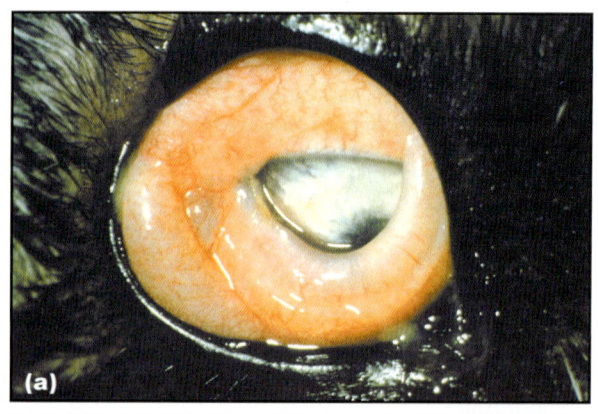

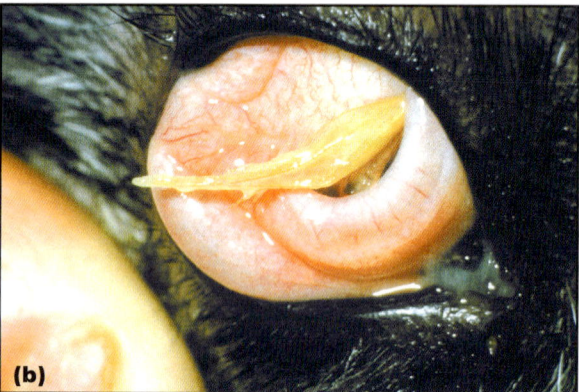

Figure 7.10 (a) The tip of a foreign body is just visible beyond the third eyelid margin. The foreign body was a large barley awn (b).

Neoplasia

Primary conjunctival neoplasia is unusual in dogs (Hendrix, 1999) but tumours may arise from the epithelial, vascular (Mughannam et al., 1997) or connective tissue elements (Figure 7.11). Melanoma, mast cell tumour, basal cell tumour, adenoma, fibroma, fibrosarcoma, haemangioma, haemangiosarcoma, angiokeratoma and viral papilloma have all been reported. Squamous cell carcinoma is rare. Secondary neoplasia is also rare, but cellular infiltration of the conjunctiva is a possible presentation of lymphoma (Figure 7.12) and systemic histiocytosis. Conjunctival involvement has also been reported in malignant angioendotheliomatosis (Kilrain et al., 1994).

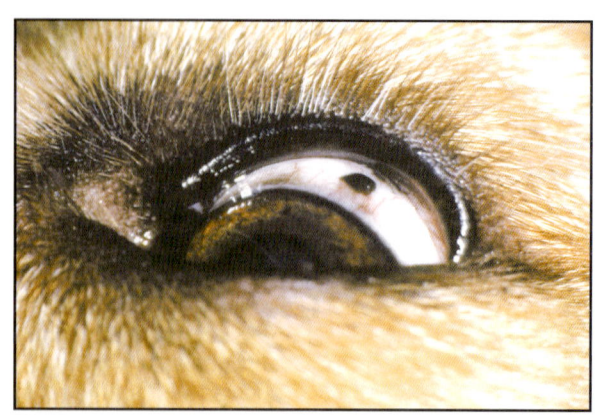

Figure 7.11 Primary conjunctival neoplasia. This angiokeratoma of the bulbar conjunctiva was removed surgically following topical local anaesthesia.

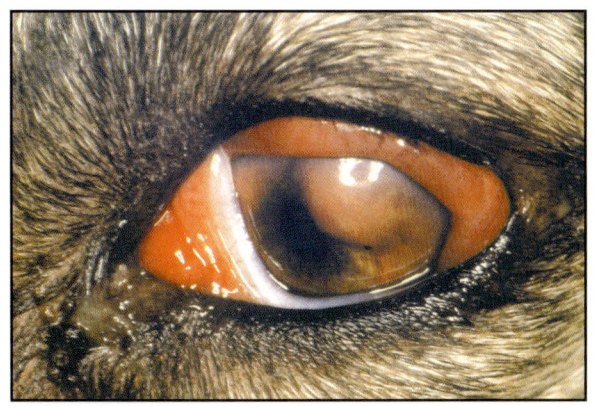

Figure 7.12 Secondary conjunctival neoplasia: conjunctival and extensive iris infiltration by lymphoma. The third eyelid is prominent because of orbital infiltration.

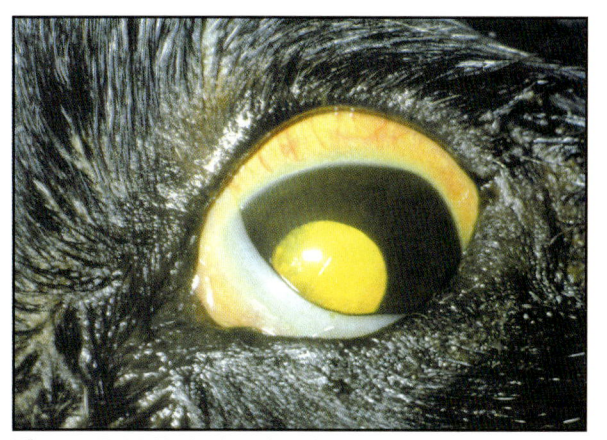

Figure 7.13 Typical conjunctival appearance in a dog with jaundice.

Histopathology should be regarded as a routine diagnostic method for conjunctival masses. In general, mast cell tumours of the conjunctiva are often benign, and conjunctival melanomas tend to be malignant.

Treatment
This is usually surgical for primary tumours, but management should be guided by the tumour's appearance and rate of growth. Small, well circumscribed, benign tumours involving only the conjunctiva can be removed under topical local anaesthesia; otherwise, general anaesthesia is required. Surgical removal can be reinforced with adjunctive therapy (e.g. cryotherapy, laser therapy or radiation therapy) at the time of surgery.

Differential diagnosis

- Dermoids should be distinguishable on the basis of their location and hair growth
- Nodular granulomatous masses may be a feature of parasitic diseases, such as onchocerciasis; conjunctival nodules may also form, rarely, in fungal diseases, such as blastomycosis
- Inflammatory diseases of the episclera and sclera that present with nodular swellings; episcleritis and scleritis are discussed in Chapter 9
- Cystic swellings including conjunctival epithelial inclusion cysts, orbital cysts and lacrimal cysts (see Chapter 6)
- Subconjunctival orbital fat prolapse, which is rare in dogs; the displaced fat can be excised and the diagnosis confirmed histologically.

Systemic disorders with conjunctival involvement
In all species, conjunctival appearance may be a useful indicator of systemic disease (Figures 7.13 and 7.14); similar changes of appearance are seen in mucous membranes at other sites. Obvious examples include the pallor of anaemia, the blue of cyanosis and the yellow of jaundice. Hyperviscosity syndromes (e.g. polycythaemia) may be associated with vascular engorgement, whereas ecchymoses and petechial haemorrhages may be indicative of platelet disorders or clotting defects.

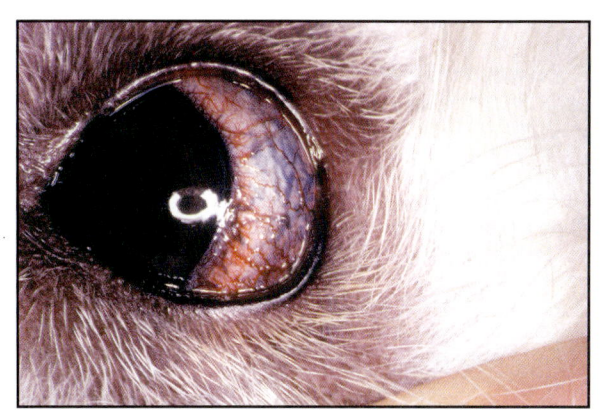

Figure 7.14 Conjunctival cyanosis and vascular congestion. Hyperviscosity was due to polycythaemia; both the polycythaemia and cyanosis were associated with congenital heart disease.

Feline conjunctival problems

Epibulbar dermoid
Epibulbar dermoids are less common in cats than in dogs and have a somewhat more variable appearance and position (Figure 7.15). They are usually unilateral. They may be inherited in the Birman (Hendy-Ibbs, 1985). Treatment is by surgical excision, as described previously for the dog.

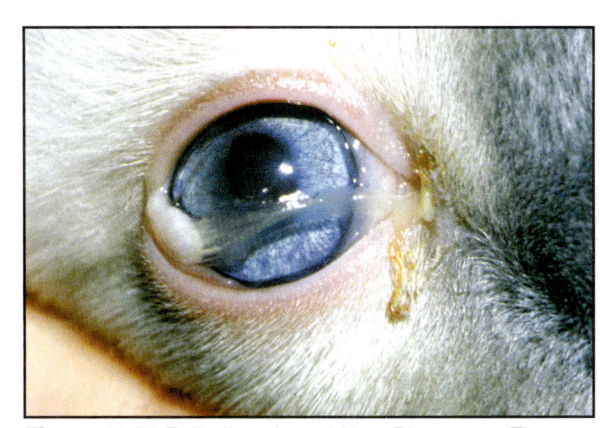

Figure 7.15 Epibulbar dermoid in a Birman cat. The dermoid also involved the lateral canthus.

Feline conjunctivitis

Aetiology

It is not always possible to differentiate the aetiology according to the ocular signs, and laboratory examination is required for precise identification, as described in Chapter 1.

Primary conjunctivitis:

- Infectious agents, notably the respiratory tract viruses (feline herpesvirus and calicivirus), chlamydia and *Mycoplasma* spp. *Chlamydophila felis* (formerly known as *Chlamydia psittaci* var. *felis*) is the organism isolated most often in the UK. The clinical significance of other bacterial isolates is not clearly defined.
- Non-infectious causes are similar to those outlined above for the dog, but they occur less frequently.

Secondary conjunctivitis: This is less common in the cat than in the dog and may follow:

- Eyelid problems such as agenesis, inflammation, neoplasia
- Tear-film abnormalities

Meibomianitis: This results in inspissation of lipid and consequent formation of chalazia when the meibomian glands rupture (Crispin, 1998). It is probably the commonest cause of lipogranulomatous conjunctivitis in cats (see Chapters 5 and 6). Release of lipid from conjunctival adipose tissue after, for example, ocular trauma, or deposition of lipids from an exogenous source cannot, however, be discounted as alternative causes (Kerlin and Dubielzig (1997).

Feline herpesvirus (FHV-1) infection: This is a significant ocular pathogen. Feline ocular herpesvirus infection has been most recently reviewed by Nasisse (1991), Glaze and Gelatt (1999) and Stiles (2000).

Clinical signs: Clinical manifestations of ocular infection vary according to the age of the animal. In neonatal kittens, ophthalmia neonatorum is typical of FHV-1 infection with secondary bacterial infection (Figure 7.16). Ophthalmia neonatorum consists of a severe conjunctivitis with ensuing epithelial necrosis, which may result in complications, such as symblepharon, corneal ulceration and corneal perforation. Endophthalmitis and panophthalmitis are also possible complications, as are a number of long-term problems associated with symblepharon formation; for example, there may be stenosis or occlusion of the lacrimal puncta, resulting in impaired tear drainage, or there may be occlusion of the lacrimal ductules, with consequent dry eye. It is particularly serious if the infection is present when the lids are still naturally fused (ankyloblepharon). Treatment in such cases must include the premature opening of the lids using blunt-tipped tenotomy scissors, as described for puppies in Chapter 5. Once the lids are opened, it is important to bathe the eyes and eyelids frequently enough to prevent recurrence and to treat any secondary bacterial infection.

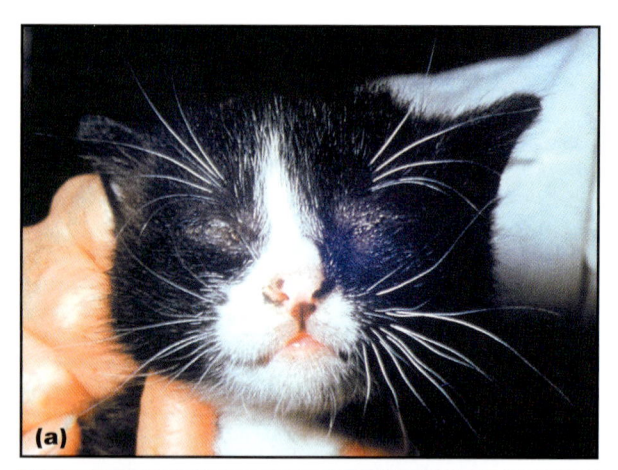

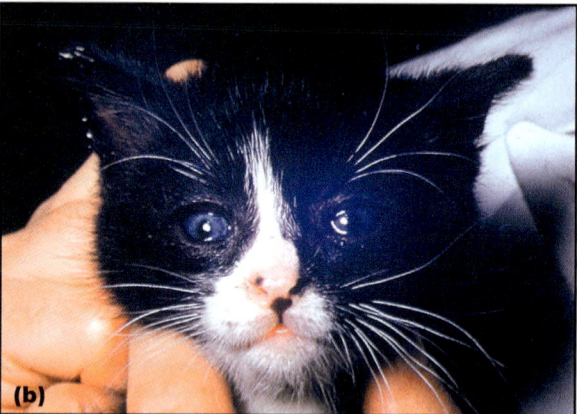

Figure 7.16 (a) Ophthalmia neonatorum associated with feline herpesvirus and secondary bacterial infection in a kitten. (b) The eyelids have been opened as a matter of urgency to excavate the pus and allow effective treatment.

In older kittens and young cats, acute, usually bilateral, conjunctivitis is the most conspicuous ocular feature, and fluorescein or rose bengal staining may reveal the pathognomonic microdendritic lesions. With acute herpes conjunctivitis there is ocular discomfort and marked chemosis, together with a discharge, which is initially serous, but later becomes purulent (Figure 7.17). In adult cats, herpetic keratitis is the commonest finding (see Chapter 8).

Chronic herpetic conjunctival disease in older cats is usually the result of reactivation of latent virus, as some 80% of affected cats become latently infected (Gaskell

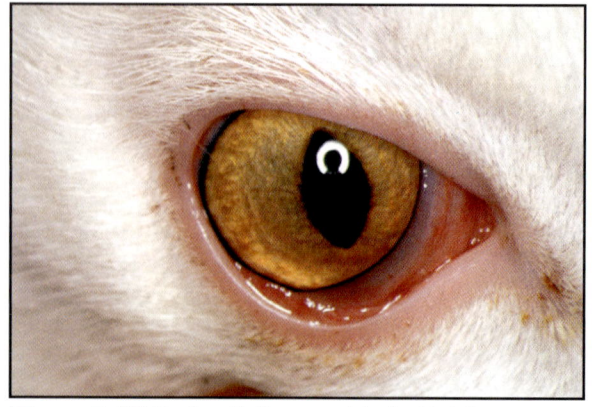

Figure 7.17 Conjunctivitis associated with feline herpesvirus infection in a young cat.

and Povey, 1977). In the chronic phase of the disease, upper respiratory infection is not usually present, although there is often a history of previous respiratory disease. The commonest manifestation is a unilateral or bilateral ocular discharge, which is often intermittent, coupled with mild conjunctival hyperaemia.

Diagnosis: The diagnosis of FHV-1 infection is usually confirmed by virus isolation, although identification of FHV-1 DNA using the polymerase chain reaction (PCR) is the most sensitive and specific technique. Samples should be collected from the oropharynx and conjunctival sac and placed in viral and chlamydial transport medium (VCTM), as described in Chapter 1.

Treatment: The treatment of acute FHV-1 infection includes provision of nursing care (removal of oculonasal discharge, nutrition and rehydration), the use of a systemic broad-spectrum antibiotic (when there is respiratory involvement) and topical tetracycline preparations to prevent secondary bacterial ocular infection. Antiviral therapy for the ocular manifestations of FHV-1 is described in Chapter 8. The prognosis for recovery from acute ocular FHV-1 infection is better than that for chronic or recurrent problems.

Feline calicivirus (FCV) infection

This is a much less common cause of viral conjunctivitis than FHV-1 and there is, in fact, some doubt as to whether FCV is a genuine conjunctival pathogen in the cat (Ramsey, 2000). Cats of any age are affected, but FCV infection is commoner and more severe in young kittens. Ocular signs may be associated with other pathogens (Figure 7.18). The clinical signs of infection largely relate to the effects of the virus on the upper respiratory tract, typically producing rhinitis and a serous nasal discharge. Vesicles, which rupture to produce clearly delineated ulcers, are commonly found in the mouth (e.g. tongue and oral mucosa). Asymptomatic carriers are common.

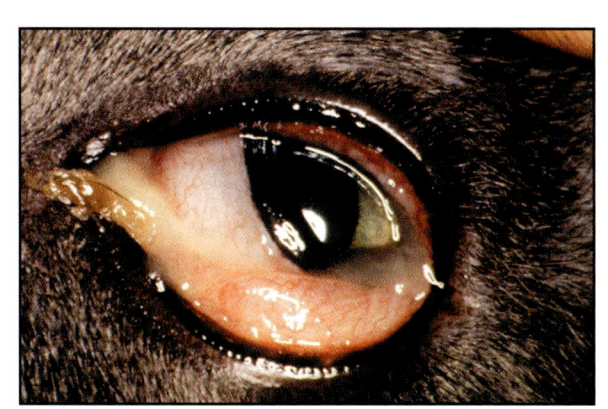

Figure 7.18 *Chlamydophila felis* and feline calicivirus were both isolated from this case of conjunctivitis.

Diagnosis: The diagnosis of calicivirus infection is usually confirmed by virus isolation. PCR provides the most sensitive and specific test for viral identification and the detection of asymptomatic carriers.

Treatment: This is mainly supportive, although systemic broad-spectrum antibiotics should also be provided, in case there is any generalized secondary bacterial infection, and topical antibiotics should be used if bacteria complicate the conjunctivitis. Calicivirus is not sensitive to the presently available antiviral drugs.

Feline *Chlamydophila felis* infection

Chlamydophila felis (formerly known as Chlamydia psittaci var. *felis)* is an obligate intracellular bacterium with a worldwide distribution. It is the most common cause of feline infectious conjunctivitis in the UK.

Clinical signs: These consist of an initial unilateral conjunctivitis which, within a few days, becomes bilateral (Figures 7.19 and 7.20). There is conjunctival chemosis and marked hyperaemia. The ocular discharge changes from serous to mucopurulent during the course of the disease. There is no corneal involvement and upper respiratory tract disease is an infrequent feature of chlamydiosis.

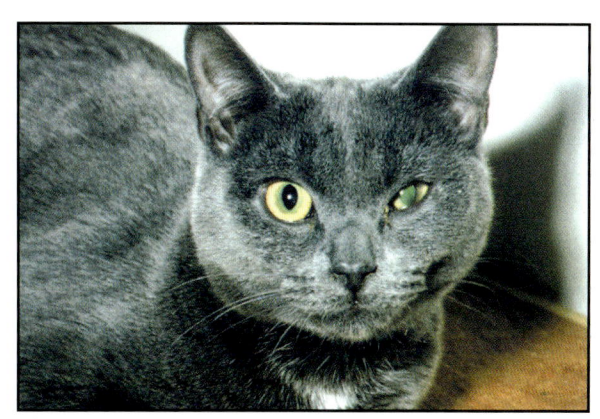

Figure 7.19 Acute conjunctivitis associated with *Chlamydophila felis* infection. Note the unilateral presentation. There was obvious discomfort.

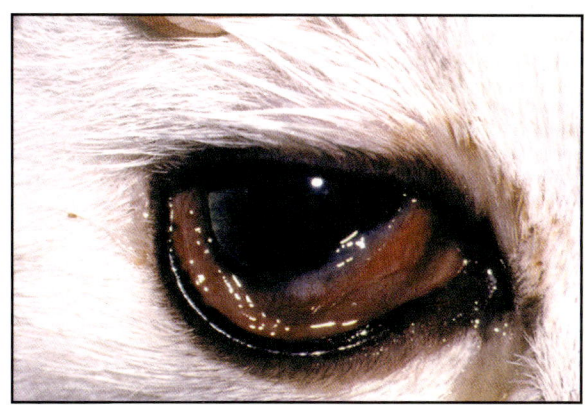

Figure 7.20 Acute conjunctivitis associated with *Chlamydophila felis* infection. There is an active hyperaemia of the conjunctival vessels, chemosis and an ocular discharge. The eye is uncomfortable.

Diagnosis: The diagnosis may be confirmed by taking conjunctival scrapings to identify intracytoplasmic inclusion bodies in the epithelial cells during the acute phase of the disease. A conjunctival swab, cytology brush or a Kimura spatula is used to obtain samples

132 The conjunctiva

from the ventral conjunctival sac for culture in VCTM and indirect fluorescent antibody or PCR testing (see Chapter 1). Serology is of limited value, in that a low antibody titre is not diagnostic of the absence of chlamydia, whereas a high antibody titre may indicate, but does not confirm, infection with chlamydia. Titres may remain high for up to a year after infection.

Treatment: This consists of systemic treatment with the tetracycline group of antibiotics. Doxycycline (5 mg/kg orally bid for 21–28 days) is the usual drug selected, and a newer-generation drug called azithromycin (see Chapter 3) requires further evaluation (Ramsey, 2000). This group of drugs should not be used in pregnant queens or kittens and clavulanic acid-potentiated amoxycillin provides a safe and effective alternative (Sturgess et al., 2001). Topical tetracycline is not always well tolerated in the cat: it may provoke a rapid hypersensitivity response initially and, if its use continues, marginal blepharitis can develop. Chlortetracycline is the only topical tetracycline preparation available for cats in the UK.

Feline *Mycoplasma* infection

Mycoplasma spp., possibly in association with primary pathogens such as FHV-1 and *Chlamydophila felis*, may be associated with feline conjunctivitis. There is increasing evidence that *Mycoplasma felis* is unlikely to be a primary pathogen (Whitley, 2000). *Mycoplasma* spp. may be isolated from the conjunctival sac of normal cats, and it is known that cats cannot be infected experimentally unless they are immunosuppressed.

Clinical signs: The initial clinical signs are blepharospasm, epiphora and conjunctival hyperaemia. Within 14 days, the most striking finding is pallor of the conjunctiva, some thickening and chemosis, and a typical pseudomembranous conjunctivitis. Confirmation of mycoplasmal conjunctivitis is difficult, as isolation requires specific *Mycoplasma* culture media, and the possibility of concurrent pathogens must also be investigated.

Treatment: *Mycoplasma* spp. are susceptible to tetracyclines given topically for 5–7 days, but there are potential disadvantages associated with the use of these drugs (see above). The clinical course is shortened to about 5 days in treated cases; without treatment, the time course is 30–60 days.

Other bacteria

The clinical significance of some bacteria (e.g. *Staphylococcus*) is uncertain, whereas *Pasteurella multocida*, transmitted in fight injuries, is clinically relevant. Bacterial conjunctivitis may occur secondary to other ocular disease (ocular, adnexal or orbital infection, keratoconjunctivitis sicca, dacryocystitis) and in cats that are stressed or immunocompromised.

Symblepharon

Symblepharon (Figures 7.21 and 7.22) is much more common in cats than in dogs. It can be the result of previous inflammation, particularly with FHV-1, but

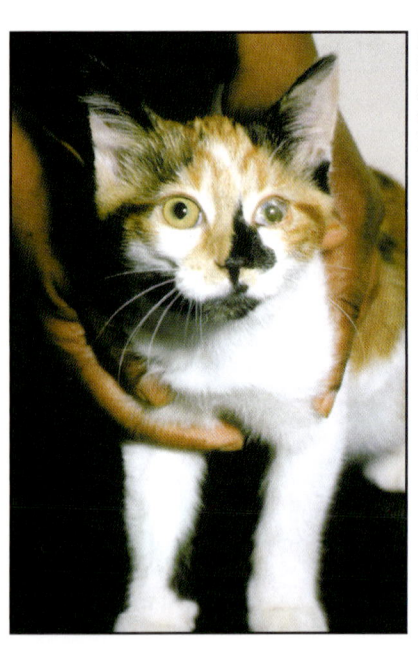

Figure 7.21 Symblepharon, affecting the left eye only in this kitten.

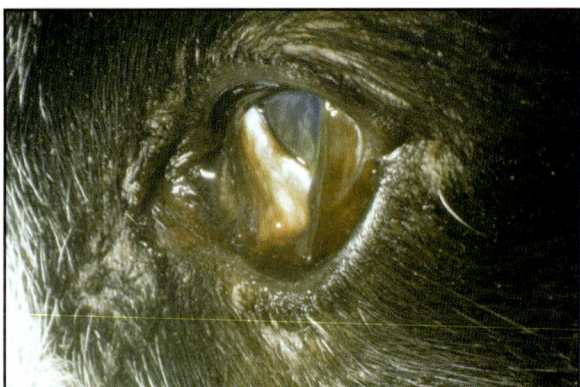

Figure 7.22 Extensive symblepharon in a young cat. Only a small area of normal cornea is visible because of the conjunctival adhesions. Note the obliteration of the ventral fornix by adhesions.

abscesses and chemical burns can also produce extensive adhesions. The severe nature of neonatal FHV-1 infection often destroys the limbal stem cell population so that ocular surface disease and aberrant healing responses compromise surgical efforts to restore normal function.

Treatment

Treatment is only necessary when problems such as reduced eyelid mobility, exposure keratopathy or impaired vision are a direct result of the symblepharon. The results of treatment are likely to be disappointing when there is pre-existing severe ocular surface disease. Whatever surgical technique is used, the most important principle is to ensure that there are no raw surfaces in contact after surgery; otherwise adhesions will re-form rapidly and more extensively than those which were present prior to surgery. There are many possible methods for surgical repair of symblepharon; the Arlt and Teale Knapp techniques have been described by Peiffer (1981). The important principles of this type of surgery are discussed by Roper-Hall (1989) and Mustardé (1991).

Trauma and foreign bodies

In cats, there is often a most spectacular chemosis as part of the clinical presentation; consequently, examination under general anaesthesia may be needed to define the extent of traumatic damage or to locate a foreign body. In other respects, these cases are handled as described for the dog.

Neoplasia

Conjunctival neoplasia is rare. Primary conjunctival tumours include papilloma, adenoma, adenocarcinoma, basal cell tumour, haemangioma, haemangiosarcoma, lymphoma, neurofibroma, neurofibrosarcoma, fibroma, fibrosarcoma and malignant melanoma. The most common neoplasm to encroach on the conjunctiva is eyelid squamous cell carcinoma (Figure 7.23). Tumours that can metastasize to the conjunctiva include lymphoma (Figure 7.24) and adenocarcinoma.

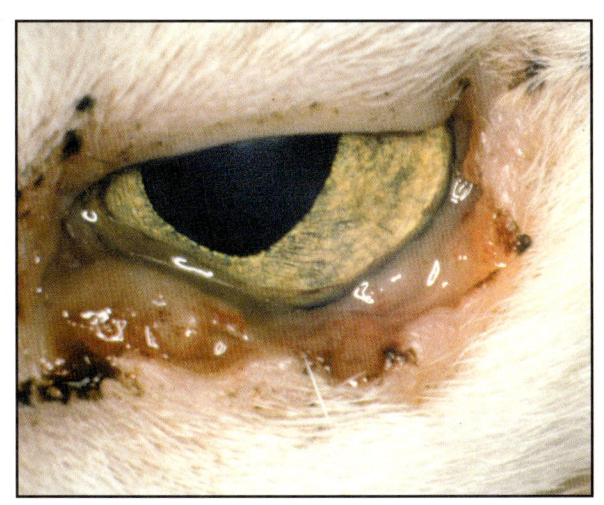

Figure 7.23 Squamous cell carcinoma has eroded the lower eyelid.

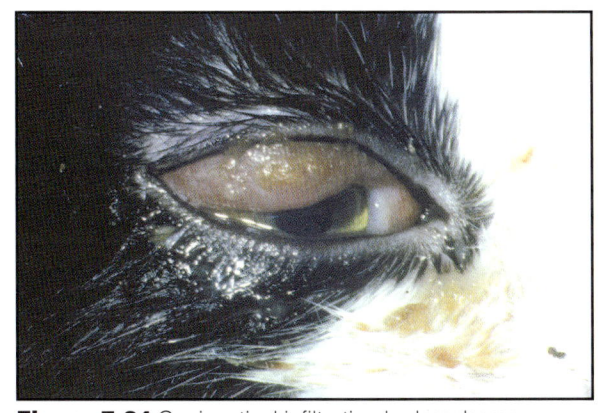

Figure 7.24 Conjunctival infiltration by lymphoma.

Management is as outlined for the dog, but with the important difference that feline tumours are usually malignant. It is, therefore, very important to perform exfoliative cytology or histopathology and to assess tumours carefully to make sure that complete excision is a realistic possibility. Squamous cell carcinomas may require a combination of surgery, radiotherapy or cryotherapy and reconstructive eyelid surgery for effective cure.

References and further reading

Bauer GA, Speiss BM and Lutz H (1996) Exfoliative cytology of conjunctiva and cornea in domestic animals: a comparison of four collecting techniques. *Veterinary and Comparative Ophthalmology* **6,** 181–186

Crispin SM (1998) Conjunctiva, limbus, episclera and sclera. In: *Feline Ophthalmology: An Atlas and Text*, ed. KC Barnett and SM Crispin, pp. 69–82. WB Saunders, London

Gaskell RM and Povey RC (1977) Experimental induction of feline rhinotracheitis virus re-excretion in FVR-recovered cats. *Veterinary Record* **100,** 128–133

Glaze MB and Gelatt KN (1999) Feline ophthalmology. In: *Veterinary Ophthalmology, 3rd edn,* ed. KN Gelatt, pp. 997–1052. Lippincott, Williams and Wilkins, Philadelphia

Hendrix DV (1999) Diseases and surgery of the canine conjunctiva. In: *Veterinary Ophthalmology, 3rd edn,* ed. KN Gelatt, pp. 619–634. Lippincott, Williams and Wilkins, Philadelphia

Hendy-Ibbs PN (1985) Familial feline epibulbar dermoids. *Veterinary Record* **116,** 13–14

Kerlin RL and Dubielzig RR (1997) Lipogranulomatous conjunctivitis in cats. *Veterinary and Comparative Ophthalmology* **7,** 177–179

Kilrain CG, Saik JE and Jeglum KA (1994) Malignant angioendotheliomatosis with retinal detachment in a dog. *Journal of the American Veterinary Medical Association* **204,** 918–921

Mughannam AJ, Hacker DV and Spangler WL (1997) Conjunctival vascular tumours in six dogs. *Veterinary and Comparative Ophthalmology* **7,** 56–59

Mustardé JC (1991) The conjunctiva. In: *Repair and Reconstruction in the Orbital Region, 3rd edn,* ed. JC Mustardé, pp. 101–108. Churchill Livingstone, Edinburgh

Nasisse MP (1991) Feline ophthalmology. In: *Veterinary Ophthalmology, 2nd edn,* ed. KN Gelatt, pp. 529–575. Lea and Febiger, Philadelphia

Peiffer RL (1981) Feline ophthalmology. In: *Veterinary Ophthalmology, 1st edn,* ed. KN Gelatt, pp. 521–568. Lea and Febiger, Philadelphia

Ramsey DT (2000) Feline chlamydia and calicivirus infections. *Veterinary Clinics of North America* **30,** 1015–1028

Ramsey DT, Ketring KL, Glaze MB, Knight B and Render JA (1996) Ligneous conjunctivitis in four Doberman Pinschers. *Journal of the American Animal Hospital Association* **32,** 439–447

Roper-Hall MJ (1989) The eyelids and reconstructive (plastic) surgery. In: *Stallard's Eye Surgery, 7th edn,* ed. MJ Roper-Hall, pp. 64–134. Wright, London

Sturgess CP, Gruffydd-Jones TJ, Harbour DA and Jones RL (2001) Controlled study of the efficacy of clavulanic acid-potentiated amoxycillin in the treatment of *Chlamydia psittaci* in cats. *Veterinary Record* **149,** 73–76

Stiles J (2000) Feline herpesvirus. *Veterinary Clinics of North America* **30,** 1001–1014

Whitley RD (2000) Canine and feline primary ocular bacterial infections. *Veterinary Clinics of North America* **30,** 1151–1167

Willis M, Bounous DI, Hirsh S, Kaswan R, Stiles J, Martin C, Rakich P and Roberts W (1997) Conjunctival brush cytology. Evaluation of a new cytological technique in dogs and cats with a comparison to conjunctival scraping. *Veterinary and Comparative Ophthalmology* **7,** 74–81

8

The cornea

Sheila Crispin

Embryology, anatomy and physiology

The cornea is derived from surface ectoderm and mesenchyme (mesoderm and neural crest). Presumptive corneal epithelium derived from the surface ectoderm which overlies the optic cup secretes an acellular primary stroma consisting of collagen fibrils and glycosaminoglycans (GAGs). Mesenchymal neural crest cells migrate between the surface ectoderm and the optic cup into the future anterior chamber to form the secondary stroma and corneal endothelium, as well as most structures of the iridocorneal angle, iris stroma and ciliary muscle (see Chapters 10 and 11). The secondary stroma consists of type I collagen fibrils and fibronectin secreted by developing keratocytes, although much of the fibronectin is lost during subsequent development (Cook, 1999).

The mature cornea is elliptical, such that the horizontal diameter is slightly bigger than the vertical diameter. Ultrasonic pachymetry has indicated that it is less than 0.7 mm in thickness in both the dog (Gilger et al., 1991) and cat (Schoster et al., 1995). It is optically clear, despite the presence of a rich network of sensory nerves, and both transmits and refracts light. Blood vessels and lymphoid tissue are conspicuously absent, but they are present in the perilimbal tissues. Normal microscopic anatomy of the canine cornea has been described by Shively and Epling (1970) and the anatomy of the feline cornea by Carrington et al. (1992). In both species it consists of an anterior epithelium and basement membrane, substantia propria (stroma), Descemet's membrane (posterior limiting lamina) and endothelium (Figure 8.1).

The corneal epithelium

This consists of an outer layer of squamous cells, a middle layer of polyhedral or wing cells and an inner, single layer of columnar cells that produce the basement membrane. The epithelium is attached to the basement membrane by hemidesmosomes, and fine fibrils link the basal epithelium, basement membrane and subepithelial stroma.

The stroma

The stroma, or substantia propria, comprises the bulk of the cornea, consisting primarily of keratocytes, regularly arranged collagen fibrils and ground substance. The fibrils are of uniform diameter and arranged in flat sheet-like bundles (lamellae) that extend across the entire width of the cornea, from limbus to limbus. The lamellae cross orthogonally (i.e. at approximately 90 degrees to each other) producing a grid iron effect in the multiple layers. The ground substance, of proteoglycans and their associated GAGs and glycoproteins, occupies the space between lamellae. The keratocytes have a slow turnover rate in normal adult cornea, but if there is a corneal insult they can become activated fibroblasts and produce the precursors of collagen and ground substance. Other cells, such as leucocytes, lymphocytes and macrophages are rare in the normal cornea, and are most likely to be found in the epithelial layers and, less frequently, the stroma.

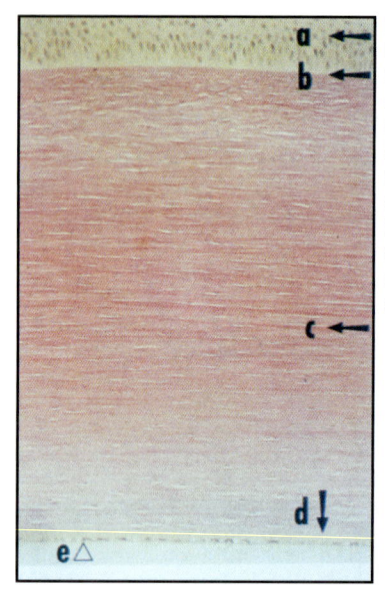

Figure 8.1 Histology of the normal canine cornea. a = anterior epithelium; b = basement membrane; c = connective tissue stroma; d = Descemet's membrane; e = endothelium.

Descemet's membrane and endothelium

The corneal endothelium produces Descemet's membrane throughout life, but its own powers of replication diminish early in life in the majority of mammals, the rabbit being one exception. When endothelial cells die, they are replaced by neighbouring cells spreading to fill the gap. Consequently, the endothelium thins and Descemet's membrane thickens as the animal ages.

The endothelium is a single layer of cells of high metabolic activity and is of crucial importance in maintaining corneal deturgescence and thus corneal clarity.

Corneal wound healing

Epithelial damage
This is repaired by corneal epithelial slide (early response) and epithelial mitosis (later response). There is also critical assistance from multipotential limbal stem cells. Phagocytic cells, notably polymorphonuclear leucocytes, gain access to the injured cornea via the limbus and the preocular tear film. Epithelial turnover in the normal eye takes about 7 days.

Stromal damage
This is repaired by the epithelial cells filling the defect, migration of cells from the limbus, and by generation from the stromal elements (fibroblasts, which produce collagen and ground substance). The type of collagen which is laid down in damaged stroma differs from the original collagen in type and orientation, so the transparency of the cornea is lost in the affected area.

Rupture of Descemet's membrane
Rupture is followed by retraction, as Descemet's membrane is elastic. Reduplication can occur from endothelial cells that slide in over the injured area.

Endothelial damage
The endothelium repairs poorly in most adult animals because of limited or absent regenerative abilities, so it can only respond to insult by spreading the single layer of cells more thinly.

Corneal response to insult

Oedema
Corneal oedema is not a specific disease but an indication of corneal damage. Discrete damage to the anterior epithelium will result in a focal area of corneal oedema (e.g. following traumatic insult), but more widespread injury, as from chemical or thermal burns, will produce more diffuse involvement.

Stromal oedema usually accompanies insult to the epithelium or endothelium. The cornea swells and becomes thicker and the optical properties of the cornea are compromized.

Damage to the corneal endothelium will affect the ability of this cell layer to keep the cornea in a relative state of deturgescence. The oedema may be localized (e.g. at the sites of adherent keratic precipitates) or diffuse (e.g. associated with a delayed hypersensitivity response in canine viral hepatitis: the classical 'blue eye').

Other causes of corneal oedema include blunt and penetrating trauma, surgical trauma (endothelial cells are easily displaced), intraocular inflammation (particularly severe inflammation, such as endophthalmitis), intraocular neoplasia and endothelial dystrophies. Glaucoma is also an important cause of corneal oedema (see Chapter 11).

Vascularization
No blood vessels are present in the normal canine and feline cornea, but corneal neovascularization is a common pathological response to corneal insult.

Superficial vessels arise from the conjunctival vessels and, in the canine eye, are readily observed as they cross the limbus; they branch dichotomously and are bright red in colour. Superficial keratitis is often associated with conjunctivitis.

Deep vessels arise from the ciliary plexus and cannot be observed until they enter the cornea. These vessels are usually short, dark and straight, occasionally they are so extensive that they form a complete circle (ciliary flush). There are many causes of deep vascularization; these include keratitis, anterior uveitis and endophthalmitis.

Vascularization may be instrumental in promoting corneal healing, and it is important to assist and not to compromise this process. Once the beneficial effects of vascularization have been achieved, the vessels narrow quite naturally and they become faint, but permanent, ghost vessels. Excessive granulation tissue or complications of healing, such as pigment deposition associated with vascularization, may be mitigated by the early use of topical corticosteroids, provided that the epithelium is intact.

Pigmentation
This may be an occasional congenital finding, usually involving the posterior cornea as a manifestation of anterior segment dysgenesis.

Acquired pigmentation is more common, usually as a nonspecific response to corneal insult involving the epithelium and stroma. This is associated with pigment proliferation and migration, as well as neovascularization. Endothelial pigmentation is most commonly seen after rupture of uveal cysts. The problems that arise from pigmentation depend on the extent and depth of pigment deposition and this, in turn, depends on the amount of pigment normally present at the limbus.

Other responses
These include cellular infiltration, degenerative changes and scarring. Corneal lipid deposition is not uncommon in dogs, but is rare in cats. Corneal calcification is encountered infrequently in cats and dogs; it can, for example, be a long-term complication of parotid duct transposition, or of dystrophic origin. Infiltration of the cornea by inflammatory cells occurs in a wide variety of conditions, and some of these are described in more detail below.

Protocol for the investigation of corneal disease

Just as it is important to follow a logical and set protocol for the examination of the whole eye, so it is crucial to apply the same logic to the investigation of corneal disease, as set out in Figure 8.2.

- Naked eye examination of the normal blink and the protective blink as part of dazzle and palpebral reflexes and menace response
- Naked eye examination of the upper and lower eyelids and the lashes – outer aspect, margin, inner aspect of eyelids
- Naked eye examination of the outer aspect of the third eyelid and its movement
- Corneal sensitivity assessment
- Corneal examination with magnification using a loupe, a magnifying lens or a slit lamp biomicroscope
- Schirmer Tear Test (usually Schirmer I, rarely Schirmer II)
- (Fluorescein break-up time)
- (Measurement of the conjunctival sac pH using standard pH test papers)
- (Application of topical local anaesthetic)
- (Examination of the inner aspect of the third eyelid)
- (Taking of swabs and scrapes for culture and sensitivity)
- Application of fluorescein stain with or without examination with magnification and blue light in darkness
- (Application of rose bengal, with or without examination with magnification)

Figure 8.2 Protocol for the investigation of corneal disease. Both eyes should be examined and the two should be compared. Investigations shown in parentheses are not a routine part of the assessment.

Developmental corneal conditions in the dog

Absence/microcornea/megalocornea

Complete absence of the cornea is extremely rare, but may be seen in association with the equally rare anomalies anophthalmos and cystic eye.

Partial absence of the cornea, or a cornea that is smaller than normal, occurs most commonly with microphthalmos. Anomalies of this type may be unilateral or bilateral, and there is usually no obvious cause, although inherited defects and the actions of teratogens should always be considered as possibilities.

Much more rarely, microcornea, a cornea that is proportionately smaller than normal for the size of the globe, is encountered, and is associated with faulty contact between the optic vesicle and the surface ectoderm during development.

Megalocornea (a cornea which is larger than normal) is rare in dogs and usually occurs in conjunction with other developmental ocular abnormalities, such as anterior segment dysgenesis severe enough to produce congenital glaucoma and buphthalmos.

There is no treatment for major defects of ocular differentiation.

Corneal opacity

Transient diffuse corneal opacity is present in young puppies when the eyes first open, but should not be apparent by the time the puppy is 4–5 weeks of age. Focal superficial opacities in the area of the palpebral fissure are also encountered in young puppies. They have usually disappeared by 4 months of age.

Permanent corneal opacities are encountered most frequently because of the presence of persistent pupillary membrane (PPM) remnants or some other form of anterior segment dysgenesis. Opacities associated with PPM are usually posterior and focal. They cause no clinical problems in the majority of animals and should be left alone.

Dermoid

A dermoid is a choristoma; these superficial skin-like masses typically involve the conjunctival, scleral and corneal temporal limbus. They are removed by superficial lamellar keratectomy, making the initial incision in clear cornea and dissecting towards the limbus. A lateral canthotomy may be needed prior to keratectomy to ensure adequate exposure of the conjunctival portion of the dermoid (see Chapter 7).

Acquired corneal conditions in the dog

Corneal dystrophies

The description 'corneal dystrophy' should be reserved for functional and morphological changes occurring bilaterally, but not necessarily symmetrically, in a previously normal cornea, and not caused by disease elsewhere in the eye or elsewhere in the body. To justify the term 'dystrophy', the condition should be of proven inheritance. In veterinary ophthalmology, a number of familial corneal dystrophies are suspected, but hard proof of inheritance is lacking for most of them at present (Crispin, 1982; Cooley and Dice, 1990).

Epithelial basement membrane dystrophy

Epithelial basement membrane dystrophy (Gelatt and Samuelson, 1982) has a variety of other descriptive names including refractory epithelial erosion, recurrent epithelial erosion and indolent ulceration. Epithelial basement membrane dystrophy is a condition which is seen with most frequency in breeds such as the Boxer and Pembroke Corgi in the UK; the mode of inheritance is unknown. Refractory epithelial erosions of less certain pathogenesis are undoubtedly a common problem in a variety of other pedigree and non-pedigree dogs and, as the management of all types of superficial erosion is similar, they will be discussed together.

Clinical findings: Epithelial basement membrane dystrophy is most common in older dogs (5–7 years) and there is no sex predisposition. Moderate pain accompanied by blepharospasm and lacrimation is typical of the clinical presentation. The appearance of the ulcer is quite characteristic in that it is always superficial, shows little if any tendency to resolve and is usually surrounded by a rim of non-adherent corneal epithelium. The affected area is fluorescein-positive (Figure 8.3). While it commonly presents as a unilateral condition, both eyes are potentially at risk in the course of the animal's life. In addition to establishing the nature of the corneal defect, it is important to check for any obvious cause or other factors which might contribute to poor healing. Inadequate tear production, distichiasis and ectopic cilia are commonly missed as causative or contributory factors.

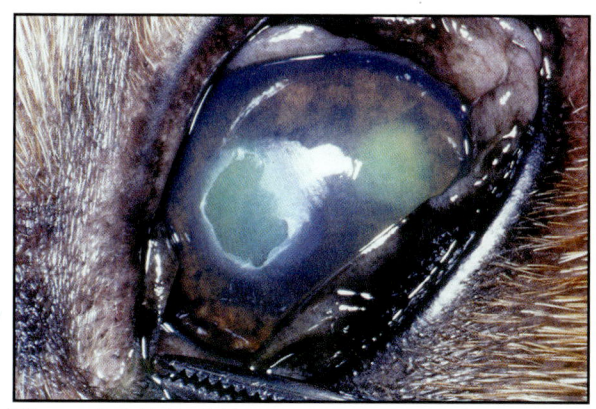

Figure 8.3 Epithelial basement membrane dystrophy in a Boxer. There are two fluorescein-positive areas. The fluorescein-positive ulcer is very superficial and the 'banked up' appearance of the epithelium at the edge of the ulcer is highly characteristic. The fluorescein staining in the oedematous area lateral to the ulcer indicates that the tight junctions between epithelial cells have been compromised, allowing fluorescein access to the underlying stroma, but frank ulceration is not yet present.

Pathology: Defects observed with microscopy in the eroded areas in affected Boxers include degeneration of basal epithelial cells, paucity of hemidesmosomes and subepithelial fibrogranular material. The basement membrane is thickened and irregular in appearance. A thin layer of abnormal hyalinized collagen in the superficial cornea may act as a further barrier to epithelial adhesion.

Treatment: In affected dogs, the mechanism of epithelial slide is apparently normal, but abnormal basement membrane material, and possibly hyalinized collagen, prevents the epithelium attaching to the underlying stroma. Treatment aims to aid the normal healing process by removing debris and encouraging epithelial attachment. The corneal erosions can be treated using chemical cauterizing agents or surgery, and these techniques have also been applied to the treatment of other types of primary persistent corneal erosion in which no underlying cause can be identified. It is most important to emphasize that it is only conditions involving simple epithelial loss that are treated by the regimes outlined below.

Chemical cauterants: Possible chemical cauterants include liquefied phenol (80% w/w phenol and 20% w/w water), pure trichloracetic acid and 6% aqueous iodine solution. These agents have antiseptic and cauterizing actions. Phenol is a most effective agent in the treatment of primary persistent corneal erosions; unfortunately, in common with other benzene derivatives, there is now some concern about its potential carcinogenic effects.

Approximately 2 ml of the cauterant selected should be decanted into a small container prior to use. A tiny pledget of cotton wool is grasped, using Halstead's mosquito forceps, and wound tightly around the closed tips. Following topical local anaesthesia (e.g. proxymetacaine hydrochloride or proparacaine hydrochloride) the cauterizing agent is applied precisely, starting at the apparent edge of the erosion (the rim of loosened epithelium) and working outwards to the true edge of the erosion (the region where the epithelium is properly attached to underlying stroma). After cautery, the eye is gently irrigated with sterile saline, although this is probably unnecessary as cauterant is applied so accurately to the affected cornea.

Surgery: Superficial keratotomy (e.g. grid and multiple punctate) and superficial keratectomy are the two most commonly used surgical treatments for primary persistent corneal erosions (Champagne and Munger, 1992; Morgan and Abrams, 1994):

- Grid keratotomy is probably the commonest approach used and may be performed under local or general anaesthesia (Gilger and Whitley, 1999). Loose epithelium is removed with a sterile dry cotton swab, using the circular motion described above for chemical cautery. A 25 gauge hypodermic needle is then used to create a grid pattern of microsurgical incisions about 1–2 mm apart and, as the needle should penetrate no further than 0.2–0.3 mm, good magnification is advisable. The grid pattern should extend 2–3 mm beyond the area of abnormal adhesion (Figure 8.4).

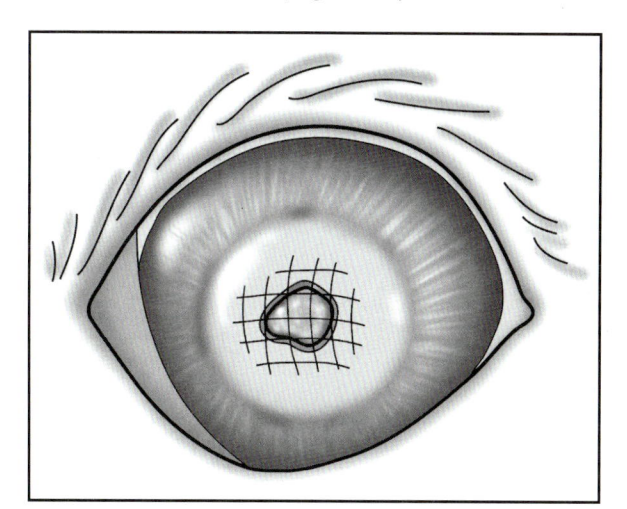

Figure 8.4 Diagram of the pattern used to perform grid keratotomy.

- Superficial keratectomy is performed under general anaesthesia, usually with the magnification provided by an operating microscope. Loose epithelium is removed with a sterile dry cotton swab, and a Beaver blade (no. 64) is used to excise superficial cornea to the same depth and extent as already described for grid keratotomy. A third eyelid flap can be used to protect the cornea after surgery. This combined approach was associated with the shortest healing time in an uncontrolled study by Stanley *et al.* (1998), which compared three methods: debridement with a sterile dry cotton swab, grid keratotomy and superficial keratectomy combined with a third eyelid flap.

Whatever approach is used, effective healing (i.e. robust epithelial cover) should have occurred within 2 weeks of treatment (Figure 8.5). If the problem does not resolve with chemical treatment, it is usually because of inadequate treatment or misdiagnosis. For example, when chemical cautery has been used, it may not have extended to the region of normal epithelial adhesion, or the dog may have some other problem, such as a tear film deficit or distichiasis. Misdiagnoses of this type can also underlie failures with surgical treatment. In addition, surgery in inexperienced hands may be associated with the immediate complication of corneal perforation and the later complication of unacceptable corneal scarring.

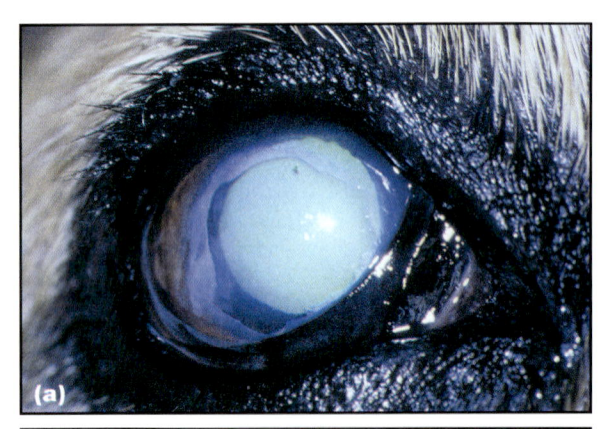

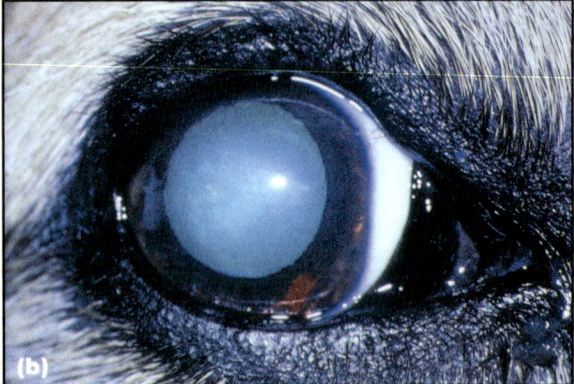

Figure 8.5 Epithelial basement membrane dystrophy in a Pembroke Corgi. (a) Prior to treatment with topical phenol. (b) Two months after treatment.

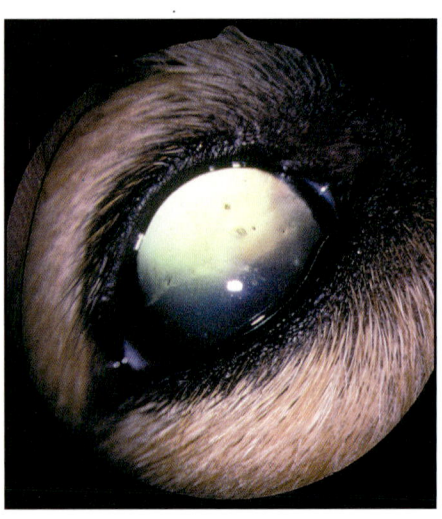

Figure 8.6 Epithelial dystrophy in a Shetland Sheepdog.

Epithelial dystrophy
A form of epithelial 'dystrophy' characterized by multiple focal grey to white ring-shaped opacities at the level of the anterior epithelium is occasionally observed in Shetland Sheepdogs (Figure 8.6); in many cases, the patients are asymptomatic. Occasionally, tiny erosions can be demonstrated with fluorescein or rose bengal, and these patients have an increased blink rate, increased lacrimation and mild ocular discomfort with a fluorescein break-up time (FBUT) of less than 10 seconds. These are features which should prompt investigation of the mucin component of the tear film. The ocular appearance is similar to human adenovirus keratitis. One report (Dice, 1984) indicated that some affected animals had low T4 levels and positive rheumatoid factors.

Treatment: As might be expected of a condition where the cause has not been established, a range of therapeutic approaches have been tried, including simple tear replacement, topical antiviral therapy, topical cyclosporin and topical corticosteroids. Debridement, keratotomy and keratectomy as already described for epithelial basement membrane dystrophy have been used to treat animals with corneal erosions.

Crystalline stromal dystrophy (central crystalline dystrophy)
This is a condition in which lipid is deposited in the corneal stroma (Crispin, 1982). It shares many features with the eponymous human condition described by Schnyder, although the mode of inheritance is uncertain in dogs. Pedigrees from affected Cavalier King Charles Spaniels and Rough Collies indicate either an autosomal dominant or multifactorial mode of inheritance as possibilities. Test matings of affected Siberian Huskies, on the other hand, have suggested a possible recessive mode of inheritance with variable expression.

Lipid deposition of this type is seen in many breeds (e.g. Rough Collie, Cavalier King Charles Spaniel, Shetland Sheepdog, Afghan Hound, Beagle, Siberian Husky, German Shepherd Dog and Samoyed). It is probably sensible to use the descriptive term corneal lipidosis if inheritance is unproven, for it is clear that systemic factors can modify the evolution of lesions of this type.

Clinical findings: The condition is most commonly seen in young adults; rarely, it is seen in puppies. It is essentially bilateral and reasonably symmetrical, although it is not uncommon for one eye to be affected in advance of the other.

The opacity is usually situated in the central or paracentral region of the cornea and is typically of crystalline appearance (Figure 8.7). Careful examination indicates that the opacity is located subepithelially in the anterior stroma of most breeds affected and the integrity of the corneal epithelium can be readily confirmed by a lack of fluorescein uptake.

In the Siberian Husky, the lipid deposition is often deeper and more extensive, so that lipid deposition can involve the posterior stroma adjacent to Descemet's membrane as well as the anterior stroma.

Conditions of the cornea 139

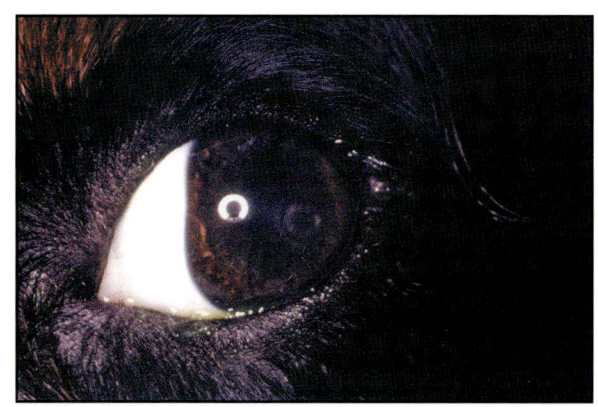

Figure 8.7 Crystalline stromal dystrophy in a Cavalier King Charles Spaniel. Fluorescein has been applied to demonstrate that the epithelium is intact. The lipid, which is visible in the central/paracentral cornea, is in the subepithelial and anterior stromal regions. The dog was normolipoproteinaemic.

There is no associated inflammation and the opacity, once formed, may remain static. On occasions, however, the opacities regress and, sometimes, they may progress, but without causing any ocular discomfort. Many of the breeds in which this condition occurs also have distichiasis, but the effects of chronic low grade mechanical trauma on an intact epithelium as a contributory factor in the pathogenesis of crystalline stromal dystrophy have not been scientifically evaluated.

In bitches, crystalline stromal dystrophy is sometimes first observed, or becomes accentuated, following oestrus, and may be associated with the transient increase in systemic lipoproteins which occurs in metoestrus. In view of this association, it is certainly worth checking the serum lipoprotein pattern of cases in which opacification is marked, or progressive, or when it is situated in the deeper cornea, as in the Siberian Husky.

Pathology: The predominant lipid is cholesterol, in both free and esterified forms, with lesser quantities of free fatty acids and phospholipids. The basic defect in this type of dystrophy appears to reside in the corneal fibroblast, which accumulates large amounts of lipid, mainly cholesterol, before dying *in situ*. The changes are largely restricted to the anterior third of the corneal stroma.

Treatment: No treatment is required in the majority of cases. Only when the opacity is progressive and dense is further investigation required, to establish the lipid and lipoprotein profile and to determine if systemic treatment is required to modify the evolution of the corneal opacity.

Corneal endothelial dystrophies

These may occur in a number of pedigree breeds of dog. However, there is, as yet, no proof of inheritance, except for the posterior polymorphous dystrophy described in the American Cocker Spaniel, which is suggested to be inherited in a dominant or incompletely dominant way. Posterior polymorphous dystrophy resembles a human corneal dystrophy of the same name. It is associated with endothelial cell abnormalities and presents clinically as multifocal posterior corneal opacities of linear and vesicular appearance, but the pathology is not usually extensive enough to produce corneal oedema. Affected dogs can be asymptomatic.

This is not the situation with the other major type of canine endothelial dystrophy, in which stromal oedema is a constant feature. Many cases progress to bullous keratopathy and loss of the normal corneal profile (keratoglobus) as decompensation occurs (Figure 8.8). This dystrophy resembles human Fuch's endothelial dystrophy, a condition in which endothelial changes also precede stromal and epithelial alterations.

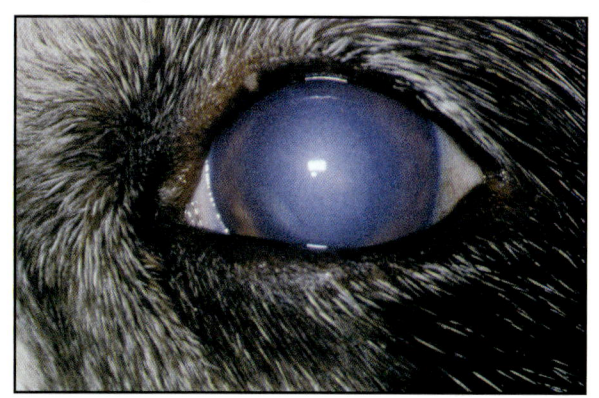

Figure 8.8 Endothelial dystrophy in an English Springer Spaniel. Mild panstromal oedema affected both eyes.

Pain can become a feature when chronic corneal erosion develops secondary to bullous keratopathy. Vision is impaired in direct proportion to the severity of the corneal oedema and the other corneal changes. Corneal decompensation is likely because of the extensive damage to the endothelium. Vascularization is not present in any but the most advanced cases.

The breeds most commonly cited as affected in the UK and USA are the Boston Terrier (mean age 7.5 years) and the Chihuahua (mean age 9.5 years). Other breeds affected in the UK include the English Springer Spaniel (often young adults) and the Boxer (usually older dogs) and, in the USA, the Dachshund is reported as a breed that can develop the problem (Martin and Dice, 1982).

Pathology: The primary abnormality in the endothelial type of dystrophy is located in the corneal endothelium; it may be detected using specular microscopy in the living animal (Gwin *et al.*, 1982). Other changes may well be of secondary importance in the pathogenesis. In most affected animals, there is degeneration of endothelial cells, so that a qualitative and quantitative reduction in endothelial cells results. It is of interest that in some cases, notably in the aged animals studied, the loss of endothelial cells appears to be a purely quantitative phenomenon; thus, the condition progresses more slowly and is often less serious than if the changes were qualitative, too.

Secondary changes include marked stromal oedema and both intercellular and intracellular epithelial oedema, so that bullous keratopathy is a common complication. Further degenerative changes in the epithelium, notably intracellular vacuolation, result in loss of epithelial cells and frank ulceration.

140 Conditions of the cornea

Treatment: Penetrating keratoplasty is the only means of restoring corneal clarity (Gilger and Whitley, 1999). Hyperosmotic preparations are often irritating and achieve only short-term reduction of corneal opacity, so they are not a practical proposition for treatment. A permanent 360 degree conjunctival flap, or the extended use of a soft contact lens may provide some symptomatic relief, but thermokeratoplasty is the best palliative treatment when bullous keratopathy is present. Thermokeratoplasty is performed under general anaesthesia using a handheld thermal cautery device that is lightly applied to multiple sites (up to 500) on the affected cornea (Gelatt and Gelatt, 1995). It is sensible to advise against breeding from affected animals.

Keratitis

Inflammation of the cornea is a common condition with a multiplicity of causes in dogs and cats. Keratitis is best classified according to aetiology, and common causes include infection, trauma, preocular tear film dysfunction, immune-mediated problems and systemic disease. A significant number of inflammatory corneal conditions are of unknown cause.

Ulcerative keratitis

The common causes of ulcerative keratitis are listed in Figure 8.9.

Aetiology	Treatment
Eyelid abnormalities (See Chapter 5)	
Absence or partial absence	Surgical correction of the primary problem
Entropion	Surgical correction of the primary problem
Neoplasia	Surgical removal if possible
Inflammation	Medical treatment, with or without surgery
Lagophthalmos (e.g. due to anatomy, nerve damage)	Correction of the primary problem
Lashes/Hairs (See Chapter 5)	
Trichiasis	Correction of the primary problem
Distichiasis	Remove distichia
Ectopic cilia	Surgical removal
Aberrant hairs e.g. nasal folds	Surgical removal
Irritants	
Heat/smoke	Systemic analgesic and topical antibiotic
Ultraviolet light	Systemic analgesic and topical antibiotic
Acids	Copious irrigation and systemic analgesic
Alkalis	Copious irrigation; refer to specialist
Preocular tear film defects (alone or in combination with other abnormalities) (See Chapter 6)	Correction of the primary problem(s)
Trauma	see text
Immune-mediated disease (See also Chapter 7)	see text
Infection	see text
Dystrophy	see text

Figure 8.9 Common causes of ulcerative keratitis in the dog.

Diagnosis: An accurate history is important and should include details of age, sex, others at risk, vaccination status, previous treatment and the duration of the clinical signs. The presence of a familial predisposition or breed tendency may be helpful.

Careful examination of the eye and adnexa with adequate magnification is essential; the equipment and protocol have been described in Chapter 1a. Topical application of fluorescein is an integral feature of the assessment of ulcerative keratitis (Figure 8.10). The important points in relation to the investigation of corneal disease are summarized in Figure 8.2.

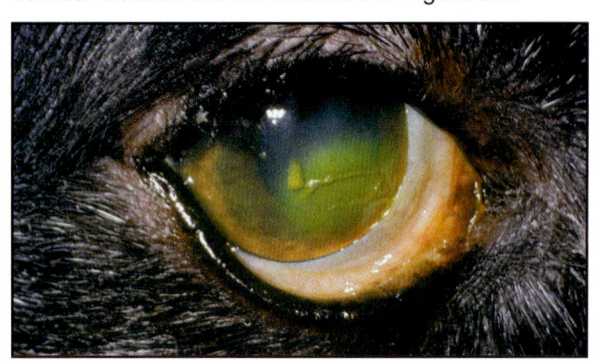

Figure 8.10 Fluorescein-stained superficial ulcer, of presumed traumatic origin, in a crossbred dog.

Clinical findings: These range from minimal ocular discomfort to severe ocular pain with photophobia, blepharospasm and excessive lacrimation or some form of ocular discharge. A number of factors may influence the degree of pain; they include the corneal sensitivity, the depth of the ulcer and whether or not there is accompanying uveitis.

Management of ulcerative keratitis: Undoubtedly, the most important factor in management strategy is to ensure that the cause of the ulcer has been identified and, if possible, removed, for this may be all that is required. Other factors relate to whether healing will be aided by medical treatment or surgical treatment, or by a combination of the two.

Primary corneal pathogens have not been identified in the dog; infection is therefore a secondary phenomenon. Topical antibiotics are used as part of the management strategy because the exposed and damaged stroma is a potential site for bacterial adherence – the first step in the production of bacterial infection.

Surgical support may be crucial in cases where the ulcer is deep, static or progressive and should always be used if there is a risk of corneal perforation as, for example, in brachycephalic dogs with prominent globes and poor corneal sensitivity. The various surgical options have been reviewed (Gelatt and Gelatt, 2001; Gilger and Whitley, 1999).

Management of superficial corneal ulceration: This type of ulceration involves the loss of epithelium with or without the anterior stroma. Uncomplicated ulcers heal quickly and without scarring if only epithelium is involved. A faint scar will persist if there has been stromal involvement. Provided the cause of the ulcer has been identified and removed, no other action is necessary (Figure 8.11). Healing can be supported by insertion of a therapeutic

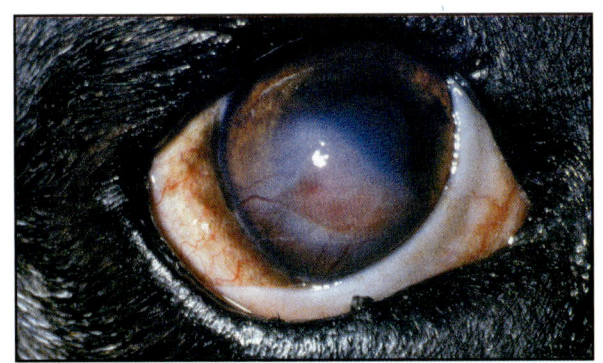

Figure 8.11 Chronic ulcerative keratitis in a Boxer, caused by a single misdirected lash on the lower eyelid. Granulation tissue indicates the chronic nature of the problem. The benign tumour located more medially was not contributing to the mechanical abrasion but was also removed when the ulcer was cured by surgical removal of the lash and its follicle.

soft contact lens, (Morgan et al., 1984), which has largely superseded the use of a third eyelid flap. The management of another type of superficial ulcer, recurrent epithelial erosion, has been described already.

Management of deep corneal ulceration: This type of ulceration involves substantial stromal loss which may extend as far as Descemet's membrane.

Surgical treatment: Deep ulceration may be an immediate result of the initial injury, or a later complication (Figure 8.12). If there is any possibility of corneal perforation, then healing must be aided by support from some form of graft, for example, a free conjunctival graft (Figure 8.13), or tissue repair material such as a porcine submucosal graft (Figure 8.14), or a conjunctival pedicle graft (Figures 8.15 and 8.16). Alternatively, corneal tissue adhesives, such as butyl-cyanoacrylate glue can be used as a non-surgical means of providing support (Refojo et al., 1971). Full thickness complications may require keratoplasty techniques, such as corneoscleral lamellar transposition (Parshall, 1973) or a lamellar graft (Brightman et al., 1989) to effect repair. A conjunctival pedicle graft is the most straightforward way of providing support, and the rotation type of pedicle graft, described in Figure 8.17, should be regarded as a routine general practice skill (Håkanson and Merideth,1987a and 1987b).

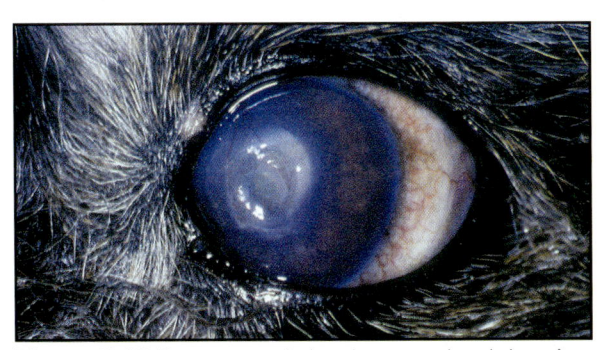

Figure 8.12 Deep corneal ulcer in a crossbred dog. A pure growth of *Pseudomonas aeruginosa* was cultured from the cornea. The dog also had diabetes mellitus: the tears are often glucose-rich in diabetic dogs and provide an ideal medium for bacterial growth.

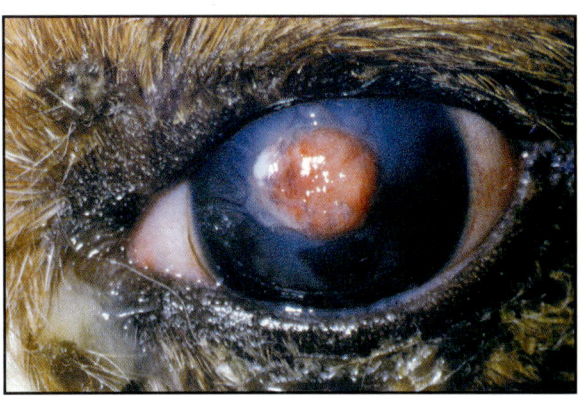

Figure 8.13 Free conjunctival graft. This is a simple way of covering a corneal defect. It is usually effected by dissecting off a piece of palpebral conjunctiva which is of the same shape as, but larger than, the defect to be covered. The graft is sutured over the defect in the same way as described for a pedicle graft. There is no need to remove the graft once the lesion has healed.

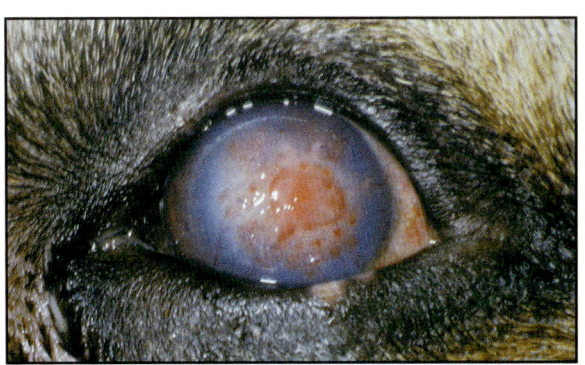

Figure 8.14 Porcine submucosa has been used to repair a deep ulcer in this dog. (Courtesy of DJ Gould.)

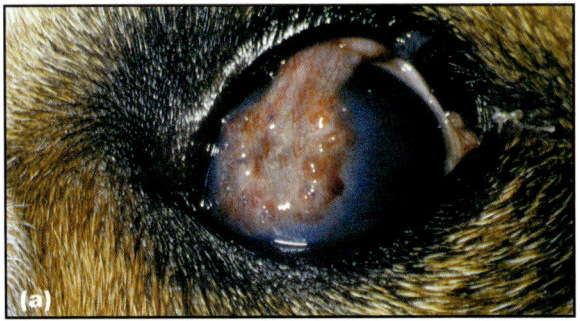

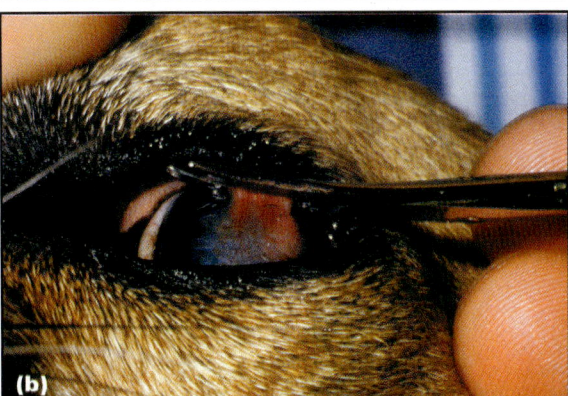

Figure 8.15 (a) Conjunctival pedicle graft. (b) Once the lesion has healed, the graft can be sectioned following the application of topical local anaesthetic. (Courtesy of DJ Gould.)

142 Conditions of the cornea

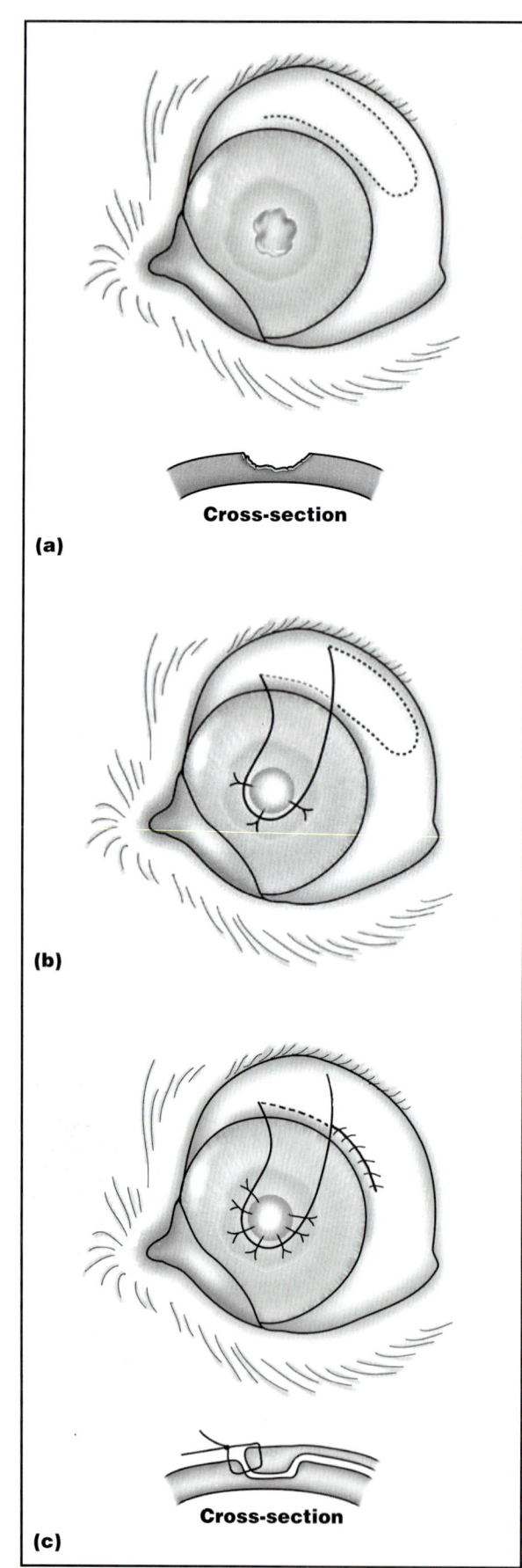

(a)

Cross-section

(b)

(c)

Cross-section

Figure 8.16 Diagrammatic representation of a conjunctival pedicle graft. For explanation see Figure 8.17.

1. Standard aseptic skin preparation is required.
2. If surgical access is poor, perform a lateral canthotomy (see Chapter 2).
3. Assess the extent of conjunctival dissection in relation to the position and size of the corneal ulcer. The graft must not be under tension when it has been placed.
4. Tent up the conjunctiva and make a small incision in the conjunctiva about 2 mm from, and at 90 degrees to, the limbus.
5. Use blunt dissection to undermine the conjunctiva in a radial fashion, so as to create a thin transparent area of conjunctiva that has been freed from underlying episcleral connective tissue (see Figure 8.16a).
6. Fashion the graft by means of two parallel radial cuts that can diverge slightly towards the base of the pedicle.
7. While the recipient bed (the ulcerated area) is being prepared, protect the graft with a surgical swab soaked in sterile saline.
8. Obtain samples for culture from the ulcer, ensuring that swabs and scrapes include material from the edge of the ulcer.
9. Clean necrotic material from the ulcerated area by sharp dissection, paying particular attention to freshening the walls of the ulcer.
10. Rotate the graft into place and trim, if necessary, to the shape of the ulcerated area (see Figure 8.16b).
11. Use 8-0 to 9-0 polyglactin 910 to suture the graft into place in the bed of the ulcer, with the first suture placed at 6 o'clock.
12. Pass the sentinel sutures (6 o'clock, 3 o'clock and 9 o'clock) through the entire thickness of the conjunctiva and into the wall of the ulcer at about two thirds of corneal thickness.
13. Once the sentinel sutures have been placed, insert other sutures in a similar fashion, approximately 1 mm apart, until the graft is firmly attached to the cornea.
14. The bulbar conjunctiva can be left open, but is usually closed with a continuous suture of 8-0 to 9-0 polyglactin 910 (see Figure 8.16c).

Figure 8.17 Surgical procedure for a rotation conjunctival pedicle graft.

Medical treatment: Although surgical treatment is indicated in a proportion of affected animals, various forms of medical therapy are required for most animals. The medical and surgical treatment options for ulcerative keratitis have been reviewed comprehensively by Kern (1990).

Topical antibiotics are needed when ulcerative keratitis with stromal loss is present and, for deep ulceration, the frequent use of fortified antibiotic solutions is the treatment of choice. Fortified antibiotic solutions provide a high concentration of antibiotic at the site of infection and have the additional advantage that they can be made up as preservative-free preparations (see Chapter 3).

Empirical treatment with collagenase inhibitors, such as fresh serum and topical and systemic tetracycline (e.g. oral doxycycline), is appropriate if there is any possibility of liquefactive stromal necrosis (corneal melting) as a result of, for example, chemical injury, the presence of excessive numbers of neutrophils, or *Pseudomonas aeruginosa* infection (see Chapter 3).

Deep corneal injuries are often accompanied by uveitis, and symptomatic treatment of this should accompany treatment of the corneal damage when this is the case. Atropine (1%) is the drug most commonly used to relieve the painful ciliary spasm (see Chapters 3 and 10).

Ocular lubricants may be helpful as, for example, when lagophthalmos or tear film problems complicate normal healing processes (see Chapter 3).

Corticosteroids should *not* be used if the corneal epithelium is defective, when active viral or mycotic keratitis is present, or when the causal agent is unknown. They may be valuable to aid resolution and minimize scarring once epithelialization has occured. Topical non-steroidal anti-inflammatories provide a safer alternative (see Chapter 3).

Local anaesthetics should never be used as part of treatment regimes. If pain is marked then systemic analgesics (see Chapters 2 and 3) should be given.

Descemetocoele

A descemetocoele is a very deep ulcer (Figure 8.18). The base of such ulcers is typically clear and the elasticity of Descemet's membrane may cause it to bulge anteriorly. Although the walls of the ulcer (stroma) will be fluorescein positive, the base (Descemet's membrane) will not take up the stain. An eye with a descemetocoele should be regarded as an ophthalmic emergency, as globe perforation is imminent.

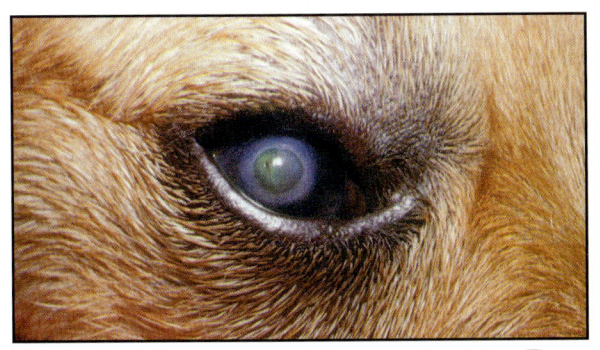

Figure 8.18 Descemetocoele in a crossbred dog. The cause was not established but it was probably related to topical corticosteroid treatment following assumed traumatic injury. There is a tiny focal full-thickness corneal penetration just lateral to the camera flash. The fluorescein staining is a consequence of subtle leakage of aqueous humour (positive Seidel test).

Management: Swabs and scrapes should be taken to obtain material for culture and sensitivity before deciding on the appropriate means of providing support for healing. Primary suture can be used to treat a small descemetocoele (<1 mm); the sutures are pre-placed using a horizontal mattress suture pattern, but, as the technique produces a high degree of astigmatism, it is seldom used. It is better to use one of the traditional means of support (e.g. a porcine intestinal submucosal graft, conjunctival graft, or lamellar corneal graft), the choice depending on the degree of complexity.

Punctate keratitis of unknown cause

There are a number of possible causes for the epitheliopathy that presents as punctate keratitis, but in many cases the cause cannot be established. The animal's facial anatomy (especially eyelid congruity), adequacy of blinking, corneal sensitivity and all components of the pre-ocular tear film should be carefully checked in such cases. In a proportion of cases, epitheliopathy will be a consequence of qualitative or quantitative tear film abnormalities (Saito and Kotani, 1999). It is also relevant to check the composition of any topical medical treatments that have been used and the length of time for which they have been applied. For example, local anaesthetic agents, preservatives and antiviral agents are all epitheliotoxic to some degree. If corneal erosions are present, it is sensible to take swabs for bacterial, and, ideally, viral culture, but the results are often equivocal or negative.

Immune-mediated keratitis

Chronic superficial keratoconjunctivitis (pannus)

Aetiology: The cause of most types of chronic superficial keratoconjunctivitis is unknown, but it is almost certainly immune-mediated in breeds such as the German Shepherd Dog. Predisposing factors include ultraviolet light, altitude and, possibly, irritative factors such as smoke.

Clinical findings: The age of onset varies, to some extent, with breed. For example, in the UK it is most likely to be diagnosed in German Shepherd Dogs of 3–5 years of age and, at this age, the condition progresses rather slowly. When younger dogs are affected, the condition progresses more rapidly. The condition is usually bilateral. Mild ocular discomfort may be present, with redness and follicular hyperplasia. Some, or all, of the conjunctiva, limbus, cornea and third eyelid may be involved (Figure 8.19). Typically, the lower lateral quadrant of the limbus and cornea is affected initially. Lipid and pigment deposition may complicate the presentation, but ulceration is rarely present.

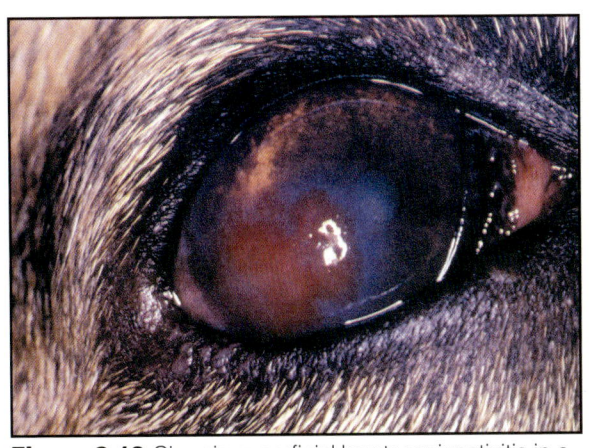

Figure 8.19 Chronic superficial keratoconjunctivitis in a German Shepherd Dog. Note the follicular hypoplasia and loss of pigment from the third eyelid as well as the typical fibrovascular corneal infiltrate.

Pathology: This is essentially a superficial fibrovascular lesion in which lymphocytes and plasma cells predominate.

144 Conditions of the cornea

Treatment: Topical cyclosporin is the treatment of choice. It is used initially twice daily and then reduced to a maintenance dose, usually once daily, for life. Corneal pigmentation usually diminishes with cyclosporin treatment, so that keratectomy is generally unnecessary.

Superficial keratectomy is occasionally indicated for removal of opacities covering the entire cornea that have not responded to medical treatment. A cruciate incision is made (approximately one third of corneal thickness) with a number 15 scalpel blade to divide the cornea into quadrants. Each separate portion is dissected back to the limbus and the quadrants are trimmed with fine scissors (Figure 8.20).

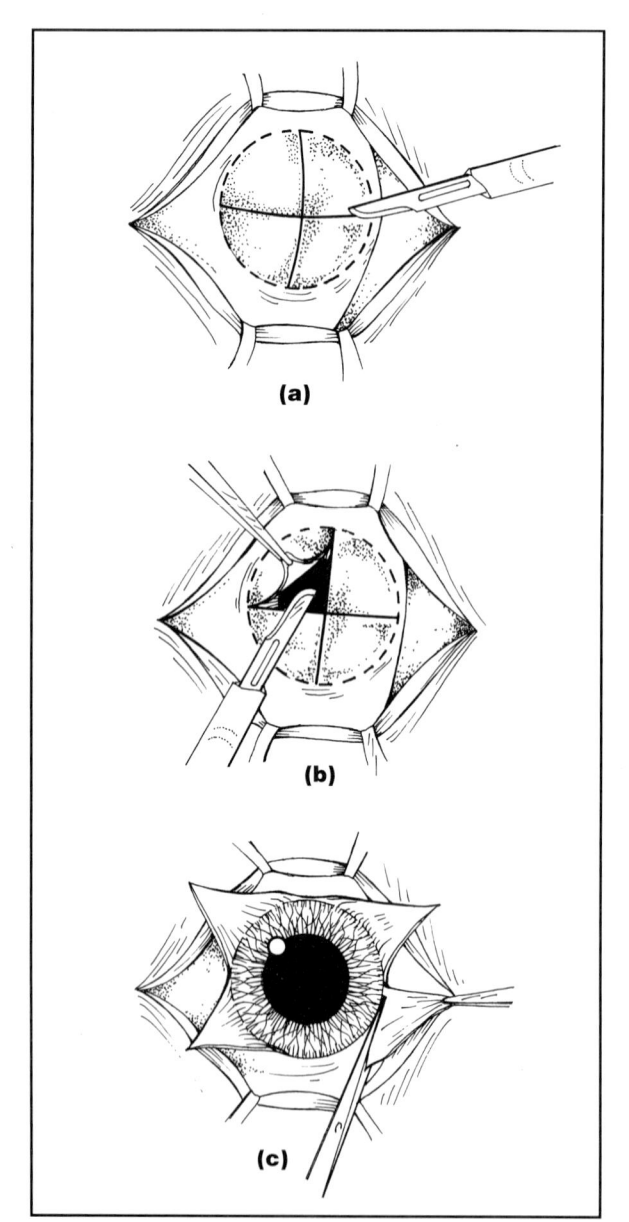

Figure 8.20 Superficial keratectomy for removal of opacities covering the entire cornea and not involving more than one third of the corneal thickness.
(a) A cruciate incision is made with a number 15 blade scalpel and divides the cornea into quadrants.
(b) Each portion is dissected back to the limbus and slightly beyond it. (c) The quadrants are trimmed with fine scissors.

Topical applications of surface-active corticosteroids (e.g. fluorometholone) can be used as a short-term alternative to cyclosporin when fibrovascular infiltration is extensive. Subconjunctival depot preparations may be needed for dogs that are difficult to treat, or for those that do not improve sufficiently on topical treatment (see Chapter 3).

Keratomalacia: Other possible immune-mediated corneal problems may present in a variety of ways, sometimes with acute and serious corneal changes that often commence in the peripheral cornea. They may be linked with systemic immune-mediated problems or may be the result of local insult (e.g. following infection with *Pseudomonas* sp.). Specialist advice should be sought (see Chapter 9).

Thermal injury

Ocular thermal injuries that include corneal damage are usually a consequence of animals becoming trapped in burning buildings. The damage to the lungs from smoke inhalation and the extent and depth of skin involvement are the major determinants of prognosis, and even survival, in such cases. The protection afforded by the eyelids usually prevents serious corneal damage, and an emollient antibiotic ointment is usually all that is required while the other injuries are managed.

Chemical injury

Chemical burns of the cornea and adnexal tissues are urgent ocular emergencies. Acids and alkalis cause immediate epithelial loss. Most acid injuries are less serious than alkali injuries, as the penetration of all but strong acids is arrested by the protein coagulation that they produce, whereas the lipid solubility of alkalis allows them to penetrate the tissues rapidly. Alkalis can therefore cause damage to external parts of the eye and adnexa, as well as internal damage to the uveal tract, lens and zonule.

Acid injuries
These may be encountered when, for example, weakly acidic spirit-based skin preparations (pH<4.5) or strongly acidic (pH 1) domestic cleaning products, such as bleach (sodium hypochlorite) and toilet cleaner (sulphuric acid), are inadvertently spilled in the eye.

Alkali injuries
These result when caustic solutions, such as ammonium hydroxide (pH 12.5), sodium hydroxide or potassium hydroxide (both pH 14), contact the eye. Lime burns (calcium hydroxide) are likely to be the result of accidental exposure when plaster, mortar, cement or whitewash is being used in the vicinity. Calcium hydroxide is unusual in that it penetrates the cornea poorly, but produces quite marked stromal opacity (Figure 8.21). On rare occasions, maliciously inflicted chemical injuries from strong acids (e.g. sulphuric acid from batteries) and alkalis (e.g. ammonia) are encountered.

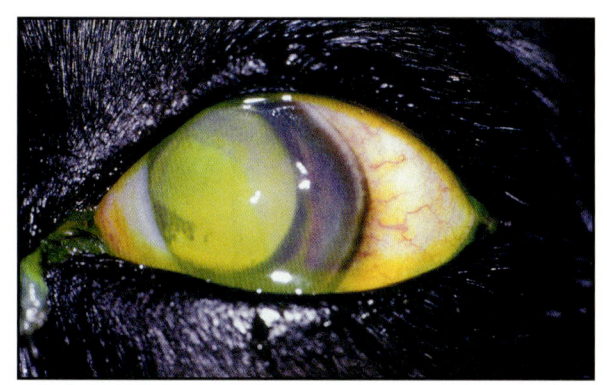

Figure 8.21 Alkali injury to the eye as a result of contact with calcium hydroxide (lime). There is corneal oedema. The diffuse staining by fluorescein is because the tight epithelial junctions have been compromised. Calcium hydroxide penetrates the eye less well than other alkalis, so the intraocular damage is less severe, but corneal stromal opacity may be marked. This dog made a complete recovery over several months.

Emergency treatment

All chemical burns should be treated immediately by copious irrigation with bland, preferably sterile, fluid. It is important to check that no particulate matter is present in the fornices. Because alkalis bind to the corneal stroma, they can continue to injure ocular structures after initial irrigation has removed all free alkali and, for this reason, it is necessary to maintain irrigation until the pH of the conjunctival sac has returned to normal (approximately pH 7.5).

The severity of the chemical injury is determined by factors such as the time of exposure, the strength and the concentration of the chemical. It is important to test the pH of both the conjunctival sac and the offending chemical whenever possible, using standard pH papers.

Subsequent treatment

This depends on the chemical involved and the severity of the injury. For injuries from weak acids, a bland ophthalmic antibiotic ointment may be all that is required for a few days after the injury. However, the management of injuries from strong acids and most alkalis is more complex and similar to that for liquefactive stromal necrosis. Early specialist advice should be sought, in order to minimize the many potential complications and provide an accurate prognosis.

Corneal trauma

The cornea may be damaged as a consequence of either blunt or penetrating trauma. Careful examination under general anaesthesia is required if the full extent of the injuries cannot be ascertained in the conscious animal, or if there is any risk of expulsive loss of the intraocular contents when the eyelids are manipulated. Blunt trauma is usually more damaging to the globe than penetrating trauma.

Blunt trauma

Blunt trauma may cause gross corneal oedema (acute hydrops) because of widespread damage to endothelial cells. The usual examination techniques must be supplemented by diagnostic imaging and the measurement of intraocular pressure in order to ascertain the full extent of ocular damage. In addition to the corneal changes, intraocular haemorrhage, disruption of the intraocular contents and loss of integrity of the ocular coats are the commonest complications.

There is no specific treatment for damage to endothelial cells, and resolution of the oedema will depend on the extent of damage to individual cells and the ability of the unaffected cells to slide over the defect.

Penetrating trauma

Clinical signs: There is an acute onset of pain, blepharospasm and lacrimation. Traumatic corneal injury should always be suspected if there is obvious third eyelid damage, especially when it is combined with a change of ocular appearance. The examination should determine the depth of the corneal injury and whether Seidel's test is required (see Chapter 1) to check for aqueous leakage. Changes that may be observed on examination of the eye include alterations in the depth and transparency of the anterior chamber, unusual appearance or position of the iris, changes in pupil shape and position and the presence of lens material in an abnormal position because the lens capsule has been ruptured. The prognosis is always guarded if extensive intraocular haemorrhage is present. Diagnostic imaging of the orbit is a sensible precaution in case radio-opaque foreign bodies, such as gunshot, are the cause of the trauma.

Treatment: Superficial oblique lacerations do not require surgical repair, but wound healing will often be enhanced if the loose flap of corneal epithelium is trimmed with fine scissors after applying topical local anaesthetic solution.

For deeper injuries, especially where full thickness damage has occurred, reconstructive surgical repair is indicated.

Gentle irrigation with sterile saline is used to prepare the ocular surface. Deep oblique lacerations are more difficult to repair than deep vertical ones and they also need very careful cleaning to remove foreign debris. Debridement should be avoided whenever possible, so as to prevent problems of wound closure and postoperative astigmatism.

If corneal penetration has occurred (Figure 8.22), the coagulated aqueous which covers the wound is carefully removed with an iris repositor or a surgical spear (e.g. cellulose surgical spears).

There may well be prolapsed iris beneath the coagulated aqueous, and this should be reposited in the anterior chamber in most cases. When the iris tissue is devitalized or contaminated, it can be excised and the bleeding controlled with wet field cautery, but this is rarely necessary.

If there is any suspicion that the lens capsule has been ruptured, it is important to make an early decision as to whether to refer the patient for specialist assessment (see Chapter 12).

Full thickness corneal wounds are repaired with 8-0 to 9-0 suture material, depending on the magnification

146 Conditions of the cornea

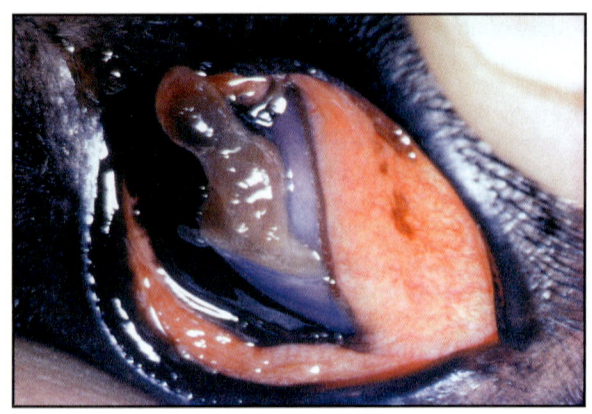

Figure 8.22 Full thickness corneal perforation in a dog as a result of a cat scratch. An iris prolapse is present beneath the coagulated aqueous. The corneal injury is extensive and oblique. There is pancorneal oedema and also hyphaema. The hyphaema makes it impossible to ascertain the full extent of the injuries on clinical examination alone.

available. Non-absorbable suture material which is removed after 4–6 weeks (e.g. 9-0 to 10-0 monofilament polyamide) can be used for small wounds in the visual axis, whereas absorbable material (e.g. 8-0 to 9-0 polyglactin) can be used in other sites and larger wounds. Primary corneal repair with simple interrupted sutures is the method of choice for a wide variety of corneal insults; the sutures should penetrate about three quarters of the corneal thickness to ensure that the wound will be watertight (Figure 8.23).

If there is difficulty in apposing the wound edges, then preplaced horizontal mattress sutures can be used, as already described under descemetocoele repair. Preplaced horizontal mattress sutures can be used to repair corneal wounds of up to 5 mm diameter, providing that the wound margins are healthy.

The anterior chamber is re-formed with a viscoelastic substance, such as sodium hyaluronate, balanced salt solution (BSS) or a small bubble of air. The medical management is as for deep corneal ulceration.

Corneal foreign bodies

The clinical signs comprise an acute onset of pain, blepharospasm and lacrimation, with the foreign body being readily visible in many instances (Figure 8.24). If the diagnosis is not made soon after the insult, some foreign bodies, particularly when they are of organic material, will evoke an inflammatory response and, in some cases, a corneal abscess results.

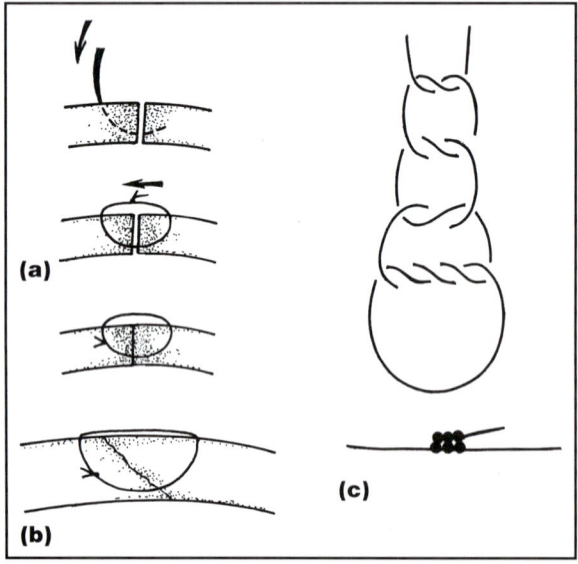

Figure 8.23 Diagrammatic representation of corneal repair. (a) Repair of a full-thickness vertical laceration to the cornea. When sufficiently fine suture material is used (e.g. 9-0 or 10-0 monofilament polyamide), the knot can be rotated into the suture track as shown. (b) Repair of a full-thickness oblique laceration; note that the suture is placed asymmetrically. (c) The correct way of tying the knot, so that an arrowhead configuration is produced which slides into the needle track more readily.

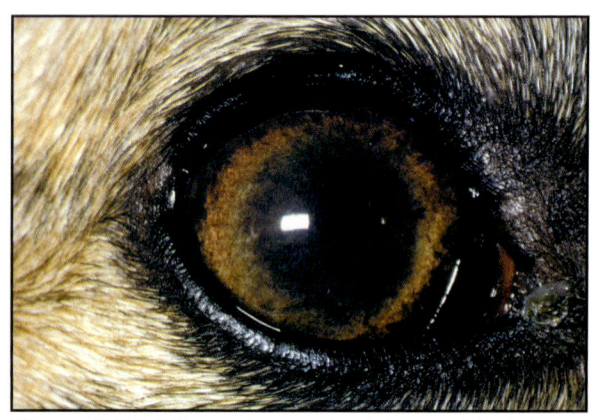

Figure 8.24 A thorn, at approximately one o'clock, has penetrated about two thirds of the corneal thickness.

Treatment

Foreign bodies require removal if they are causing, or are capable of causing, corneal irritation. Organic foreign bodies are the commonest types necessitating this approach. Superficial foreign bodies are easily removed with a surgical spear or similar, or a foreign body spud (Figure 8.25a). Deeply embedded foreign bodies should be approached more circumspectly, and it is usually necessary to incise the overlying layers with a razor blade fragment or similar. Gentle undermining of the edges of the incision assists access to the foreign body which can then be removed with a foreign body needle (Figure 8.25b), hypodermic needle or forceps, usually following the line of entry in reverse. When forceps are used, it is particularly important to avoid inadvertently pushing the foreign body further into the tissues. In chronic cases where an abscess has formed, it is best to excise the entire abnormal area, together with a rim of normal tissue.

Lipid deposition in the cornea

Corneal lipidoses, which include possibly inherited dystrophies such as crystalline stromal dystrophy, are bilateral depositions of lipid in an apparently normal cornea (see earlier). They represent the commonest type of corneal lipid deposition. The plasma lipid and lipoprotein profile may be normal in these dogs, but the evolution of the lesion can be modified by systemic dyslipoproteinaemia.

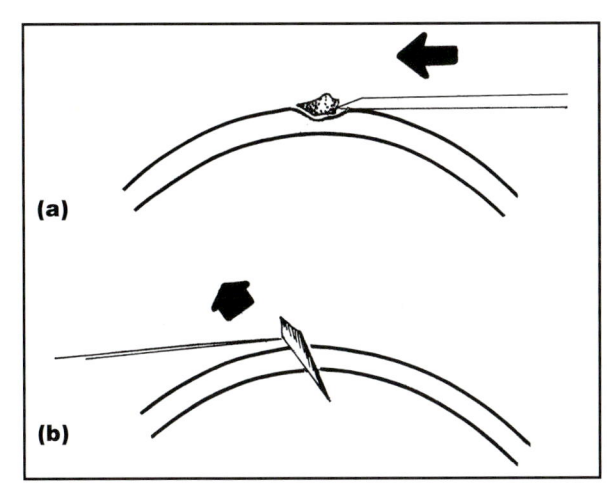

Figure 8.25 Removal of foreign bodies. (a) Removal of a superficial foreign body with a foreign body spud. (b) Removal of a penetrating foreign body with a foreign body needle.

Lipid keratopathy
This is the deposition of lipid within the cornea. It may be unilateral or bilateral, and the appearance is very variable because a range of ocular abnormalities may be associated with its pathogenesis. Vascularization is a constant feature of lipid keratopathy and it may precede, or follow, the predominantly stromal lipid deposition. Lipid keratopathy may be a complication of many types of anterior segment disease (Figure 8.26), and hypotony is an exacerbating factor. The majority of affected animals have plasma hyperlipoproteinemia, but the alterations can be quite subtle and require lipoprotein analysis rather than measurement of total lipids (Crispin, 1987).

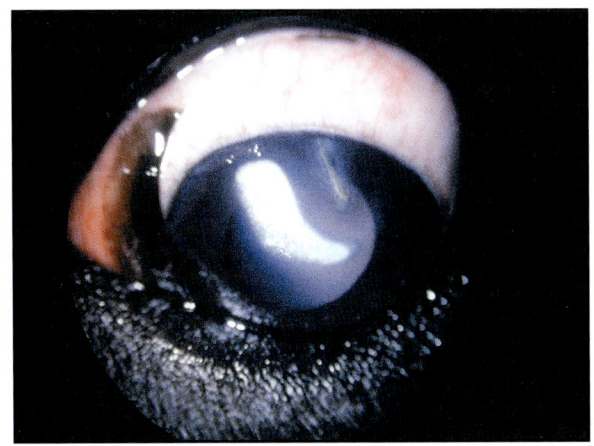

Figure 8.26 Unilateral lipid keratopathy in a Boxer, associated with a foreign body (splinter of wood) that had been present for some weeks. The dog was normolipoproteinaemic at the time of referral.

Arcus lipoides corneae (corneal arcus)
This is a bilateral condition which, in dogs, represents peripheral corneal accumulation of lipid as a result of excessive insudation of plasma lipids (Figure 8.27). The condition in dogs is always associated with plasma hyperlipoproteinaemia, usually secondary to a problem such as hypothyroidism (Crispin and Barnett, 1978).

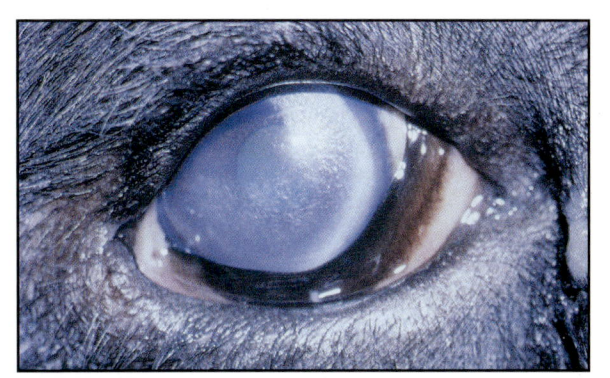

Figure 8.27 Arcus lipoides corneae in a Rottweiler with primary acquired hypothyroidism. The dog had hyperlipoproteinaemia: total plasma cholesterol 7.1 mmol/l and total plasma triglycerides 1.1 mmol/l.

Neurotrophic keratopathy
Damage to the trigeminal nerve results in corneal desensitization and neurotrophic keratopathy, which may present initially as punctate epithelial erosions in the interpalpebral area of the cornea, and later as more obvious corneal oedema and ulceration. This type of keratopathy is difficult to recognize in the early stages, as corneal sensitivity varies widely in different breeds of dog.

Exposure keratopathy
Exposure keratopathy may result from abnormal eyelid anatomy or movement, or because of abnormal size and position of the globe itself. For example, symblepharon formation or other cicatricial lid disorders will restrict the normal excursion of the eyelids.

Facial nerve paresis can result in neuroparalytic keratopathy, although active retraction of the globe by the unaffected retractor oculi muscles (cranial nerve VI) tends to protect the cornea when the VIIth nerve is dysfunctional. However, this is not the case in brachycephalic breeds, as they have a shallow orbit and poor excursion of the nictitating membrane.

Exposure keratopathy is more likely to develop if there is proptosis or globe enlargement (Figure 8.28). The clinical features vary according to the severity of the underlying problem and range from discrete punctate erosions to gross ulceration, infection and perforation.

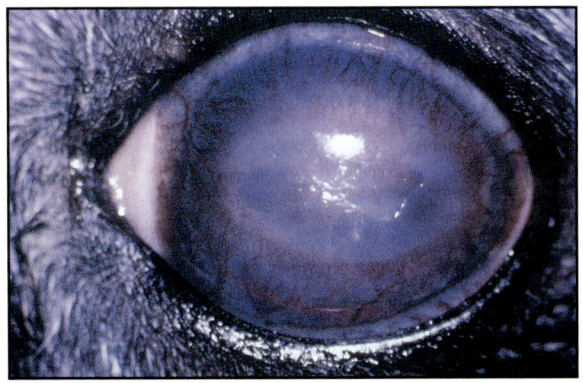

Figure 8.28 Exposure keratopathy associated with globe enlargement in a Giant Schnauzer. There had been a previous uveitis complicated by secondary glaucoma (IOP >60 mmHg). The globe is now permanently enlarged and painful, and requires removal.

Neoplasia

Primary corneal neoplasia
This is extremely rare. The majority of tumours that involve the cornea arise from the limbus and these are described, together with pseudotumours and inflammations in this region, in Chapter 9. Of those that are specifically corneal tumours, the most commonly reported are intraepithelial squamous cell carcinomas and papillomas, and there are single case reports of a corneal epithelioma and a corneal adenocarcinoma.

Intraepithelial squamous cell carcinoma presents as a roughened pinkish-white mass. Viral papillomas are regarded as the commonest primary corneal tumour of young dogs, and appear similar to the more common oral and eyelid papillomas. Both intraepithelial squamous cell carcinoma and corneal papilloma can be excised by keratectomy, and surgery can be combined with either radiotherapy or cryotherapy.

Differential diagnosis is important, as it is much more likely that solitary corneal masses that do not involve the limbus are epithelial inclusion cysts or reactions to implanted foreign material.

Secondary corneal neoplasia
This is also extremely rare; lymphoma is the tumour most likely to infiltrate the cornea or to produce corneal signs associated with ocular infiltration, such as oedema and neovascularization. Similar corneal signs may be a consequence of generalized systemic diseases, such as histiocytosis and leishmaniasis, as well as a variety of intraocular tumours, so careful examination of the whole dog and intraocular imaging are needed.

Other conditions of the canine cornea

Calcium keratopathy
Calcium may be deposited in the cornea because of local 'dystrophic' factors, usually associated with chronic inflammation, or as an ocular manifestation of systemic calcium metabolism abnormality, when it is called metastatic calcification. Calcium deposition may be one of the long-term complications of parotid duct transposition.

The calcium is usually deposited in a subepithelial position and the corneal epithelium must be removed if treatment with chelating agents such as EDTA is to be effective. Determination of the underlying cause and its removal, are also crucial in terms of preventing additional calcium deposition.

Epithelial inclusion cyst
The pathogenesis of inclusion cysts is not well understood, although, in many cases, a history of prior corneal insult would suggest that implantation of epithelial cells in deeper cornea is the likely cause (Bedford et al., 1990). The appearance is typical, consisting of a well circumscribed whitish focal stromal lesion and absence of an inflammatory component (Figure 8.29), which allows it to be differentiated readily from a corneal abscess. Inclusion cysts are best removed by complete excision. Histology demonstrates that inclusion cysts are lined by non-keratinized squamous epithelium.

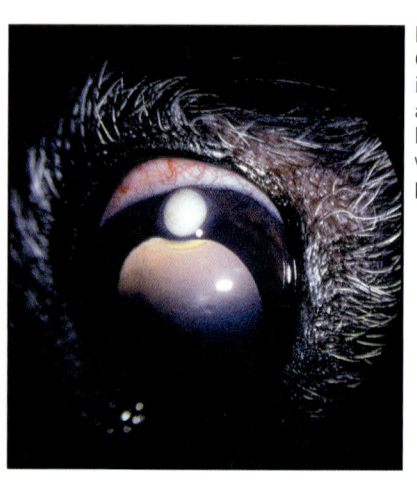

Figure 8.29 Corneal epithelial inclusion cyst in a Miniature Poodle. There was no history of previous trauma.

Florida keratopathy (Florida 'spots')
A keratopathy typified by non-painful focal grey white corneal opacities may be encountered in a variety of species, including the dog and cat, in the Southeastern United States and the Caribbean. Affected animals do not exhibit any signs of ocular discomfort, there are no indications of ocular inflammation and the epithelium is intact. The cause is unknown, but as it is self-limiting, there is no necessity to provide empirical treatment. On the basis of positive acid-fast staining in the corneal stroma, atypical mycobacterial infection has been suggested as a possible cause in a single case report in a dog (Fischer and Peiffer, 1987).

Developmental corneal conditions in the cat

Absence/microcornea/megalocornea
The unusual nature of problems of this type has been discussed previously for the dog; the situation is similar in the cat. In the cat, the effects of infectious agents (e.g. feline herpesvirus) should be considered when litters are born with multiple ocular anomalies which include corneal abnormality.

Poor differentiation of the limbus with associated microcornea may be seen in animals suffering from metabolic disorders of collagen.

Corneal opacity
Transient diffuse corneal opacity is present in young kittens when the eyes first open, but should have disappeared by the time the kitten is 4 weeks of age.

Permanent corneal opacities are, as in dogs, most frequently encountered because of persistent pupillary membrane remnants, or some other form of anterior segment dysgenesis (see Chapter 9).

Neurometabolic disease
Corneal clouding (Figure 8.30) is a feature of a number of neurometabolic (lysosomal) storage diseases (mucopolysaccharidosis, mannosidosis, gangliosidosis). Specific enzyme deficiencies lead to the accumulation of abnormal products within lysosomes and extracellularly. Diagnosis is made on clinical grounds (nervous and ocular signs), enzyme analysis and from microscopic examination of biopsy material.

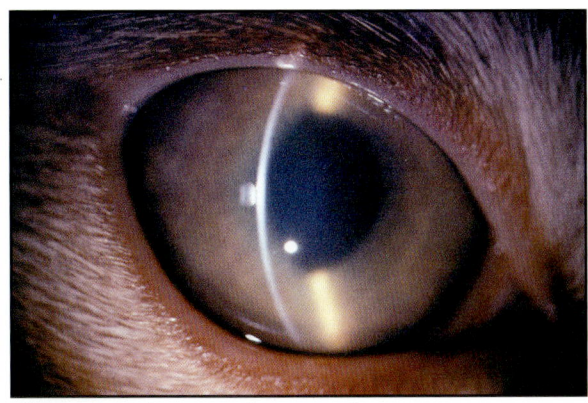

Figure 8.30 Lysosomal storage disease: mucopolysaccharidosis in a 3-month-old domestic shorthair cat. Abnormal accumulation of mucopolysaccharides in the corneal cells results in corneal clouding.

Acquired corneal conditions in the cat

Corneal dystrophies

Endothelial dystrophy

A progressive, bilateral and severe endothelial dystrophy is occasionally encountered in domestic cats. Affected animals are usually closely inbred, but the mode of inheritance is unknown. Abnormalities are limited to the cornea.

Clinical findings: Stromal oedema may be detected as early as 3 or 4 weeks of age, beginning centrally and spreading towards the limbus, but with perilimbal sparing. Keratoconus and keratoglobus are frequent complications (Figure 8.31).

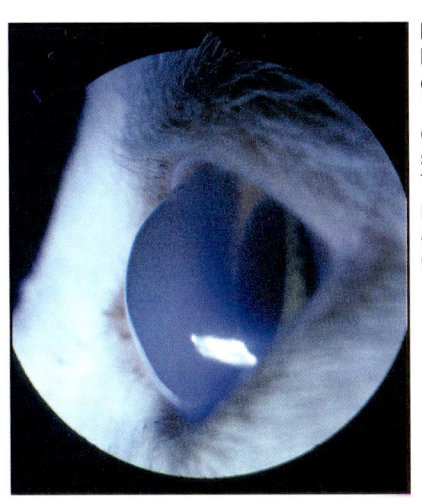

Figure 8.31 Endothelial dystrophy in an 11-month-old domestic shorthair cat. The corneal profile has altered (keratoglobus).

Pathology: The earliest microscopic change is probably in the central corneal endothelium. The cytoplasm of the endothelial cells becomes vacuolated, a change which is especially marked in the region between Descemet's membrane and the nuclei of the endothelial cells. Towards the limbus, the endothelial cells are of normal appearance.

There is stromal oedema and an increase in stromal thickness. The corneal epithelium shows no abnormality early on in the disease, but later it becomes thinner than normal with a reduced number of layers; a change of corneal profile is clinically evident at this stage.

Treatment: Penetrating keratoplasty is the treatment of choice (Bahn *et al.*, 1982).

Keratitis

Ulcerative keratitis

Aetiology: This is frequently of traumatic origin, especially from cat scratches. Otherwise, the possible causes are similar to those for the dog, with the notable exception of eyelid and cilia abnormalities, which are less common in cats, apart from those associated with developmental eyelid defects, such as colobomas.

Persian and Himalayan cats are brachycephalic, and have the same characteristic as brachycephalic dogs of reduced corneal sensitivity (Blocker and van der Woerdt, 2001). In these breeds of cat, ulcerative keratitis may be more difficult to manage, as corneal perforation is a possible complication.

Infection is a real possibility following claw or bite injuries in the cat, so a course of topical antibiotic is required, with a spectrum of activity that includes *Pasteurella multocida* (e.g. chloramphenicol).

Clinical findings: Usually an acute onset of pain, blepharospasm and excessive lacrimation are seen; the condition is most commonly unilateral.

Superficial lesions (Figure 8.32) may be more painful than those more deeply situated. Careful examination with magnification should enable the extent and depth of ulceration to be determined. Deeper lesions have a characteristic crater-like appearance. Descemet's membrane may be visible when a full stromal defect is present. The elasticity of this layer in the cat may result in a spectacular descemetocoele.

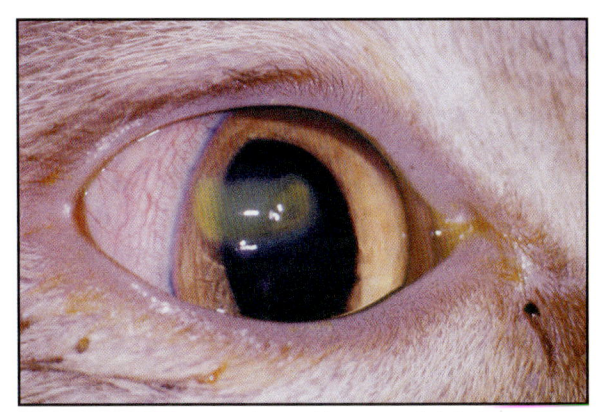

Figure 8.32 Fluorescein-positive superficial ulcerative keratitis of traumatic origin (cat scratch) in a cat. The loose piece of epithelium was trimmed (using tenotomy scissors) after application of local anaesthetic. Topical antibiotic cover (chloramphenicol ointment) was provided. The injury healed uneventfully.

The examination may be aided by the use of topical local anaesthetic, although, if extensive damage is present or full thickness penetration suspected, it is better to examine the cat under general anaesthesia. On occasions, there may be such marked chemosis

150 Conditions of the cornea

that examination under general anaesthesia is required to establish the extent of the injuries. In addition to corneal damage, there may be damage to the limbus and sclera (Figure 8.33). The extent of any scleral injury may be hidden by the overlying conjunctiva, and subconjunctival exploration under general anaesthesia will be required in such cases.

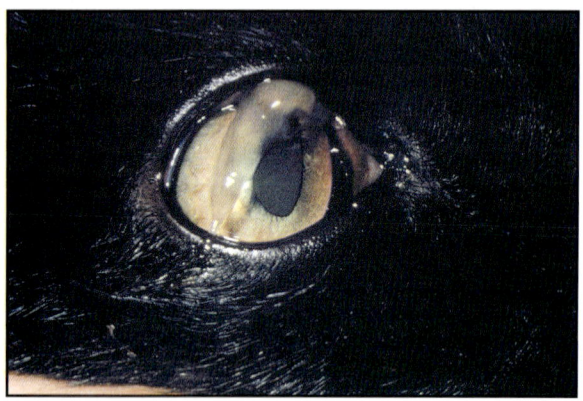

Figure 8.33 Penetrating injury as a result of a cat scratch. Coagulating aqueous is the most obvious feature. The claw had entered obliquely and damaged the limbus, sclera and ciliary body, as well as the cornea and iris. Injuries of this type can only be assessed properly at the time of microsurgery. Primary repair was performed and the eye healed uneventfully.

Treatment: Establish and eliminate the cause, as already described for the dog.

Superficial corneal ulceration

As in dogs, there appears to be a form of recurrent epithelial erosion that may represent an epithelial basement dystrophy. Background factors of importance that may influence the efficacy of treatment include infection with feline herpesvirus (Figure 8.34) and eyelid and tear film abnormalities. Epithelial erosion, without other complicating factors, can be treated by the removal of abnormal epithelium, and by placing a conjunctival pedicle graft if sequestrum formation is feared as a complication.

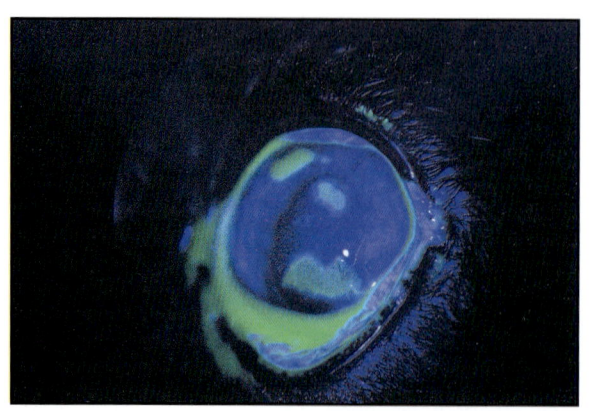

Figure 8.34 Recurrent epithelial erosion photographed with blue light to show the multiple fluorescein-positive areas. Erosions of this type are often related to underlying feline herpesvirus infection.

Deep corneal ulceration

This may be an immediate result of an injury or a later complication (Figure 8.35). The approach adopted in the management of deep corneal ulcers is as already described for the dog.

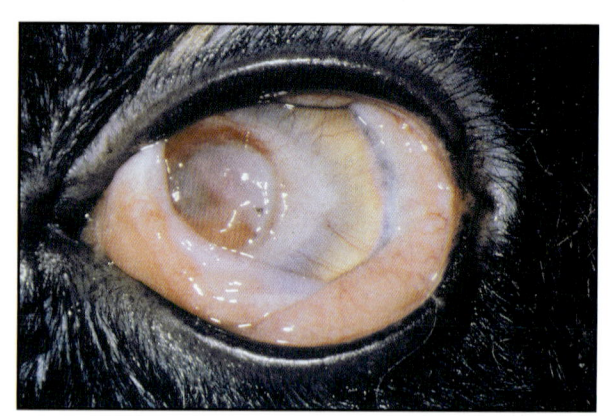

Figure 8.35 Central ulceration in a domestic shorthair cat. A third eyelid flap had been used to provide support for healing an ulcer but the ulcer was more extensive and deeper when the flap was taken down. The complication was probably the result of mechanical irritation from sutures that had penetrated the full thickness of the third eyelid.

Herpetic keratitis

Aetiology: Feline herpesvirus (FHV-1), the virus responsible for feline rhinotracheitis, has already been described as a cause of ophthalmia neonatorum and conjunctivitis, but it is also a cause of herpetic keratitis. In adults, herpetic keratitis often represents reactivation of latent virus, and is not necessarily associated with upper respiratory tract disease (Nasisse, 1990).

Clinical findings: Mild blepharospasm with lacrimation or a serous ocular discharge are common. The keratitis consists of discrete superficial punctate opacities in the early stages as the virus invades and replicates in the corneal epithelial cells which then die. Dendritic ulcers are pathognomonic for herpetic keratitis when identified and consist of linear branching erosions (Figure 8.36). Irregular, but superficial, geographic ulcers are formed when the small ulcers enlarge and coalesce, producing the typical appearance of superficial erosions (see Figure 8.37).

Rose bengal is useful for demonstrating subtle lesions, but it should be remembered that it is more irritating to the eye than fluorescein, so it is better to use fluorescein first and to view it in the dark with a blue light source, before resorting to rose bengal. In addition to the cytopathic effects on the corneal epithelium, suppression of local immune responses probably enables the virus to gain access to the corneal stroma. Stromal keratitis mediated by an immune response to the viral antigen results.

Chronic stromal keratitis (Figure 8.37) may result in sight-threatening corneal scarring and the other possible herpes-related complications such as keratoconjunctivitis sicca (see Chapter 6), and symblepharon (see Chapter 7) may also be present in affected animals.

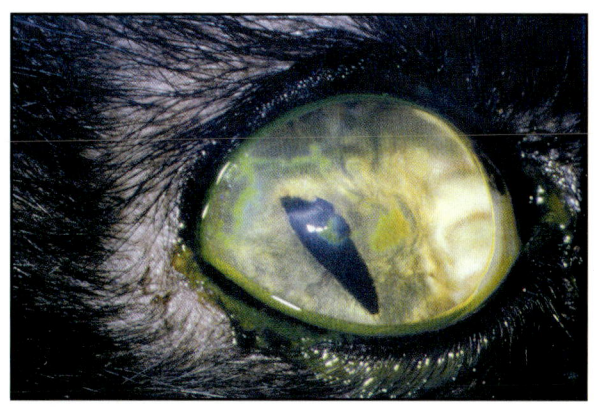

Figure 8.36 Superficial dendritic ulcers, stained with fluorescein, in acute feline herpesvirus infection.

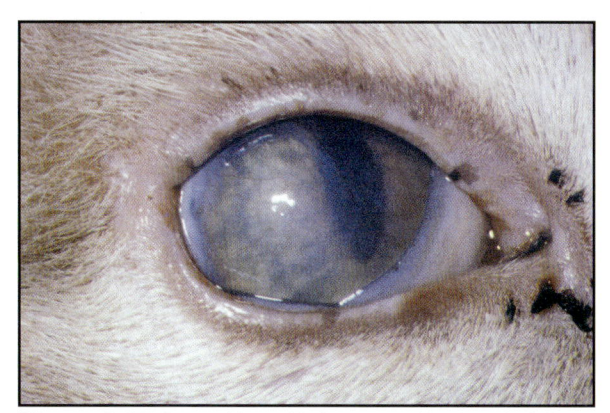

Figure 8.37 Stromal keratitis in a cat with chronic feline herpesvirus infection. The cat was also FIV-positive.

A number of affected cats are positive for FIV or FeLV infection, suggesting that, in these cases, herpetic keratitis may be an example of an essentially opportunist infection in an immunocompromised host.

Diagnosis: The diagnosis of ocular feline herpesvirus was reviewed by Nasisse and Weigler in 1997. It is based on the clinical findings and confirmed by laboratory analysis of corneal scrapings (see Chapter 1). Unfortunately, virus isolation is reliable only in the early course of infection, so negative results do not allow the diagnosis of feline herpesvirus infection to be ruled out. Serology helps in confirming exposure; active infection may be present if the titre exceeds 1 : 200.

Treatment: Herpetic keratitis responds unpredictably to topical antiviral agents (see Chapter 3). In practice, it is the acute superficial forms of herpetic keratitis that are most likely to respond favourably to treatment, and antiviral treatment should be given for at least 2 weeks and continued for at least a week after the clinical signs have resolved.

Chronic cases with stromal involvement appear to be resistant to antiviral therapy. Topical corticosteroids may reduce post-herpetic scarring when there is stromal involvement, but they should only be used in the treatment of chronic cases in conjunction with antiviral agents; on their own they may exacerbate the condition.

Immunotherapy has a possible role in the management of herpetic keratitis, but there have been no controlled clinical trials to assess the efficacy of this approach in the cat. The use of human interferon-α and vaccine are being evaluated at present.

Encouraging results from *in vitro* investigations of L-lysine have been extrapolated to the clinical situation, and 250–500 mg orally daily may have a part to play in either reducing or preventing the severity of recurrent FHV-1 infection.

Finally, mechanical removal of affected corneal epithelium might assist in the treatment of epithelial keratitis, whereas lamellar keratectomy or even penetrating keratoplasty might be of value in the treatment of stromal keratitis.

Clinical course: In practice, many cases relapse because of persistent conjunctival infection, or reactivation of a latent viral infection. Reactivation of latent virus is triggered by many forms of stress, intercurrent disease and corticosteroid administration.

Vaccination: The prevention of feline herpesvirus infection by routine vaccination is obviously the most satisfactory long-term aim, although, at present, vaccination does not necessarily prevent infection, and is unlikely to be of value in already infected animals or chronic carriers.

Other forms of feline keratitis

Mycobacterial keratitis: This may be caused by typical or atypical forms of mycobacteria. It presents as an infiltrative corneal opacity of roughened appearance. It is a rarely diagnosed condition, although the presence of acid-fast organisms can be readily confirmed from corneal samples stained with Ziehl–Neelson carbol–fuchsin. It should be differentiated from neoplastic infiltration, notably squamous cell carcinoma and lymphoma, both of which can be confirmed by microscopical examination of scrapings or biopsy specimens.

Mycotic keratitis: There are sporadic reports of mycotic keratitis in cats, usually emanating from those parts of the world where the climate is supportive of fungal growth. Mycotic keratitis is usually associated with long-term corticosteroid or antibiotic usage, or some other form of immunosuppression, and is very rarely seen in the UK, unless the animal has been imported from an endemic zone.

Corneal trauma

Surgical repair

As in the dog, the aim is primary repair. The cat is an excellent candidate for ocular surgery and the prognosis for most injuries is excellent. The techniques adopted are as described for the dog, with the caveat that complex penetrating injuries that have damaged the lens may be complicated by intraocular sarcoma formation some time later (see Chapter 12).

Foreign bodies

The ocular signs range from minimal ocular discomfort to obvious pain and marked chemosis. In general, the reaction to foreign material is much less florid than that encountered in dogs. Corneal foreign bodies are slightly less common in cats than dogs, but malicious injuries (e.g. involving firearms) are more frequently encountered, and it is sensible to perform routine skull radiography in all cases of unexplained ocular trauma.

Corneal sequestration

Aetiology

This is a condition of unknown cause that has many descriptive names – corneal necrosis, corneal sequestration, corneal sequestrum, corneal mummification, focal degeneration, corneal nigrum, keratitis nigrum, primary necrotizing keratitis, isolated black lesion and chronic ulcerative keratitis. It is unique to the cat, and it is of particular interest in that there is both a breed disposition (e.g. Colourpoint, Persian, Siamese, Birman) and a tendency for the condition to appear after previous corneal insult (trauma, feline herpesvirus infection) in all breeds, be they pedigree or non-pedigree. The condition has been reviewed comprehensively by Startup (1988), Pentlarge (1989) and Morgan (1994).

Clinical findings

Corneal sequestration is usually unilateral, although the other eye may be affected at a later date; rarely are both eyes affected at the same time. The pigmented material is almost certainly derived from the tear film. In many respects, sequestrum formation may be regarded as a complication of corneal healing after epithelial or stromal loss.

It is sensible to conduct a comprehensive examination, to exclude complicating factors such as medial entropion, tear film abnormalities and infection. The appearance of the lesion is often so striking that the necessity for complete examination is forgotten.

About 55% of affected cats are positive for feline herpesvirus (FHV-1 DNA) when corneal scrapings are assayed using the sensitive polymerase chain reaction (Nasisse et al., 1996).

The lesion is of somewhat variable appearance, ranging from an ill-defined darkening of the corneal stroma to a clearly demarcated black plaque (sequestrum) which is usually raised above the level of the corneal epithelium (Figures 8.38 and 8.39). The different appearances probably relate to the different underlying causes of the initiating corneal insult, as well as to different stages in the evolution of the opacity.

A discrete zone of oedema or frank ulceration may surround the sequestrum, and there is usually obvious neovascularization. In most cases, the corneal sequestrum is eventually sloughed, but this is a process that may take many months and, if ulceration is present, there will be chronic discomfort for the patient and risk of additional complications such as corneal perforation. In breeds with poor ocular anatomy, such as the Persian cat, undue delay before surgical intervention would be unacceptable.

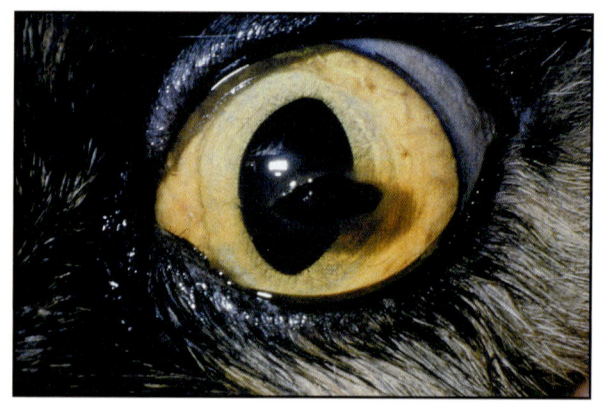

Figure 8.38 Corneal sequestration in a Persian cat, associated with medial lower eyelid entropion.

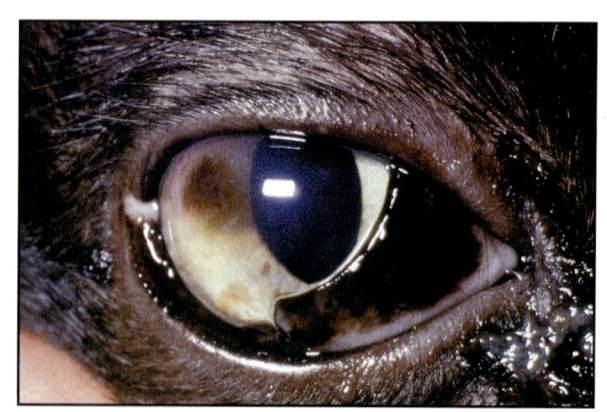

Figure 8.39 Corneal sequestration associated with epithelial erosion. There is a defect in the margin of the third eyelid because of traumatic injury some years previously. The erosion may be a complication of low-grade exposure keratopathy.

Pathology

The most obvious findings are coagulative necrosis and non-specific inflammatory cells.

Treatment

This will depend on the ocular anatomy, the extent and progression of the condition and the amount of discomfort which is present. The time course is reduced considerably if the lesion is removed surgically, so this is usually the treatment of choice.

Keratectomy combined with a graft, usually a conjunctival pedicle graft or one of porcine intestinal submucosa (Featherstone et al., 2001), gives good results. Corneoconjunctival transposition is also an effective surgical treatment (Andrew et al., 2001). It is rarely, if ever, necessary to perform lamellar keratoplasty or penetrating keratoplasty, unless the sequestrum is deep enough to warrant this approach. Inevitably, there is some corneal scarring when the sequestrum involves the stroma, but this is scarcely apparent with time.

After surgery, the patient is usually given a 5-day course of topical antibiotic. Recurrence is unusual with careful case selection and surgery.

If the sequestrum is superficial and causing no discomfort, it may be left to slough and the cat may be treated by applying a therapeutic soft contact lens, or simply using topical tear replacement solutions.

Eosinophilic (proliferative) keratoconjunctivitis

Aetiology
The cause of this condition is unknown (Morgan et al., 1996; Paulsen et al., 1996; Prasse and Winston, 1996). It has been compared with the eosinophilic granuloma complex but many cats have only ocular involvement and skin lesions are absent. Circulating eosinophilia is sometimes present, and in one study allergic bronchitis and eosinophilic enteritis were reported. Feline proliferative keratoconjunctivitis is remarkably similar to human vernal keratoconjunctivitis and shares some similarities with chronic superficial keratoconjunctivitis in dogs. PCR assay has demonstrated that 76% of corneal scrapings are positive for FHV-1 DNA in affected cats (Nasisse et al., 1996).

Clinical findings
The condition is usually unilateral initially, but without effective treatment it frequently progresses to affect both eyes. Typical corneal changes include diffuse oedema, neovacularization, minute erosions and plaque formation; the dorsolateral quadrant is most often affected. The plaques are of bizarre and irregular form, frequently whitish in colour and sometimes resembling cottage cheese. Similar plaques may be found on adjacent bulbar and palpebral conjunctiva. Chronicity is associated with patchy depigmentation, low-grade inflammation, small granulomas and eyelid thickening (Figure 8.40). Ocular discomfort and a low-grade ocular discharge are usually present.

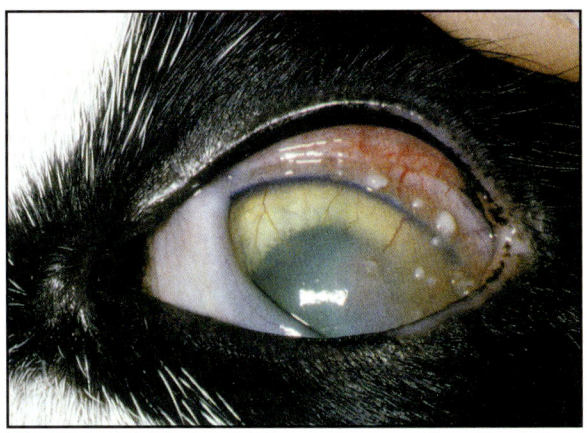

Figure 8.40 Characteristic appearance of proliferative keratoconjunctivitis. Note the patchy loss of pigment on the eyelid margin and the superficial white plaques on the conjunctiva and cornea. The extent of corneal changes such as vascularization and cellular infiltration varies between cases.

Diagnosis
The diagnosis is usually made from the characteristic clinical signs and can be confirmed by exfoliative corneal cytology (using Wright or Giemsa stains). Epithelial cells, eosinophils, mast cells, lymphocytes and neutrophils are typical. The white plaques are composed of nuclear debris from disrupted cells, eosinophils and eosinophilic granules (Prasse and Winston, 1996).

Treatment
The condition responds to topical corticosteroid or cyclosporin therapy, and also to corticosteroids or megoestrol acetate given by mouth. All these drugs have potentially undesirable side-effects (see Chapter 3). Treatment may achieve remission rather than cure, and this means that caution must be exercised in the long-term treatment of eosinophilic keratoconjunctivitis. In practice, therefore, the aim is to achieve control with the safest drug used as infrequently as possible. Topical corticosteroids, such as betamethasone sodium phosphate, prednisolone sodium phosphate, dexamethasone and fluorometholone are used initially, followed by maintenance with cyclosporin, to achieve this. The effectiveness of topical corticosteroids puts in doubt the clinical significance of the high detection rate of FHV-1 DNA with PCR, which may more truly reflect the sensitivity of the technique, rather than the presence of clinically relevant herpetic keratitis.

Acute bullous keratopathy
This unusual, intriguing, but potentially devastating condition is of unknown aetiology; theories include acute hypersensitivity reactions to insect stings and bites (Glover et al., 1994). Acute onset panstromal oedema may result in rapid corneal decompensation, sometimes complicated by perforation. The commonest treatment approach is provision of corneal support by means of a conjunctival graft.

Florida keratopathy
As outlined earlier, this is an unusual keratopathy of unknown cause. Corneal histology in the cat has indicated lipid-staining granules, particularly in the region of the epithelial basement membrane.

Lipid deposition
The cat is rarely affected by corneal lipid deposition. Lipid keratopathy occurs sporadically, usually following corneal injury, and can indicate previously unsuspected hyperlipoproteinemia, usually chylomicronaemia. *Arcus lipoides corneae* is very rare and crystalline stromal dystrophy has never been described in this species.

Neurotrophic keratopathy and exposure keratopathy
These problems have already been described in the dog. The cat is not as likely to develop problems of exposure keratopathy because of anatomical malformation, but may develop a severe exposure keratopathy following removal of the third eyelid, or in association with problems such as glaucoma when the globe is markedly enlarged. Facial nerve (VII) paresis and paralysis can follow otitis interna or aural surgery, especially bulla osteotomy. Postsurgical paresis is usually temporary and, as in the dog, the globe can be actively retracted by the retractor oculi muscles (supplied by cranial nerve VI), thus mitigating the effects of facial nerve dysfunction.

References and further reading

Andrew SE, Tou S and Brooks DE (2001) Corneoconjunctival transposition for the treatment of feline corneal sequestra: a retrospective study of 17 cases (1990–1998). *Veterinary Ophthalmology* **4**, 107–111

Bahn CF, Meyer RF, MacCallum DK, Lillie JH, Lovett EK, Sugar A, and Martonyi CL (1982) Penetrating keratoplasty in the cat. *Ophthalmology* **89**, 687–699

Bedford PGC, Grierson I and McKechnie NM (1990) Corneal epithelial inclusion cyst in the dog. *Journal of Small Animal Practice* **31**, 64–68

Bistner SI, Aguirre G and Shively JN (1976) Hereditary corneal dystrophy in the Manx cat: a preliminary report. *Investigative Ophthalmology* **15**, 15–26

Blocker T and van der Woerdt A (2001) A comparison of corneal sensitivity between brachycephalic and Domestic Short-haired cats. *Veterinary Ophthalmology* **4**, 127–130

Brightman AH, McLaughlin SA and Brogdon JD (1989) Autogenous lamellar corneal grafting in dogs. *Journal of the American Veterinary Medical Association* **195**, 469–475

Carrington SD, Crispin SM and Williams DL (1992) Characteristic conditions of the feline cornea. In: *The Veterinary Annual, 32nd Issue*, ed. M-E Raw and TJ Parkinson, pp. 83–96. Blackwell Scientific, Oxford

Champagne ES and Munger RJ (1992) Multiple punctate keratotomy for the treatment of recurrent epithelial erosions in dogs. *Journal of the American Animal Hospital Association* **28**, 213–216

Cook CS (1999) Ocular embryology and congenital malformations. In: *Veterinary Ophthalmology, 3rd edn*, ed. KN Gelatt, pp. 3–30. Lippincott, Williams and Wilkins, Philadelphia

Cook CS, Sulik KK and Wright WW (1995) Embryology. In: *Paediatric Ophthalmology and Strabismus*, ed. KW Wright, pp. 3–13. Mosby, St Louis

Cooley PL and Dice PF (1990) Corneal dystrophy in the dog and cat. *Veterinary Clinics of North America: Small Animal Practice* **20**, 681–692

Crispin SM (1982) Corneal dystrophies in small animals. In: *The Veterinary Annual, 22nd Issue*, ed. CSG Grunsell and FWG Hill, pp. 298–310. JohnWright and Sons, Bristol

Crispin SM (1987) Lipid keratopathy in the dog. In: *The Veterinary Annual, 27th Issue*, ed. CSG Grunsell, FWG Hill and M-E Raw, pp. 196–208. Scientechnica, Bristol

Crispin SM (1988) Crystalline stromal dystrophy in the dog: histochemistry and ultrastructure of the cornea. *Cornea* **7**, 149–161

Crispin SM (1989) Lipid deposition at the limbus. *Eye* **3**, 240–249

Crispin SM (1998) Cornea. In: *Feline Ophthalmology: An Atlas and Text*, ed. KC Barnett and SM Crispin, pp. 83–103. WB Saunders, London

Crispin SM and Barnett KC (1978) Arcus lipoides corneae secondary to hypothyroidism in the Alsatian. *Journal of Small Animal Practice* **19**, 127–142

Dice PF (1984) Corneal dystrophy in the Shetland Sheepdog. *Transactions of the American College of Veterinary Ophthalmologists* **15**, 211–242

Featherstone HJ, Sansom J and Heinrich CL (2001) The use of porcine small intestinal submucosa in ten cases of feline corneal disease. *Veterinary Ophthalmology* **4**, 147–153

Fischer CA and Peiffer RL (1987) Acid-fast organisms associated with corneal opacities in a dog. *Transactions of the American College of Veterinary Ophthalmologists* **18**, 241–243

Gelatt KN and Gelatt JP (2001) *Small Animal Ophthalmic Surgery*. Butterworth-Heinemann, Oxford

Gelatt KN and Samuelson DA (1982) Recurrent corneal erosions and epithelial dystrophy in the Boxer dog. *Journal of the American Animal Hospital Association* **18**, 453–460

Gilger BC and Whitley RD (1999) Surgery of the cornea and sclera. In: *Veterinary Ophthalmology, 3rd edn*, ed. KN Gelatt, pp. 675–700. Lippincott, Williams and Wilkins, Philadelphia

Gilger BC, Whitley RD, McLaughlin SA, Wright JC and Drane JW (1991) Canine corneal thickness measured by ultrasonic pachymetry. *American Journal of Veterinary Research.* **52**, 1570–1572

Glaze MB and Gelatt KN (1999) Feline ophthalmology. In: *Veterinary Ophthalmology, 3rd edn*, ed. KN Gelatt, pp. 997–1052. Lippincott, Williams and Wilkins, Philadelphia

Glover TL, Nasisse MP and Davidson MG (1994) Acute bullous keratopathy in the cat. *Veterinary and Comparative Ophthalmology* **4**, 66–70

Gwin RM, Polack FM, Warren JK, Samuelson DA and Gelatt KN (1982) Canine corneal endothelial cell dystrophy: specular microscopic evaluation, diagnosis and therapy. *Journal of the American Animal Hospital Association* **18**, 471–479

Håkanson NE and Merideth RE (1987a) Conjunctival pedicle grafting in the treatment of corneal ulcers in the dog and cat. *Journal of the American Animal Hospital Association* **23**, 641–648

Håkanson NE and Merideth RE (1987b) Further comments on conjunctival pedicle grafting in the treatment of corneal ulcers in the dog and cat. *Journal of the American Animal Hospital Association* **24**, 602–605

Kern TJ (1990) Ulcerative keratitis. *Veterinary Clinics of North America: Small Animal Practice* **20**, 643–666

Martin CL and Dice PF (1982) Corneal endothelial dystrophy in the dog. *Journal of the American Animal Hospital Association* **18**, 427–336

Morgan RV (1994) Feline corneal sequestration: a retrospective study of 42 cases (1987–1991). *Journal of the American Animal Hospital Association* **30**, 24–28

Morgan RV and Abrams KL (1994) A comparison of six different therapies for persistent erosions in dogs and cats. *Progress in Veterinary and Comparative Ophthalmology* **4**, 38–43

Morgan RV, Abrams KL and Kern TJ (1996) Feline eosinophilic keratitis: a retrospective study of 54 cases (1989–1994). *Progress in Veterinary and Comparative Ophthalmology* **6**, 131–134

Morgan RV, Bachrach A and Ogilvie GK (1984) An evaluation of soft contact lens usage in the dog and cat. *Journal of the American Animal Hospital Association* **20**, 885–888

Nasisse MP (1990) Feline herpesvirus ocular disease. *Veterinary Clinics of North America: Small Animal Practice* **20**, 667–680

Nasisse MP (1991) Feline ophthalmology. In: *Veterinary Ophthalmology, 2nd edn*. ed. KN Gelatt, pp. 529–575. Lea and Febiger, Philadelphia

Nasisse MP and Guy JS (1989). Feline ocular disease and the rhinotracheitis virus. *Veterinary Medicine Report* **1**, 155

Nasisse MP, Luo H, Wang YJ, Glover TL and Weigler BJ (1996) The role of feline herpesvirus-1 (FHV-1) in the pathogenesis of corneal sequestration and eosinophilic keratitis. *Proceedings of the American College of Veterinary Ophthalmologists* **27**, 80

Nasisse MP and Weigler BJ (1997) The diagnosis of ocular feline herpesvirus infection. *Veterinary and Comparative Ophthalmology* **7**, 44–51

Parshall CJ (1973) Lamellar corneal-scleral transposition. *Journal of the American Animal Hospital Association* **9**, 220–277

Paulsen ME, Lavach JD, Severin GA and Eichenbaum JD (1987) Feline eosinophilic keratitis: a review of 15 clinical cases. *Journal of the American Animal Hospital Association* **23**, 63–69

Pentlarge VW (1989) Corneal sequestration in cats. *Compendium on Continuing Education for the Practising Veterinarian* **11**, 24–29

Prasse KW and Winston SM (1996) Cytology and histopathology of feline eosinophilic keratitis. *Veterinary and Comparative Ophthalmology* **6**, 74–81

Refojo MF, Dohlman CH and Koliopoulos J (1971) Adhesives in ophthalmology: a review. *Survey of Ophthalmology* **15**, 217–236

Saito A and Kotani T (1999) Tear production in dogs with epiphora and corneal epitheliopathy. *Veterinary Ophthalmology* **2**, 173–178

Schoster JV, Wickman L and Stuhr C (1995) The use of ultrasonic pachymetry and computer enhancement to illustrate the collective corneal thickness profiles of 25 cats. *Veterinary and Comparative Ophthalmology* **5**, 68–73

Shively JN and Epling G (1970) Fine structure of the canine cornea. *American Journal of Veterinary Research* **13**, 713–717

Stanley RG, Hardman C and Johnson BW (1998) Results of grid keratotomy, superficial keratectomy and debridement for the management of persistent corneal erosions in 92 dogs. *Veterinary Ophthalmology* **1**, 233–238

Startup FG (1988) Corneal necrosis and sequestration in the cat: a review and record of 100 cases. *Journal of Small Animal Practice* **29**, 476–486

Stiles J (2000) Feline herpesvirus. *Veterinary Clinics of North America: Small Animal Practice* **30**, 1001–1014

Whitley RD (1991) Canine cornea. In: *Veterinary Ophthalmology, 2nd edn*, ed. KN Gelatt, pp. 307–356. Lea and Febiger, Philadelphia

Whitley RD and Gilger BC (1999) Diseases of the canine cornea and sclera. In: *Veterinary Ophthalmology, 3rd edn*, ed. K.N. Gelatt, pp. 635–673. Lippincott, Williams and Wilkins, Philadelphia

Wyman M (1979). Ophthalmic surgery for the practitioner. *Veterinary Clinics of North America: Small Animal Practice* **9**, 311–348

9

The sclera, episclera and corneoscleral limbus

David T. Ramsey

Introduction

Primary disorders of the sclera, episclera and corneoscleral limbus are encountered infrequently in dogs, and are extremely rare in cats. Many ocular diseases have a predisposition to begin, or to be detected, near the corneoscleral limbus, but they are considered to be primary diseases of the cornea, conjunctiva or anterior uvea and affect the corneoscleral limbus, episclera or sclera secondarily. These diseases will be mentioned briefly here, but are covered in detail in other chapters in this text. Because of the very low incidence of scleral, episcleral and limbal diseases in cats, this chapter will primarily consider diseases of these ocular tissues in dogs; however, diseases affecting these ocular tissues in cats, species differences and species exclusions will also be discussed.

Anatomy

Sclera

The sclera comprises the largest component of the dense fibrous tunic of the globe. It terminates anteriorly at a pigmented zone of transition, where it joins the peripheral corneal stroma at the corneoscleral limbus and, posteriorly, at the lamina cribrosa and dura mater of the optic nerve. It is composed primarily of type I collagen fibres that are arranged in bundles and orientated randomly, in comparison with the precisely arranged and oriented parallel collagen bundles in the corneal stroma. Elastic fibres and fibroblasts are interspersed among the collagen bundles.

The sclera is approximately 0.3–0.4 mm thick at the posterior pole and 0.12–0.2 mm thick at the equator of the globe in the dog; these values are 0.13–0.6 mm and 0.09–0.2 mm, respectively, in the cat (Martin and Anderson, 1981). The colour of the sclera is, in part, dependent upon its stromal thickness. When sufficiently thick, the sclera reflects light, making it appear white. The underlying choroid may be partially visible through a sclera that is thin (e.g. in young animals and animals with buphthalmic globes), giving the sclera a pale blue colour. The normal sclera may appear ivory to yellow in colour in elderly animals. The coloration may be abnormal, for example, if the animal is jaundiced, or when it contains an abnormally increased lipid content.

Vasculature

The sclera is modestly vascularized in the dog and cat. Anterior ciliary arteries anastomose with the superficial vascular plexus in the superficial sclera. Venous drainage of blood occurs primarily through the scleral venous plexus, located within the mid-sclera; this anastomoses with the angular aqueous plexus in the deep sclera, to drain aqueous humour.

Episclera

Anatomically, the episclera is considered to be part of the sclera, and consists of a thin fibroelastic structure composed of collagen, fibroblasts, melanocytes, proteoglycans and glycoproteins (Pearlstein, 1997). It is a highly vascular tissue; it coalesces with Tenon's fascia, that overlies it, and it is loosely adherent to the underlying sclera.

Vasculature

It is very important to differentiate episcleral injection from conjunctival injection; this indicates whether serious deep ocular or systemic disease (signified by episcleral vascular injection), or superficial ocular disease (signified by conjunctival vascular injection) is present. The vasculature of the episclera tends to move in the same direction as the underlying sclera during eye movements or eyelid manipulations and cannot be displaced from its normal position using a cotton swab. The vasculature of the overlying bulbar conjunctiva, however, is freely moveable over the surface of the episclera with eyelid manipulations or movement of the globe and can be displaced from its normal position using a cotton swab.

Disorders of the episclera are more common than those of the sclera or the corneoscleral limbus.

Corneoscleral limbus

The corneoscleral limbus is an anatomical transition zone between the two tissues composing the fibrous tunic of the globe (i.e. the stroma of the cornea and that of the sclera), and the epithelia of the conjunctiva and cornea. The limbus appears grossly as a 1 mm wide poorly defined pigmented area, encircling the peripheral cornea. Melanocytes are scattered sparsely throughout this zone of transition, and traverse the limbus obliquely, from the deep to superficial stroma between the cornea and sclera. A population of corneal epithelial stem cells are also present at the limbus. The sclera, near its insertion with the cornea at the limbus, projects axially and extends beyond the root of the iris, thereby creating an overhanging scleral shelf.

The sclera, episclera and corneoscleral limbus

Developmental abnormalities

Thin sclera
The sclera is often thin in young dogs of various breeds and also in young cats; thin sclera has an opalescent light blue colour, as the underlying anterior uveal tissue is partially visible through it. If the sclera remains blue during maturity, concomitant signs suggestive of a hereditary defect in collagen synthesis (joint hyperextensibility, skin fragility and hyperelasticity) should be checked for. Complete ophthalmic and physical examinations are indicated.

Dermoid
A dermoid is a choristoma, i.e. a growth of tissue composed of elements that are not normally present in the affected area. Ocular dermoids are located most commonly near the ventrotemporal corneoscleral limbus and affect the conjunctiva, cornea and sometimes the eyelids. Dermoids are usually raised above the surface, and contain dermal appendages (e.g. hair, sebaceous glands). Canine breeds most frequently reported with dermoids include the Miniature Dachshund, Dalmatian, Dobermann Pinscher and St Bernard. Predisposed feline breeds include the Burmese, Birman and Domestic Shorthair. Affected animals do not usually have clinical signs until they are 2–4 months of age, when ocular irritation or ulceration may become evident. Lamellar keratectomy (and conjunctivectomy of affected tissue) is curative.

A dermoid is pictured in Chapter 7.

Congenital staphyloma of the sclera with ectasia
A staphyloma is defined as focal thinning and protrusion of the fibrous tunic of the globe that is lined with uveal tissue.

Congenital posterior staphylomas are more common than congenital anterior staphylomas. They are most frequently associated with Collie eye anomaly, but are also seen with multiple ocular abnormalities in Australian Shepherd Dogs and, sporadically, in cats. An anterior staphyloma may involve a focal area of sclera, and may resemble limbal melanoma when it is located at or near the corneal limbus and is thin enough to allow extreme protrusion of uveal tissue (Figure 9.1). Dyscoria may occur with an anterior staphyloma, and other intraocular abnormalities may coexist with anterior or posterior scleral staphylomas.

Most lesions are static, and require no treatment. When ectatic protrusion of an anterior staphyloma causes distortion of the palpebral fissure, surgical correction is effected by direct apposition of the defect if it is less than 3 mm wide, or by using a scleral autograft or xenograft, or commercially available intestinal submucosa or microporous mersilene.

Multifocal staphylomas are frequently present in a cystic eye (Figure 9.2). In such instances, malformation of intraocular tissues is usually present, and the eye is usually blind.

Congenital posterior staphylomas (colobomas) are pictured in Chapter 14.

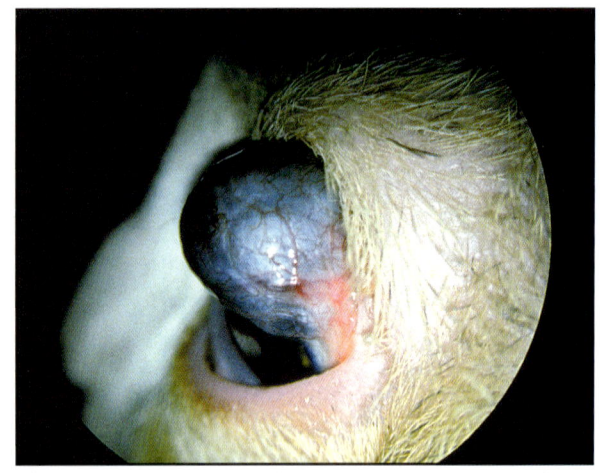

Figure 9.1 The left eye of a cat with a staphyloma of the dorsal limbus and perilimbal sclera. The sclera is thin and protrudes anteriorly and dorsally, causing entropion of the upper central eyelid. Note the dark blue colour, resulting from anterior uveal tissue lining the staphyloma.

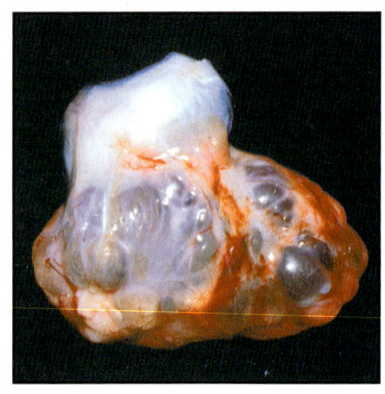

Figure 9.2 An enucleated cystic eye of a dog. There are multiple, intercommunicating, thin-walled cysts that extend from the posterior sclera.

Sclerocornea
Peripheral or total scleralization of the cornea, and a corneal curvature less than the scleral curvature, are the hallmarks of sclerocornea (Figure 9.3). Variable degrees of corneal opacification occur with overlying episcleral and conjunctival vascularization, and a poorly defined or absent corneoscleral limbus. Sclerocornea results from a congenital absence of the limbal anlage.

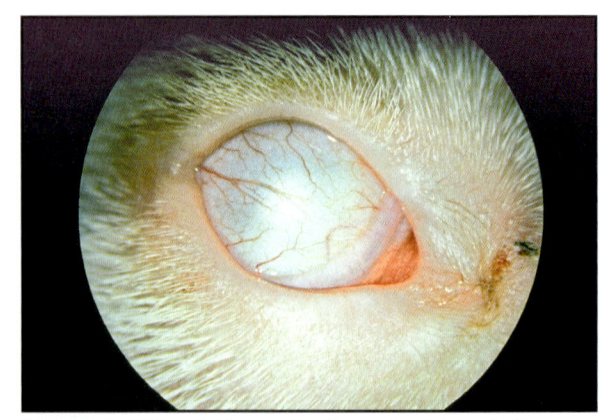

Figure 9.3 The right eye of a 6-month-old Australian Shepherd Dog with total sclerocornea. The corneoscleral limbus is absent, and conjunctival tissue overlies the sclerocornea. The margin of the nictitating membrane can be seen ventronasally.

During normal embryogenesis the limbal anlage is responsible for inducing neural crest-derived mesenchymal cells to undergo limbal differentiation into normal cornea and sclera and allows corneal curvature to exceed scleral curvature. Scleralization begins from the periphery and progresses toward the central cornea, and either the peripheral cornea, or the entire cornea, may be affected. Associated intraocular malformations are commonly present with sclerocornea.

Acquired abnormalities

The most common acquired abnormalities are classified as inflammatory; however, other abnormalities include immune-mediated, degenerative, traumatic and neoplastic diseases.

Inflammatory diseases

Primary inflammatory diseases affecting the episclera are relatively uncommon, and occur more frequently in dogs than in cats. However, inflammatory episcleral diseases occur more frequently than all other abnormalities of the sclera and corneoscleral limbus in dogs and cats. Most of the more common inflammatory diseases that affect the limbus occur secondary to diseases which primarily affect or begin near the peripheral cornea (e.g. chronic superficial keratitis in dogs, eosinophilic keratoconjunctivitis in cats) or the conjunctiva. In such instances, the limbus becomes involved as an 'innocent bystander', as a result of extension of the inflammatory process from neighbouring tissues. Readers are referred to Chapters 7, 8 and 10; these discuss inflammatory diseases of the conjunctiva, cornea and anterior uvea, respectively.

Episcleritis

Episcleritis is categorized clinically as nodular or simple (Pearlstein, 1997). Both forms usually appear within the interpalpebral fissure, at or near the corneoscleral limbus. Signs of ocular pain are not common in the history. Nodular episcleritis is recognized more frequently and appears as a well demarcated raised area (Figure 9.4), whereas simple episcleritis lacks a discrete, raised nodule and may be somewhat more diffuse (Figure 9.5). With the nodular form, the nodule is firm, but it is moveable over the surface of the sclera when displaced with a cotton swab. Less frequently, several nodules may be clustered together or may occur in different sectors. With both simple and nodular episcleritis, the disease may be unilateral or bilateral. The cornea is usually affected adjacent to the lesion and there is an accompanying congestion of the superficial episcleral and conjunctival vasculature; the deep layer of the episclera and the sclera are usually unaffected. Necrosis of the nodule does not occur. Collagen degeneration is a typical histological feature of nodular episcleritis.

One study showed a predilection for the disease of American Cocker Spaniels and Golden Retrievers (Deykin et al., 1997). The disease has not been reported in cats.

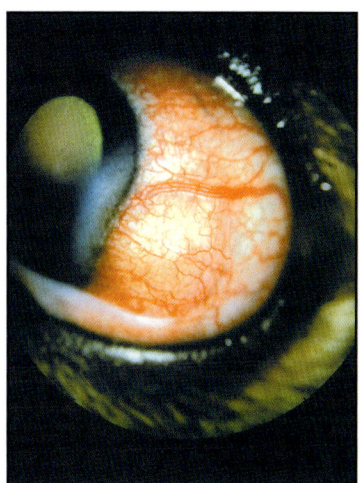

Figure 9.4 Nodular episcleritis is present at the ventrolateral perilimbal region in this 9-year-old female American Cocker Spaniel. Note the hyperaemic, well demarcated nodule. The overlying conjunctiva is hyperaemic and corneal oedema is present near the mass.

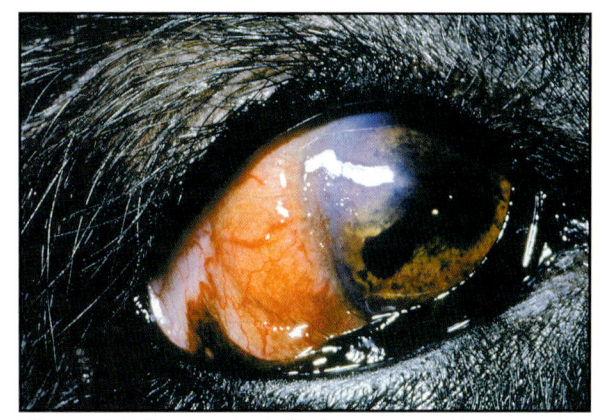

Figure 9.5 Simple episcleritis is present in this 6-year-old male American Cocker Spaniel. The lateral episclera is diffusely thickened and hyperaemic, but a discrete nodule is absent. Note the corneal oedema near the affected episclera.

Treatment: Simple episcleritis responds favourably to topical treatment with corticosteroids, compared with nodular episcleritis, in which topical corticosteroid treatment as the sole treatment may not result in resolution of the inflammation. Alternative medical treatment options include oral administration of corticosteroids, azathioprine, or a combination of tetracycline and niacinamide (Rothstein et al., 1997). Cryosurgery and surgical removal may also be used, if medical treatment is not effective.

Nodular episclerokeratitis

A plethora of terms has been used for nodular episclerokeratitis, including nodular granulomatous episclerokeratitis (Paulsen et al., 1987), nodular granulomatous episcleritis, ocular nodular faciitis (Bellhorn and Henkind, 1967), ophthalmic nodular faciitis (Gwin et al., 1977), fibrous histiocytoma (Latimer et al., 1983), idiopathic granulomatous disease (Collins et al., 1992), proliferative keratoconjunctivitis (Blogg, 1977; Wheeler et al., 1989), proliferative episcleritis (Peiffer et al., 1976), histiocytic sclerokeratitis, limbal granuloma, non-necrotizing scleritis and limbal pseudotumour (Whitley and Gilger, 1999).

A histological review of tissues acquired from dogs with clinical diagnoses of the aforementioned diseases shows a similar inflammatory picture in all of them; this consists of histiocytes, lymphocytes and plasma cells. It is likely that different stages of the disease process may represent a continuum of a single disease, and this may have contributed to the multitude of names for similar nodular diseases affecting the episclera and cornea.

Clinical features: Nodular episclerokeratitis occurs most frequently in the Collie, Collie crosses and Shetland Sheepdogs. It is more common in some geographical locations.

The disease is bilateral and is typified by singular or multiple raised well delineated pink fleshy-appearing mass(es) that arise at or near the corneoscleral limbus and infiltrate the episclera and peripheral corneal stroma (Figure 9.6). Corneal ulceration is not a feature of this disease and affected dogs do not demonstrate signs of ocular pain. Masses may also be present on the eyelids, nictitating membrane, lateral labial commissure of the mouth and, rarely, in the anterior chamber, as they arise from the iris (Dugan *et al.,* 1993).

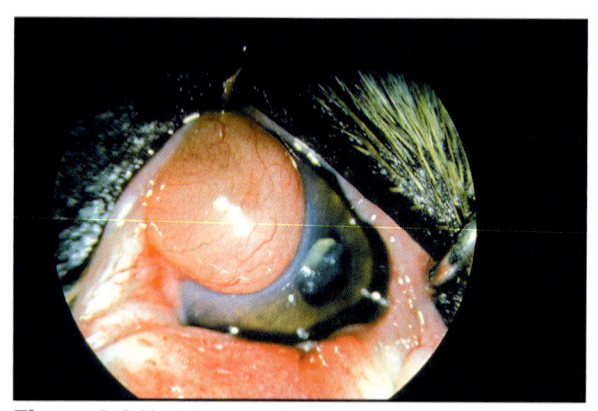

Figure 9.6 Nodular granulomatous episclerokeratitis is present in this 2-year-old Collie. A large raised well delineated pink fleshy-appearing mass extends from the limbus into the clear cornea, and typifies the clinical appearance of the disease. A thin band of corneal oedema frequently surrounds the part of the mass infiltrating the cornea.

Treatment: Medical therapy includes treatment with orally administered corticosteroids, azathioprine, tetracycline and niacinamide, or cyclophosphamide. Beta-irradiation, intralesional corticosteroid injection, surgical removal, cryosurgery and lamellar corneoconjunctival transposition have also been advocated.

Scleritis

Inflammation of the sclera is exceedingly rare in dogs and has not been reported as a primary entity in cats. Spaniels (particularly American Cocker Spaniels) are predisposed. In humans, scleritis is frequently associated with other immune-mediated and/or systemic diseases, but this is rare in the dog. Scleritis may occur as an idiopathic event, or may be secondary to local infection of adjacent ocular tissues (e.g. fungal granuloma of the uvea extending into the sclera). It is categorized arbitrarily, based on the anatomical location of the inflammation (anterior scleritis *versus* posterior scleritis) and the presence or absence of necrosis (non-necrotizing granulomatous scleritis *versus* necrotizing granulomatous scleritis).

Anterior scleritis: The most common form of scleritis reported in dogs is non-necrotizing granulomatous anterior scleritis. A well defined nodule is not usually present but, if present, is immobile. The eye is painful, and the superficial and deep episcleral vasculature, as well as the overlying conjunctival vasculature, are congested. The affected sclera may be a deep purple or red colour. Peripheral corneal infiltrates may be present when the anterior sclera in close proximity to the cornea is affected.

Posterior scleritis: Posterior scleritis is usually more diffuse, and is much more difficult to diagnose definitively. When posterior scleritis is a consideration, but thickening of the sclera is not obvious on fundoscopic examination, scleral depression should be used to enable complete visualization of the peripheral fundus. Flat or bullous exudative retinal detachment and altered tapetal reflectivity may be present. Concurrent anterior and/or posterior uveitis and retinitis is common (Deykin *et al.,* 1997). When the fundus appears unremarkable, the use of ocular ultrasonography may assist with making the diagnosis. Ultrasonographically, the sclera appears markedly thickened and hyperechoic, and concomitant choroidal and intraconal anterior orbital hyperechogenicity may be present.

Necrotizing scleritis: Necrotizing granulomatous scleritis may result in perforation of the globe (scleromalacia perforans, Figure 9.7) but, clinically, this is a rare form of scleritis in dogs. It is interesting to note that, based on the results of a recent histological study of scleritis in dogs, collagenolysis is common and the necrotizing form of scleritis predominates (Deykin *et al.,* 1997).

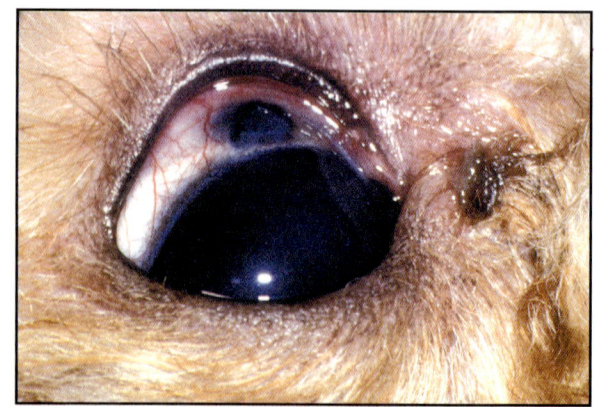

Figure 9.7 Necrotizing granulomatous scleritis resulted in perforation (scleromalacia perforans) in this Poodle.

Treatment: Treatment with orally administered (and topically administered, for anterior scleritis) corticosteroids and azathioprine may result in resolution of scleritis but as a general rule, the response to treatment is less favourable than that of episcleritis.

Subconjunctival granuloma

Focal granulomatous inflammation at the site of injection is common following subconjunctival injection with depot corticosteroid (Fischer, 1979, Håkanson et al., 1991). Such granulomas occasionally become large, raised, and ivory to yellow in colour, and remain freely moveable over the sclera (Figure 9.8). The depot vehicle is thought to be responsible for the formation of the granuloma. Treatment is seldom necessary as most post-injection granulomas resolve spontaneously.

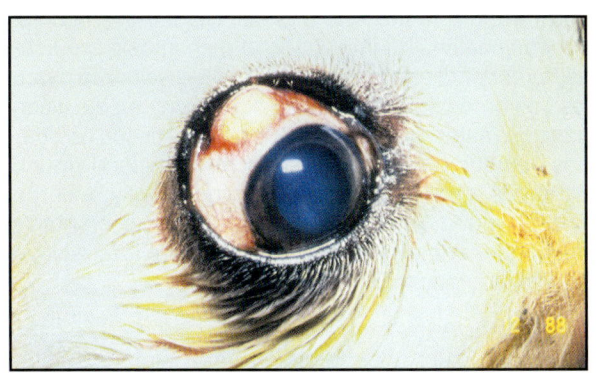

Figure 9.8 A focal, raised, ivory-coloured granuloma is present at the dorsal perilimbal region in this mixed breed dog. The conjunctiva and episclera around the granuloma are hyperaemic. A subconjunctival injection of depot corticosteroid was administered one month before this photograph was taken.

Abscess

Abscess of the limbus, sclera or peripheral cornea is detected infrequently. In the author's experience, scleral or limbal abscesses occur most commonly as a result of infection (primarily fungal) of adjacent ocular tissues (e.g. the anterior uvea). Peripherally located intrastromal corneal epithelial inclusion cysts are frequently mistaken for peripheral corneal abscesses, but they lack the characteristic features of severe stromal oedema, neovascularization, conjunctival and episcleral hyperaemia and ocular pain. Intrastromal inclusion cysts are also very well delineated, unlike stromal abscesses.

Ulcerative limbal keratitis

Limbal ulcers are uncommon and are believed to be attributable to immune-mediated inflammation since, histologically, Langerhans cells (antigen-presenting cells) are seen to be localized peripherally in the cornea. The typical clinical appearance of ulcerative limbal keratitis is peripheral ulceration of the cornea with a pronounced steep sloping gutter that always faces toward the limbus (Figure 9.9). The elimination of infectious keratitis with collagenolysis, as a differential consideration, is difficult. The practitioner should contemplate referring such cases to a specialist for a diagnostic evaluation, before treatment is started.

Neoplastic diseases

Nodular inflammatory diseases affecting the perilimbal episclera are commonly mistaken for neoplasia, but limbal, episcleral and scleral neoplasia is uncommon in dogs, and very rare in cats. The dorsotemporal area is reportedly the most common location for neoplasms affecting these tissues, but any area may be affected.

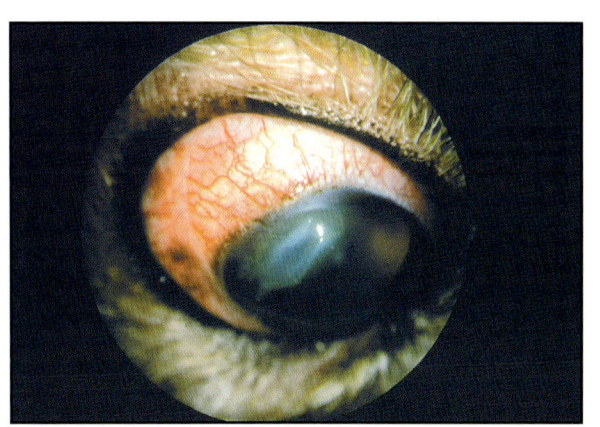

Figure 9.9 Limbal ulcerative keratitis in a 4-year-old American Cocker Spaniel. The typical clinical appearance is seen here: there is peripheral ulceration of the cornea, with a pronounced steep sloping gutter that always faces toward the limbus. Vascularization extends to the ulcer, and corneal oedema surrounds the lesion.

Melanocytoma

Neoplasms arising from limbal melanocytes are the most common limbal neoplasms in dogs and cats (Figure 9.10). The term 'melanocytoma' is favoured over use of the previous term 'melanoma', based on its histological appearance and biological behaviour.

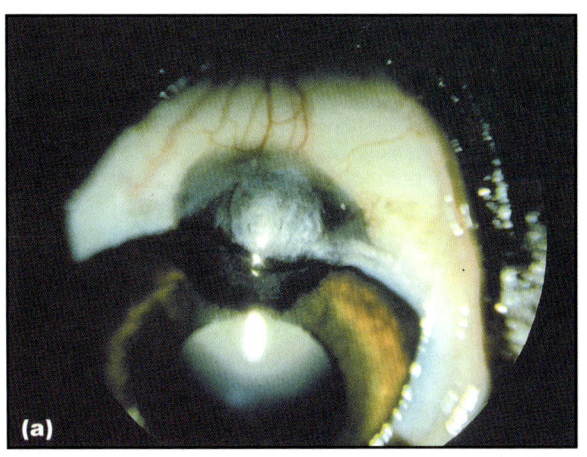

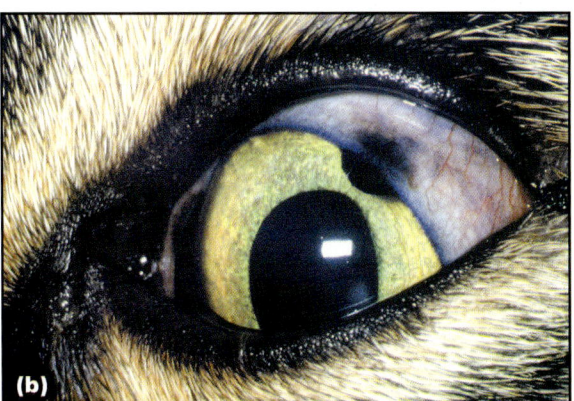

Figure 9.10 (a) A limbal melanocytoma in this dog appears as a well circumscribed, raised, darkly pigmented mass arising from the corneoscleral limbus and extending into the sclera and cornea. The overlying bulbar conjunctiva is normal, and can be moved freely over the mass. (b) A well circumscribed limbal melanocytoma in a cat. (Courtesy of SM Crispin.)

The term 'epibulbar melanocytoma' has been used synonymously for 'limbal melanocytoma', based on the location in which it occurs. Limbal melanocytoma arises from the limbus and extends from the limbus into the perilimbal sclera and corneal stroma. The mass is usually dark, well circumscribed and raised, but the overlying bulbar conjunctiva moves freely over scleral extension of the mass. The primary differential considerations for limbal melanocytoma include anterior uveal melanoma with extrascleral extension, limbal melanoma and staphyloma.

Gonioscopy: When the diagnosis is not immediately obvious, gonioscopy should be performed to differentiate these disease entities. When limbal melanocytoma is sufficiently large, focal appositional angle closure may be evident by gonioscopic examination.

Clinical features: Two different forms of clinical course are seen in dogs. The neoplasm is characterized by rapid growth rate in young dogs. In elderly dogs the neoplasm grows slowly or remains static (Martin, 1981). In cats, the clinical course of limbal melanocytoma appears to be similar to that in the dog (Harling *et al.*, 1986; Patnaik and Mooney, 1988). However, in contrast to dogs, limbal melanocytoma is very uncommon. Limbal melanoma is also very rare in cats; a single case report has documented metastasis of a limbal melanoma early in the course of disease in a cat (Betton *et al.*, 1999).

Treatment: When a rapid rate of growth has been documented in a young dog, treatment by cryosurgery, free-hand corneoscleral graft (Martin, 1981; Wilkie and Wolf, 1991), nictitating membrane graft (Blogg *et al.*, 1989), or laser photocoagulation (Sullivan *et al.*, 1996) may be warranted. Periodic monitoring for evidence of growth in older dogs is recommended (Martin, 1981).

Ocular melanosis

A familial condition that occurs in middle-aged to elderly Cairn Terriers leads to melanocyte deposition in the episclera (Figure 9.11) and iridocorneal angle; this frequently results in secondary glaucoma (Petersen-Jones, 1991). Melanosis of the perilimbal episclera should alert the clinician to consider referral to a specialist, for complete ophthalmic examination and treatment.

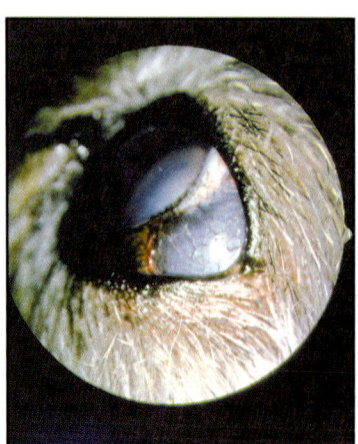

Figure 9.11
A middle-aged Cairn Terrier with ocular melanosis. Note the large pigmented, raised lesion involving the ventral sclera and episclera adjacent to the limbus. (Courtesy of SM Petersen-Jones.)

Other neoplastic diseases

Other, less common, primary neoplasms that begin at, or infiltrate, the limbus include fibrosarcoma, schwannoma, squamous cell carcinoma (Ward *et al.*, 1992), haemangioma and haemangiosarcoma. The most common secondary neoplasm affecting the corneoscleral limbus is lymphoma. Surgical excision and adjuvant laser photocoagulation or beta-irradiation is recommended.

Traumatic diseases

Blunt trauma to the sclera is common; if this occurs, subconjunctival haemorrhage and chemosis are usually present. Perforating trauma to the sclera is much less common than perforating corneal injury, but it can have devastating consequences. Uveal tissue or vitreous humour may be incarcerated in the scleral wound if there is a conjunctival wound lying directly over the scleral wound. Alternatively, the overlying conjunctiva may appear only hyperaemic, while there is extensive scleral laceration.

Examination

Whenever blunt or perforating scleral injury occurs, a thorough ophthalmic examination is indicated. The globe should be examined, to determine if shape and size are normal, and intraocular pressure should be measured. Abnormalities of pupillary shape, and a difference in the plane of the iris relative to the cornea are common when perforating injury to the anterior sclera occurs. Furthermore, aqueous humour may flow out from the wound, resulting in ocular hypotony. A step defect in the corneoscleral limbus is the hallmark of a full-thickness corneoscleral wound that crosses perpendicular to the limbus.

It is of paramount importance to determine the full extent of the scleral injury before surgical correction is attempted.

Treatment

When a large defect is present, simply creating and placing a conjunctival flap is inappropriate, because rigid support of the weakened sclera is necessary. When a small area of sclera is involved, rigid support can be achieved by creating a square or triangular partial-thickness scleral flap adjacent to the wound. Care must be used to remove conjunctival tissue from the surgical area. A conjunctival incision should be located toward the periphery of the scleral wound, and the conjunctiva reflected, so that the two wounds do not directly overlie each other. Incarcerated vitreous or uveal tissue should be excised using wet-field cautery, and necrotic sclera should be excised. The base of the flap should be oriented parallel to the defect, so that the flap can be reflected over the wound, and sutured in position to healthy sclera surrounding the defect. When the defect is sizeable, the use of autologous tissue is not recommended. Homologous sclera from a cadaver donor, or, alternatively, biosynthetic collagen matrix manufactured from intestinal submucosa, may be used as onlay grafts over the defect. Interrupted sutures of 9-0 or 10-0 nylon or polyglactin should be placed at half-thickness in sclera, with the suture knots orientated away from the limbus, if possible. Conjunctiva is then repositioned to cover the scleral surgical area and the incision is closed using 9-0 polyglactin in a continuous pattern. Topically and systemically administered antibiotics, corticosteroids and nonsteroidal anti-inflammatory drugs, and topically administered mydriatic drugs, are necessary after surgery.

Degenerative diseases

Scleral thinning

Acquired thinning of the sclera occurs, most commonly, secondary to chronic glaucoma, due to buphthalmos or scleritis, or secondary to trans-scleral laser cyclophotocoagulation (Figure 9.12). When glaucoma occurs in juvenile dogs and cats, buphthalmos can occur rapidly, because of sparse and immature scleral and corneal collagen. The sclera may appear a light blue in colour, as the underlying uveal tissue becomes partially visible through the thinned sclera.

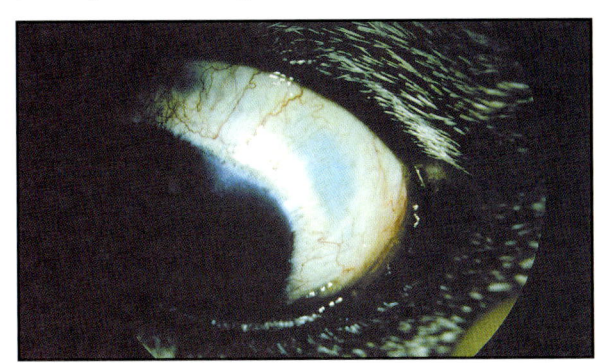

Figure 9.12 Focal areas of scleral thinning are present in this dog that had laser cyclophotocoagulation surgery for glaucoma performed several months previously. The focal areas appear dark in colour because the underlying uveal tissue is partially visible through thinned areas.

Symblepharon

When symblepharon involves the peripheral cornea, the limbus may be obliterated and, therefore, not visible to the examiner. This occurs most frequently in cats, secondary to infection with feline herpesvirus-1. Treatment is usually contraindicated, because of the high likelihood of symblepharon recurring after corrective surgery.

References

Bellhorn RW and Henkind P (1967) Ocular nodular faciitis in a dog. *Journal of the American Veterinary Medical Association* **150**, 212–213

Betton A, Healy LN, English RV and Bunch SE (1999) Atypical limbal melanoma in a cat. *Journal of Veterinary Internal Medicine* **13**, 379–381

Blogg JR (1977) Proliferative keratoconjunctivitis in the Collie. *Proceedings of the 8th Annual Meeting of the American College of Veterinary Ophthalmologists*, 89–90

Blogg JR, Dutton AG and Stanley RG (1989) Use of third eyelid grafts to repair full-thickness defects in the cornea and sclera. *Journal of the American Animal Hospital Association* **25**, 505–512

Collins BK, Macewan EG, Dubielzig RR and Swanson JF (1992) Idiopathic granulomatous disease with ocular adnexal and cutaneous involvement in a dog. *Journal of the American Veterinary Medical Association* **201**, 313–316

Deykin AR, Guandilini A and Ratto A (1997) A retrospective histopathologic study of primary episcleral and scleral inflammatory disease in dogs. *Veterinary and Comparative Ophthalmology* **7**, 245–248

Dugan SJ, Ketring KL, Severin GA and Render JA (1993) Variant nodular granulomatous episclerokeratitis in four dogs. *Journal of the American Animal Hospital Association* **29**, 403–409

Fischer CA (1979) Granuloma formation associated with subconjunctival injection of a corticosteroid in dogs. *Journal of the American Veterinary Medical Association* **174**, 1086–1088

Gwin RM, Gelatt KN and Peiffer RL (1977) Ophthalmic nodular faciitis in the dog. *Journal of the American Veterinary Medical Association* **170**, 611–614

Håkanson N, Shiveley JN and Meredith RE (1991) Granuloma formation following subconjunctival injection of triamcinolone in two dogs. *Journal of the American Animal Hospital Association* **27**, 89–92

Harling DE, Peiffer RL, Cook CS and Belkinn PV (1986) Feline limbal melanoma: four cases. *Journal of the American Animal Hospital Association* **22**, 795–802

Latimer CA, Wyman M, Szymanski C and Winston SL (1983) Azathioprine in the management of fibrous histiocytoma in two dogs. *Journal of the American Animal Hospital Association* **19**, 155–158

Martin CL (1981) Canine epibulbar melanomas and their management. *Journal of the American Animal Hospital Association* **17**, 83–90

Martin CL and Anderson BG (1981) Ocular anatomy. In: *Veterinary Ophthalmology*, 1st edn, ed. KN Gelatt, p.12. Lea & Febiger, Philadelphia

Patnaik AK and Mooney S (1988) Feline melanoma: a comparison of ocular, oral and dermal neoplasms. *Veterinary Pathology* **25**, 105–112

Paulsen ME, Lavach JD, Snyder SP, Severin GA and Eichenbaum JE (1987) Nodular granulomatous episclerokeratitis in dogs: 19 cases. *Journal of the American Veterinary Medical Association* **190**, 1581–1587

Pearlstein ES (1997) Episcleritis. In: *Cornea*, ed. JH Krachmer *et al.*, pp. 1473–1478. Mosby Year Book Publishing, St. Louis

Peiffer RL, Gelatt KN and Gwin RM (1976) Use of corneoscleral homograft to treat proliferative episcleritis in the dog. *Veterinary Medicine for the Small Animal Clinician* **71**, 1273–1278

Petersen-Jones SM (1991) Abnormal ocular pigment deposition associated with glaucoma in the Cairn Terrier. *Journal of Small Animal Practice* **32**, 19–22

Rothstein E, Scott DW and Riis RC (1997) Tetracycline and niacinamide for the treatment of a sterile pyogranulomatous/granuloma syndrome in a dog. *Journal of the American Animal Hospital Association* **33**, 540–543

Sullivan TL, Nasisse MP, Davidson MG and Glover TL (1996) Photocoagulation of limbal melanoma in dogs and cats: 15 cases (1989–1993). *Journal of the American Veterinary Medical Association* **208**, 891–894

Ward DA, Latimer KS and Askren RM (1992) Squamous cell carcinoma of the corneoscleral limbus in a dog. *Journal of the American Veterinary Medical Association* **200**, 1503–1506

Wheeler CA, Blanchard GL and Davidson H (1989) Cryosurgery for treatment of proliferative keratoconjunctivitis in five dogs. *Journal of the American Veterinary Medical Association* **195**, 354–357

Whitley RD and Gilger BC (1999) Diseases of the canine cornea and sclera. In: *Veterinary Ophthalmology*, 3rd edn, ed. KN Gelatt, pp.635–673. Lippincott, Williams & Wilkins, Philadelphia

Wilkie DL and Wolf ED (1991) Treatment of epibulbar melanocytoma in a dog, using full-thickness eyewall resection and synthetic graft. *Journal of the American Veterinary Medical Association* **198**, 1019–1022

10

The uveal tract

Sheila Crispin

Introduction

The uveal tract (Figure 10.1) consists of the iris, ciliary body and choroid. It is derived from mesenchyme (neural crest of neuroectodermal origin and mesoderm). Embryogenesis of congenital malformations of the eye has been reviewed by Cook (1995, 1999). Melanocytes of neural crest origin are scattered throughout the uveal tract and produce the characteristic pigment. In addition to the specialized muscular functions of the iris and ciliary body, the uveal tract is concerned with the nutrition of the eye. The choriocapillaris vessels supply the outer retina, and the aqueous humour is a source of nutrients for the cornea, lens and other adjacent tissues.

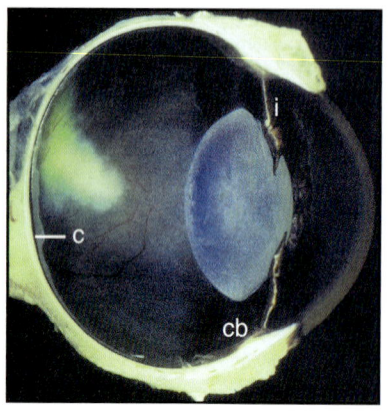

Figure 10.1 The uveal tract. Gross specimen of canine globe. c, choroid: between sclera (white) and retina; cb, ciliary body; i, iris (Courtesy of JRB Mould.)

This chapter is primarily concerned with disorders of the anterior uvea (iris and ciliary body), but there are occasions when both the anterior uvea and the posterior uvea (choroid) are involved, and these are also included. Conditions of the canine anterior uvea have been reviewed by Collins and Moore (1999) and those of the feline anterior uvea by Crispin (1998) and Glaze and Gelatt (1999). Posterior uveal disorders affecting the fundus are described in Chapter 14.

In this chapter developmental conditions of the uvea will be considered concurrently for the dog and cat while acquired problems will be considered separately by species.

Anatomy and physiology of the iris

On gross examination the anterior surface of the iris is grossly divisible into a central (pupillary) zone and a peripheral (ciliary) zone, separated by the collarette. The pupillary zone is usually darker than the ciliary zone, but this distinction is less clear in cats than in dogs.

Histologically the iris consists of an anterior border layer, the stroma and sphincter muscle, and the posterior epithelial layers and the dilator muscle. The cellular anterior border layer is a modification of the loosely arranged stroma that lies beneath it. The iris sphincter muscle is located in the pupillary portion of the stroma. Two layers of epithelial cells form the posterior part of the iris. The anterior epithelium consists of an epithelial apical portion and a muscular basal portion, the iris dilator muscle, which projects into the iris stroma. The posterior surface of the iris consists of very heavily pigmented epithelial cells. Iris musculature and the epithelial layers are of neuroectodermal origin, whereas the stroma is of mesodermal origin. Iris colour depends on the number of melanocytes in the stroma and the thickness of the anterior border layer.

There is some variation of iris capillary permeability between species. Feline iridal capillaries, for example, are apparently more permeable to molecules the size of serum proteins than are those of humans (Bellhorn, 1991). Furthermore, the morphology of the iridal capillaries of immature cats differs from that of adults, suggesting that the vessels are 'leakier' in kittens.

Control of pupil size

The iris is designed to function as the lens aperture of the eye, and the opposing actions of the sphincter and dilator muscles regulate the amount of light entering the eye through the pupil. The sphincter muscle circles the iris at the pupillary zone, allowing the pupil shape in the dog to change from a large circle to a smaller circle. In the cat the smooth muscle fibres not only encircle the pupil but also criss-cross dorsal and ventral to the pupil, and extend to the periphery of the iris; this arrangement allows the feline pupil to constrict to a vertical slit. Constriction is mediated by the parasympathetic branches of the oculomotor nerve. The dilator muscle, which controls pupillary dilation, consists of radially oriented fibres that pass from close to the pupil towards the root of the iris. Dilation is mediated by postganglionic sympathetic nerves.

Although the most important pupillary function in domestic animals is to regulate the amount of light entering the eye, constriction of the pupil also serves to increase the depth of focus for near vision and to minimize optical aberrations.

Anatomy and physiology of the ciliary body

The ciliary body is located posterior to the iris and anterior to the choroid. It is approximately triangular in cross-section, with its base facing the anterior chamber and its apex blending with the choroid. Topographically the ciliary body can be divided into two zones: an anterior pars plicata and a posterior pars plana. The pars plana extends to the edge of the retina, a zone known as the ora ciliaris retinae.

Histologically the ciliary body consists of the ciliary processes, ciliary body muscles and the deep aspect of the iridocorneal angle (see Chapter 11). Its stroma, ciliary muscles and blood vessels are of mesenchymal origin. The inner non-pigmented epithelium and the outer pigmented epithelium are anterior continuations of the neuroretina and retinal pigment epithelium, respectively, both originating from neuroectoderm.

The ciliary body has important metabolic functions. It is involved in the production and drainage of aqueous humour (see Chapter 11), serves to anchor the zonular fibres of the lens, and is also concerned with accommodation. However, as the ciliary muscles are poorly developed in domestic animals, accommodation may be regarded as a subsidiary function.

The blood–aqueous 'barrier' to free diffusion of molecules is formed by the tight junction between non-pigmented epithelial cells. Breakdown of the blood–aqueous barrier occurs in many conditions, including inflammation, trauma and vascular disease. Interventions such as paracentesis and surgery also cause breakdown, as does topical administration of drugs such as pilocarpine. Typically, the aqueous humour becomes turbid (aqueous flare) because of leakage of plasma proteins into the anterior and posterior chambers. Fibrinogen and other proteins render the aqueous 'plasmoid', as its protein content approaches that of normal plasma, and when inflammation is severe fibrin clots may form. The cellular component varies according to the underlying aetiology. A preponderance of white blood cells is termed hypopyon; a preponderance of red blood cells is called hyphaema.

Anatomy and physiology of the choroid

The choroid is situated between the sclera and retina. It is highly vascularized and its stroma contains elastic fibres and collagen fibres, fibrocytes and many melanocytes. The choroid in dogs and cats consists of, from the outside to the inside:

- The suprachoroidea of heavily pigmented connective tissue that links the choroid with the lamina fusca of the inner sclera
- Large vessels consisting mainly of large veins and less prominent arteries
- Medium-sized vessels beneath the large vessels and, internal to these vessels in most dogs and cats, a cellular tapetum (tapetum cellulosum) located in the dorsal choroid. The tapetum increases visual sensitivity by reflecting light back through the photoreceptors, but at some loss to visual acuity. The medium-sized vessels link with the choriocapillaris via smaller emissary vessels, which pass at right angles to connect the two. In the tapetal region these linking vessels, predominantly capillaries, are often very obvious; because of their star-like apppearance when viewed end-on with an ophthalmoscope they are termed the 'stars of Winslow'
- Highly fenestrated capillaries, collectively termed the choriocapillaris, forming the innermost layer of choroidal vessels
- A basal complex known as Bruch's membrane, consisting of connective tissue and the basement membranes of the choriocapillaris and retinal pigment epithelium.

The retina depends on both choroidal and retinal vessels for nutrition. The energy needs of the outer retina are met by diffusion of glucose and oxygen from the richly vascular choroid; specifically the permeable capillaries of the choriocapillaris. There is a very high rate of blood flow through the choroid so that oxygen extraction for each millilitre of blood is very low and the outer retina is exposed to near arterial levels of oxygen.

Developmental anomalies and abnormalities of the anterior uveal tract in the dog and cat

Deficiencies of pigmentation

Heterochromia
Difference in colour between the two irides (heterochromia iridis) or within the same iris (heterochromia iridum) may be either developmental or acquired; the latter is usually the result of previous inflammation (see below) but can be a side effect of some drugs (e.g. echothiopate iodide). Ocular heterochromia may be the only manifestation of colour dilution, or may be part of more widespread colour dilution, especially in merle animals.

Subalbinism and albinism
These refer to partial and complete absence of normal pigmentation, respectively. Subalbinism, typified by a blue iris, is reasonably common in dogs (Figure 10.2) and cats, but true albinism, in which the iris is usually pink, has not been reported.

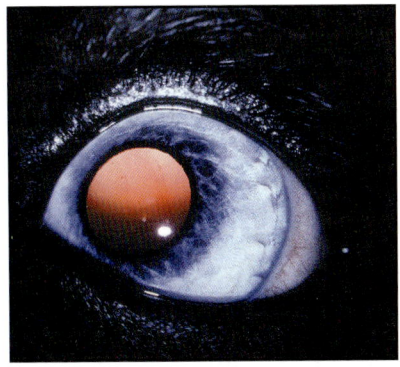

Figure 10.2 Subalbinotic iris in a Border Collie. Note the pinkish-red fundus reflex, which indicates that the fundus is also subalbinotic and atapetal.

164 The uveal tract

A range of ocular abnormalities may be encountered in merle animals (Figure 10.3). Mildly affected animals have heterochromia irides and iris hypoplasia (incomplete iris development), often with abnormal pupil position (correctopia) and shape (dyscoria). Persistent remnants of the pupillary membrane and iris colobomas (see below) are also common. Severe ocular defects, often multiple in nature, are more likely to be encountered in animals homozygous for the merle trait; these include microphthalmos, retinal dysplasia, optic nerve hypoplasia and cataracts. Affected animals are also likely to be congenitally deaf. The combination of a white coat, blue eyes and deafness in animals is analogous to human Waardenburg's syndrome.

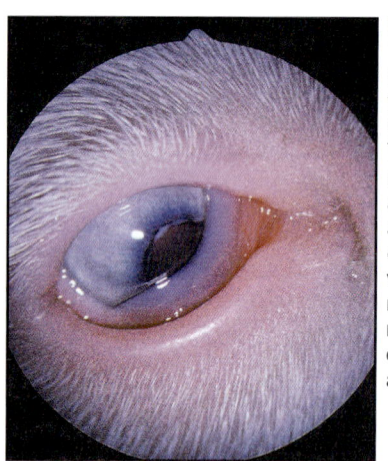

Figure 10.3 There are multiple ocular anomalies in this merle Border Collie puppy. The eye is microphthalmic and there is anterior segment dysgenesis. The whole litter of this merle x merle mating had gross ocular abnormalities.

Chédiak–Higashi syndrome is an autosomal recessive disorder of Blue-smoke Persian cats. Ocular manifestations include photophobia, cataract, iris hypoplasia and ocular hypopigmentation. Systemic manifestations include increased susceptibility to infections and bleeding tendencies, and affected cats show cutaneous hypopigmentation.

Aniridia and iris hypoplasia

Aniridia, a complete absence of the iris, is very rare and in most cases of apparent aniridia a rudimentary iris base is present. Iris hypoplasia and iris colobomas are less rare and most commonly encountered as a manifestation of colour dilution. Although iris hypoplasia may be a partial thickness or full thickness defect, the latter defects are usually termed colobomas.

Coloboma

When a portion of the anterior uvea fails to develop, the resulting condition is known as a colobomatous defect (Figure 10.4). Typical colobomas occur in the region of the optic (choroidal) fissure at the 6 o'clock position and are a result of abnormal closure of the optic fissure. Colobomas that occur away from the 6 o'clock position are termed atypical. Colobomatous defects within the body of the iris constitute pseudopolycoria (multiple holes in the iris but without any encircling sphincter muscle), as distinct from polycoria (where there is more than one pupil each with a proper iris sphincter). A notch coloboma is apparent when the pupillary margin is defective.

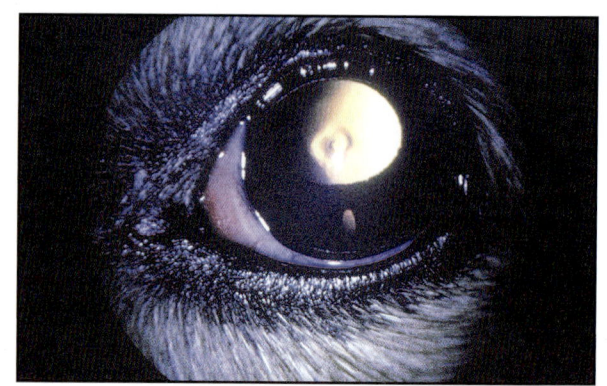

Figure 10.4 Typical coloboma (6 o'clock) in a Shetland Sheepdog. The reason for referral was the corneal ulcer, which is apparent dorsal to the coloboma.

Iris colobomas in the cat may be seen in association with eyelid agenesis (see Chapter 5), when they are usually in the 6 o'clock position.

Colobomas of the ciliary body are usually associated with absence of the lens zonule and indentation of the equator of the lens. Ciliary body dysplasia is another rare developmental defect of this region and affected animals present with microphthalmos, cataract and lens subluxation.

Anterior segment dysgenesis

Faulty differentiation of the mesenchyme of the anterior segment may produce a range of rare defects, primarily involving the cornea, drainage angle and iris of the dog and cat (Williams, 1993). Anterior segment dysgenesis (ASD) may be one aspect of multiple ocular defects, which are more common in dogs than in cats. ASD with microphthalmos and retinal dysplasia is thought to be inherited as an autosomal recessive trait in the Dobermann (Lewis et al., 1986). Peripheral defects that involve the canine drainage angle are the most clinically important type of ASD; goniodysgenesis is described in Chapter 11.

Persistence of remnants of the embryonic pupillary membrane

Persistent pupillary membrane (PPM) represents a failure of the normal process of atrophy of the mesodermal vascular arcades and their associated mesenchymal tissue. There are a myriad of possible clinical appearances in the dog (Figure 10.5) and cat (Figure 10.6). The remnants are usually short strands that

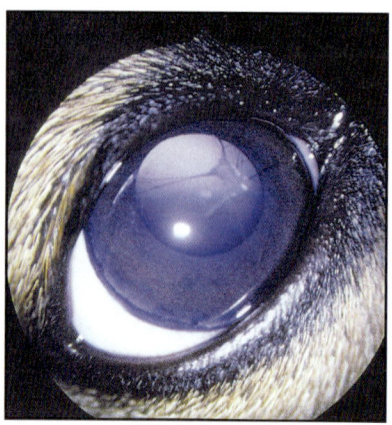

Figure 10.5 Persistent pupillary membrane in a young Jack Russell Terrier. The remnants are extending anteriorly to the cornea and posteriorly to the lens, producing discrete opacities at the point of contact in both structures.

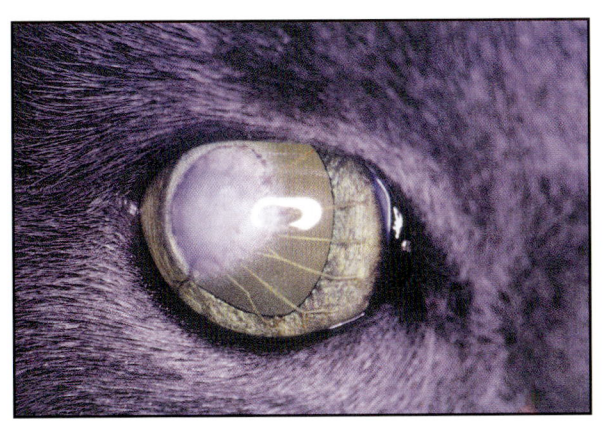

Figure 10.6 Persistent pupillary membrane in a cat. Some of the vascular remnants (tunica vasculosa lentis anterioris) are still patent and there is discrete haemorrhage in the opaque region of the posterior cornea in consequence.

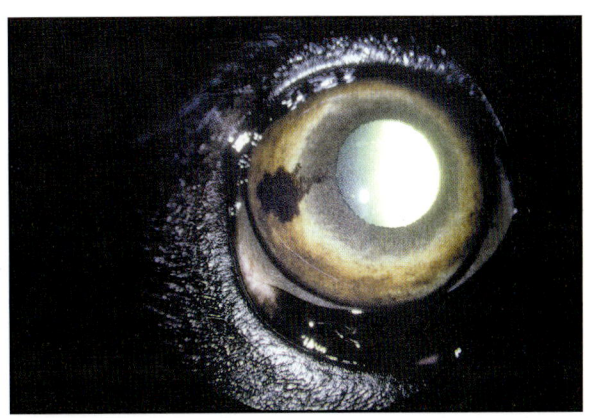

Figure 10.7 Benign melanosis in a Labrador Retriever. This is a breed in which iris melanoma is over-represented, so it is important to keep all changes of iris pigmentation under review.

originate from the collarette region of the iris; the strands may run circumferentially, span the pupil or pass posteriorly to the anterior lens capsule or anteriorly to the posterior cornea. They should be distinguished from synechiae, which more typically involve the pupillary margin and follow ocular insults such as penetrating injury or iritis. While PPM remnants are a relatively common and apparently isolated finding of no clinical significance in many breeds of dog, there is a familial tendency in other breeds (e.g. Pembroke Welsh Corgi, English Mastiff) and they may be inherited in the Basenji. In breeds in which multiple ocular defects have been reported (e.g. English Cocker Spaniel, Old English Sheepdog) PPM remnants are one of the abnormalities that may be found.

Uveal cysts

Uveal cysts are infrequently recognized as of developmental origin, probably beause they may initially be hidden from view behind the iris, attached to posterior uveal tissue and small enough to escape notice. In both dogs and cats they originate from the pupillary posterior pigmented epithelium of the iris (embryonic marginal sinus region) and from the ciliary body epithelium and are generally of no clinical significance. If the cysts progressively enlarge and detach from the posterior uveal tissue they will pass through the pupil into the anterior chamber where they are obvious; the degree of pigmentation is quite variable. Treatment is not usually required. Further details are given below.

Acquired abnormalities of the canine anterior uvea

Iris pigmentation

Benign melanosis
Discrete foci of pigment are sometimes observed on the surface of the iris in normal dogs. Discrete pigment proliferation of these areas, with consequent increase in size, may occur as a phenomenon of ageing and is usually of no clinical significance (Figure 10.7). More widespread pigment proliferation, however, should be regarded with suspicion, whether it is limited to one sector of the iris or is more diffuse, for it may be indicative of iris neoplasia (see later).

Diffuse ocular melanosis associated with proliferation of melanocytes may occur in the Cairn Terrier; affected dogs are middle-aged or older. It is possible that this condition is a form of benign iris melanoma (see later). Secondary glaucoma occurs because melanocytes accumulate in the iridocorneal angle and intrascleral venous plexus (see Chapter 11).

Ectropion uveae
This is not unusual and represents eversion of the posterior pigment epithelium of the iris. Strictly speaking, it occurs because shrinkage of the anterior surface of the iris allows the dark posterior pigment to become visible at the pupillary border. Ectropion uveae is most commonly observed following previous iris inflammation, and small cystic swellings may also be apparent. It should be noted that the posterior pigment epithelium will also be more obvious at the pupillary border in animals with colour dilution and in such cases is a developmental anomaly rather than an acquired abnormality.

Pre-iridal fibrovascular membranes
Neovascularization of the iris surface occurs when angiogenic factors stimulate production of blood vessels by the iris stroma. The release of angiogenic factors occurs secondary to pre-existing disease such as intraocular neoplasia, chronic uveitis and long-standing retinal detachment; factors such as hypoxia and ischaemia are implicated. These abnormal blood vessels may be a source of haemorrhage into the anterior chamber, resulting in the formation of peripheral anterior synechiae and subsequent secondary glaucoma.

Iris atrophy
Iris atrophy can occur as a feature of ageing. Senile iris atrophy is seen most commonly in breeds such as the Miniature and Toy Poodle, but it can also follow trauma, chronic uveitis and glaucoma. The atrophy can be quite extensive, resulting in full thickness defects (Figure

10.8). Loss of the sphincter muscle is associated with poor pupil constriction, and photophobia may also be present because of inability to respond appropriately to bright light.

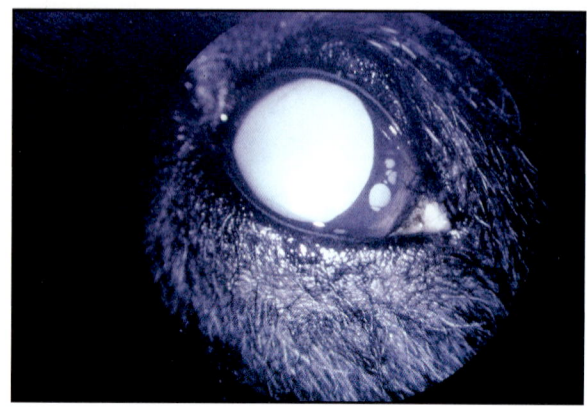

Figure 10.8 Senile iris atrophy in a Miniature Poodle. The dog also had generalized progressive retinal atrophy and secondary cortical cataract.

Iridociliary cysts

While iridociliary cysts can be developmental, they may not become obvious until the animal is an adult. Uveal cysts are a common finding in dogs. They may be a consequence of uveitis or appear as an apparent feature of ageing in breeds such as the Labrador Retriever. The cysts may be single or multiple (Figure 10.9) and commonly arise from the posterior pigment epithelium of the iris and the ciliary body epithelium. Their size is variable. They occasionally rupture and remnants may be identified on the anterior face of the lens or the posterior surface of the cornea. It is important to distinguish uveal cysts from primary tumours of the iris and ciliary body and from metastatic tumours. Intact cysts are often free floating and can be transilluminated with a bright light, even when they are heavily pigmented. In the majority of cases no treatment is required as animals seem quite unperturbed by their presence, although multiple cysts that obstruct the visual axis can be treated with a variety of techniques, of which laser therapy is the only non-invasive method. The situations in which cyst removal is advocated have been reviewed by Slatter (2001).

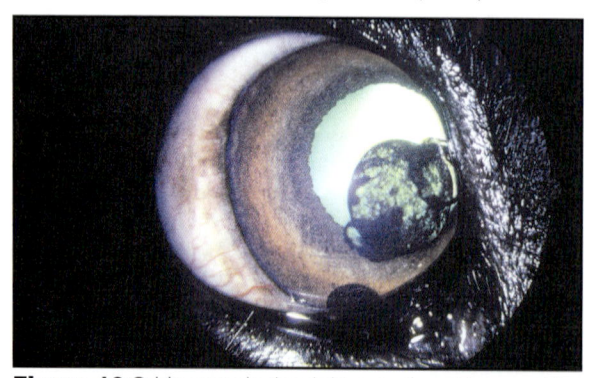

Figure 10.9 Iris cysts in the right eye of an 11-year-old Labrador Retriever. There are two intact cysts: one is very large and readily transilluminated; the other is smaller and much darker and cannot be transilluminated. The remnants of two cysts that have ruptured are visible adhering to the posterior cornea.

There are some exceptions to the general rule that cysts are innocuous; e.g. in the Great Dane (Slatter, 1990; Spiess *et al.*, 1998) and Golden Retriever, iridociliary cysts may lead to the development of glaucoma. In the Golden Retriever iridociliary cysts have also been associated with anterior uveitis and secondary glaucoma (Deehr and Dubielzig, 1998; Sapienza *et al.*, 2000). Pigment deposition on the anterior lens capsule has been noted as a key feature, and pre-iridal fibrovascular membranes are a common histopathological finding. Iridociliary cysts may be thin-walled and vacuolated or thick-walled; they may contain hyaluronic acid or, occasionally, blood.

Synechiae

Synechiae are adhesions that form as a result of iris inflammation; they should be differentiated from persistent pupillary membrane. There are a great number of possible causes:

- Anterior synechiae – adherence of the iris to the cornea – are a common complication of corneal penetrating injuries (Figure 10.10)
- Posterior synechiae – adherence of the iris to the anterior lens capsule – are a common sequel to iritis (Figure 10.11)
- Peripheral anterior synechiae involve the iridocorneal angle and are usually a complication of inflammation (see Chapter 11).

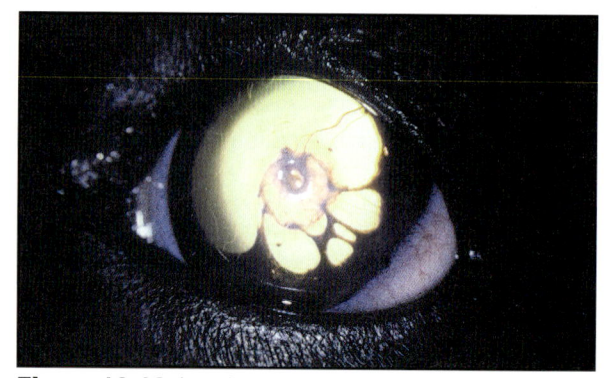

Figure 10.10 Anterior synechiae in an adult Border Collie, following traumatic penetrating injury from a cat claw as a puppy. Note the darkened iris, indicating previous uveitis, and the deep corneal facet.

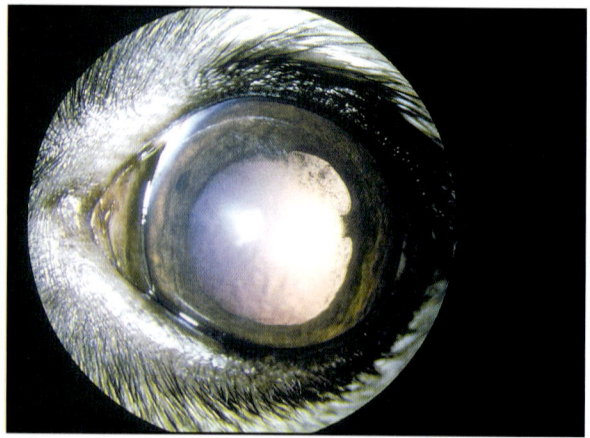

Figure 10.11 Posterior synechiae and iris rests (pigment deposits on the anterior lens capsule) in a Fox Terrier with panuveitis.

Uveitis

- Anterior uveitis may primarily involve the iris (iritis) or both the iris and the anterior part of the ciliary body (iridocyclitis)
- Intermediate uveitis predominantly involves the posterior part of the ciliary body (pars planitis)
- Posterior uveitis primarily involves the choroid (choroiditis), but close association of the retina means that inflammation of both choroid and retina is the usual situation
- Panuveitis is inflammation of the entire uveal tract: iris, ciliary body and choroid.

To provide a complete overview of uveitis, all parts of the uveal tract will be considered in this section, which should be read in conjunction with the sections on inflammatory chorioretinopathies in Chapter 14.

Clinical features

The clinical features of uveitis (Figure 10.12) vary according to the time for which it has been present, the cause of the inflammation and the extent of uveal tract involvement. In general, acute uveitis (Figure 10.13) is likely to be a painful condition associated with a red eye and should be differentiated from other causes of red eye (see Appendix). Bilateral uveitis usually indicates systemic involvement, but one eye may be affected before the other and the ocular changes will not be symmetrical when both eyes are involved. Bilateral uveitis should be differentiated from other generalized diseases that present with uveal involvement (Martin, 1999).

Diagnosis

The standard ophthalmic examination (see Chapter 1) can be supplemented in a number of simple ways to help in the assessment and diagnosis of uveitis cases (Figure 10.14). It is essential to attempt to find the cause of the uveitis in order both to provide specific treatment and to reduce the risk of significant complications (Figure 10.15).

General
Pain
Photophobia
Lacrimation
Visual impairment
Decreased intraocular pressure
Anterior
Perilimbal hyperaemia or ciliary injection (red eye)
Aqueous flare
Swollen iris with loss of fine detail
Miosis
Posterior
Vitreous opacities
Chorioretinitis

Figure 10.12 Salient clinical features of acute uveitis in the dog.

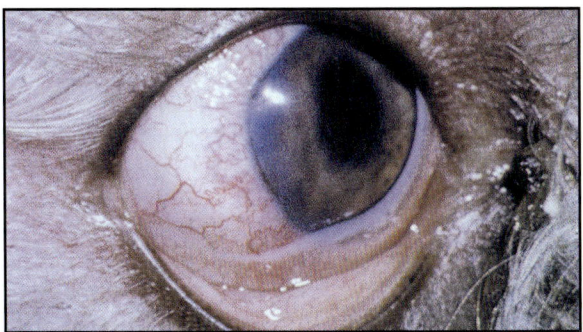

Figure 10.13 Acute canine uveitis in a cross-bred dog presented with pain, photophobia, blepharospasm and lacrimation. Perilimbal hyperaemia is obvious and aqueous flare is present as well as keratic precipitates in the anterior chamber. The iris is swollen and there is loss of surface detail. The pupil is irregular and moderately constricted (miotic) and response to a bright light was poor. An intraocular pressure of 7 mmHg was recorded with a Mackay–Marg tonometer. The intensity of the anterior segment inflammation prevented examination of the posterior segment initially, but after a few hours of intensive treatment this was possible. Vitritis, chorioretinitis and optic neuritis confirmed a panuveitis. Both eyes were involved.

- Complete physical examination
- Neurological examination (the extent may vary)
- Complete ophthalmic examination of both eyes with magnification, indirect and direct ophthalmoscopy
- Shining a beam of light directly across the anterior chamber from a number of different directions to gain an estimate of the position and thickness of the iris and the depth of the anterior chamber
- Shining a narrow beam of light, ideally from a slit lamp, to check for aqueous flare or other abnormalities of the anterior segment, such as the position and state of the pupil
- (Transillumination, with or without ultrasonography, to distinguish solid masses from fluid-filled masses)
- (Diagnostic imaging techniques, e.g. radiography, ultrasonography and, possibly, magnetic resonance imaging)
- (Routine haematology, blood biochemistry and, possibly, specific diagnostic tests)
- (Serodiagnosis)
- (Identification of the cause by sampling (e.g. for culture), aspiration cytology or biopsy followed by histology)
- (Paracentesis to obtain samples for cytology and histology)
- (Tonometry)
- (Gonioscopy)

Figure 10.14 Approach to a case of canine uveitis. Investigations shown in parentheses are not a routine part of the assessment.

- Unmanageable pain
- Increased intraocular pressure (secondary glaucoma)
- Blindness
- Corneal oedema / vascularization
- Hypopyon / hyphaema
- Synechiae (anterior, peripheral anterior / posterior)
- Pupillary seclusion / iris bombé
- Pupillary occlusion / iris rests
- Iris cysts / ectropion uveae
- Iris neovascularization, colour change / atrophy
- Irregular / immobile pupil
- Cataract / lens luxation
- Permanent vitreous opacities / vitreous liquefaction / intraocular haemorrhage
- Retinal detachment
- Chorioretinal degeneration / pigment proliferation
- Optic neuritis / atrophy
- Endophthalmitis / panophthalmitis
- Globe enlargement (hydrophthalmos) / shrinkage (phthisis bulbi)

Figure 10.15 Possible complications of canine uveitis.

Causes

There are many causes of uveitis. Common types include: reflex uveitis; infectious uveitis; uveitis associated with toxicity; uveitis associated with corneal insult; traumatic uveitis; lens-associated uveitis; immune-mediated uveitis; and uveitis associated with neoplasia. There are also occasions when the cause of the uveitis cannot be determined or the association with other factors is not well defined. Uveitis can be broadly categorized as exogenous (the result of an external ocular insult) or endogenous (arising from within the eye or the result of haematogenous spread from elsewhere), although there is, inevitably, considerable overlap on occasions. Uveitis in the dog and cat has been reviewed by Håkanson and Forrester (1990). The following, which emphasizes the aetiology and management of anterior uveitis, should be read in conjunction with the section on posterior uveitis in Chapter 14. There are a number of recent reviews of relevance: canine viral infections (Willis, 2000b); rickettsial infections (Stiles, 2000); systemic bacterial infections (Dziezyc, 2000); systemic fungal infections (Krohne, 2000); protothecosis (Hollingsworth, 2000); and toxoplasmosis (Davidson, 2000).

Reflex uveitis

Reflex uveitis is the transient and usually mild uveitis that can follow a corneal or ocular surface insult in all species. Reflex uveitis is mediated by an axon reflex within the trigeminal nerve.

Infectious uveitis

Viral

Infectious canine hepatitis: This is the most important viral cause of uveitis. Two distinct phases of endogenous inflammation may be distinguished: (1) a mild and usually transient uveitis that occurs during the acute phase of clinical illness; and (2) a severe kerato-uveitis that occurs some 1–3 weeks after infection. Typically, intraocular pressure (IOP) is lower than normal and there are often substantial numbers of keratic precipitates, or frank hypopyon. The single most striking ocular sign, however, is corneal oedema ('blue eye') as a result of an Arthus reaction (delayed hypersensitivity response), which damages the corneal endothelium (Figure 10.16). In the majority of cases the corneal oedema is unilateral. If the corneal damage is extensive enough, there may be an alteration of corneal profile (keratoglobus or keratoconus) and bullous keratopathy can develop. When kerato-uveitis is severe there is the possibility of secondary glaucoma in a small number of cases, and the resulting substantial rise in IOP may produce permanent globe enlargement (hydrophthalmos), especially in young dogs. Phthisis bulbi is a less common sequel to intense kerato-uveitis. In some animals there is slow resolution of the corneal oedema which clears from the limbus towards the centre over a period of weeks. On occasions, however, the corneal opacity is permanent. Treatment is symptomatic and supportive.

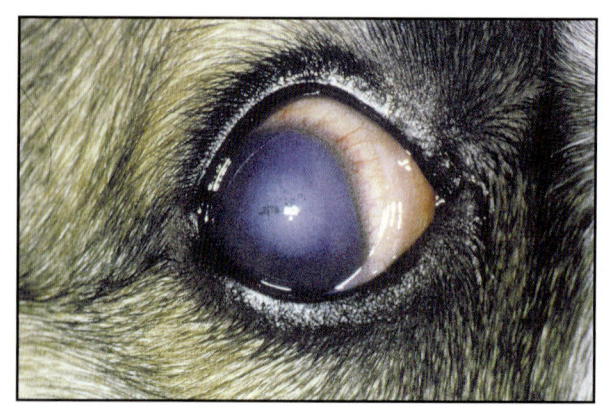

Figure 10.16 Corneal oedema ('blue eye') associated with canine viral hepatitis in a young crossbred dog. Although there is panstromal oedema, it is possible to see some details of the underlying anterior chamber, iris and pupil, and these were readily observed when the dog was examined with a focal bright light in darkness.

Canine herpesvirus: This is an occasional cause of neonatal death in litters of puppies. Ocular signs include severe panuveitis, kerato-uveitis and chorioretinitis, and survivors may be blind or severely visually impaired (Figure 10.17).

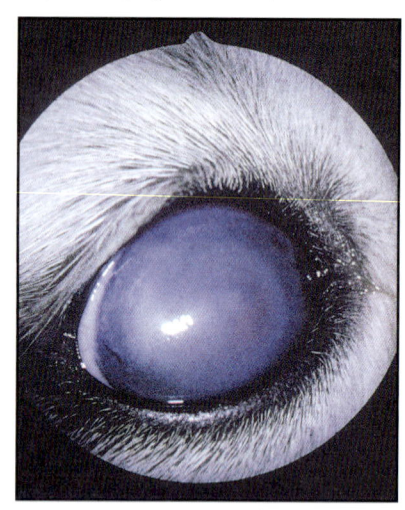

Figure 10.17 Uveitis in a puppy, associated with neonatal infection with canine herpesvirus. Both eyes were involved. Despite the gross corneal opacity, it is possible to see haemorrhage in the region of the pupillary aperture.

Canine distemper virus: This is an uncommon cause of anterior uveitis, whereas retinochoroiditis is a frequent finding, especially in dogs with neurological signs (see Chapter 14).

Rickettsial

Monocytic ehrlichiosis or tropical canine pancytopenia *(Ehrlichia canis)*, Rocky Mountain spotted fever *(Rickettsia rickettsii)* and infectious cyclic thrombocytopenia *(Ehrlichia platys)* have all been reported as causes of uveitis in tropical and subtropical zones.

Monocytic ehrlichiosis is the most important disease in this group. It is not endemic in the UK, although there is a single case report of a subclinically infected dog being imported (Gould *et al.*, 2000). Whilst some dogs eliminate the organism after the acute phase of infection, others become subclinically infected and chronic disease can develop years later. All these tick-borne rickettsial diseases are associated with vasculitis and thrombocytopenia. Serious bleeding problems, especially epistaxis and ocular haemorrhage, are most likely to be associated with monocytic ehrlichiosis, and this infection should be considered in the differential diagnosis of intraocular haemorrhage.

Doxycycline is the standard drug for treating acute rickettsial infections (5 mg/kg twice daily for 14 days). Subclinical infections are less successfully treated and Stiles (2000) has reviewed the treatment options, of which imidocarb dipropionate (5 mg/kg i.m. once, repeated after 14–21 days) is probably the treatment of choice. The uveitis is treated symptomatically. Unfortunately, ocular complications such as severe ocular haemorrhage, retinal detachment and secondary glaucoma are common to both monocytic ehrlichiosis and Rocky Mountain spotted fever.

Bacterial

Leptospirosis: A number of potential serovars are involved and the kidney is usually the main target organ in dogs. Leptospires cause both vasculitis and endotheliitis; renal failure and/or disseminated intravascular coagulation are possible life-threatening complications. There is some debate as to whether uveitis is actually a feature of acute infection or is more likely after a latent period following previous acute infection. The diagnosis is usually confirmed from the clinical signs, urinalysis and serology. Acute leptospiral infection can be treated with penicillin and its derivatives; tetracyclines can be used for follow-up therapy to eliminate the carrier state. Alternatively, doxycycline can be used for treatment of the acute infection and as follow-up therapy. Supportive care is required for the renal disease. The zoonotic implications of infection must be explained to the owner.

Brucellosis: This may present as a low-grade recurrent uveitis. Confirmation of the diagnosis is based on serological testing and, ideally, blood culture. *Brucella canis* is not seen in the UK. Canine brucellosis is not an easy condition to treat (Dziezyc, 2000). The zoonotic implications and difficulties of treating the disease effectively should be explained to the owner.

Lyme disease: Borreliosis is a tick-borne multisystem disease that typically presents with lameness and lymphadenopathy. *Borrelia burgdorferi* sensu stricto is the primary isolate in the USA, and borreliosis has been implicated as an occasional cause of canine uveitis (Cohen *et al.*, 1990), although there is some doubt as to the association. There are no confirmed reports of uveitis associated with borreliosis in the UK. Definitive diagnosis is difficult, as is treatment (Dziezyc, 2000). Treatment options include antibiotics such as doxycycline and the tetracylines.

Systemic bacterial infection: Uveitis may occur, although it is the posterior uvea that is most likely to be involved (see Chapter 14). Examples include salmonellosis as well as bacteraemia associated with pyorrhoea and endocarditis. Occasionally, direct introduction of pathogens such as *Pasteurella multocida* from a penetrating injury may be associated with abscessation and bacteraemia. Hypopyon may be one of the ocular manifestations in such cases (Figure 10.18). Diagnosis may sometimes be inferred from the history and clinical signs. Some or all of clinical biochemistry, haematology and serodiagnosis can be helpful. Occasionally, the causative organism can be isolated from the affected area or from blood culture, in which case specific antibiotic treatment can be selected for systemic administration.

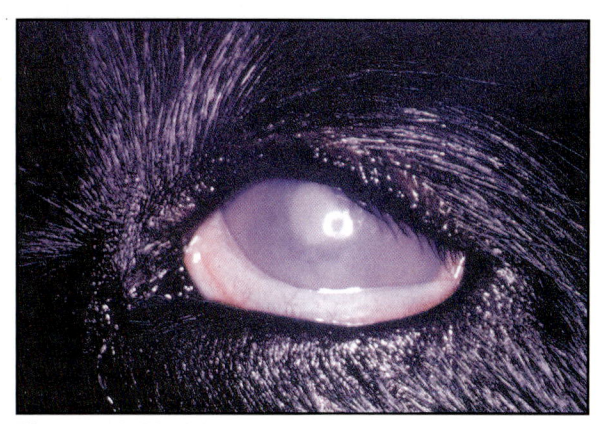

Figure 10.18 Unilateral hypopyon as a feature of septicaemia in a Border Collie that had received serious bite injuries to its left front leg in a dog fight.

Yeasts, fungi and algae

In certain parts of the world mycotic uveitis is common and algal uveitis may also be encountered. These problems are encountered rarely in animals that have been imported into the UK. For information on canine systemic fungal infections and protothecosis, the reviews by Krohne (2000) and Hollingsworth (2000) should be consulted.

Infection by inhalation is a common primary route for the systemic mycoses. Ocular involvement may occur via haematogenous dissemination, although meningoencephalitis can also be associated with ocular signs, and lymphatic spread may also occur. Ocular involvement is often the most obvious feature. Lesions are typically granulomatous or pyogranulomatous in type. Examples of systemic mycoses include blastomycosis, cryptococcosis, coccidioidomycosis, geotrichosis, aspergillosis and histoplasmosis.

Protothecosis is a rare disease caused by colourless algae that are widely distributed in nature, but only *Prototheca zopfii* (disseminated infection) and *P. wickerhamii* (cutaneous syndrome) have been implicated as pathogens.

Diagnosis of mycotic and algal diseases is based on the clinical signs, identification of the causative organisms in tissue aspirates (including oculocentesis) and biopsies. Direct microscopic examination is used to examine imprints and aspirates, and histopathology and microscopy for biopsy samples. Fungal culture may be required but should not be performed when the organism is highly contagious (e.g. the mycelial phase of coccidioidomycosis). Serological testing can be useful, except that positive results may indicate previous exposure rather than infection in endemic regions.

The uveal tract

Treatment of mycotic disease is a long-term proposition and expensive (see Chapter 3) and should continue for at least 2 months after resolution of the clinical disease. Relapses are common.

Parasites

Leishmaniasis: There are reports of leishmaniasis in dogs from all parts of the world, especially the Mediterranean area. Leishmaniasis is caused by a diphasic protozoan parasite. Old World leishmaniasis is caused by *Leishmania donovani infantum* and New World leishmaniasis by *L. donovani chagasi.* Clinical disease develops in a high proportion of infected dogs after an incubation period of several months to several years. The clinical signs of disseminated leishmaniaisis include chronic emaciation and non-pruritic skin disease and a variety of periocular lesions, including blepharitis (see Chapter 5). Leishmaniasis may also be associated with a range of ocular lesions (Peña *et al.*, 2000) including conjunctivitis, keratitis, scleritis, keratouveitis and uveitis (Figure 10.19). The parasite depresses T cell immunity and this may enable opportunistic infections (e.g. demodicosis) to develop. Increased B cell activity associated with autoantibody and immune complex formation is also a feature.

Diagnosis is based on the history of visiting an endemic area, the clinical signs and serology. Identification of the causative organism in lymph node or bone marrow aspirates or from biopsy specimens provides confirmation. Leishmaniasis is an endemic problem in many parts of the world but may also occur in dogs that have been imported to the UK. It is a difficult condition to treat effectively as the relapse rate is high. The zoonotic implications should be discussed before considering treatment.

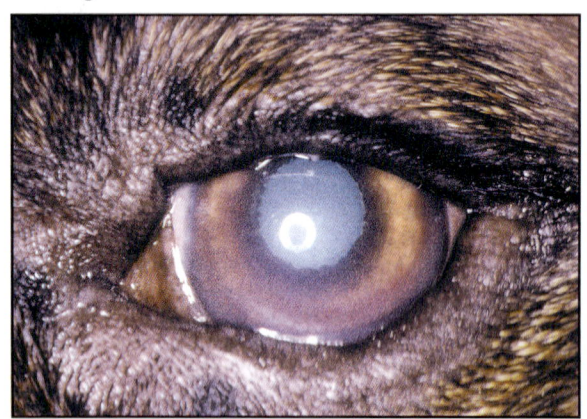

Figure 10.19 Kerato-uveitis in a Boxer with leishmaniasis. The slightly crenulated appearance of the pupillary margin is indicative of ectropion uveae.

Toxoplasmosis: *Toxoplasma gondii* infection is unusual in dogs and most of the ocular lesions encountered in clinical practice are associated with chronic and subclinical infection. The ocular manifestations are varied: both the anterior and posterior uvea may be involved; less commonly, there is extraocular myositis, scleritis and optic neuritis. Concurrent disease is usually present on the rare occasions when generalized toxoplasmosis develops.

Serological testing may be indicative of active infection if a four-fold increase in antibody levels can be demonstrated in paired serum samples. The definitive diagnosis is by histopathological identification of the organism.

Toxoplasmosis is treated with oral clindamycin 12.5 mg/kg twice daily for 3–4 weeks. In addition, symptomatic treatment of the uveitis will be required, including topical corticosteroids (1% prednisolone acetate) for animals with anterior uveitis and systemic prednisolone for those with posterior uveitis and/or optic neuritis. Both topical and systemic corticosteroid treatment is needed if panuveitis is present.

Neosporosis: *Neospora caninum* infection shares a number of similarities with toxoplasmosis, although differentiation is possible as the two organisms do not cross-react serologically. Most cases occur in very young dogs, and ascending paralysis is the classic clinical presentation; any accompanying uveitis is generally mild. Treatment is as for toxoplasmosis.

Migrating helminth larvae: These may provoke uveitis of differing intensities. For example, canine toxocariasis, angiostrongylosis and filariasis have all been reported as causes of uveitis. The ocular manifestations of toxocariasis are varied and it is the posterior segment that is primarily involved (see Chapter 14). Working Border Collies demonstrate a high incidence of chorioretinopathy lesions associated with toxocariasis.

Angiostrongylus vasorum is a nematode that infects dogs via their ingestion of the intermediate snail host found in Europe and parts of Africa. Aberrant larvae that reach the eye may provoke a range of responses, from minimal to severe granulomatous uveitis. The most spectacular ocular manifestation is undoubtedly the free nematode or nematodes within the vitreous or anterior chamber (Figure 10.20).

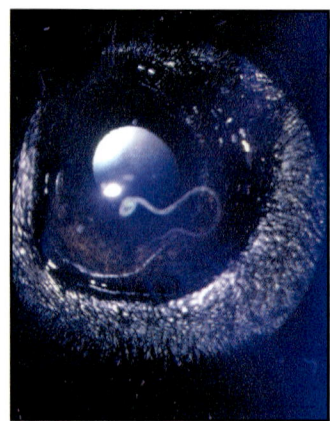

Figure 10.20 *Angiostrongylus vasorum* in the anterior chamber of a crossbred dog. The worm was immobilized with echothiopate iodide and evacuated through a small corneal incision by slowly injecting viscoelastic material through a second corneal incision on the opposite side of the cornea.

Dirofilaria immitis is the most commonly reported intraocular parasite of dogs in North America. Ocular manifestations include a consistent anterior uveitis with varying degrees of corneal oedema. It is also possible to detect aberrant dirofilaria in the anterior chamber of some cases.

In addition to systemic treatment (e.g. subcutaneous ivermectin 200 μg/kg is effective against *A. vasorum* but should not be used in Collies), it is usual to remove the free nematode from the anterior chamber after first immobilizing it with a topical cholinesterase inhibitor (e.g. echothiopate iodide). The simplest technique is to make two small limbal incisions opposite each other and to inject a small quantity of viscoelastic material through one incision so as to expel the parasite through the other incision.

Myiasis: Intraocular dipteran larvae that may penetrate the eye through the conjunctiva are also a potential cause of uveitis. Ophthalmomyiasis interna may present as anterior uveitis in the acute phase of invasion but is more likely to be an incidental finding in the chronic stage when fundus examination reveals typical curvilinear criss-crossing tracts (see Chapter 14).

Uveitis associated with toxicity

Uveitis can be initiated by circulating toxins and is thus associated with a variety of conditions that result in toxaemia or sepsis. The commonest associations are with dental disease and pyometritis.

Uveitis associated with corneal insult

Transient reflex uveitis associated with corneal insult has been described earlier; sustained uveitis will accompany deep keratitis and more serious corneal injury (see Chapter 8). Hypopyon may be present as a feature of deep keratitis.

In dogs the uveitis that follows penetrating or blunt traumatic injury may become complicated by secondary problems such as glaucoma (soon after the injury), cataract and phthisis bulbi (both some time after the injury). Endophthalmitis (severe intraocular inflammation which does not extend beyond the sclera) or panophthalmitis (severe intraocular inflammation which also involves the ocular coats, Tenon's capsule and even the orbital tissues themselves) are also possible following traumatic injury, particularly from bites and scratches. Traumatic injuries to the anterior uvea are discussed in more detail below.

Uveitis associated with lens damage

Lens-induced uveitis has been reviewed recently by van der Woerdt (2000) and occurs when there is a breakdown of the normal T cell tolerance to lens proteins. It is usually a consequence of traumatic rupture of the lens capsule such as a penetrating claw injury (Figure 10.21) or a gunshot wound. The release of antigenic lens protein initiates a phacoclastic uveitis, irrespective of any accompanying damage to the uveal tract. Phacoclastic uveitis is usually very intense in dogs and may become complicated by the development of persistent uveitis, glaucoma or fulminating endophthalmitis (see Chapter 4); sometimes the damaged eye becomes phthitic. Small puncture wounds in the lens capsule can seal and such cases can be managed medically, but when there is likely to be extensive or sustained release of lens contents, surgery to remove the antigenic lens protein, usually by phacoemulsification, should be undertaken without delay. Because the examination and assessment of lens damage can be difficult, early referral is advised.

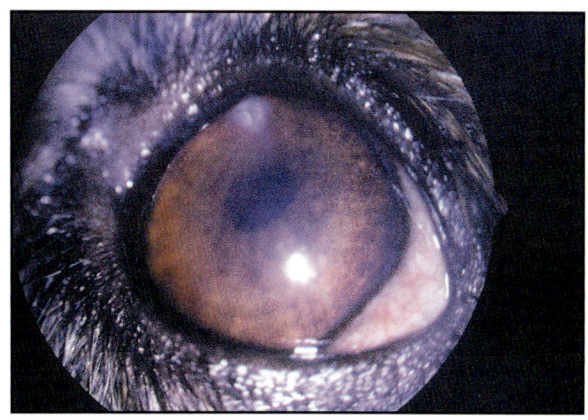

Figure 10.21 Phacoclastic uveitis in a Border Terrier as a result of a penetrating injury from a cat claw. The site of corneal penetration is obvious dorsally. The flocculent, slightly dark material in the anterior chamber close to the pupil is lens material.

Slow leakage of soluble lens protein though an intact lens capsule, associated for example with hypermature cataracts, produces a low-grade or phacolytic uveitis that may be treated symptomatically (Figure 10.22).

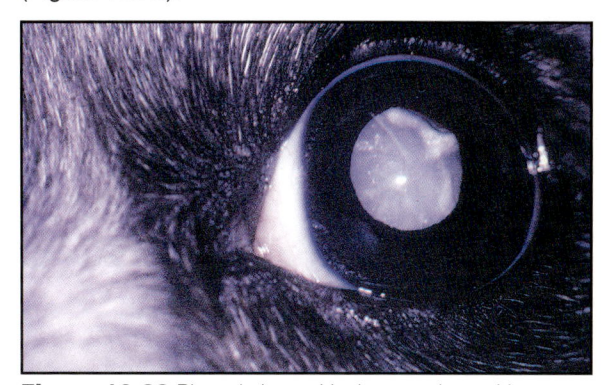

Figure 10.22 Phacolytic uveitis: low-grade uveitis associated with a hypermature cataract in a diabetic Border Collie. The iris colour has darkened and there is some loss of fine surface detail.

Immune-mediated uveitis

The initiation, perpetuation, or recurrence of uveitis may be immune mediated in many species. In dogs, panuveitis associated with depigmentation of the lids, muzzle, rhinarium and skin and whitening of the hair (uveodermatological syndrome; UDS) has been compared with the Vogt–Koyanagi–Harada syndrome in humans; in both species the disease is a possible example of an autoimmune reaction against melanocytes. UDS is seen particularly in young Chow-Chows, Japanese Akitas, Golden Retrievers, Samoyeds, Siberian Huskies and Shetland Sheepdogs, although a range of other breeds can be affected. It presents as an acute, usually bilateral, panuveitis that may precede, or follow, mucocutaneous involvement, skin depigmentation (vitiligo) and whitening of the hair (poliosis) (Figures 10.23 and 10.24). In addition to the inflammatory changes in the uvea, other intraocular changes are common, and complications include retinal detachment, glaucoma and cataract formation. Even with early and aggressive treatment the prognosis is guarded.

172 The uveal tract

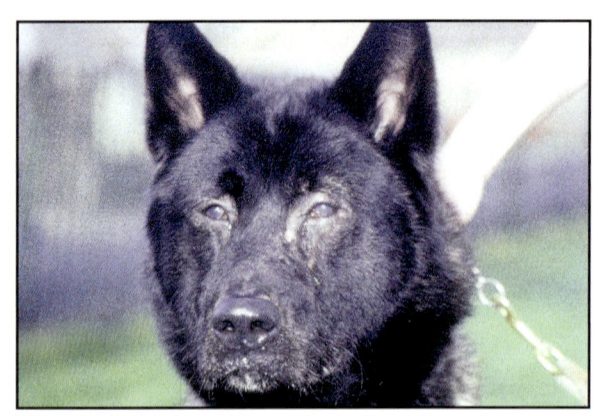

Figure 10.23 Uveodermatological syndrome in a Japanese Akita. There has been some loss of pigment from the eyelids, muzzle and rhinarium. Ocular pain, blepharospasm, lacrimation and photophobia accompanied the panuveitis.

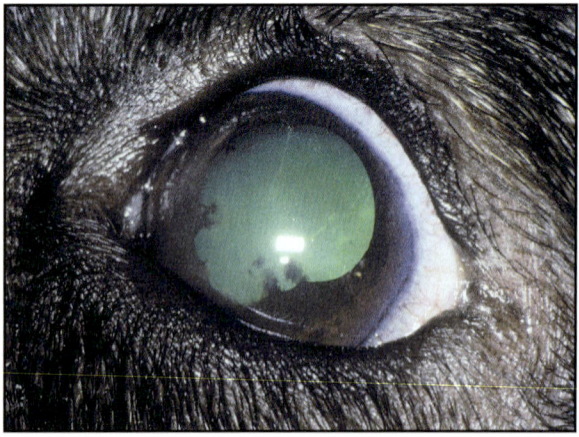

Figure 10.24 Uveodermatological syndrome in a Japanese Akita showing the typical appearance of an eye that has undergone repeated attacks of iritis. The pupil is irregular and dilated, posterior synechiae are present and iris surface detail is poor. There is a rather dull green tapetal reflex. The recurrent attacks had also involved the posterior segment. Secondary glaucoma has complicated the presentation.

Diagnosis is based on the characteristic clinical signs and may be aided by skin biopsy, as the primary disease process is associated with destruction of dermal, as well as uveal, melanocytes.

Treatment should be started as early as possible and maintained long term, using a combination of immunosuppressive doses of systemic corticosteroids (e.g. oral prednisolone 2 mg/kg/day initially, with gradual reduction to the lowest dose that prevents recurrence) and immunosuppressive drugs such as oral azathioprine at a dose of 2 mg/kg/day, reducing after 3–5 days. The uveitis must also be treated locally with topical applications of corticosteroid (prednisolone acetate 1% some five times daily for the first 5–10 days) and atropine 1% (as frequently as necessary to achieve and maintain pupil dilation).

If there is any suspicion of secondary glaucoma developing, the animal should be hospitalized and the IOP monitored (see Chapter 11). Because of the potential for both ocular complications and undesirable side effects from the systemic treatment, the patient should be checked regularly (see Chapter 3).

Uveitis associated with neoplasia

Primary and secondary ocular tumours can release neoplastic cells that induce an inflammatory response from the uveal tract to which immune-mediated mechanisms may contribute. The inflammatory response can be marked if there is tumour necrosis. In addition, intraocular tumours of all kinds, both primary and secondary, can mimic uveitis ('masquerade syndrome'). It is important to perform very careful assessment of all uveitis cases in view of these associations, and ultrasonography can be of particular value as a diagnostic aid. Primary and secondary neoplasia involving the anterior uvea is described in greater detail below.

General principles of treatment for canine uveitis

The cause should be eliminated and specific treatment used whenever possible, as outlined for the conditions described above. For example, systemic antibiotics will be required if bacterial septicaemia is present. Supportive therapy may also be required as, for instance, in nursing patients with canine viral hepatitis. Symptomatic treatment is needed for the uveitis whatever the cause and usually consists of anti-inflammatory agents and mydriatic cycloplegics (see Chapter 3).

Corticosteroids: Topical or systemic corticosteroids are the commonest type of anti-inflammatory agent used in uveitis. Subconjunctival corticosteroids are less common in routine treatment. As a general rule, corticosteroids should be avoided when corneal ulceration is present and should be used with caution in the treatment of uveitis resulting from viral or mycotic infection.

Topical corticosteroids: Prednisolone acetate 1% is currently the preparation of choice for anterior uveitis. Initially, one drop is applied to the eye up to five times daily and treatment should be tapered off over a period of 5–10 days when the uveitis has resolved.

Subconjunctival corticosteroids: Subconjunctival injections are painful, so this route is used less commonly than others (see Chapter 3). The advantage of these preparations is that one injection lasts for 2–3 weeks. The disadvantages, aside from the pain of injection, include the risk of accidental ocular penetration, variable intraocular concentrations, and occasional granuloma formation at the site of injection. Dexamethasone acetate and betamethasone phosphate with acetate (0.75–2.0 mg per eye according to size of the dog), are suitable preparations.

Systemic corticosteroids: Oral prednisolone is indicated for the treatment of intermediate and posterior uveitis. Both topical and oral corticosteroids will be required for the treatment of panuveitis and for immune-mediated types of uveitis. As a general rule, higher dose rates are selected when immunosuppression is the prime purpose of treatment (2 mg/kg prednisolone every 12 hours), and lower dose rates may be used when anti-inflammatory effects are primarily required (1 mg/kg prednisolone every 12 hours). Treatment should be tapered off and not stopped abruptly when the condition has resolved.

Non-steroidal anti-inflammatory drugs (NSAIDs)

Topical NSAIDs: Those available as topical preparations include indomethacin 0.1–1.0%, diclofenac sodium 0.1%, flurbiprofen sodium 0.03% and ketorolac trometamol 0.5%. These drugs are mainly used in cataract surgery but also have an important anti-inflammatory role in situations where corticosteroids would be contraindicated (see above and Chapter 3). In the UK, ketorolac trometamol is commonly selected for this purpose.

Systemic NSAIDs: These drugs inhibit prostaglandin synthesis through their inhibition of the prostaglandin endoperoxide synthase or cyclo-oxygenase (COX) pathway. They can be used on their own if systemic corticosteroids are contraindicated, or they may be combined with systemic corticosteroids if the patient can be closely supervised (see Chapter 3). Their side effects include inhibition of platelet function and gastrointestinal haemorrhage, and the risk of gastrointestinal haemorrhage is considerably increased when they are used in combination with corticosteroids. Most of the side effects of NSAIDs are a consequence of COX-1 inhibition (COX-1 is one of the two prostaglandin endoperoxide synthase isoenzymes involved), so NSAIDs that selectively block only COX-2, such as carprofen (2 mg/kg orally twice daily), are the preferred choice. Many commonly used NSAIDs like acetylsalicylic acid, phenylbutazone and flunixin meglumine inhibit both COX-1 and COX-2.

Cytotoxic drugs: These preparations have powerful immunosuppressive effects and are used, on occasion, to treat cases of presumed immune-mediated disease, including uveitis. Azathioprine, a purine analogue, is the most commonly used agent in this group and is often used in conjunction with corticosteroids (see Chapter 3). Side effects of therapy include vomiting and diarrhoea, bone marrow suppression and, occasionally, acute hepatic necrosis, so it is important to monitor the blood cell count and liver function during the course of treatment. The action of azathioprine is limited to helper T lymphocytes. Methotrexate, a folic acid analogue, might have a greater potential, as it suppresses both B and T cell functions, but it has not yet been evaluated in the treatment of canine ocular inflammatory disease.

Mydriatic cycloplegics: Usually 1% atropine alone is sufficient, but 10% phenylephrine can also be used for recalcitrant cases when pupillary dilation is difficult to achieve (see Chapter 3). Caution should be exercised when there is a risk of secondary glaucoma, a particular hazard in the dog (see Chapter 11). The patient's progress should be monitored closely and the aim is to eliminate pain (by relaxing ciliary spasm) and to reduce the risk of synechiae formation. Once the pupil has dilated, mydriatic cycloplegics can be applied only as often as is necessary to maintain this state.

Anterior uveal trauma

In any case of suspected ocular trauma it is crucial to examine both eyes and their adnexae. If an eye is too painful to approach, or if there is potential for loss of the intraocular contents, examination should be performed under general anaesthesia. Radiography of the skull is required if bony damage is suspected. The periocular region should be checked first for signs of bruising, contusion, laceration and penetrating injury. Examination of the globe should follow, to ascertain whether there are any indications of globe penetration, with the caveat that whilst corneal injury may be obvious, damage to the sclera may be obscured by the eyelids and conjunctiva. If the globe is intact then topical local anaesthetic can be instilled to allow more complete examination, and a gentle stream of warm sterile saline can be used to remove any debris or discharge. Extraocular and intraocular haemorrhage makes precise assessment of the damage more difficult and must be supplemented by accurate measurement of IOP and diagnostic imaging, usually ultrasonography. In the majority of cases careful examination of the eye will demonstrate an altered appearance, described in more detail below.

Penetrating injuries

Focal penetrating injuries of the ocular tunics may seal spontaneously without complication, so that surgical intervention is not required and symptomatic treatment for any accompanying uveitis is all that is necessary. Fluorescein can be applied to check for aqueous leakage using Seidel's test (see Chapter 1). The anterior segment and anterior vitreous should be assessed carefully with magnification, ideally using a slit lamp as this instrument allows easier assessment of corneal and iris damage, aqueous flare, blood and other cells within the aqueous, as well as lens subluxation, luxation, penetration or rupture. The ocular fundus and vitreous should be examined with indirect and direct ophthalmoscopy, supplemented by ultrasonography if the ocular media are partially or completely opaque. Extensive injuries associated with, for example, aqueous or vitreous loss, uveal prolapse, aqueous flare, a shallow or absent anterior chamber, distortion or loss of the pupil, lens displacement or damage and hyphaema or intraocular haemorrhage, usually require prompt specialist assessment to see if microsurgical intervention is required (Figure 10.25). If the lens has

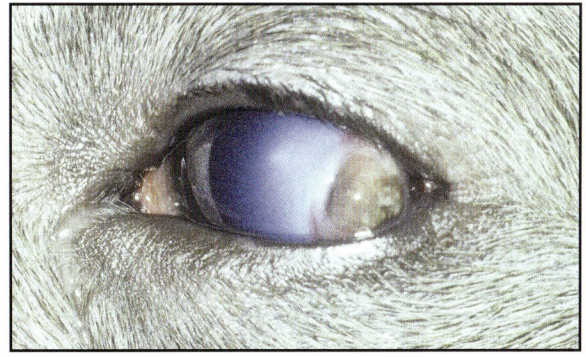

Figure 10.25 Whippet puppy with a large iris prolapse laterally as a consequence of a penetrating injury caused by a cat claw. By viewing the anterior chamber from different angles, using a focal light source in the dark, it was possible to visualize the anterior displacement of the iris in the affected region.

been penetrated, producing leakage of lens protein, it is better to remove the lens contents before phacoclastic uveitis ensues (see above). The IOP should be checked initially and for some days following surgery. Repair of traumatic penetrating injury to the globe is discussed briefly in Chapter 2.

Blunt ocular trauma

Blunt ocular trauma (Figure 10.26) usually produces more severe intraocular damage than does penetrating injury (see Chapter 8), particularly if the blow is severe enough to rupture the globe (Figure 10.27a). The prognosis for cases of blunt ocular trauma associated with globe rupture is very poor. In dogs, the ocular coats tend to split posteriorly (Figure 10.27b), so that routine examination procedures may fail to detect the extent of the injuries, although ultrasonography can be diagnostic.

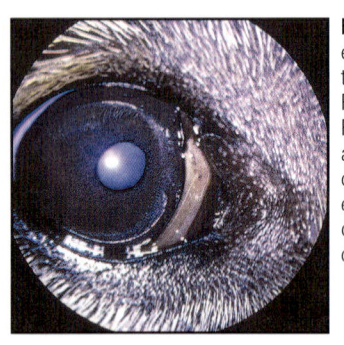

Figure 10.26 The effects of blunt trauma to the eye. This Labrador Retriever x Golden Retriever had been hit accidentally with a golf club some 3 months earlier. Note the very dark iris and secondary cataract.

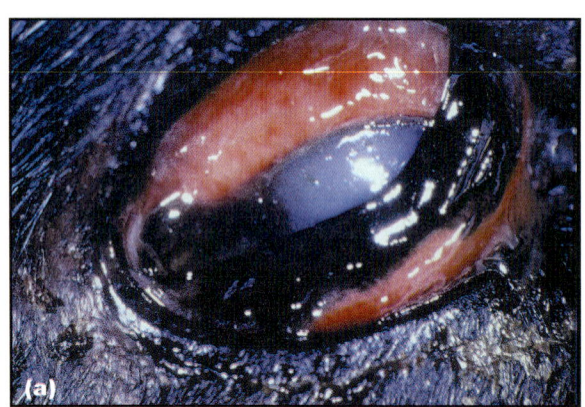

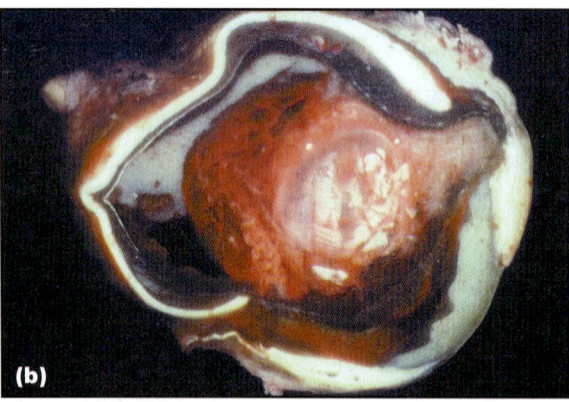

Figure 10.27 An eye that has suffered severe blunt trauma. (a) There is severe chemosis and conjunctival haemorrhage, diffuse corneal oedema, a large iris prolapse laterally and intraocular haemorrhage. (b) Gross pathology specimen sectioned in the region of the iris prolapse. The ocular tunics have ruptured and intraocular haemorrhage fills the eye. (Courtesy of JRB Mould.)

Intraocular haemorrhage is the result of bleeding from uveal and/or retinal vessels and is a common sequel to both blunt and penetrating injuries. Hyphaema usually resorbs rapidly in uncomplicated cases; therefore, although it is possible to evacuate hyphaema using viscoelastic material, it is unwise to attempt this if unskilled in microsurgery or if there is any possibility of recurrent haemorrhage. Tissue-type plasminogen activator (tPA), which has the capacity to lyse intraocular fibrin clots, is not usually indicated in the management of hyphaema associated with acute trauma. Such hyphaema is usually unilateral; bilateral hyphaema is more likely to indicate systemic disease.

Foreign bodies

Intraocular foreign bodies may also be a cause of uveitis; the clinical signs and the treatment required depend upon the nature, size, entry site and location of the foreign body as well as the extent of associated tissue damage and the intensity of uveal inflammation (Figure 10.28).

As with corneal foreign bodies, the nature of the foreign material defines the ocular response. Unfortunately, a number of foreign bodies reach the anterior chamber because of failed attempts to remove them from the cornea. Organic and reactive inorganic material should be removed, but not necessarily via the point of entry as this may cause additional trauma if objects are of awkward shape; such foreign bodies can be removed using a limbal-based incision.

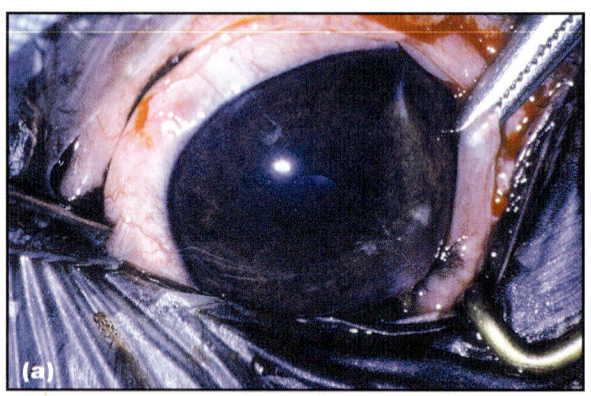

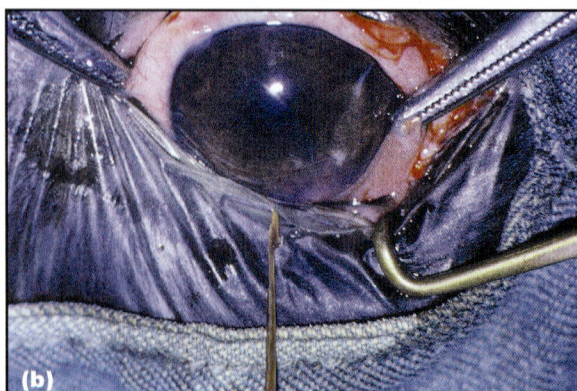

Figure 10.28 (a) A piece of bracken, 13 mm long, had penetrated the cornea and iris, and was mainly positioned between the posterior iris and the anterior lens. There was surprisingly little intraocular reaction, although the eye was uncomfortable. The bracken was removed (b) and the patient made an uneventful recovery.

Differential diagnosis of intraocular haemorrhage

While trauma is a common reason for intraocular haemorrhage, there are a great many other reasons and these should be differentiated (Figure 10.29). Although the underlying aetiology of uveitis may be difficult, if not impossible, to establish in many cases, this does not mean that symptomatic treatment should be given in default of diagnosis. The pathophysiology, diagnosis and treatment of hyphaema has been reviewed by Komaromy *et al.* (1999a,b).

Developmental conditions
Persistent hyperplastic primary vitreous or hyaloid vessels
Severe retinal or vitreoretinal dysplasia
Collie eye anomaly
Acquired conditions
Blunt and penetrating injuries to the globe
Uveitis and vasculitis
Neoplasia
Chronic glaucoma
Systemic hypertension
Coagulopathies (inherited and acquired)
Platelet disorders, both quantitative and qualitative (inherited and acquired))
Hyperviscosity syndrome
Retinal tear or detachment

Figure 10.29 Differential diagnosis of intraocular haemorrhage.

Lipaemic aqueous

Triglyceride-rich lipid in the aqueous humour may be an ocular manifestation of systemic hyperlipoproteinaemia and presents as a 'pseudouveitis'. The turbidity of the triglyceride-enriched aqueous may be confused with aqueous flare and there is often mild ocular reddening. There may well be innate differences in susceptibility to this problem, as the permeability of iridal capillaries can differ at different ages and between species. Other factors of relevance include the observation that systemic hyperlipoproteinaemia may be associated with dilation and hyperaemia of vessels in the region of the limbus and deep scleral plexus, and affected vessels will be more pemeable than normal. In addition, a pre-existing uveitis as part of primary ocular disease will be associated with breakdown of the blood–aqueous barrier and lipid will enter the anterior chamber when there is concurrent systemic hyperlipoproteinaemia. The lipid is only visible if triglyceride levels are abnormally high (>25 mmol/l); raised cholesterol levels are not associated with changes in aqueous appearance. If there is triglyceridaemia alone the aqueous appears turbid, but if chylomicrons are also raised the aqueous may appear milky white. For example, in Miniature Schnauzers with primary chylomicronaemia, or in any breed with secondary chylomicronaemia, chylomicron-rich aqueous is a possible ocular manifestation (Figure 10.30), although lipaemia retinalis (see Chapter 14) is likely to be more common. Secondary causes of hyperlipoproteinaemia, in which triglycerides are markedly raised, have similar potential ocular manifestations; the commonest association is with diabetes mellitus.

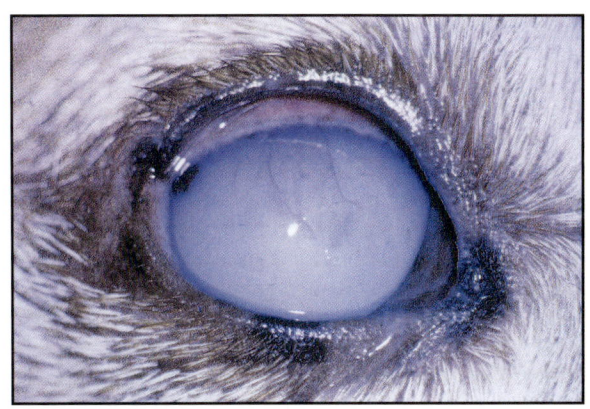

Figure 10.30 Miniature Pinscher with chylomicronaemia associated with diabetes mellitus. There was a pre-existing low-grade keratouveitis of the right eye only. The dog also had bilateral cataracts. Total plasma cholesterol concentration was 5.2 mmol/l and total plasma triglycerides 8.4 mmol/l in a blood sample taken approximately 18 hours after the lipid-laden aqueous had been noticed by the owner.

Canine uveal neoplasia

Useful reviews of canine uveal neoplasia can be obtained from Gwin *et al.* (1982), Bussanich *et al.* (1987), Dubielzig (1990), Duncan and Peiffer (1991), Dubielzig *et al.* (1998) and Collins and Moore (1999).

Primary neoplasia

The majority of primary tumours of the uveal tract arise from the iris and ciliary body rather than from the choroid and are usually benign with little tendency to metastasize.

Melanoma: Melanoma (Figure 10.31) is the commonest primary intraocular neoplasm (Wilcock and Peiffer, 1986), and the majority of anterior uveal melanomas are unilateral and benign. There is a single case report of a bilateral ciliary body melanoma (Roperto *et al.*, 1993). Melanomas arising from the choroid, the commonest origin in humans, are rare in the dog (Collinson and Peiffer, 1993). While the behaviour pattern is invariably benign, melanomas can cause secondary intraocular disease such as glaucoma. Rarely, primary uveal melanomas may metastasize to distant sites and

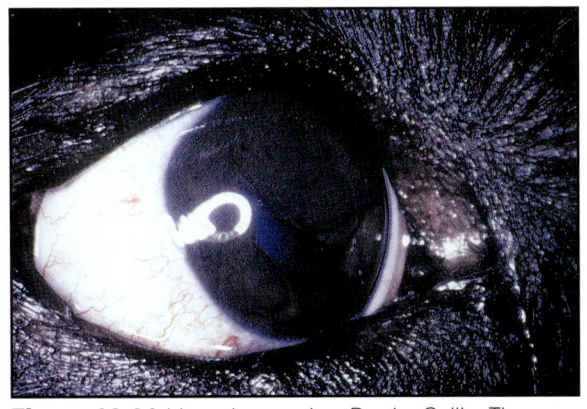

Figure 10.31 Iris melanoma in a Border Collie. These tumours usually have a benign course, and this one is only beginning to cause problems because it is compromising aqueous drainage.

there is a single report of metastasis to other sites (bone, synovium and spinal canal) and the fellow eye (Render et al., 1997). It is also possible for melanomas in sites other than the eye, notably the mouth and skin, to metastasize to the eye. From unpublished data collated under the British Veterinary Association/ Kennel Club/International Sheepdog Society Eye Scheme, primary iris melanoma appears to be over-represented in the Labrador Retriever in the UK; Cook and Lannon (1997) have reported on the inherited nature of the tumour in this breed in the USA.

Other: Ciliary body adenoma (Figure 10.32) and adenocarcinoma are the most commonly reported canine primary ciliary body tumours and are usually unilateral. All other primary anterior uveal tumours are rare; they include fibrosarcoma, medulloepithelioma, haemangioma, haemangiosarcoma and leiomyosarcoma.

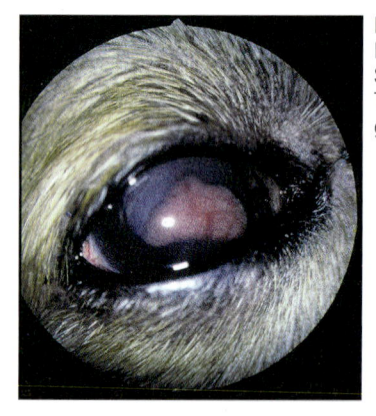

Figure 10.32 Ciliary body adenoma in a Shetland Sheepdog. These tumours are generally benign.

Diagnosis: This is based on the history and clinical appearance, together with ancillary aids such as transillumination of the eye, gonioscopy and ultrasonography. Thoracic radiography is indicated to screen for pulmonary metastatic disease, and abdominal ultrasonography may also be needed on occasions. Aspirates may provide diagnostic cytology, but interpretation can be difficult. Needle biopsy and histology of the tumour is more likely to provide an accurate diagnosis. Similarly, if there is lymphadenopathy, then lymph node biopsy is appropriate.

Management: Individual assessment should determine if the tumour should simply be kept under careful observation or whether it is possible to perform laser ablation or local excision, or if removal of the whole eye is the treatment of choice. Whatever approach is used, the tissues should always be submitted for histopathology. Neodymium:yttrium, aluminium garnet (nd:YAG) laser therapy has been reviewed in the treatment of primary canine intraocular tumours by Nasisse et al. (1993). Diode laser photocoagulation also appears to be a safe and effective method of treating isolated pigmented iris masses in the dog (Cook and Wilkie, 1999).

Secondary neoplasia

Secondary neoplasia involving the uveal tract is not infrequent. Lymphoma (Figure 10.33) is the most common secondary tumour to affect the eye and orbit. The

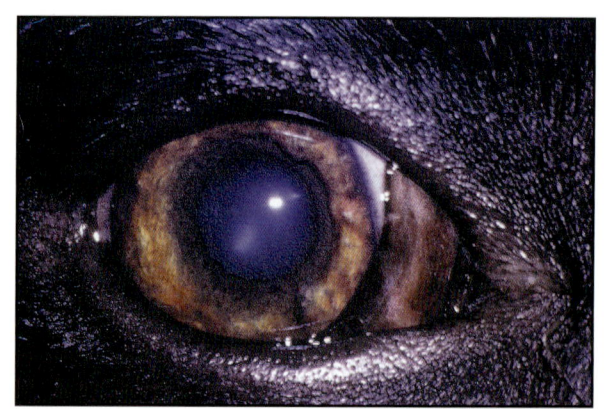

Figure 10.33 Early infiltration of the iris caused by lymphoma in a German Shepherd Dog. This is the commonest secondary tumour to involve the eye. Generalized lymphadenopathy is usually obvious on physical examination.

ocular involvement is second only to lymphadenopathy as the most frequently diagnosed clinical sign, and Krohne et al. (1994) cited significant involvement of the eye in 37% of the dogs in their prospective study.

Haemangiosarcoma (Figure 10.34) is probably the next most common secondary tumour and, like lymphoma, may present with hyphaema as the most obvious ocular feature. Other metastatic tumours include adenocarcinoma, fibrosarcoma, rhabdomyosarcoma, osteosarcoma, phaeochromocytoma, seminoma, transmissable venereal tumour and, as described earlier, malignant melanoma (Collins and Moore, 1999).

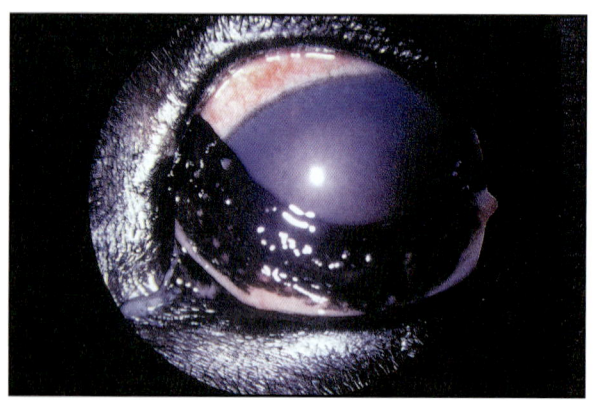

Figure 10.34 Ocular metastasis from splenic haemangiosarcoma in a German Shepherd Dog. Bilateral haemorrhage was the reason for referral, but the tumour had already spread to numerous sites. The spleen was grossly enlarged and readily palpable.

Diagnosis: This is based on the history, ocular signs, clinical signs, haematology and biochemistry profiles and appropriate tests (e.g. lymph node and bone marrow biopsy) where indicated. The ocular manifestations are variable; there is not only infiltration of the uveal tract by the tumour, but there will be associated generalized abnormalities such as anaemia, thrombocytopenia and disseminated intravascular coagulation, that can all present with ocular manifestations.

Treatment: This depends upon the extent and type of tumour. Chemotherapy is the approach adopted for disseminated tumours judged to be treatable. Malignant lymphoma is the commonest and responds well to chemotherapy.

Other diseases
A number of other disorders may involve the uveal tract.

Histiocytosis: This is an example of an immunoproliferative disease with a clinical presentation that is often remarkably similar to malignant lymphoma (Figure 10.35); the same chemotherapy protocol is used for management.

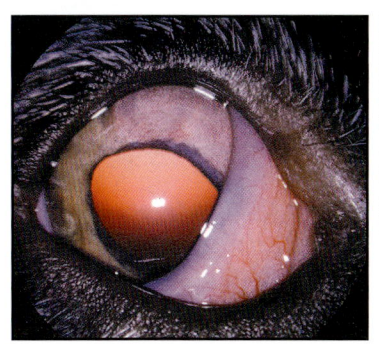

Figure 10.35 Systemic histiocytosis in a Border Collie. The iris and third eyelid were infiltrated and there was a mild generalized lymphadenopathy.

Granulomatous meningoencephalitis: This is an inflammatory disease in which there is proliferation of reticuloendothelial cells. It involves the central nervous system, optic nerves and globes. The ocular manifestations typically involve the posterior segment (see Chapter 14), although anterior uveitis may be observed on occasions.

Acquired abnormalities of the feline anterior uvea

Acquired iris atrophy, iridociliary cysts, ectropion uveae and changes of iris colour may be incidental findings in adult cats. While such degenerative changes can be age related, they may also be encountered as part of a disease process. Changes of iris colour should always be evaluated carefully. Darkening of the iris is most likely to be a consequence of previous inflammation but can be associated with neoplasia, particularly diffuse iris melanoma. The uveal tract may be a useful indicator of systemic disease (Stiles, 1999).

As the iris of the cat is usually less heavily pigmented than that of the dog, the iris vasculature, both normal and abnormal, is easier to identify. Pre-iridal fibrovascular membranes are a frequent finding in cats with chronic uveitis. Glaucoma is a possible complication of feline uveitis (Wilcock *et al.*, 1990); indeed, anterior uveitis and ocular neoplasia accounted for most of the cases of secondary glaucoma in a series reported by Blocker and van der Woerdt (2001).

Uveitis

Causes
There are similar categories of uveitis in the dog and cat, but in general the clinical signs are less florid in the cat and it is often easier to establish the aetiology. Feline uveitis has been reviewed by Davidson *et al.* (1991) and Chavkin *et al.* (1992). As in the dog, exogenous causes include ocular insults such as trauma and ulcerative keratitis; endogenous causes include infectious agents, lens-induced, neoplasia and idiopathic.

The clinical presentation of many endogenous cases of feline uveitis is chronic rather than acute (Figure 10.36). The clinical signs of acute uveitis are similar to those already described for the dog and include pain, photophobia, blepharospasm, lacrimation, inflammation-induced hyperaemia of visible vessels, aqueous flare, hyphaema, miosis, low IOP and a swollen iris with loss of iris detail. As the iris of the cat is generally less pigmented, and the anterior chamber is deeper, it is possible to observe details not readily apparent in the dog; for example, pre-iridal fibrovascular membranes may be a very striking feature of chronic uveitis in the cat. Choroiditis, optic neuritis and intraocular haemorrhage are less commonly reported, partly because of the difficulties of examining the posterior segment when there are anterior segment abnormalities and a miotic pupil. It may be possible to make a more accurate assessment of the posterior segment after administering a topical mydriatic cycloplegic.

Anterior
Eye is not obviously inflamed and there may be no redness
Presence of aqueous flare, keratic precipitates, mutton fat precipitates or hypopyon
Presence of swollen iris, vasculitis, pre-iridal fibrovascular membranes, iris nodules, synechiae, ectropion uveae or darkened iris
Pupil may be of normal size and shape or of irregular appearance
Normal or slightly sluggish pupillary reaction to bright light
Anterior lens capsule opacities
Intermediate
Inflammatory cells on posterior lens capsule, pars plana and anterior vitreous ('snowflake' opacities and 'snow-banking', typical of intermediate uveitis or pars planitis)
Posterior
Vitreous opacities
Chorioretinitis
Retinal haemorrhage or detachment
Optic neuritis

Figure 10.36 Salient clinical features of chronic uveitis in the cat.

Infectious uveitis

Systemic viral disease

Feline infectious peritonitis: FIP is a common cause of feline uveitis and and has been reviewed most recently by Andrew (2000). It is more common in younger than in older cats and also in pedigree cats kept in multi-cat households. Systemic signs of this invariably fatal disease include non-specific signs of illness such as lethargy, pyrexia, inappetence, weight loss and progressive neurological dysfunction (Kline *et al.*, 1994).

The ocular manifestations of FIP (Figure 10.37) are

most readily appreciated on examination of the anterior segment, but the posterior segment is also frequently involved. Bilateral ocular involvement is common, although the two eyes may be of different appearance. The classic underlying pathology is perivascular pyogranulomatous inflammation and breakdown of the blood–aqueous barrier. Inflammatory cells and plasma proteins, such as fibrin, leak into the aqueous or vitreous, giving rise to aqueous flare, keratic precipitates and hypopyon in the anterior chamber, or vitritis when cells infiltrate the vitreous. Vasculitis is always present and may be associated with microhaemorrhages and even frank hyphaema; fibrin-rich aqueous is a common finding. Fundus examination may reveal vasculitis, focal or diffuse areas of chorioretinitis, with accompanying retinal oedema and, sometimes, haemorrhage and retinal detachment. If plasma protein levels are sufficiently increased the retinal vasculature, especially the venules, will reflect the systemic hyperviscosity.

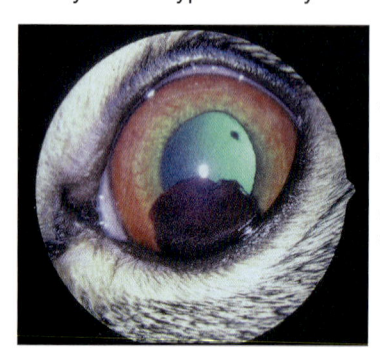

Figure 10.37 Extensive vasculitis, neovascularization of the iris and hyphaema in a cat with FIP. The haemorrhage has clotted and the fibrin content will be high.

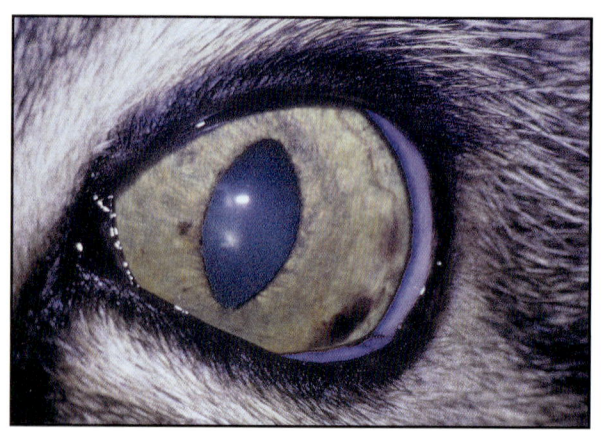

Figure 10.38 Feline leukaemia–lymphoma complex. Hyphaema associated with chronic anaemia is the most prominent ocular sign in this cat; a number of microhaemorrhages are apparent, escaping from the greater arterial circle. The other eye was more severely affected.

It is difficult, if not impossible, to confirm the diagnosis in the live animal; a provisional diagnosis is often made on the basis of the history and clinical signs and the exclusion of other diseases. Serodiagnosis may be misleading as a number of coronaviruses can infect cats, though few cause clinical disease. Evidence from experimental studies indicates that frequent and rapid mutations of feline enteric coronavirus may produce pathogenic FIP phenotypes (Poland et al., 1996). Antibody levels will not indicate whether a pathogenic strain of coronavirus is involved; many healthy cats have high anti-coronavirus titres and, conversely, some cats with FIP have low or even zero anti-coronavirus titres. The laboratory and diagnostic techniques used to determine titres can also produce different results. Effusions are not usually a feature of cats with ocular involvement, although protein analysis is a helpful diagnostic aid when they are. Clinicopathological changes, such as raised total proteins, hyper-gammaglobulinaemia, lymphopenia and a coronavirus antibody titre >160, taken in conjunction with other clinical findings, are strongly suggestive of FIP in cats with non-effusive disease (Sparkes et al., 1994).

Feline leukaemia virus: FeLV is a retrovirus with a worldwide distribution. It most commonly affects male cats aged 1–6 years and with an outdoor lifestyle. The ocular manifestations are broadly divisible into those related to the haemorrhage that accompanies severe anaemia (Figure 10.38) and those associated with neoplasia (Figure 10.39). Uveitis is not universal, but may be immune-mediated or a non-specific reaction to cellular infiltration. FeLV-infected cats may present with a wide range of non-specific clinical signs, and most cats with persistent viraemia usually die of an FeLV-related illness within 2–3 years of infection. Commercially available assays for the detection of viral antigen provide confirmation of FeLV infection but do not prove that the disease present was induced by FeLV. Feline leukaemia virus and feline immunodeficiency virus have been reviewed most recently by Willis (2000a).

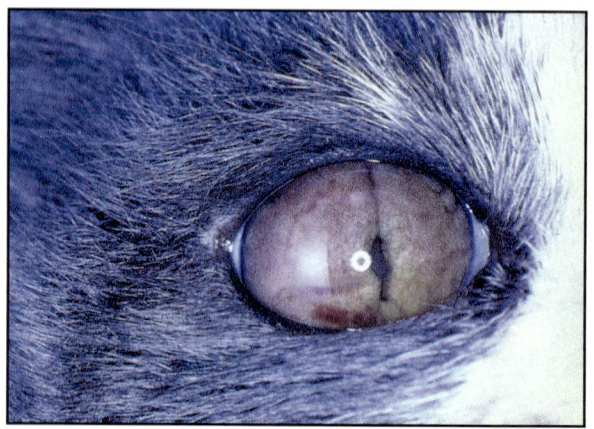

Figure 10.39 Feline leukaemia–lymphoma complex. There is lymphomatous infiltration of the iris. The pupil is distorted and the anterior chamber is shallow because of the swollen iris.

Feline immunodeficiency virus: FIV has been associated with a range of ocular manifestations, which are generally observed during the immunodeficient (late) stage of infection (Figure 10.40). There is a latency of some years between infection and clinical illness for most strains of FIV, so it is older free-roaming, usually male, cats that are most likely to present with a range of non-specific signs. Detection of antibodies against FIV indicates exposure and correlates closely with persistent infection, but FIV seropositivity does not correlate well with immunodeficiency or disease caused by the virus. Opportunistic infections such as toxoplas-

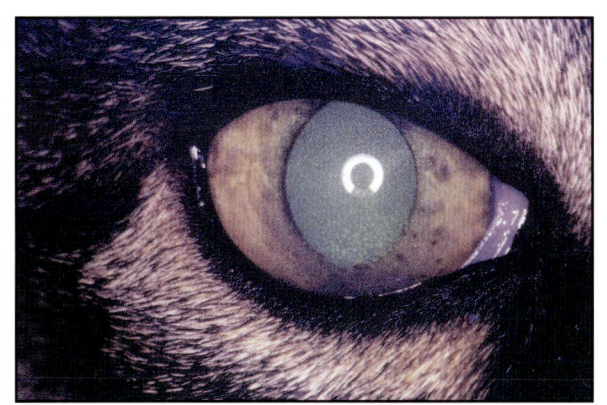

Figure 10.40 Chronic uveitis in FIV infection. The iris is rather dull. Keratic precipitates adhering to the ventral corneal endothelium are the most obvious feature.

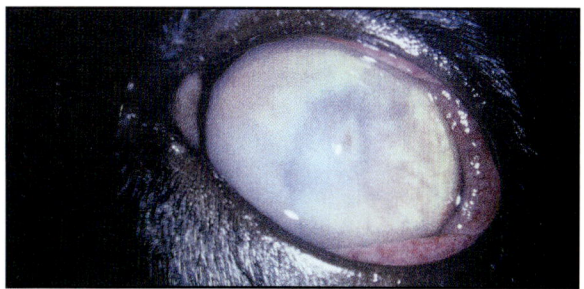

Figure 10.41 An original penetrating cat scratch injury was not treated in this cat, and infection (note the hypopyon) and uveitis resulted. The situation has become further complicated because extensive posterior synechiae have formed, resulting in secondary glaucoma. The IOP (Mackay–Marg tonometer) was >70 mmHg.

mosis (see later) are responsible for many of the ocular syndromes associated with FIV. Other associations with infectious disease have been reported; e.g. FIV infection prolonged the duration of clinical signs resulting from experimental infection with *Chlamydiophila felis* (O'Dair *et al.*, 1994). There is also some evidence that infection with a secondary pathogen accelerates the clinical progression of FIV infection. There is also a possible association between FIV and malignancy.

Treatment of the uveitis associated with FeLV, FIV and FIP tends to be symptomatic and supportive. Treatment of systemic illness is palliative rather than curative; thus, cats with FIV may be given a good quality of life for a considerable time after the diagnosis has been made if their accompanying medical problems are managed carefully. Different chemotherapy protocols have been used with variable success in the treatment of FeLV-infected cats. Palliative treatment of FIP is sometimes undertaken with a view to improving quality of life for the remaining period

Feline herpesvirus-1: FHV-1 may be a potential cause of uveitis, and specific antibodies and DNA have been detected in the aqueous humour of cats (Maggs *et al.*, 1999).

Bacterial

Bartonellosis: This is a common infection in cats and there is increasing evidence that *Bartonella* spp. may be a cause of uveitis (Lappin and Black, 1999; Lappin *et al.*, 2000). Doxycycline is used for systemic treatment, together with local treatment of the uveitis.

Mycobacteria: Typical and atypical mycobacterial infections are rare; ocular manifestations include both anterior and posterior uveitis, most typically choroiditis. The organisms produce a classic granulomatous response, sometimes combined with caseous necrosis. Retinal detachment and extensive tuberculous vitreal infiltration were described by Formston (1994). Affected animals may present with a variety of clinical signs in addition to ocular involvement; most typically, however, there is weight loss despite a healthy, even ravenous, appetite.

Intraocular infection: Local injury, usually as a result of a fight, may result in direct intraocular inoculation of bacteria (e.g. *Pasteurella multocida*), and this type of trauma is a relatively common cause of uveitis (Figure 10.41). Treatment consists of topical atropine, together with topical and systemic antibiotics such as newer generation penicillins (see Chapter 3).

Mycoses

Mycotic infections may occur in countries with suitable climatic conditions. Uveitis has been reported in cats as a consequence of cryptococcosis, coccidioidomycosis, blastomycosis, histoplasmosis and candidiasis, but these are unlikely to be seen in the UK unless the animal has been imported. Cryptococcosis is the most commonly encountered systemic fungal infection of cats in the UK and should be considered a differential diagnosis in imported animals with fever, respiratory tract disease, subcutaneous nodules, central nervous system disease and intraocular inflammation, most typically involving the fundus (see Chapter 14). Treatment of cryptococcosis can be successful (Mikicuik *et al.*,1990). Feline systemic fungal infections have been reviewed recently by Gionfriddo (2000). Diagnosis and treatment are along the lines outlined above for the dog, and the prognosis is similarly guarded.

Parasites

Toxoplasmosis: The cat is the definitive host for *Toxoplasma gondii*, and toxoplasmosis appears to be a common cause of uveitis in cats, but it is important to emphasize that the presence of infection is not necessarily synonymous with disease as many infections remain subclinical (Dubey and Beattie, 1988). In neonatal kittens bred from specific pathogen-free queens, chorioretinitis was the most consistent finding attributable to different strains of *T. gondii* infection (Powell and Lappin, 2001). Systemic toxoplasmosis varies in severity, and cats with suspected infection should be checked for concurrent FIV, FeLV and FIP. There is a range of possible clinical signs in adult cats (Dubey and Carpenter, 1993), but the uveal tract is the most likely site for ocular involvement. Feline ocular toxoplasmosis has been the subject of recent reviews (Davidson and English, 1998; Davidson, 2000).

180 The uveal tract

Ocular lesions are rare in primary disease but frequently occur in secondary chronic toxoplasmosis. Lesions may be unilateral or bilateral. Anterior uveitis is probably the commonest ocular manifestation (Lappin et al., 1992) although the pathogenesis is not fully understood (Davidson, 2000). The appearance is clinically indistinguishable from other forms of infectious uveitis. Intermediate uveitis or pars planitis may also be encountered and is associated with typical snowflake opacities, sometimes with snowbanking behind the lens and in the anterior vitreous (Figure 10.42). Retinal lesions consist of multifocal or, occasionally, generalized chorioretinitis that may be granulomatous or non-granulomatous. There may be associated serous (bullous) retinal detachments. Old inactive focal chorioretinopathies may coexist with active lesions.

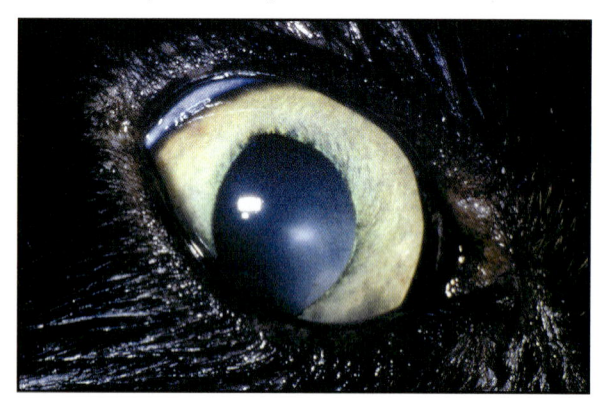

Figure 10.42 Uveitis associated with toxoplasmosis. Note the keratic precipitates on the posterior cornea and the 'snow-banking' typical of pars planitis, comprising inflammatory cells in the anterior vitreous and adherent to the posterior lens capsule.

Diagnosis is based on the clinical signs, serology, exclusion of other infections (e.g. FeLV, FIV and FIP) and response to appropriate therapy. Standard testing involves the detection of *T. gondii*-specific antibodies (IgM, IgG and IgA) (Lappin et al., 1989). Detection of IgM antibodies at a titre of >1:64 is the most reliable indicator of active infection, as IgM levels rise early in the course of infection, but it should be noted that serology is not diagnostic as some healthy cats have very high serum antibody titres and some clinically ill cats have low serum antibody titres. The best laboratory-based indicator of clinical disease may be the use of the PCR for the detection of *T. gondii* in the aqueous humour of cats with uveitis (Lappin et al., 1996).

Oral clindamycin hydrochloride is normally selected for the treatment of toxoplasmosis (12.5 mg/kg orally for 14–21 days). In common with any other currently available anti-toxoplasmal drug, it will not eliminate the organism completely, and so relapse is likely.

Dirofilariasis: This is less common in cats than in dogs. As the infection is usually self-limiting and the treatment not without risk of fatality, it is usually managed symptomatically.

Uveitis associated with neoplasia

As in the dog, both primary and secondary neoplasia can involve the uveal tract and either mimic uveitis or be associated with uveitis. Anterior uveal neoplasia in the cat is discussed below.

Uveitis associated with trauma

Blunt or penetrating injuries to the globe can be associated with uveitis, as described for the dog. The reaction of the feline eye is not necessarily as intense but the intraocular damage can be greater because of the close orbital fit. Management is similar to that outlined for the dog except for injuries associated with lens penetration. Traumatic injuries to the anterior uvea are described below.

Lens damage

Penetrating injury: Uveitis may result from direct lens trauma, including gunshot wounds. In cats it is often possible to control acute-onset lens-associated uveitis with symptomatic treatment. Cataract, often focal in appearance initially but becoming more diffuse with time, may form as the only obvious legacy of previous penetrating lens injury. However, quite unlike the situation in the dog, the release of lens epithelium is thought to be associated with the development of poorly differentiated intraocular spindle cell sarcoma in later life, although an origin from ciliary body epithelial cells cannot be discounted (Dubielzig et al., 1994).

Blunt injury: This can also be a cause of cataract, which may follow many months after the original injury. In such cases, characteristic darkening of the iris is often the only legacy of an earlier uveitis.

Idiopathic and other forms of uveitis

Idiopathic lymphocytic–plasmacytic uveitis: This is thought to be an example of local immune-mediated disease (Wilcock et al., 1990; Peiffer and Wilcock, 1991). The uveitis (Figure 10.43) may be unilateral or bilateral and affects older cats (Davidson et al., 1991; Gemensky et al., 1996). As a lymphocytic–plasmacytic response is not unusual in cats with chronic disease, it is possible that this type of uveitis is indicative of the poor sensitivity of diagnostic tests rather than a specific disease entity. The long-term prognosis for affected eyes is poor as the condition is only partially controlled by anti-inflammatory and immunosuppressive therapy.

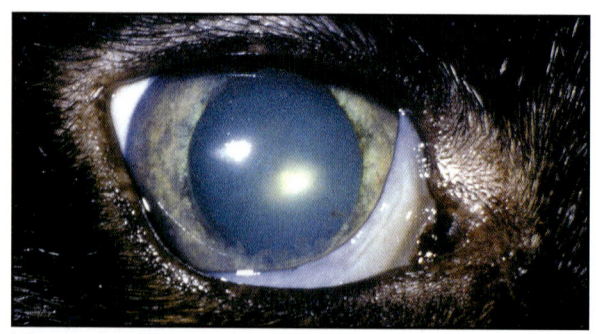

Figure 10.43 Idiopathic uveitis in a 12-year-old Domestic Shorthair. Note the dull metallic appearance of the iris and keratic precipitates adherent to the posterior cornea. The precipitates are almost hidden by the third eyelid.

Complications include loss of vision, cataract, glaucoma and lens luxation. It is also possible that long-term use of corticosteroids increases the incidence of complications like glaucoma.

Polyarteritis nodosa: This is an immune-mediated necrotizing arteritis with widespread and debilitating effects that can include panuveitis.

Treatment
The treatment principles are as already outlined for the dog, except that flunixin meglumine is not licensed for use in cats. Oral acetylsalicylic acid can be used with caution at a total dose of 80 mg every 48–72 hours. Oral phenylbutazone can also be used.

Anterior uveal trauma

Penetrating injuries
The majority of penetrating injuries in the cat are the result of cat scratches. The commonest bacterium introduced into the eye is *Pasteurella multocida*; in addition to treatment for uveitis, topical antibiotic therapy with chloramphenicol solution is required to avoid complications of intraocular infection. Hypopyon is common, and endophthalmitis may complicate untreated cases (Figure 10.44).

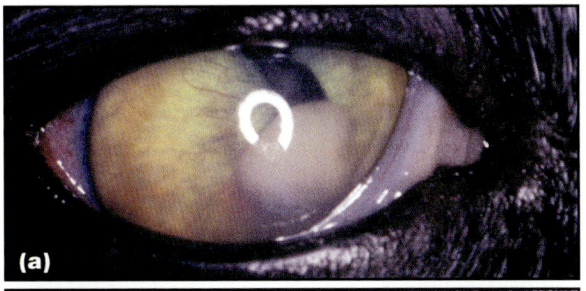

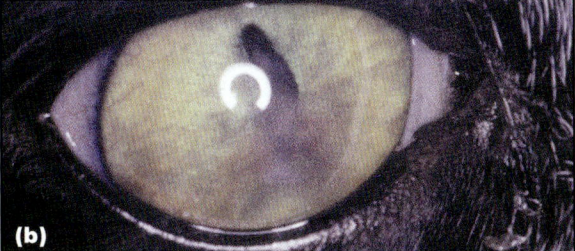

Figure 10.44 Acute penetrating injury as the result of a fight. (a) Hypopyon makes it difficult to see the site of corneal penetration. (b) Once the hypopyon starts to resolve, the site of the penetration can also be seen at 6 o'clock.

Malicious injury is a not uncommon cause of penetrating ocular injury in the cat, and it is always sensible to consider non-accidental trauma when the cause of penetrating injury is not obvious. Radiography of the skull, or even the whole cat, is the easiest way of confirming gunshot wounds.

Penetrating injuries associated with such complications as extensive haemorrhage, loss of aqueous or vitreous humour, a shallow or absent anterior chamber, prolapse or incarceration of the iris, distortion of the pupil or lens damage may require microsurgical repair (Figure 10.45). The prognosis is excellent in most cats, provided that treatment is prompt and that lens penetration has not occurred.

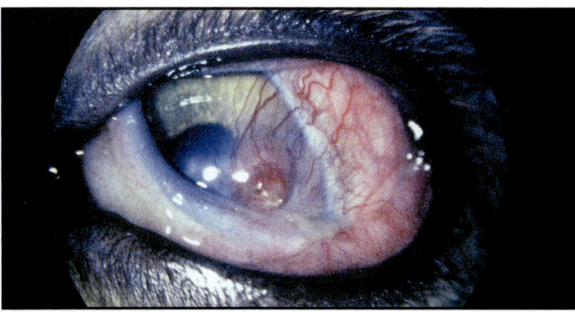

Figure 10.45 Penetrating injury from a cat scratch some weeks earlier. Prolapsed iris has become incarcerated into the corneal wound and there is constant leakage of aqueous humour. Although the damage would have been simpler to repair at the time of the injury, surgical repair should not be delayed further as the prognosis is excellent.

Blunt ocular trauma
Blunt trauma to the globe can be very damaging in the cat, related partly to the close orbital fit. Direct impact injuries can produce globe rupture. Assessment is as for the dog.

Differential diagnosis of intraocular haemorrhage
Intraocular haemorrhage can occur because of trauma, severe uveitis, neoplasia, systemic hypertension and haematological problems, including severe anaemia and thrombocytopenia.

Foreign bodies
Intraocular foreign bodies may also be a cause of uveitis; in general they produce less serious inflammation in cats than in dogs and inert foreign bodies may be better left *in situ*.

Lipaemic aqueous
The secondary causes of hypertriglyceridaemia reviewed briefly earlier are common to the dog and cat and, in both species, can result in lipaemic aqueous. A genetic lipoprotein lipase deficiency resulting in primary chylomicronaemia has been reported in the cat (Jones *et al.*, 1983). A transient turbidity of the aqueous may be observed as a feature of a possible primary hypertriglyceridaemia in young Burmese cats (Figure 10.46). Affected animals become less susceptible as they grow older, and this may simply reflect the leakier nature of iridal capillaries in immature cats as opposed to adults (Bellhorn, 1991).

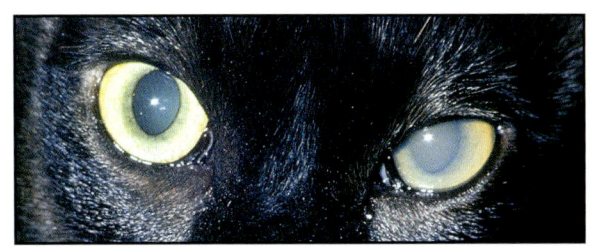

Figure 10.46 Lipaemic (triglyceride-rich) aqueous in a young Burmese cat. Systemic hypertriglyceridaemia was responsible for this 'pseudouveitis', and the ocular appearance returned to normal soon after the triglyceride levels normalized.

Feline uveal neoplasia

Comprehensive reviews of feline ocular neoplasia have been published by Williams *et al.* (1981), Håkanson *et al.* (1990), Dubielzig (1990) and Glaze and Gelatt (1999).

Primary neoplasia

Melanoma: As in the dog, the commonest primary intraocular tumour in the cat is melanoma; it is fairly rare and more malignant than its canine counterpart and can be melanotic or amelanotic, localized (Figure 10.47) or diffuse (Figure 10.48). Atypical primary ocular melanomas, originating multifocally from any portion of the uvea, have also been reported (Harris and Dubielzig, 1999).

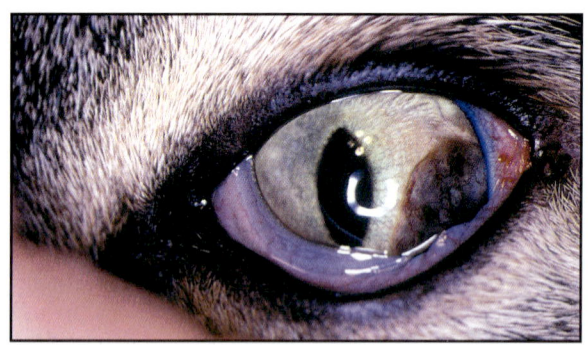

Figure 10.47 Discrete iris melanoma in a cat. (Courtesy of JP Oleshko.)

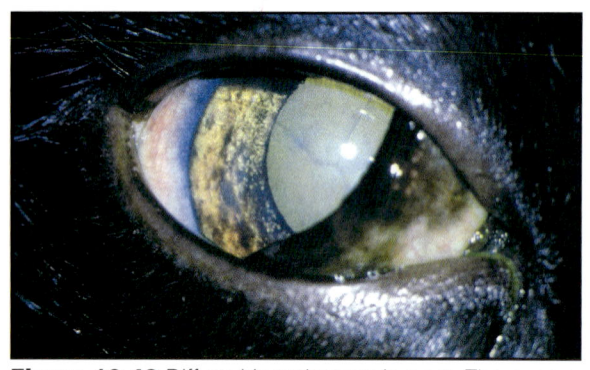

Figure 10.48 Diffuse iris melanoma in a cat. The owners had become aware of a gradual change of iris colour over 18 months.

Diffuse iridal melanomas appear to arise from diffusely transformed cells on the surface of the iris which, over time, infiltrate the stroma. Transformation from iris melanosis to iris melanoma can take several months to a few years and is one of the reasons why it is difficult to give unequivocal advice as to how best to manage these cases. Initially there is a change of iris colour and appearance, a consequence of multiple patches of hyperpigmentation which are superficial in location. The patches develop a typical velvety sheen and become slightly raised. Pupil shape and mobility are affected once the transformed cells infiltrate the stroma and the iris becomes thicker. Abnormal melanocytes may be shed, and the iridocorneal angle becomes involved. Secondary glaucoma with globe enlargement can result when the tumour has infiltrated the iridocorneal angle.

Once the tumour has infiltrated the iris and ciliary body the potential for metastasis is higher and survival time is shortened. Histopathological features helpful in predicting potential for metastatic spread include a high mitotic index, the location of neoplastic cells and the extent of ocular involvement. Metastasis occurs in more than half the cases, usually after a long latency (Duncan and Peiffer, 1991) and up to 3 years after enucleation of the globe. Kalishman *et al.* (1998) suggested that early enucleation is important if premature death, from presumed metastastic spread, is to be avoided.

Other: Primary ciliary body neoplasms include adenoma (Figure 10.49), adenocarcinoma and possibly leiomyoma, but these are all rare. They originate from the pars plicata and may produce secondary glaucoma.

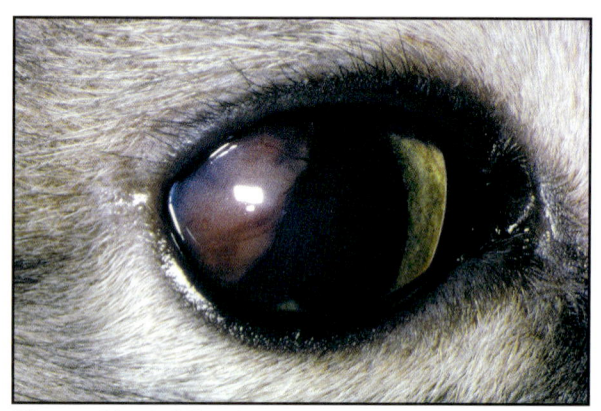

Figure 10.49 Ciliary body adenoma that has invaded the anterior chamber in a Domestic Shorthair.

The cat is unusual in having the potential to develop intraocular spindle cell sarcoma following ocular trauma, and this can occur several years after the initial damage (Figure 10.50). Håkanson *et al.* (1990) reviewed the literature relating to intraocular spindle cell sarcoma in the cat and Dubielzig *et al.* (1994) reported on the morphological features, which indicated that lens epithelial cells or ciliary body epithelial cells might be the neoplastic cell of origin.

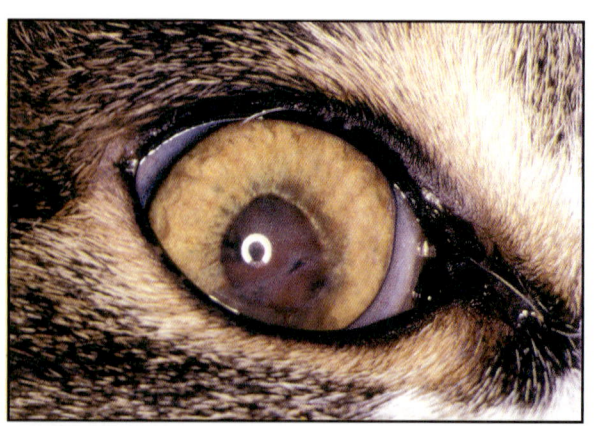

Figure 10.50 Poorly differentiated sarcoma following previous trauma some years earlier. There was evidence of previous full-thickness corneal perforation and the pupil was opaque (leucocoria). Ultrasonography indicated a solid intraocular mass and histopathology confirmed the clinical diagnosis.

Diagnosis: This is essentially as already outlined for the dog.

Management: Enucleation is usually the treatment of choice for primary uveal tumours in cats, provided there is no sign of distant metastases to organs such as liver and lungs. Severely traumatized non-visual eyes should also be removed and traumatized visual eyes kept under very careful review because of the risk of subsequent sarcoma. Orbital exenteration is the correct approach for cats that develop post-traumatic sarcomas, but the prognosis is poor in such cases and a high proportion of cats die from tumour-related complications within months of surgery. All eyes that are removed should be submitted for histopathology.

Secondary neoplasia

Lymphoma: This is the commonest secondary neoplasm affecting the eye and orbit of the cat (Figure 10.51), and the uveal tract is commonly involved. There is a spectrum of clinical appearances and it is not usually possible to differentiate lymphoma from other feline problems affecting the uveal tract on ocular signs alone when uveitis is the main feature of the presentation (see earlier). Lymphoma should, however, be high on the list of differential diagnoses when there is a defined white to pink mass in the anterior chamber, or gross infiltration of the iris. The histopathological features have been reviewed by Corcoran *et al.* (1995). General physical examination may locate abnormalities in other parts of the body, and the diagnosis is usually confirmed from a positive FeLV-antigen test, biopsy of non-ocular tumour masses or bone marrow biopsy, although not all cats with lymphoma are FeLV-positive.

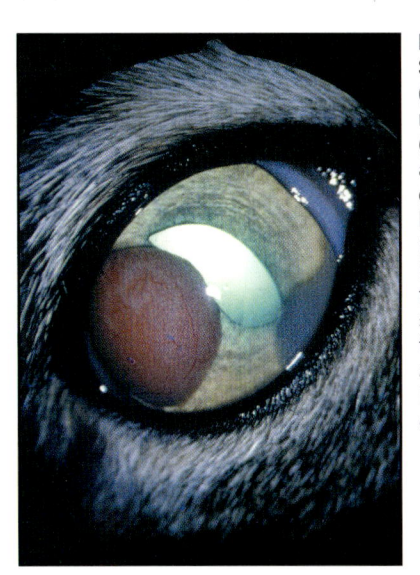

Figure 10.51 Solid tumour (laterally) and neoplastic cells (ventrally) in the anterior chamber of a cat with lymphoma. The pupil is distorted by the solid tumour and subtle aqueous flare was apparent on slit-lamp examination.

Other: Metastatic carcinomas of the uveal tract should also be considered as a cause of secondary uveal neoplasia, and arise from a number of primary sites. Metastatic ocular squamous cell carcinomas have been reported, as have adenocarcinomas from the uterus and mammary gland. The prognosis is usually grave.

References

Andrew SE (2000) Feline infectious peritonitis. *Veterinary Clinics of North America: Small Animal Practice* **30**, 987–1000

Bellhorn RW (1991) An overview of the blood–ocular barriers. *Progress in Veterinary and Comparative Ophthalmology* **1**, 205–217

Blocker T and van der Woerdt A (2001) The feline glaucomas: 82 cases (1995–1999). *Veterinary Ophthalmology* **4**, 81–85

Bussanich NM, Dolman PJ, Rootman J and Dolman CL (1987) Canine uveal melanomas: series and literature review. *Journal of the American Animal Hospital Association* **23**, 415–422

Chavkin MJ, Lappin MR, Powell CC, Roberts SM, Parshall CJ and Reif JS (1992) Seroepidemiologic and clinical observations of 93 cases of uveitis in cats. *Progress in Veterinary and Comparative Ophthalmology* **2**, 29–36

Cohen ND, Carter CN, Thomas MA, Angulo AM and Eugster AK (1990) Clinical and epizootiologic characteristics of dogs seropositive for *Borrelia burgdorferi* in Texas: 110 cases (1988). *Journal of the American Veterinary Medical Association* **197**, 893–898

Collins BK and Moore CP (1999) Diseases and surgery of the canine anterior uvea. In: *Veterinary Ophthalmology, 3rd edn*, ed. KN Gelatt, pp. 755–795. Lippincott, Williams and Wilkins, Philadelphia

Collinson PN and Peiffer RL (1993) Clinical presentation, morphology, and behaviour of primary choroidal melanomas in eight dogs. *Progress in Veterinary and Comparative Ophthalmology* **3**, 158–164

Cook CS (1995) Embryogenesis of congenital eye malformations. *Veterinary and Comparative Ophthalmology* **5**, 109–123

Cook CS (1999) Ocular embryology and congenital malformations. In: *Veterinary Ophthalmology, 3rd edn*, ed. KN Gelatt, pp. 3–30. Lippincott, Williams and Wilkins, Philadelphia

Cook CS and Lannon A (1997) Inherited iris melanoma in Labrador Retriever dogs. *Transactions of the American College of Veterinary Ophthalmologists* **28**, 106

Cook CS and Wilkie DA (1999) Treatment of presumed iris melanoma in dogs with diode laser photocoagulation: 23 cases. *Veterinary Ophthalmology* **2**, 217–225

Corcoran KA, Peiffer RL and Koch SA (1995) Histopathologic features of feline ocular lymphosarcoma: 49 cases (1978–1992). *Veterinary and Comparative Ophthalmology* **5**, 35–41

Crispin SM (1998) Uveal tract. In: *Feline Ophthalmology: an Atlas and Text*, ed. KC Barnett and SM Crispin, pp. 122–143. WB Saunders, Philadelphia

Davidson MG, Nasisse MP, English RV, Wilcock BP and Jamieson V (1991) Feline anterior uveitis: a study of 53 cases. *Journal of the American Animal Hospital Association* **27**, 77–83

Davidson MG and English RV (1998) Feline ocular toxoplasmosis. *Veterinary Ophthalmology* **1**, 71–80

Davidson MG (2000) Toxoplasmosis. *Veterinary Clinics of North America: Small Animal Practice* **30**, 1051–1062

Deehr AJ and Dubielzig RR (1998) A histopathological study of iridociliary cysts and glaucoma in Golden Retrievers. *Veterinary Ophthalmology* **1**, 153–158

Dubey JP and Beattie CP (1988) Toxoplasmosis in cats. In: *Toxoplasmosis of Animals and Man*, ed. JP Dubey, pp. 117–124. CRC Press, Boca Raton

Dubey JP and Carpenter JL (1993) Histologically confirmed clinical toxoplasmosis in cats – 100 cases (1952–1990). *Journal of the American Veterinary Medical Association* **203**, 1556–1566

Dubielzig RR (1990) Ocular neoplasia in small animals. *Veterinary Clinics of North America: Small Animal Practice* **20**, 837–848

Dubielzig RR, Hawkins KL, Toy KA, Rosebury WS, Mazur M and Jasper TG (1994) Morphologic features of feline ocular sarcomas in 10 cats: light microscopy, ultrastructure, and immunohistochemistry. *Veterinary and Comparative Ophthalmology* **4**, 7–12

Dubielzig RR, Steinberg H, Garvin H, Deehr AJ and Fischer B (1998) Iridociliary epithelial tumours in 100 dogs and 17 cats: a morphological study. *Veterinary Ophthalmology* **1**, 223–231

Duncan DE and Peiffer RL (1991) Morphology and prognostic indicators of anterior melanomas in cats. *Progress in Veterinary and Comparative Ophthalmology* **1**, 25–32

Dziezyc J (2000) Canine systemic bacterial infections. *Veterinary Clinics of North America: Small Animal Practice* **30**, 1103–1118

Formston C. (1994) Retinal detachment and bovine tuberculosis in cats. *Journal of Small Animal Practice* **35**, 5–8

Gemensky A, Lorimer D and Blanchard G (1996) Feline uveitis: a retrospective study of 45 cases. *Proceedings of the American College of Veterinary Ophthalmologists* **27**, 19

Gionfriddo JR (2000) Fungal infections. *Veterinary Clinics of North America: Small Animal Practice* **30**, 1029–1050

Glaze MB and Gelatt KN (1999) Feline Ophthalmology. In: *Veterinary Ophthalmology, 3rd edn*, ed. KN Gelatt, pp. 997–1051. Lippincott, Williams and Wilkins, Philadelphia

Gould DJ, Murphy K, Rudorf H and Crispin SM (2000) Canine monocytic ehrlichiosis presenting as acute blindness 36 months after importation into the UK. *Journal of Small Animal Practice* **41**, 263–265

Gwin RM, Gelatt KN and Williams LW (1982) Ophthalmic neoplasms in the dog. *Journal of the American Animal Hospital Association* **18**, 853–866

Håkanson N and Forrester SD (1990) Uveitis in the dog and cat. *Veterinary Clinics of North America: Small Animal Practice* **20**, 715–735

Håkanson N, Shively JN, Reed RE and Merideth RE (1990) Intraocular spindle cell sarcoma following ocular trauma in a cat: case report and literature review. *Journal of the American Animal Hospital Association* **26**, 63–66

Harris BP and Dubielzig RR (1999) Atypical primary ocular melanoma in cats. *Veterinary Ophthalmology* **2**, 121–124

Hollingsworth SR (2000) Canine protothecosis. *Veterinary Clinics of North America: Small Animal Practice* **30**, 1091–1102

Jones BR, Wallace EA, Harding DRK, Hancock WS and Campbell CH (1983) Occurrence of idiopathic familial hyperchylomicronaemia in a cat. *Veterinary Record* **112**, 543–547

Kalishman JB, Chappell R, Flood LA and Dubielzig RR (1998) A matched observational study of survival in cats with enucleation due to diffuse iris melanoma. *Veterinary Ophthalmology* **1**, 25–29

Kline KL, Joseph RJ and Averill DR (1994) Feline infectious peritonitis with neurologic involvement: clinical and pathological findings in 24 cats. *Journal of the American Animal Hospital Association* **30**, 111–118

Komaromy AM, Brooks DE, Kallberg ME, Andrew SE, Ramsey DT and Ramsey CC (1999a) Hyphema Part I: pathophysiologic considerations. *Compendium on Continuing Education for the Practicing Veterinarian* **21**, 1064–1069

Komaromy AM, Brooks DE, Kallberg ME, Andrew SE, Ramsey DT and Ramsey CC (1999b) Hyphema Part II: diagnosis and treatment. *Compendium on Continuing Education for the Practicing Veterinarian* **22**, 74–79

Krohne SG, Henderson NM, Richardson RC and Vestre WA (1994) Prevalence of ocular involvement in dogs with multicentric lymphoma: prospective evaluation of 94 cases. *Veterinary and Comparative Ophthalmology* **4**, 127–135

Krohne SG (2000) Canine systemic fungal infections. *Veterinary Clinics of North America: Small Animal Practice* **30**,1063–1090

Lappin MR, Greene CE, Winston S, Toll SL and Epstein ME (1989) Clinical feline toxoplasmosis: serologic and therapeutic management of 15 cases. *Journal of Veterinary Internal Medicine* **3**, 139–143

Lappin MR, Marks A, Greene GE, Collins J, Carman J, Reif JS and Powell CC (1992) Serologic prevalence of selected infectious diseases in cats with uveitis. *Journal of the American Veterinary Medical Association* **201**, 1005–1009

Lappin MR, Burney DP, Dow SW and Potter TA (1996) Polymerase chain reaction for the detection of *Toxoplasma gondii* in aqueous humour of cats. *American Journal of Veterinary Research* **57**, 1589–1593

Lappin MR and Black JC (1999) *Bartonella* spp. infection as a possible cause of uveitis in a cat. *Journal of the American Veterinary Medical Association* **214**, 1205–1207

Lappin MR, Kordick DL and Breitschwerdt EB (2000) *Bartonella* spp. antibodies and DNA in aqueous humour of cats. *Journal of Feline Medicine and Surgery* **2**, 61–68

Lewis DG, Kelly DF and Sansom J (1986) Congenital microphthalmia and other developmental abnormalities in the Dobermann. *Journal of Small Animal Practice* **27**, 559–566

Maggs DJ, Lappin MR and Nasisse MP (1999) Detection of feline herpesvirus-1-specific antibodies and DNA in the aqueous humour of cats. *American Journal of Veterinary Research* **60**, 932–936

Martin CL (1999) Ocular manifestations of systemic disease. Part 1: the dog. In: *Veterinary Ophthalmology, 3rd edn*, ed. KN Gelatt, pp. 1401–1448. Lippincott, Williams and Wilkins, Philadelphia

Mikicuik MG, Fales WH and Schmidt DA (1990) Successful treatment of feline cryptococcosis with ketoconazole and flucytosine. *Journal of the American Animal Hospital Association* **26**, 199–201

Nasisse MP, Davidson MG, Olivero DK, Brinkmann M and Nelms S (1993) Neodymium:YAG laser treatment of primary canine intraocular tumours. *Progress in Veterinary and Comparative Ophthalmology* **3**, 152–157

O' Dair HA, Hopper CD, Gruffydd-Jones TJ, Harbour DA and Waters L (1994) Clinical aspects of *Chlamydia psittaci* infection in cats infected with feline immunodeficiency virus. *Veterinary Record* **134**, 365–368

Peiffer RL and Wilcock BP (1991) Histopathological study of uveitis in cats: 139 cases (1978–1988). *Journal of the American Veterinary Medical Association* **198**, 135–138

Peña MT, Roura X and Davidson MG (2000) Ocular and periocular manifestations of leishmaniasis in dogs: 105 cases (1993–1998). *Veterinary Ophthalmology* **3**, 35–41

Poland AM, Vennema H, Foley JE and Pedersen NC (1996) Two related strains of feline infectious peritonitis virus isolated from immunocompromised cats infected with a feline enteric coronavirus. *Journal of Clinical Microbiology* **34**, 3180–3184

Powell CC and Lappin MR (2001) Clinical ocular toxoplasmosis in neonatal kittens. *Veterinary Ophthalmology* **4**, 87–92

Render JA, Ramsey DT and Ramsey CC (1997) Contralateral uveal metastasis of malignant anterior uveal melanoma in a dog. *Veterinary and Comparative Ophthalmology* **7**, 263–266

Roperto F, Restucci B and Crovace A (1993) Bilateral ciliary body melanomas in a dog. *Progress in Veterinary and Comparative Ophthalmology* **3**, 149–151

Sapienza JS, Francisco J, Domenech S and Prades-Sapienza A (2000) Golden Retriever uveitis: 75 cases (1994–1999). *Veterinary Ophthalmology* **3**, 241–246

Slatter DH (1990) *Fundamentals of Veterinary Ophthalmology, 2nd edn*. WB Saunders, Philadelphia

Slatter DH (2001) *Fundamentals of Veterinary Ophthalmology, 3rd edn*, p330. WB Saunders, Philadelphia

Sparkes AH, Gruffydd-Jones TJ and Harbour DA (1994) An appraisal of the value of laboratory tests in the diagnosis of feline infectious peritonitis. *Journal of the American Animal Hospital Association* **30**, 345–350

Spiess BM, Bolliger JO, Guscetti F, Haessig M, Lackner PA and Ruehli MB (1998) Multiple ciliary body cysts and secondary glaucoma in the Great Dane: a report of nine cases. *Veterinary Ophthalmology* **1**, 41–45

Stiles J (1999) Ocular manifestations of systemic disease. Part 2: the cat. In: *Veterinary Ophthalmology, 3rd edn*, ed. KN Gelatt, pp. 1448–1473. Lippincott, Williams and Wilkins, Philadelphia

Stiles J (2000) Canine rickettsial infections. *Veterinary Clinics of North America: Small Animal Practice* **30**,1135–1150

van der Woerdt A (2000) Lens-induced uveitis. *Veterinary Ophthalmology* **3**, 227–234

Wilcock BP and Peiffer RL (1986) Morphology and behaviour of primary ocular melanomas in 91 dogs. *Veterinary Pathology* **23**, 418–424

Wilcock BP, Peiffer RL and Davidson MG (1990) The causes of glaucoma in cats. *Veterinary Pathology* **27**, 35–40

Williams LW, Gelatt KN and Gwin R (1981) Ophthalmic neoplasms in the cat. *Journal of the American Animal Hospital Association* **17**, 999–1008

Williams DL (1993) A comparative approach to anterior segment dysgenesis. *Eye* **7**, 607–616

Willis AM (2000a) Feline leukaemia virus and feline immunodeficiency. *Veterinary Clinics of North America: Small Animal Practice* **30**, 971–986

Willis AM (2000b) Canine viral infections *Veterinary Clinics of North America: Small Animal Practice* **30**, 1119–1134

11

Glaucoma

Peter Renwick

Introduction

Glaucoma in domestic animals presents as a group of well recognized pathological changes involving the globe. These may result from one or more of a number of ocular disorders whose common end point is prolonged elevation of the intraocular pressure above normal limits.

Disturbance to the optic nerve head, in terms both of its microcirculation and of the axoplasmic flow in its retinal ganglion cell axons, is the earliest and most significant effect of glaucoma. These changes are accompanied by retinal necrosis, which occurs as the result of a reduction in choroidal vascular perfusion, and this effect is greatest initially in the non-tapetal fundus. In an uncontrolled situation, these events may progress to complete and irreversible blindness in the affected eye.

The outlook for vision in cases of glaucoma is always guarded, and it remains one of the most challenging and potentially frustrating conditions for the clinician to manage. Early recognition of the problem followed by prompt, appropriate therapy is essential if sight is to be preserved.

Physiological control of intraocular pressure

The intraocular pressure (IOP) is dependent on a number of factors including ocular rigidity and the volume of aqueous humour in the anterior segment of the eye. Constant production and drainage of aqueous is required to maintain both a formed globe and a steady state of physiological IOP. The aqueous is optically clear under normal conditions, a property important for visual function. Its continual flow is vital for the delivery of nutrients to, and removal of waste products from, the avascular structures it bathes, i.e. the lens, cornea and trabecular meshwork (a major part of the drainage apparatus of the eye).

Aqueous is produced from the processes of the ciliary body (Figure 11.1), primarily by the mechanism of active secretion and, to a lesser degree, by ultrafiltration. The ciliary processes are highly vascular, possess a double epithelial layer, and have a large surface area to facilitate their secretory function.

Once produced, aqueous traverses the posterior chamber, passes through the pupil and enters the anterior chamber (Figure 11.1). In order to maintain a steady IOP, aqueous must then drain out of the eye at the same rate at which it is produced. The majority of aqueous outflow in dogs and cats occurs through the drainage structures at the junction of the iris base and the corneoscleral tissue (Figure 11.2). This region is often termed the drainage angle (iridocorneal angle, filtration angle).

The major structures of the drainage apparatus are the pectinate ligament (Figure 11.3) and the ciliary cleft, which contains the sponge-like tissue of the trabecular meshwork. The bulk of the aqueous drains across these structures to the avascular aqueous plexus and thence to the scleral venous circulation (so-called 'conventional' outflow). In addition, an 'unconventional' uveoscleral outflow route involves aqueous passing into the ciliary cleft and gaining access to the scleral venous circulation via the choroid and suprachoroidal space, bypassing the aqueous plexus. This route is believed to comprise approximately 15% of the total aqueous outflow in normal dogs and around 3% in normal cats.

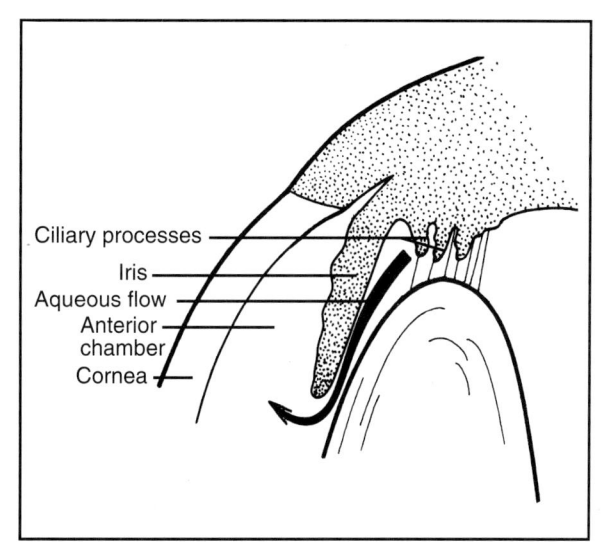

Figure 11.1 Aqueous humour is produced by the processes of the ciliary body and flows through the pupil into the anterior chamber.

Glaucoma

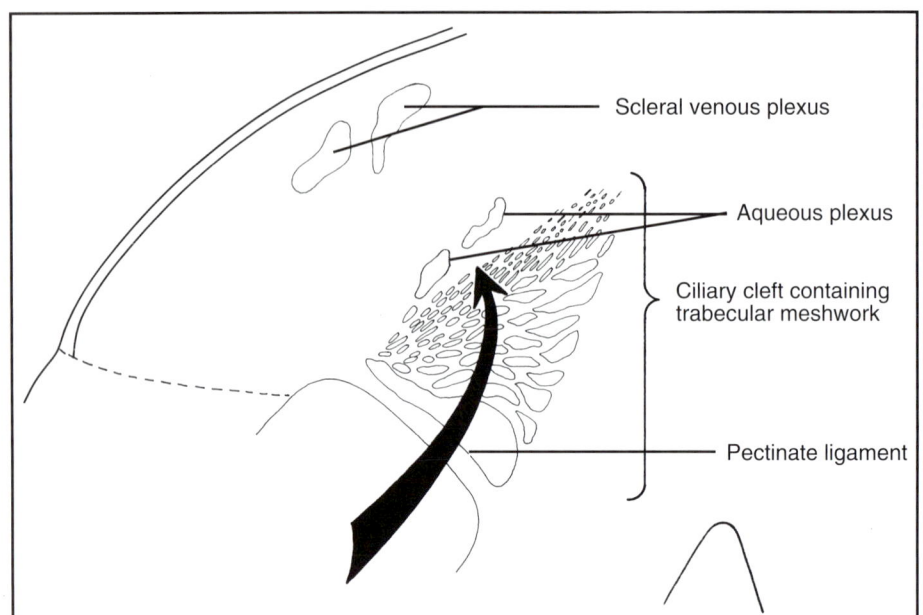

Figure 11.2 Drainage of aqueous occurs primarily through the pectinate ligament and trabecular meshwork into the aqueous plexus, and thence to the scleral venous circulation.

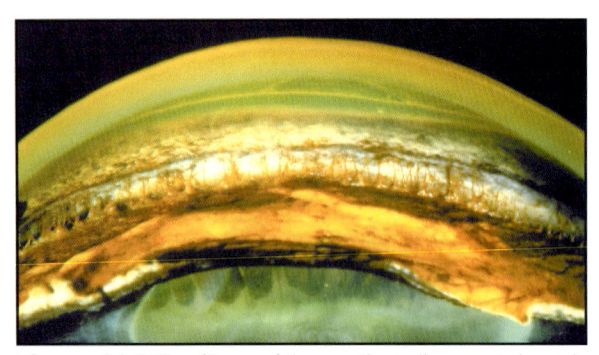

Figure 11.3 The fibres of the pectinate ligament viewed from within the anterior chamber. (Courtesy of JRB Mould)

Normal variations

The IOP in normal dogs measured by applanation tonometry is generally found to be between 10 and 25 mmHg. Various factors may influence the reading obtained (Figure 11.4). In assessing a suspected case of glaucoma, it is important to bear in mind the possible physiological parameters that may influence IOP. For example, measured IOP can rise to around 30 mmHg when pressure is applied to the neck and immediately fall to <20 mmHg once the grip on the patient is relaxed.

- Instrumentation used for measurement of IOP
- Age of dog – the IOP is reported to decrease with ageing
- Position of patient – a head-back posture increases IOP
- Degree of restraint – vigorous restraint increases IOP
- Forced lid opening and pressure on the globe increase IOP
- Breed of dog – e.g. terrier breeds have been shown to have fluctuating IOPs
- Possibly other factors, such as obesity and arterial blood pressure

Figure 11.4 Factors influencing intraocular pressure in normal dogs.

Diagnostic tools

The basic approach to examination is outlined in Chapter 1a. The following section deals with the use of instruments specifically aimed at determining IOP (tonometry) or examining the drainage apparatus (gonioscopy).

Tonometry

Almost all patients with glaucoma have elevated IOP on presentation. Measurement of IOP is therefore fundamental to making the diagnosis. It is also a very useful aid in the diagnosis and management of cases of uveitis, as the IOP often falls as a result of anterior segment inflammation. Various methods of IOP estimation are available.

Digital tonometry

This technique involves placing the forefinger on the upper eyelid, over the globe, and applying pressure to estimate how hard the eye feels. This can be carried out simultaneously on both eyes for comparison. It is a crude technique at best, and may be thoroughly misleading in some instances, even in experienced hands. In cases where the eye is markedly soft or hard the abnormality will be detected but in less extreme cases no reliance can be placed on the method. Additionally, digital tonometry is of no value in monitoring a case once therapy has commenced, as it is far too insensitive. The diagnosis and management of glaucoma cases using only digital tonometry as a means of estimating IOP cannot be recommended.

Schiøtz tonometers

The Schiøtz tonometer is readily available and relatively cheap. All practitioners should own, and be familiar with the use of, this instrument. It estimates IOP by the use of a weighted plunger, which indents the eye to a degree that is inversely proportional to the IOP (Figure 11.5). The nearer to zero the reading on the scale, the higher is

Glaucoma 187

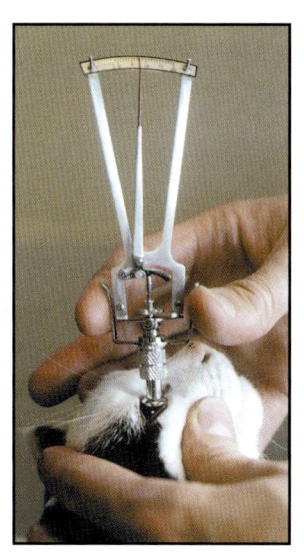

Figure 11.5 After applying topical anaesthetic (e.g. proxymetacaine), the patient is restrained with the head back, so that the cornea lies in the horizontal plane (unfortunately this position causes a physiological increase in IOP). The plunger is placed vertically on the central cornea on several occasions until several similar readings have been obtained. Care must be taken to keep the footplate away from the third eyelid, and the plunger must be resting freely on the globe with no hindrance from the remainder of the instrument.

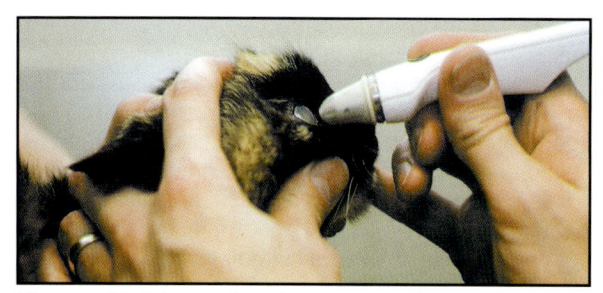

Figure 11.6 An applanation tonometer in use. The instrument is tapped gently several times on the corneal surface. An averaged value of the IOP is given by a digital readout on the instrument, along with an indication of the estimated accuracy of the reading.

the IOP, especially if a greater weight has been placed on the plunger. The scale reading is converted to one of IOP using a standardized chart for human eyes that is supplied with the instrument, as this is reasonably accurate for use in both dogs and cats (Miller and Pickett 1992a,b). To increase reliability and accuracy, it is advisable to perform several readings and to repeat them using a different weight on the plunger. An averaged value may then be obtained. The IOP should always be measured in the opposite eye, even if it has a clinically normal appearance.

There are disadvantages in using the Schiøtz tonometer:

- Aligning the instrument correctly on the globe can be difficult
- Difficulty in restraining some patients may artefactually increase IOP
- Indentation tonometry is inherently subject to a degree of inaccuracy
- Should not be used after recent intraocular surgery
- Corneal oedema or other abnormalities such as scarring may render the reading inaccurate
- A dirty instrument can be highly inaccurate.

It is very important to keep the tonometer meticulously clean by dismantling and cleaning it after every session of use.

Applanation tonometers

There are a number of tonometers available that operate on the principle of measuring the force required to flatten or 'applanate' a small area of cornea (Figure 11.6). The force required is proportional to the IOP. Applanation tonometers tend to be the most accurate in clinical use (Gelatt *et al.*, 1977). They can be used with the dog or cat in a normal standing position, they are less influenced by some of the factors such as ocular rigidity which affect indentation tonometers, and they can be used after intraocular surgery. While these instruments are expensive, their purchase by progressive small animal practices is encouraged.

Gonioscopy

Gonioscopy is a technique that allows visual inspection of the opening to the ciliary cleft. It is not normally possible to see the drainage structures using routine ophthalmic examination techniques, except to some extent in cats, where a limited and somewhat distorted view of the pectinate ligament can be obtained by viewing through the cornea at an oblique angle.

The technique of gonioscopy depends upon the use of a contact lens of some type (Figures 11.7 and 11.8). In the absence of a goniolens, a condensing lens pressed against the cornea offers a less satisfactory alternative.

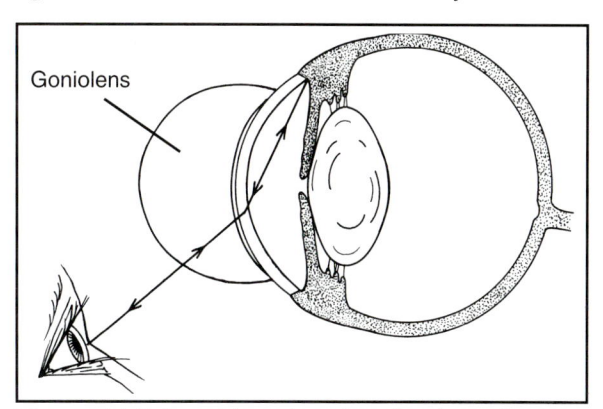

Figure 11.7 A goniolens alters the refraction at the corneal surface, allowing light that would normally be internally reflected to travel from the drainage angle to the viewer's eye.

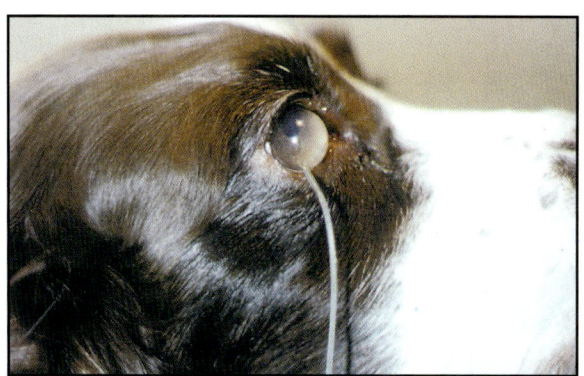

Figure 11.8 A goniolens is applied to a topically anaesthetized cornea and employs a negative pressure, created by a column of saline within the attached silicone tubing, to maintain adherence of the lens to the globe. An improved view may be obtained by filling the chamber of the lens with artificial tears prior to placement on the cornea.

188 Glaucoma

Magnification (e.g. a direct ophthalmoscope, slit-lamp biomicroscope or fundus camera) is then used to inspect the structures of the iridocorneal angle (Figure 11.9). The viewer may see: indications of pectinate ligament abnormalities, such as goniodysgenesis; collapse of the ciliary cleft and pectinate ligament; or other changes in the area, such as infiltration by neoplastic tissue, the presence of inflammatory swelling or deposits, or fibrovascular tissue ingrowth.

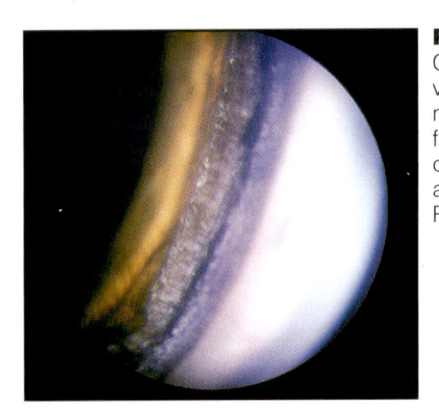

Figure 11.9 Gonioscopic view of the normal pectinate fibres and ciliary cleft entrance in a Labrador Retriever.

Gonioscopy is indicated in any case of glaucoma where the cause of the IOP elevation is not immediately apparent. It is also a necessity when primary inherited glaucoma is suspected, particularly when an outwardly normal fellow eye may be inspected for abnormalities of the iridocorneal angle. This can be helpful in determining the diagnosis of glaucoma (the glaucomatous globe may be unsuitable for gonioscopy due to the presence of corneal opacity), and it also gives useful information regarding the potential for predisposition to glaucoma in the normotensive globe.

The technique is not straightforward. The goniolens can be difficult to retain on the eye and the view obtained is not always clear, especially if the lens becomes contaminated with meibomian gland secretion or other debris. The positioning of the lens can be critical and slight alterations in this or in the viewing angle can lead to artefactual changes in the appearance of the entrance to the ciliary cleft. Practice is required in order to perform gonioscopy and interpret the findings reliably.

Gonioscopy is a very important technique for the diagnosis and management of glaucoma. If the clinician is presented with a case of suspected or confirmed glaucoma and the necessary equipment or expertise is lacking, then immediate referral should be considered.

Clinical signs of glaucoma

The presenting signs of glaucoma vary, depending on a number of factors:

- Speed of onset
- Degree of elevation of IOP
- Duration of the problem
- Underlying cause
- Age of the animal (young animals have more distensible globes).

Special features of glaucoma in cats are discussed further at the end of this chapter. It is very important to appreciate that many of the clinical signs of glaucoma are common to numerous other ophthalmic disorders, and the importance of a careful comprehensive clinical examination in making a diagnosis of glaucoma cannot be overemphasized.

For convenience, the signs will be considered under the headings of 'acute' and 'chronic' but this division is somewhat arbitrary and not always clear-cut in a clinical setting. For example, some chronic cases may not be presented until an acute exacerbation draws the problem to the owner's attention.

Acute glaucoma

The major signs seen most often in the face of an acute rise in IOP are summarized in Figure 11.10.

Pain:
  Increased lacrimation
  Blepharospasm
  Enophthalmos or third eyelid prolapse
  Head shyness

Corneal oedema: especially with acute rise in IOP > 40–50 mmHg

Corneal vascularization:
  Deep 'brush-border' appearance in acute cases
  May advance towards the central cornea at a rate of up to 1 mm per day

Mydriasis: mid-dilated unresponsive pupil

Episcleral congestion: often accompanied by conjunctival congestion

Vision loss: may not be noticed by the owner if the problem is unilateral

Figure 11.10 Clinical signs of acute glaucoma.

Pain
In severe and very acute cases, especially where the IOP is above 40–50 mmHg, the degree of discomfort may be so severe as to cause yelping, head shyness and marked depression and/or inappetence. Blepharospasm, globe retraction with consequent third eyelid prolapse, increased lacrimation and epiphora may also result from discomfort. The signs may be less apparent in cases where the increase in IOP is less dramatic. The pain associated with glaucoma does not respond well to NSAIDs, and controlling the IOP is the main aim in affording pain relief.

Corneal oedema
The whole cornea may take on a 'steamy', bluish appearance, especially with a sudden elevation of IOP to >40–50 mmHg. The normal optical clarity of the cornea depends upon a number of factors. One of the most important is the state of deturgescence. This is primarily the result of the action of a pump mechanism in the corneal endothelial cells. Active transport of solutes from the cornea into the aqueous humour causes movement of water out of the corneal stroma down the resulting diffusion gradient. A marked

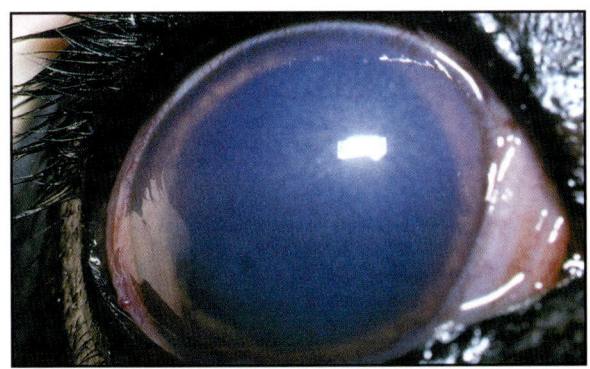

Figure 11.11 Acute-onset primary glaucoma due to goniodysgenesis in a Basset Hound. The high IOP interferes with the corneal endothelial pump mechanism, leading to the development of corneal oedema.

elevation of IOP interferes with this phenomenon and oedema ensues (Figure 11.11). This sign is not found consistently; it tends to be less marked at low levels of IOP elevation and in chronic cases.

Corneal vascularization

In acute cases, a fringe of blood vessels may invade the deep cornea from the limbus, usually through 360 degrees. The vessels may take on a 'brush-border' densely packed appearance at their leading edge, due to the fact that they are constrained by the surrounding stromal collagen lamellae (Figure 11.12). Such vascularization is most commonly seen in association with marked corneal oedema and where the glaucoma is secondary to uveitis.

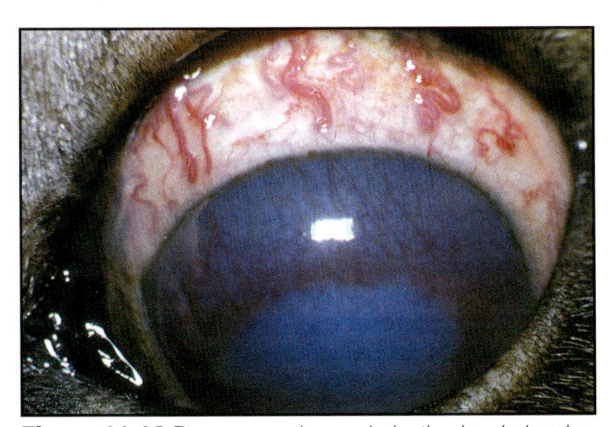

Figure 11.12 Deep corneal vascularization in a Labrador Retriever with primary glaucoma due to goniodysgenesis. The vessels have invaded the cornea through 360 degrees and exhibit a 'brush-border' appearance at the leading edge. Deep vessels cannot be seen to cross the limbus in dogs (compare with Figure 11.19).

Mydriasis

A dilated or moderately dilated, poorly responsive pupil results from pressure-induced paresis or paralysis of the iris sphincter muscle. The absence of a direct pupillary light reflex under such circumstances must not be presumed to equate with loss of vision; instead, other features should be used to gauge the presence or absence of vision. Mydriasis is not an invariable finding in glaucomatous globes, and in some cases of uveitis-induced glaucoma the pupil may even be constricted.

Episcleral congestion

Episcleral congestion (Figure 11.13) is a commonly encountered and useful diagnostic indicator in glaucoma cases. The engorged episcleral vessels run at right angles to the limbus, are frequently set against the white background of the sclera, and do not move in association with movement of the overlying lids and conjunctiva. The conjunctival vessels may also be distended, in which case the tissue between the episcleral vessels will appear hyperaemic. The conjunctival vessels may be blanched rapidly by the application of topical 10% phenylephrine drops, allowing the episcleral vessels (which blanche less readily) to be assessed more accurately. It is important to appreciate that not all cases with episcleral congestion have glaucoma and *vice versa* (Figure 11.14).

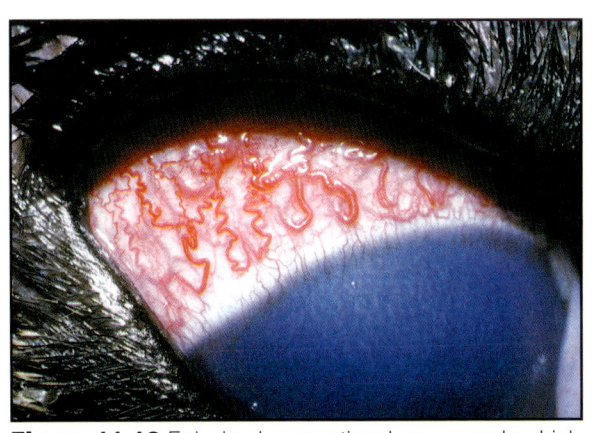

Figure 11.13 Episcleral congestion: large vessels which do not move with the conjunctiva are seen against the scleral background.

- Glaucoma
- Uveitis or endophthalmitis or panophthalmitis
- Episcleritis (often localized in dogs)
- Retrobulbar space-occupying lesion, e.g. abscess, neoplasia
- Hyperviscosity syndromes
- Excitement

Figure 11.14 Differential diagnosis of episcleral congestion or hyperaemia.

Vision loss

Loss of vision initially occurs as a result of damage to the ganglion cell axons in the region of the optic nerve head, and this is accompanied in some acute-onset cases by retinal necrosis, especially within the non-tapetal fundus. In addition, the levels of glutamate within the vitreous and retina increase, and this in turn leads to retinal ganglion cell death due to 'excitotoxicity', mediated, at least in part, by an influx of calcium into the cells (Brooks *et al.*, 1999). In acute cases, the eye may become blind within hours of the onset of glaucoma, and these changes rapidly become irreversible.

Whilst an observant owner may detect loss of vision in one eye, it is unlikely that partial visual field loss in only one eye will be noticed. By virtue of this fact, glaucoma affecting only one eye tends to present relatively late in the course of the disease and it is generally an alteration in appearance of the eye rather than altered vision which prompts presentation. It is also relatively easy for the clinician to overlook the very important question of whether an abnormal, possibly glaucomatous, eye is visual or not, especially if the owners have not reported any historical evidence of blindness. A positive effort must therefore be made both during history taking and during the examination to establish whether or not the eye is visual (Figure 11.15). This can not only assist in making a diagnosis but also has a major impact on the future management of the case.

- Loss of menace response in the affected eye
- Loss of dazzle reflex to bright light shone into the affected eye
- Loss of consensual pupillary light reflex – no constriction of pupil in fellow eye when affected eye illuminated in a dimly lit room
- Re-dilation of the pupil in the affected eye on a swinging flashlight test
- Absence of tracking response to cotton wool ball with fellow eye patched
- Inability to negotiate a maze with fellow eye patched

Figure 11.15 Clinical signs of unilateral blindness in glaucoma.

Those animals that have already lost vision in one eye will tend to present as soon as the second eye is clinically affected.

In the early stages of vision loss, optic nerve head damage and retinal ganglion cell dysfunction are potentially reversible, at least to some degree. In those cases which present with a very high IOP or once the eye has been blind for more than a few days (even hours in some instances), the prospects for the return of vision, even when the IOP is restored to normal, become more remote. It is therefore imperative that cases of acute onset glaucoma are diagnosed accurately and as early in the course of the disease as the presentation allows.

Genuine acute-onset glaucoma in those cases where there is the potential for preserving or restoring vision constitutes an ocular emergency. For those clinicians not fully familiar with both the diagnosis and therapy of the condition, it is advisable to offer urgent referral to a specialist.

Chronic glaucoma

Chronic glaucoma may arise as a sequel to an unsuccessfully controlled or misdiagnosed episode (or episodes) of an acute-onset nature, or it may develop insidiously and first present at a point where the eye is already showing signs of gross abnormality.

Many of the signs seen in acute glaucoma will also be present to a greater or lesser degree in more chronic cases, although some (e.g. pain and corneal oedema) will tend to become less marked with increasing chronicity. In addition to the signs of acute glaucoma, chronic cases will demonstrate various combinations of the signs summarized in Figure 11.16.

Globe enlargement:
  Stretching of the ocular tunics leads to many of the other changes listed below
  Once the globe has enlarged, the prognosis is often very poor and enucleation is frequently indicated
  Every attempt should therefore be made to diagnose glaucoma well before this stage is reached

Corneal neovascularization:
  Often superficial branching vessels (unlike the 'brush-border' of acute cases)
  Vessels may bring pigment into the superficial cornea

Corneal ulceration: due to exposure or inadequate blink (lagophthalmos)

Descemet's streaks (Haab's striae): grey streaks in the cornea resulting from breaks in Descemet's membrane due to stretching

Equatorial staphyloma: scleral thinning seen as a bluish transilluminating bulge behind the limbus

Iris atrophy:
  Thinning allows easy transillumination or holes may develop
  More commonly results from ageing or uveitis

Lens subluxation/luxation with aphakic crescent or penumbra: must be differentiated from primary lens luxation

Cataract

Intraocular haemorrhage: more commonly seen in other disease states (see text)

Optic disc cupping: posterior bowing of the optic disc due to scleral weakness at this point (the lamina cribrosa)

Retinal and optic nerve head atrophy

Phthisis bulbi

Figure 11.16 Signs of glaucoma associated with chronicity.

Globe enlargement

Enlargement of the globe (hydrophthalmos, buphthalmos) occurs due to pressure-induced stretching of the ocular tunics. It is often marked in young animals as they possess less rigid globes than adults. Many of the signs of chronic glaucoma are the result of stretching of the globe.

Buphthalmos (Figure 11.17) must be differentiated from exophthalmos, in which a normal-sized eye is pushed forward by a retrobulbar space-occupying process such as abscess or neoplasia (Figure 11.18).

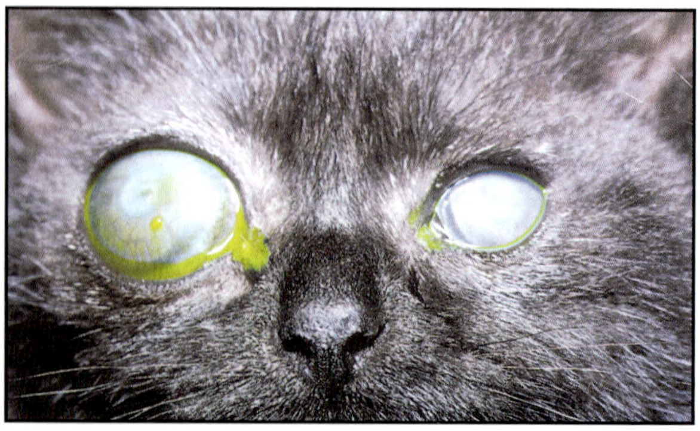

Figure 11.17 Buphthalmos in a kitten with congenital glaucoma.

Glaucoma

Feature	Buphthalmos	Exophthalmos
Third eyelid position	Pushed back towards medial canthus	Often prolapsed across globe
Corneal diameter	Increased	Normal
Pupil appearance	Often mid-dilated and unresponsive	Variable – may be normal
Lens position	Often subluxated – aphakic crescent and stretched zonular fibres visible	Normal
Optic disc appearance	Cupped	Disc may be swollen or congested – not cupped
Oral examination	Normal	Swelling may be seen caudal to last molar tooth
Intraocular pressure	Increased	Normal in most cases

Figure 11.18 Differentiation of buphthalmos from exophthalmos.

Corneal changes

The corneal diameter increases as the globe enlarges. Blood vessels may invade the cornea from the limbus, often in a superficial, arborizing pattern (Figure 11.19). Pigment is frequently deposited, having gained access to the cornea via the invading vessels. As the globe enlarges, the ability to blink and distribute the tear film becomes compromised. This, in turn, affects corneal health and may ultimately result in areas of epithelial irregularity and even frank ulceration, particularly of the central cornea.

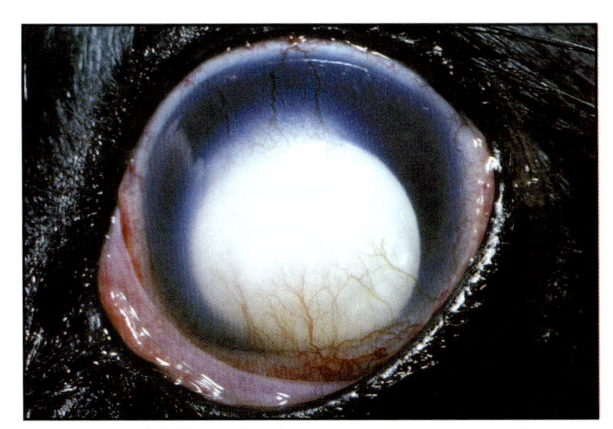

Figure 11.19 Superficial vascularization in chronic glaucoma. The vessels are branching and can be seen to cross the limbus. The lens in this case has luxated and become cataractous secondary to globe enlargement.

Grey opacities may develop within the cornea, due to a number of factors. These include:

- Disturbance to the normally regular arrangement of the collagen lamellae, e.g. by oedema or blood vessels
- Scar tissue formation, e.g. following ulceration
- Thickening/keratinization of the corneal epithelium secondary to exposure

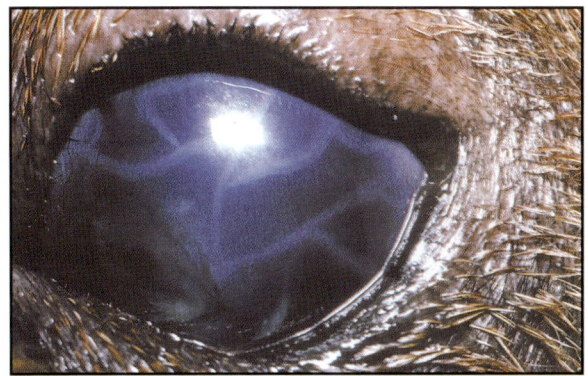

Figure 11.20 A Chow-Chow with chronic glaucoma secondary to previous anterior uveitis. Descemet's streaks (Haab's striae) can be seen; they are breaks in Descemet's membrane which result from stretching of the ocular tunics.

- Breaks in Descemet's membrane caused by stretching of the cornea; the grey streaks are also known as Haab's striae (Figure 11.20).

Equatorial staphyloma

Scleral thinning and stretching may become marked at the equator of the globe, leading to the development of outward protrusion. This is seen as a bluish bulge some distance behind the limbus and is often obscured by the eyelids (Figure 11.21). The swelling must be differentiated from a solid mass; this may achieved by transillumination – light shines through a staphyloma, due to thinning of the tissues.

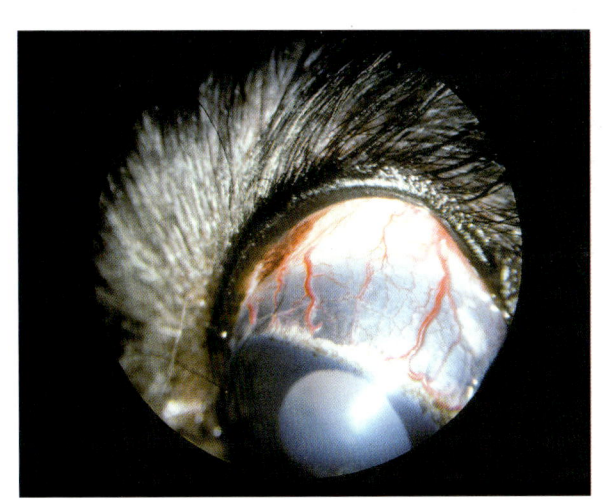

Figure 11.21 Equatorial staphyloma. Occasionally pressure-induced thinning of the sclera may cause a bluish swelling posterior to the limbus. In contrast to a neoplastic mass, a staphyloma can be transilluminated due to thinning of the tissues. (Courtesy of PGC Bedford.)

Lens changes

Luxation or subluxation: Enlargement of the globe results in stretching and tearing of the zonular fibres that support the lens. This results in subluxation and, in some instances, eventual luxation of the lens (see Figure 11.19).

The lens may come to lie in the anterior or posterior segment of the eye and is frequently seen to retain part

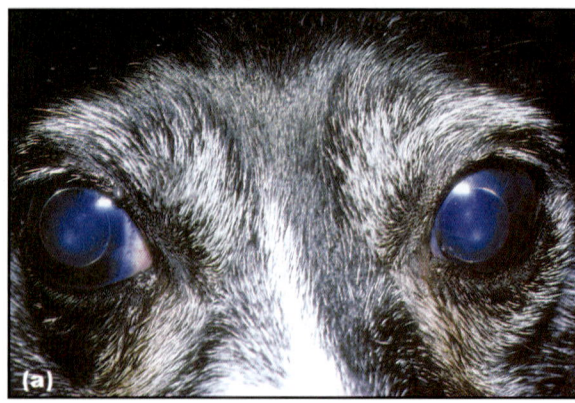

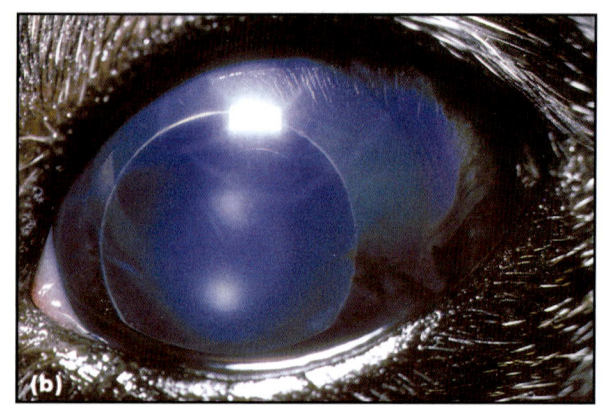

Figure 11.22 Primary open-angle glaucoma in a Collie cross. (a) Both lenses are suspended near the visual axis by the remaining zonular fibres. (b) The refractile lens equator can be seen, and adjacent to this is an aphakic crescent. The cornea also shows signs of breaks in Descemet's membrane and corneal pigmentation as a consequence of gross buphthalmos.

of the zonular attachments around its equator (Figure 11.22). An aphakic crescent develops in cases of lens subluxation where the lens comes to occupy a position away from the visual axis. The crescent is bordered by the pupil margin on one side and the equator of the lens on the other. The fundus can be viewed through the aphakic region, either by using close direct ophthalmoscopy (with the lens in the ophthalmoscope set to approximately +12 dioptres), or by using a focal light source and naked eye examination, which will often allow a limited view of the retinal vessels. In some cases with marked globe enlargement, the lens may remain approximately within the visual axis, and a complete aphakic ring or penumbra may be seen between the lens equator and the pupillary margin.

Luxation or subluxation of the lens may affect aqueous humour dynamics and further increase the degree of glaucoma present.

Lens luxation may also develop as a primary event and it is therefore very important to determine whether the lens luxation is the cause or effect of glaucoma (see below).

Cataract: Lens opacities often develop in chronic glaucoma cases, especially where luxation has occurred. These probably result from alterations to lens nutrition and a build-up of toxic products within the eye. The delivery of nutrients to, and removal of metabolic waste products from, the lens is hampered by alterations in aqueous humour dynamics. In addition, it is known that toxic levels of products such as glutamate build up in the posterior segment in glaucomatous globes.

Cataractous lenses may also cause glaucoma through a variety of mechanisms (see below).

Intraocular haemorrhage

Gross haemorrhage within the globe may develop as a result of glaucoma, but it may also be related to the cause of the elevated IOP. Its presence may render accurate diagnosis of the cause of the glaucoma difficult, or impossible if it is present at the first assessment of the case. Some of the differentials which should be considered are shown in Figure 11.23.

- Trauma/surgery
- Intraocular neoplasia
- Uveitis
- Bleeding diathesis – numerous causes
- Systemic hypertension
- Retinal detachment – numerous causes
- Congenital abnormalities
    - Collie eye anomaly
    - Retinal dysplasia
    - Persistent hyaloid artery
    - Persistent hyperplastic primary vitreous
- Chronic glaucoma

Figure 11.23 Causes of intraocular haemorrhage.

Optic disc cupping

Cupping of the optic disc is the phenomenon in which the optic nerve head becomes bowed outwards (Figures 11.24 and 11.25). This is a result of the effect of raised IOP on the relatively weak lamina cribrosa (the perforated region of the sclera that allows optic nerve fibres to exit from the globe) and the loss of optic nerve fibres due to glaucoma.

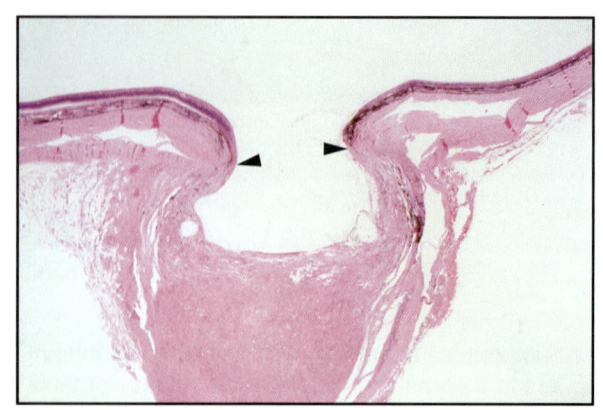

Figure 11.24 Histological section of a globe with chronic glaucomatous damage. The optic disc is cupped. Arrowheads mark the margins of the disc. (Courtesy of JRB Mould)

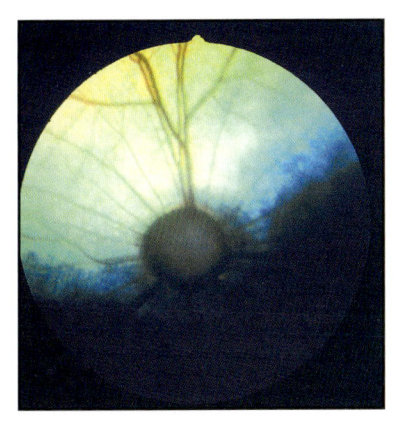

Figure 11.25 Primary open-angle glaucoma in a crossbred dog. The optic disc is severely cupped. The retinal vessels drop down into the rim of the cup and are lost to view when the focus is in the plane of the retina.

Optic disc cupping is perhaps most readily appreciated using stereoscopic indirect ophthalmoscopy, which gives a three-dimensional view of the fundus. However, it is also possible to gain an impression of the degree of cupping by using a direct ophthalmoscope. The retina is first brought into focus by dialling up the required lens in the ophthalmoscope (this may be a negative lens due to globe enlargement), and then the centre of the optic disc is focused upon by dialling in a negative lens of greater dioptre. The difference in the lens settings required gives an indication of the degree of optic disc cupping (each additional dioptre is approximately equivalent to 0.3 mm of cupping).

Retinal and optic nerve atrophy

With chronicity, the optic disc undergoes changes in its ophthalmoscopic appearance in addition to those of cupping. Typically, it takes on a chalky appearance due to loss of vasculature, and it may also become darkened due to loss of myelinated nerve fibres.

Tapetal hyper-reflectivity is another potential ophthalmoscopic finding. It results from retinal thinning, which allows increased reflection of light back from the tapetum (which lies within the choroid). In glaucoma patients this is often seen initially as shiny fan-shaped bands extending out from the optic disc. The bands represent so-called 'watershed' lesions and result from pressure-induced effects on zones of choroidal vasculature (supplying the outer layers of the retina). As the disease progresses, the extent of tapetal hyper-reflectivity increases and the retinal vessels (supplying the inner retinal layers) become attenuated (Figure 11.26).

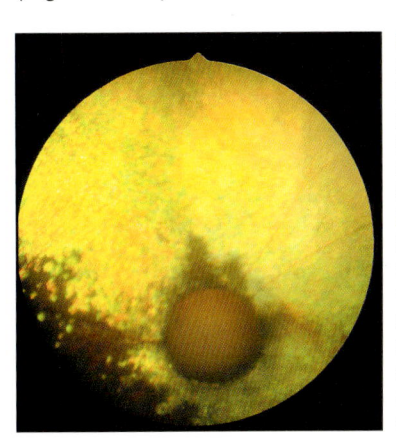

Figure 11.26 Chronic changes in long-standing glaucoma due to goniodysgenesis in an English Springer Spaniel. The tapetal fundus is hyper-reflective and the retinal vessels are severely attenuated. In addition, the optic disc is severely cupped.

Phthisis bulbi

It is important to note that in some cases signs of chronic glaucoma may be present although the IOP at the time of examination is found to be normal. This occurs when a previously raised IOP has caused pressure-induced atrophy of the ciliary processes, thus reducing aqueous production. In extreme cases this may lead to a reduction in the size of the globe or phthisis bulbi.

Classification and causes of glaucoma

Glaucoma can be classified in a number of ways. In addition to whether the presenting signs are acute or chronic, it is possible to consider glaucoma in terms of its underlying cause:

- Primary glaucoma – two major types:
  - Goniodysgenesis ('closed-angle' glaucoma)
  - Primary 'open-angle' glaucoma
- Secondary glaucoma; numerous conditions may lead to a reduction in aqueous outflow
- Congenital glaucoma, present perinatally for whatever reason; rare in veterinary practice.

Primary glaucoma

In cases of primary glaucoma, there is no other recognized antecedent ocular disease process and, almost invariably, there is the potential for elevation of the IOP to become bilateral.

A number of breeds worldwide have been demonstrated to be predisposed to the development of primary glaucoma. In some of these, the disease has been demonstrated to have a hereditary basis. The breeds vary between countries but those recognized as more commonly affected are listed in Figure 11.27.

Goniodysgenesis	
English Cocker Spaniel	Flat-coated Retriever
American Cocker Spaniel	Golden Retriever
English Springer Spaniel	Great Dane
Welsh Springer Spaniel	Welsh Terrier
Basset Hound	Dandie Dinmont Terrier
Bouvier des Flandres	Siberian Husky
Labrador Retriever	Samoyed
Open-angle glaucoma	
Norwegian Elkhound	
Beagle	

Figure 11.27 Breeds disposed to primary glaucoma.

Acute primary 'closed-angle' glaucoma

Goniodysgenesis is the commonest cause of primary glaucoma in dogs in the UK. The breeds in which it is most frequently seen are listed in Figure 11.27. In these cases there is a developmental bilateral abnormality of the pectinate ligament (Martin, 1975; Bedford, 1980). Instead of the normal structure seen in Figure 11.9, the dysplastic ligament comprises sheets of tissue which may be so extensive in some cases as to be perforated only by intermittent flow holes (Figure 11.28).

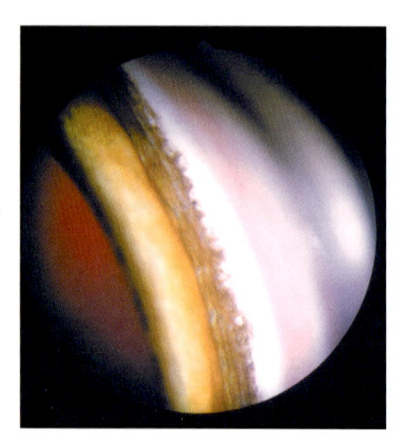

Figure 11.28 Gonioscopic view of goniodysgenesis in an English Springer Spaniel (the fellow eye of the dog in Figure 11.26). The pectinate ligament comprises a sheet of tissue with only intermittent flow holes (compare with Figure 11.9).

The entrance to the ciliary cleft, spanned by the pectinate ligament, may also be narrowed (Ekesten, 1993). In early life, these limited channels allow sufficient passage of aqueous for the maintenance of a normotensive globe. After a variable period, usually in middle age, although earlier in adulthood in the Welsh Springer Spaniel (Cottrell and Barnett, 1988), the flow becomes further compromised and glaucoma develops, often with an acute onset. However, the precise mechanisms whereby aqueous drainage ultimately fails are not fully understood. Not surprisingly, those individuals that exhibit the greatest degree of pectinate ligament dysplasia have been shown to be most likely to develop clinical signs of glaucoma (Read et al., 1998).

Any dog of a breed listed in Figure 11.27 that presents with a sudden onset of a red or painful eye should be suspected of having closed-angle glaucoma, until proven otherwise. It is mandatory to carry out IOP measurement and gonioscopy in such a case. In addition, as goniodysgenesis is a bilateral condition, the opposite eye is predisposed to developing glaucoma in the future. This may well influence case management and is very important information with respect to client education.

Chronic primary 'open-angle' glaucoma

Primary open-angle glaucoma is the type seen in Norwegian Elkhounds, and occasionally other breeds and crossbred dogs in the UK, and in a laboratory strain of Beagle in the USA. Much research has been carried out on the condition in the Beagle, particularly because of its relevance to the similar, very common, disease in humans, but its importance in the clinical setting is limited. The condition is thought to develop as a result of the build-up of certain types of glycosaminoglycans (mucopolysaccharides) within the trabecular meshwork, leading to an increase in the resistance to aqueous outflow (Gum et al., 1993).

The condition is bilateral and is insidious in onset. Patients are often presented relatively late in the course of the disease, with enlarged globes and poor vision in both eyes. However, the optic nerve head appears to tolerate these prolonged, often marked, elevations of IOP better than in acute-onset forms of glaucoma. In some cases, useful vision can be retained through to the late stages of the disease, despite the presence of sometimes massive buphthalmos.

Secondary glaucoma

Secondary glaucoma is the most commonly encountered type of glaucoma in both dogs and cats. It develops when antecedent ocular pathology reduces the circulation and drainage of aqueous, leading to increased IOP.

Aqueous flow in secondary glaucoma may be impeded at the pupil or at the filtration angle (pectinate ligament and ciliary cleft structures). The site at which the major obstruction to aqueous circulation occurs may vary from one case to another.

There are numerous possible causes of secondary glaucoma (Figure 11.29).

- Primary lens luxation: most common in terrier breeds
- Lens luxation secondary to hypermature cataract
- Uveitis, including lens-induced uveitis due to lens rupture or hypermature cataract
- Intraocular haemorrhage in neoplasia
- Ocular melanosis (Cairn Terriers); formerly described as pigmentary glaucoma
- Multiple iris cysts and uveitis (Golden Retrievers)
- Intumescence (swelling) of a cataractous lens, especially in diabetes
- Fibrovascular membrane formation in the drainage angle, secondary to retinal detachment, uveitis or neoplasia
- Vitreous prolapse after surgical lens extraction

Figure 11.29 Causes of secondary glaucoma.

Primary lens luxation

Primary lens luxation (see Chapter 12) is commonly seen in the terrier breeds and occasionally the Border Collie in the UK. It has been described in the Shar Pei in the USA (Lazarus et al., 1998) and has recently been seen in an imported stud dog of this breed in the UK.

The lens may luxate into the anterior chamber, carrying vitreous humour with it. The flow of aqueous is then impeded, both by any prolapsed vitreous which comes to overlie the entrance to the ciliary cleft, and by the lens occupying a large proportion of the anterior chamber. The presence of vitreous or lens within the pupil may further exacerbate the rise in IOP by causing pupillary block. Glaucoma may also be seen in cases where a luxated lens is resting within the posterior segment, and even in some instances where the lens is only subluxated. Once the IOP has been elevated for any length of time, the ciliary cleft may collapse and this change can rapidly become permanent due to the development of peripheral anterior synechiae. These are adhesions of the iris base to corneoscleral tissue which effectively obliterate the ciliary cleft.

In some cases, it may be difficult to decide whether lens luxation is a cause or an effect of glaucoma. This distinction may well have a profound influence on case management and will, to a certain extent, influence the prognosis. Establishing the order of events depends upon a careful assessment of the signalment, history and clinical findings. Gonioscopy, especially of the opposite eye, may give valuable information in this regard.

Uveitis

Inflammation of the uveal tract may result in secondary glaucoma through a variety of mechanisms:

- Accumulation of inflammatory debris within the structures of the filtration angle
- Damage to and swelling of the trabecular meshwork structures as a direct result of involvement in the inflammatory process (the ciliary cleft is composed of uveal tissue)
- The development of posterior synechiae (adhesions between iris and lens). If these become sufficiently extensive, then aqueous will be unable to flow from the posterior to the anterior chamber. This leads to a build-up of aqueous behind the iris which then bulges forward – so-called 'iris bombé' (Figures 11.30 and 11.31). Initially the obstruction to aqueous flow may be restricted to the pupil but, with time, the forward displacement of the iris leads to collapse of the ciliary cleft. At this stage, the IOP will remain elevated, even if the posterior synechiae are broken down, or an alternative drainage channel is created through the iris
- Fibrin clot material in the anterior chamber, impeding aqueous outflow
- Fibrovascular membrane formation over the pectinate ligament
- Peripheral anterior synechiae. These may develop in disease states associated with inflammation, e.g.
  - iris bombé, intumescent cataract or a luxating lens pushing the iris base forward
  - anterior uveitis combined with a dilated pupil, e.g. with excessive use of atropine
  - as a result of loss of the anterior chamber due to globe rupture.
- A syndrome of severe uveitis and multiple iris cyst formation leading to glaucoma has been described in Golden Retrievers (Deehr and Dubielzig, 1997).

When dealing with any case of uveitis, it is important to monitor IOP, whether glaucoma is initially present or not. Both uveitis and glaucoma may present as a red, painful eye of cloudy appearance. Tonometry is essential to distinguish the two conditions. In addition, even initially uncomplicated uveitis may later become complicated by glaucoma and this may be overlooked until the situation is irreversible, unless a policy of routine IOP measurement is adopted in the handling of uveitis patients.

Neoplasia

Neoplasia (see Chapter 10) may induce glaucoma by a variety of means:

- Direct involvement of the drainage angle in the neoplastic process
- A build-up of neoplastic cells from the aqueous within the trabecular meshwork
- Secondary blood-aqueous barrier breakdown, leading to debris within the trabecular meshwork
- Stimulation of fibrovascular membrane formation as a result of the release of angiogenic substances (Peiffer et al., 1990).

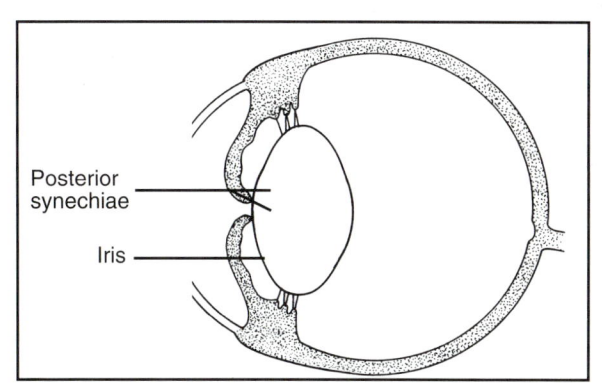

Figure 11.30 Iris bombé results when 360-degree posterior synechiae prevent flow of aqueous through the pupil.

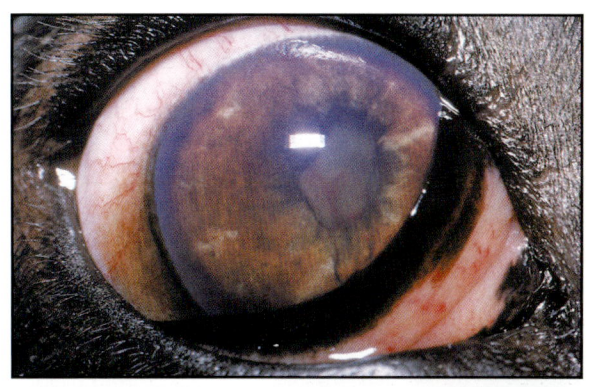

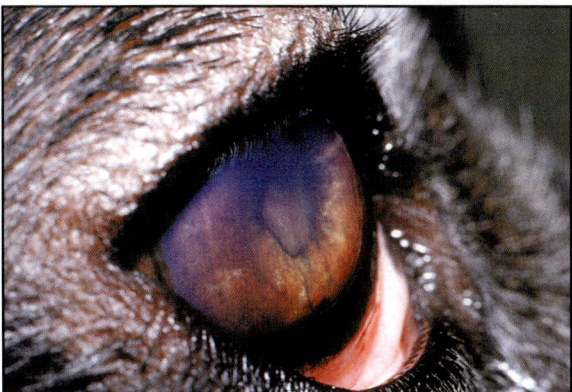

Figure 11.31 A Labrador Retriever hit in the eye by a golf ball 2 weeks previously. Glaucoma has developed as a result of uveitis, and there has been consequent iris bombé formation. A cataract is also present, and a small amount of haemorrhage can be seen in the pupil. The side view shows the iris bulging forward.

The commonest intraocular neoplasms are primary uveal melanoma (Figure 11.32), primary ciliary body adenoma/adenocarcinoma and lymphoma (usually with systemic involvement). Secondary intraocular neoplasia is also an occasional cause of glaucoma, the commonest type in dogs being mammary adenocarcinoma.

The diagnosis of intraocular neoplasia, especially when it is complicated by glaucoma, may not be straightforward. The cornea may exhibit marked oedema, neovascularization and pigmentation, all of which serve to obscure the view of the intraocular structures. Should any doubt exist as to the presence of an intraocular neoplasm, further investigations are required (Figure 11.33).

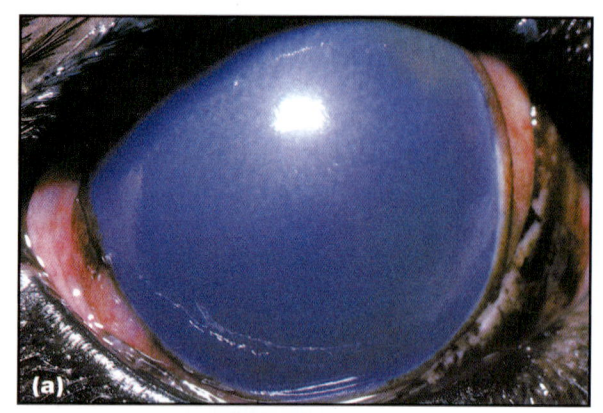

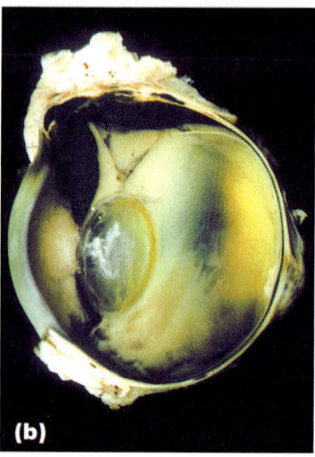

Figure 11.32
A 9-year-old Boxer presenting with a history of signs of pain and a recent blue discoloration of the cornea (a). The diagnosis was one of glaucoma secondary to anterior uveal melanoma. The cross-section (b) shows that the bulk of the melanoma lies in the dorsal iris and ciliary body, but there is ring spread to involve the entire anterior uvea. (b, courtesy of JRB Mould)

- Full physical examination
- Ultrasonography of globe or orbit
- Radiography of chest or abdomen
- Ultrasonography of abdomen
- Blood samples (for haematology and biochemistry)
- Aqueous/vitreous centesis for cytological examination (probably best reserved for blind eyes)
- Enucleation and histopathology

Figure 11.33 Investigation of glaucoma where neoplasia is suspected.

Intraocular haemorrhage

This may occur for a number of reasons (see Figure 11.23). Even extensive haemorrhage may not lead to glaucoma, but in some instances the presence of blood and fibrin clots compromises aqueous outflow sufficiently to cause a rise in IOP. Trauma cases often retain a low IOP in the face of severe intraocular haemorrhage; this may be the result of concomitant ciliary body damage leading to a marked reduction in aqueous production.

In addition to being a potential cause of increased IOP, intraocular haemorrhage may occur as a result of glaucoma in some chronic cases.

Ocular melanosis

This condition (previously called 'pigmentary glaucoma' or 'abnormal pigment deposition'), which affects Cairn Terriers, involves the accumulation of pigment in the anterior segment structures including the ciliary cleft (Petersen-Jones, 1991). This may lead to an insidious onset of glaucoma in middle-aged and older dogs. Large quantities of pigment are visible in the anterior chamber and the sclera, especially ventrally (Figure 11.34). Pigment accumulation can also be seen in the tapetal fundus and not infrequently over the region of the optic disc.

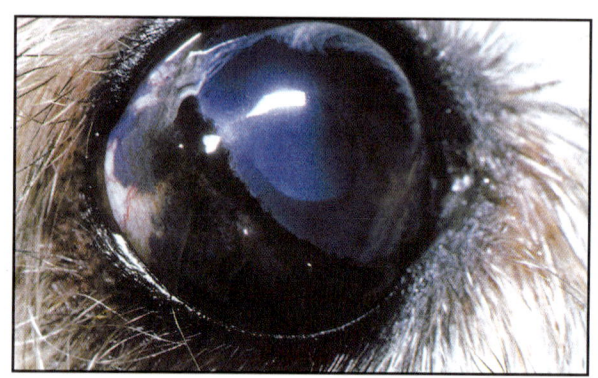

Figure 11.34 Ocular melanosis in a Cairn Terrier.

Glaucoma secondary to lens pathology

In addition to primary lens luxation (see above), glaucoma may develop as a sequel to a variety of pathological changes involving the lens:

- Lens-induced uveitis, due to leakage of antigenic lens proteins into the aqueous humour
  - Secondary to mature/hypermature cataract
  - As a result of traumatic lens rupture
- Luxation of a hypermature cataractous lens
- Swelling (intumescence) of the lens. This is a rare cause of glaucoma
- Retinal detachment secondary to cataract, leading to fibrovascular membrane formation within the drainage angle.

Vitreous prolapse

Large quantities of vitreous may enter the anterior chamber as a result of intraocular surgery (usually intracapsular lens extraction) or following lens luxation. Obstruction of aqueous flow subsequently occurs, either at the pupil or within the filtration angle. If vitreous presents in the anterior chamber during lens surgery, vitrectomy is necessary and will reduce the likelihood of the subsequent development of glaucoma.

Therapeutics

The major aim in glaucoma management is to lower the IOP to a level at which vision no longer deteriorates. Setting a target IOP of 20 mmHg or less should help to reduce the persistence of neurodestructive mechanisms that may otherwise continue to cause vision loss even after a grossly elevated IOP has been corrected.

Glaucoma therapy can be divided into medical and surgical approaches, although in many instances a combination of both will be required. In general terms, a reduction in IOP may be achieved either by reducing the production of aqueous or by increasing the facility of aqueous outflow. Examples of both of these mechanisms are to be found in the various medical and surgical approaches to glaucoma management.

The management strategy in any individual case will depend on a number of factors, including:

- The degree of vision present and the likelihood of its return. This is partly dependent on the duration of the condition. In acute-onset cases of only a few hours or days duration, where blindness is apparent, some return of vision may be achieved with rapid normalization of IOP. Long-standing cases where the patient is blind are unlikely to see again, even with vigorous treatment. Signs of chronicity, e.g. buphthalmos and Descemet's streaks, do not necessarily preclude the presence of some useful vision. Young animals and patients with primary open-angle glaucoma may develop signs of globe enlargement well before optic nerve damage has caused total blindness. A careful evaluation of vision in any patient presenting with glaucoma is vital when formulating a treatment plan
- The underlying cause of the problem. For example, the approach to a case with uveitis that has led to secondary glaucoma will be entirely different from that to one where neoplasia is the underlying cause. In some instances, the management of the opposite eye is as important as that of the globe with elevated IOP, e.g. in goniodysgenesis
- The gonioscopic findings. Medical therapy in uveitis or open-angle cases may be satisfactory if the appearance of the drainage structures suggests that a potentially adequate pathway remains for aqueous outflow. If gonioscopy shows pectinate ligament dysplasia due to goniodysgenesis, then medical therapy alone may well be insufficient to achieve even short-term control of IOP. In many cases, especially those of a chronic nature, increased IOP generally results in the iris base being displaced anteriorly, leading to the development of peripheral anterior synechiae. Peripheral anterior synechiae and ciliary cleft collapse are often found, even at the first presentation of glaucoma in domestic animals. They result in a severe reduction in the facility of aqueous outflow, and in such circumstances surgical therapy may be required to regain sustained control of IOP
- Initial response to therapy. If medical therapy is attempted and the initial response is excellent, the necessity for surgical intervention may become less urgent
- If the opposite eye is blind or absent, the need to preserve vision in the glaucomatous eye becomes more pressing to the majority of owners
- The age of the animal. Major surgery may be less justifiable in elderly patients
- Financial considerations and the ease of access to a specialist.

Medical therapy

Osmotic diuretics

Acute glaucoma with high IOP (>40–50 mmHg) of very recent onset warrants the immediate use of osmotic diuretics to achieve a rapid reduction in IOP, especially if blindness is present. The drug in common use is intravenous mannitol (for dosage see Figure 11.35). Oral glycerol may be supplied for emergency home use in dogs known to have a predisposition to primary glaucoma.

Care must be taken when using these drugs, as they can cause a rapid loss of body fluid. In certain cases this may induce prerenal azotaemia and even renal failure. If there is any doubt as to the renal function of a patient, it should be assessed before therapy commences.

While a rapid response may be seen with the use of mannitol, the effect is likely to be short lived and further action will be required to achieve long-term control of IOP medically and/or surgically.

Therapeutic agent	Class of agent	Dosage
Mannitol 10% or 20% solution	Osmotic diuretic	1–2 g/kg i.v. over 20–30 min
Glycerol 50%	Osmotic diuretic	1–2 ml/kg orally
Dorzolamide hydrochloride 2% drops	Carbonic anhydrase inhibitor	three or four times a day
Brinzolamide drops 10 mg/ml	Carbonic anhydrase inhibitor	two or three times a day
Acetazolamide tablets or solution	Carbonic anhydrase inhibitor	Tablets: 10–25 mg/kg orally twice a day Solution: same dose i.v or i.m.
Dichlorphenamide	Carbonic anhydrase inhibitor	5–10 mg/kg orally two or three times a day
Methazolamide	Carbonic anhydrase inhibitor	5–10 mg/kg orally two or three times a day
Latanoprost drops	Prostaglandin analogue	once or twice a day
Pilocarpine 1% drops	Miotic	two or three times a day
Demecarium bromide	Miotic	once or twice a day
Timolol 0.5% drops	β-Adrenergic blocker	once or twice a day
Metipranolol 0.3% drops	β-Adrenergic blocker	twice a day
Levobunolol 0.5% drops	β-Adrenergic blocker	once or twice a day
Betaxolol 0.25% drops	β-Adrenergic blocker	twice a day

Figure 11.35 Medical treatments used in glaucoma.

Carbonic anhydrase inhibitors

Carbonic anhydrase inhibitors decrease the production of aqueous humour. Initially, at least, their effect can be so dramatic as to reduce the IOP by up to 50%. The therapeutic action of these agents is independent of their diuretic effects when used systemically. They are traditionally the mainstay of longer-term medical management of canine glaucoma.

The drugs of this class currently available in the UK are acetazolamide, which is used systemically, and dorzolamide and brinzolamide, which are topical preparations. Of these, the topical agents are the drugs of choice in dogs, as they appear to be as effective as acetazolamide but without the side-effects encountered with the use of systemic carbonic anhydrase inhibitors (Figure 11.36). Acetazolamide can be obtained in intravenous form for emergency use, although mannitol is more often used in these circumstances. Dichlorphenamide and methazolamide are systemic carbonic anhydrase inhibitors which can be used for the reduction of IOP in dogs; they appear to have a lower incidence of side-effects than acetazolamide. They are not currently available in the UK. For dosages, see Figure 11.35.

- Potassium depletion
- Metabolic acidosis
- Diuresis
- Anorexia
- Gastrointestinal disturbances (vomiting and diarrhoea)

Figure 11.36 Side-effects of systemic carbonic anhydrase inhibitors. Cats are particularly susceptible – use dorzolamide or brinzolamide where possible.

Prostaglandin analogues

Latanoprost is a prostaglandin pro-drug. It has recently become available for topical treatment of glaucoma and acts by causing an increase in the uveoscleral outflow of aqueous. Although this unconventional route is responsible for only 15% of aqueous drainage in the normal dog, latanoprost can have a profound effect on IOP (at least initially), even where the entrance to the ciliary cleft appears to be severely compromised gonioscopically. The drug is applied once or sometimes twice daily, usually in addition to dorzolamide. It causes miosis in dogs and cats, and the intensity of pupil constriction can cause discomfort. The prolonged use of latanoprost may result in increased iris pigmentation in some species, although this has not been reported in dogs, and its use in cases with uveitis is not recommended.

Miotics

Miotics, such as pilocarpine, have their major indication for use in primary open-angle glaucoma. They cause an increase in aqueous outflow through their action on the ciliary muscles by opening up the trabecular meshwork. In cases where the ciliary cleft is permanently collapsed or in cases of goniodysgenesis, there is little likelihood that these agents will prove effective. As these changes predominate in the canine glaucomas, the routine use of miotics is probably not indicated. Miotics may be beneficial for patients in which the drainage angle remains open, but with the advent of agents such as dorzolamide and latanoprost, their use is rarely warranted. The use of miotics is contraindicated in cases of uveitis.

Pilocarpine is a direct-acting parasympathomimetic which is generally used as a 1% solution applied two or three times a day. It may cause local irritation.

Demecarium bromide is commonly used as a miotic, but it is not currently available in topical ophthalmic form in the UK. It is an anti-cholinesterase and a potent indirect-acting parasympathomimetic. It may cause the formation of iris cysts in long-term use.

β-Adrenergic blockers

β-Adrenergic blockers are used topically to reduce aqueous production (they may also increase outflow). Their effect at the concentrations commercially available is limited (Gum et al., 1991), and as a result they are normally used in combination with a carbonic anhydrase inhibitor such as dorzolamide.

Timolol maleate is the most commonly used of these agents. Metipranolol, levobunolol and betaxolol are other β-blockers available. Betaxolol causes less marked cardiac side-effects (bradycardia) than timolol as a result of its reduced β_1-blocking activity.

α-Adrenergic agents

Sympathomimetics such as adrenaline 1% and the pro-drug dipivefrin are probably best avoided in the treatment of canine and feline glaucoma. They cause unwanted pupillary dilation, which may compromise aqueous outflow in all but open-angle glaucoma. It may be possible to reduce the pupillary effects by using these drugs in combination with a miotic such as pilocarpine.

Apraclonidine is an α_2-adrenergic agonist which is used in the short-term management of primary open-angle glaucoma in humans. It may be beneficial in some canine patients with primary open-angle glaucoma, but its effect is inconsistent, and it can cause bradycardia.

Atropine

The use of atropine is contraindicated in all cases of glaucoma except those caused by early iris bombé. A potentially devastating cause of glaucoma, iris bombé must be dealt with very aggressively – ideally within hours of onset. In these circumstances, attempting to dilate the pupil may break down posterior synechiae, allowing aqueous humour to escape from the posterior chamber. Topical 10% phenylephrine may be used in addition to atropine in these circumstances in order to maximize the desired mydriatic effect.

Tissue plasminogen activator

Tissue plasminogen activator (TPA) causes the production of plasmin from plasminogen, and this in turn results in the lysis of fibrin. Among other indications for its use, TPA may be injected intracamerally when significant quantities of fibrin are contributing to an increase in IOP. With the patient under a general anaesthetic, a small quantity (0.1–0.2 ml) of aqueous is removed by paracentesis and an equivalent volume of fluid containing 25–50 µg of TPA is injected into the anterior chamber. Clot lysis is normally complete within a few hours of injection.

Prophylactic treatment

There may be some benefit of prophylactic medical therapy in dogs with goniodysgenesis. These cases often present with glaucoma in one eye and an apparently normal opposite eye. However, gonioscopy reveals the essentially bilateral nature of goniodysgenesis and in these cases the onset of glaucoma in the contralateral eye may be delayed with the long-term use of topical dorzolamide or latanoprost.

Neuroprotection

The major means by which the optic nerve head and the retinal structures can be protected from the effects of glaucoma is by lowering IOP. However, other therapeutic strategies for neuroprotection are being developed, particularly with regard to improving survival of retinal ganglion cells and their axons. Cytotoxic levels of glutamate within the retina in glaucomatous eyes lead to an excessive influx of calcium into the retinal ganglion cells, and the systemic use of calcium channel blockers such as diltiazem and amlodipine may therefore offer a neuroprotective effect to the retinal ganglion cells (Gelatt and Brooks, 1999).

Other drugs currently under investigation may help to reduce the rate of cell death in the retina in glaucoma patients, while others may encourage regeneration of already damaged neural elements.

Surgical therapy

In many instances, particularly of primary glaucoma, medical therapy alone is not sufficient to reduce IOP to a safe level. The decision-making process as to when to undertake surgery and what procedures may be indicated is not necessarily straightforward. If the patient is a potential surgical candidate, early (and sometimes urgent) referral to a specialist should be considered.

Surgical approaches to glaucoma are aimed at either reducing aqueous production or creating an alternative pathway for aqueous drainage. The main techniques currently available for treating glaucoma are summarized in Figure 11.37.

Lens extraction:
In cases of primary lens luxation
Infrequently indicated where lens luxation is secondary to glaucoma

Procedures reducing aqueous production:
Laser cyclophotocoagulation
Cyclocryotherapy

Procedures increasing aqueous outflow:
Drainage implant surgery
Scleral trephination and peripheral iridectomy

Enucleation

Figure 11.37 Surgical techniques for management of glaucoma.

Lens extraction

In the event of primary lens luxation, removal of the lens may be sufficient to allow return to a normal IOP, especially when the condition is detected and treated promptly. In longer-standing cases, however, irreversible damage to the drainage apparatus may occur in the form of peripheral anterior synechiae. Additional surgical treatment is then likely to be required to reduce the IOP to a safe level.

When lens luxation is secondary to glaucoma, lentectomy is rarely indicated as the eye is often blind by this time; enucleation may be a better approach in these circumstances. However, if the eye is still visual, lentectomy combined with other glaucoma surgery may offer the best chance of controlling IOP and retaining useful vision.

Techniques for reducing aqueous production

These procedures involve destruction of a proportion of the ciliary body sufficient to bring IOP down to within normal limits. Surgical cyclodestruction can be achieved through laser cyclophotocoagulation, cryotherapy or diathermy. These techniques were initially employed as an alternative to enucleation in blind eyes but have become more frequently used in sighted eyes. A potential drawback of cyclodestruction is that many of the intraocular structures rely on aqueous circulation for maintenance of healthy function; significantly reducing aqueous production may therefore produce undesirable 'knock-on' effects.

Laser cyclophotocoagulation: The commonest type of laser in veterinary use for the treatment of glaucoma is the diode laser (Figure 11.38). The treatment is delivered through the sclera and the laser energy is absorbed by the pigmented tissue of the ciliary body (Figure 11.39). This causes coagulative necrosis of the ciliary processes and surrounding tissues, resulting in a reduction of aqueous production.

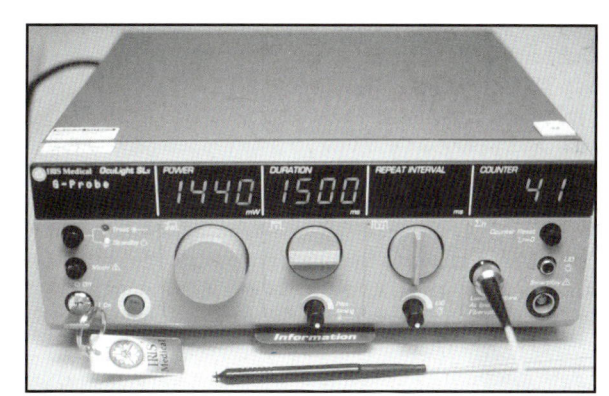

Figure 11.38 A diode laser unit.

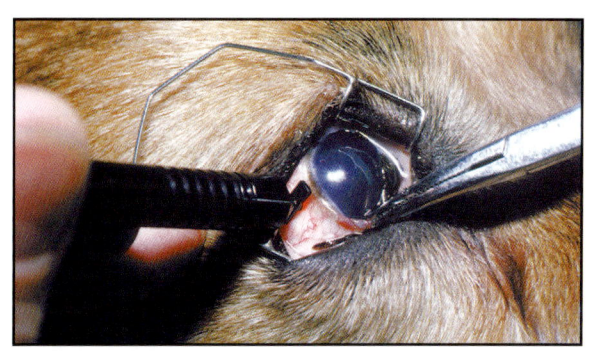

Figure 11.39 Laser cyclophotocoagulation. The globe has been rotated so that the 9 o'clock position is away from the laser beam.

The protocols in use vary but usually approximately 30–40 treatments are delivered trans-sclerally at multiple sites about 3–4 mm behind the limbus and avoiding the 3 and 9 o'clock positions (to prevent damage to the long posterior ciliary arteries). The total energy delivered is about 80 joules.

In a large series of cases of dogs with glaucoma, IOP was reduced to 30 mmHg or less in approximately 50% of patients one year after diode laser cyclophotocoagulation, although only 20% retained vision (Cook *et al.*, 1997). The complications of laser cyclophotocoagulation are listed in Figure 11.40. Laser cyclophotocoagulation has the advantages of being non-invasive and relatively quick to perform. However, management in the postoperative period can be problematical and the equipment is expensive.

- Immediate pressure spike after procedure; often requires aqueous paracentesis
- Intraocular fibrin formation/uveitis
- Intraocular haemorrhage
- Corneal ulceration
- Keratoconjunctivitis sicca
- Cataract formation
- Inadequate control of IOP
  Procedure may require repeating
  Poorly pigmented eyes absorb less energy and respond less well
- Excessive drop in IOP, leading to phthisis bulbi

Figure 11.40 Complications of laser cyclophotocoagulation.

Cyclocryotherapy: Freezing of the ciliary body through the sclera can be carried out to reduce IOP. The cryoprobe is placed over the ciliary body 5 mm from the limbus and the area is frozen until the ice ball extends to the limbus. This procedure is repeated at approximately eight sites around the globe, avoiding the 3 and 9 o'clock positions. The IOP often increases for several days after the procedure, and it therefore tends to be reserved for blind eyes, in which it is used as an alternative to enucleation.

Pharmacological ablation of the ciliary body: In blind eyes this can be achieved by the intravitreal injection of gentamicin (Moller *et al.*, 1986). However, many treated patients will eventually require enucleation, primarily due to the complications of severe uveitis and pain. The technique is not recommended and should definitely not be used in cats, as they may develop intraocular sarcoma in response to chronic inflammation and trauma (Dubielzig *et al.*, 1990). Enucleation is a more satisfactory surgical approach to end-stage glaucoma.

Techniques for increasing aqueous outflow

The best prospects for retaining vision are generally offered by techniques that improve aqueous outflow. The techniques used in dogs all aim to create an outflow for aqueous that bypasses the drainage apparatus.

Scleral trephination and peripheral iridectomy: This technique involves the formation of a drainage hole through the sclera and entering the anterior chamber (Bedford, 1977). This allows aqueous to flow from the anterior chamber into a subconjunctival bleb from which it is absorbed (Figure 11.41). A peripheral iridectomy adjacent to the sclerostomy site prevents it from becoming plugged with iris tissue and allows passage of aqueous from the posterior chamber to the anterior chamber (useful in cases of iris bombé). However, due to complications such as uveitis, and scarring of both the sclerostomy and the subconjunctival bleb, the technique frequently fails after a few months.

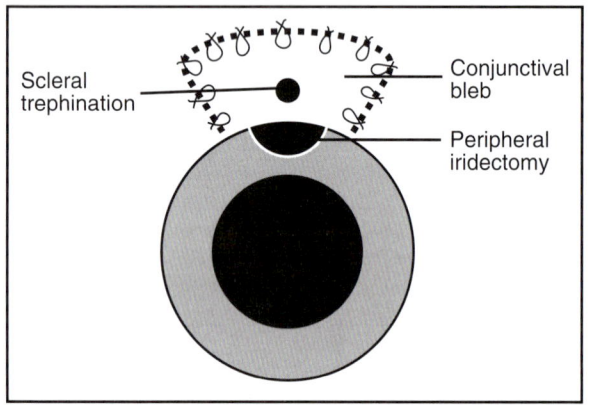

Figure 11.41 Scleral trephination and peripheral iridectomy. Aqueous flows from the anterior chamber through the trephine hole and is absorbed from a subconjunctival bleb.

Drainage implant surgery: The use of drainage implants for the treatment of selected canine glaucoma patients has gained popularity in recent years, as these devices reduce the likelihood of early postoperative failure often seen with techniques such as scleral trephination (Gelatt *et al.*, 1987, 1992; Bedford, 1989).

The use of various implant types has been reported (Garcia *et al.*, 1998), the commonest in use in the UK being the Joseph implant. A large silicone strap retained under the rectus muscles and covered by conjunctiva is joined to a silicone tube which enters the anterior chamber at the limbus (Figure 11.42). Other implants available include the Molteno, Ahmed and Krupin–Denver devices, which have smaller strap arrangements and various inbuilt valves.

The placing of a drainage implant is a major procedure and should only be performed by clinicians familiar with this type of surgery. Complications include:

- Postoperative uveitis
- Blockage of the tubing with fibrin in the immediate postoperative period. This often requires intracameral injection of TPA
- Implant loosening or loss
- Scarring of the filtering bleb, reducing aqueous absorption. This may be reduced by the interoperative use of antifibroblastic agents (e.g. mitomycin C, 5-fluorouracil). Failure often occurs at the 6–12-month stage due to scarring.

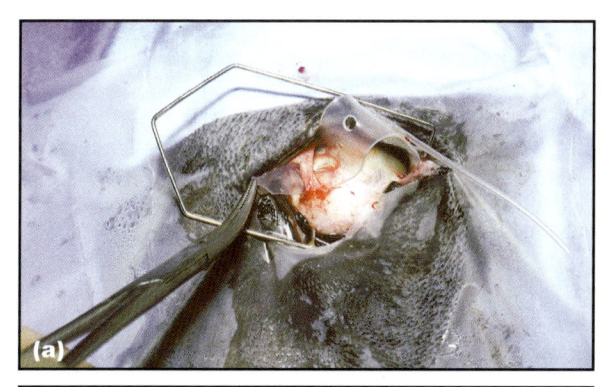

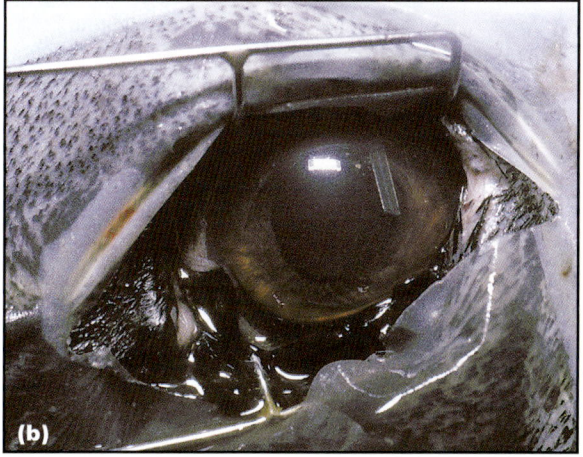

Figure 11.42 (a) A Joseph implant being placed in the left eye of a Flat-coated Retriever with primary glaucoma due to goniodysgenesis. The strap is passed under the rectus muscles and sutured in position. (b) The Joseph implant tubing in the anterior chamber at the end of the procedure.

Implant surgery and laser cyclophotocoagulation currently offer the best prospects of medium- to longer-term control of IOP, particularly in dogs with primary glaucoma. Both procedures may ultimately fail, although both can be repeated if necessary. Both carry the risk of complications, and patient management in the immediate postoperative period can be challenging. It is not uncommon for patients to have both laser cyclophotocoagulation and drainage implant surgery during the course of their glaucoma management, and there is some suggestion that combined therapy may offer advantages in terms of long-term IOP control when compared with either procedure used alone (Bentley *et al.*, 1999). In most instances, superior postoperative IOP control is afforded by continued lifelong medical therapy.

Enucleation

Despite attempts at therapy, glaucoma cases may ultimately become end-stage and enucleation may be indicated. In some patients, this may be required bilaterally. Indications for enucleation include:

- A blind eye that requires unacceptable medication or surgery to control IOP
- Intractable pain
- Buphthalmos with persistent complications due to exposure
- Primary neoplasia.

In the author's view, any irreversibly blind eye where the IOP cannot readily be kept below 40 mmHg should be enucleated on the grounds that it may be causing the patient undetected discomfort. Many owners will report an improvement in their animal's demeanour postoperatively under such circumstances.

Glaucoma in cats

The majority of the previous discussion is applicable to both dogs and cats, but some features of feline glaucoma are worthy of note.

Aetiology

Primary glaucoma is rarely seen in cats but it appears sporadically in any breed (Ridgway and Brightman, 1989; Wilcock *et al.*, 1990). There is currently no evidence of hereditary primary glaucoma such as is seen in dogs, although it has been suggested that the Siamese may be predisposed (Peiffer, 1981; Brooks, 1990). However, secondary glaucoma is not uncommon in cats and most frequently occurs as a result of uveitis or neoplasia (Wilcock *et al.*, 1990; Blocker and Van der Woerdt, 2001). Iris melanoma and intraocular lymphoma are the commonest tumours to cause glaucoma in the cat (Figure 11.43).

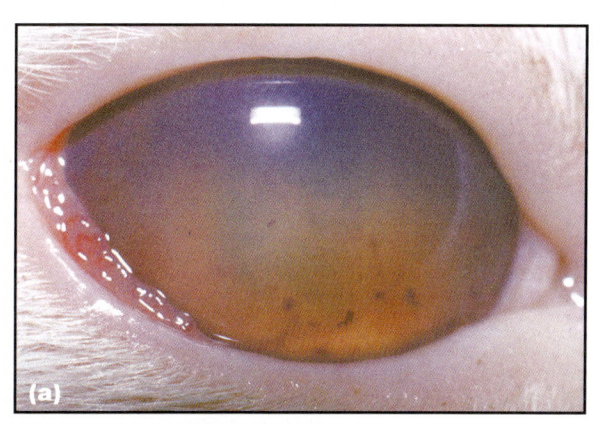

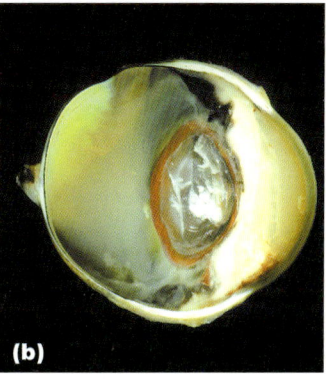

Figure 11.43 (a) Glaucoma secondary to lymphoma in an FeLV-positive domestic short-haired cat. (b) The cross-section of the globe shows that the iris is heavily infiltrated by lymphoma tissue. The aqueous appears cloudy due to the effect of fixative in the presence of high protein levels. (b, courtesy of JRB Mould)

In glaucoma secondary to uveitis, the signs of the underlying disease can be extremely subtle in cats, and careful inspection of both eyes using slit-lamp biomicroscopy may be necessary to establish that the glaucoma is indeed secondary to inflammation. Uveitis cases should be investigated for potential systemic disease (see Chapter 10).

One major difference between feline and canine glaucoma is the low incidence of primary lens luxation in cats (Olivero et al., 1991). Lens luxation associated with glaucoma in a cat is usually secondary to an underlying uveitis (sometimes with resultant cataract formation) or globe enlargement, or a combination of the two.

Other causes of secondary glaucoma in cats include trauma and intraocular haemorrhage (frequently secondary to systemic hypertension).

Clinical signs

Feline glaucoma is very commonly insidious in onset. Signs of pain, corneal oedema and episcleral injection are frequently much less marked than in dogs. Alteration to the ophthalmoscopic appearance of the optic nerve head is less marked in cats with chronic glaucoma than in dogs, due to the normally smaller and darker appearance of the unmyelinated optic disc in cats. The first presenting signs may include suspected vision loss (although cats are extremely good at adapting to blindness) or, more often, a change in the appearance of the eye due to mydriasis, buphthalmos, uveitis or tumour (Figure 11.44). Any uveitis case on long-term management should be carefully monitored for the possibility of glaucoma development, and this can only be achieved by regularly measuring the IOP. This is of particular importance, as topical steroids have been shown to cause elevation of the IOP in normal cats (Zhan et al., 1992).

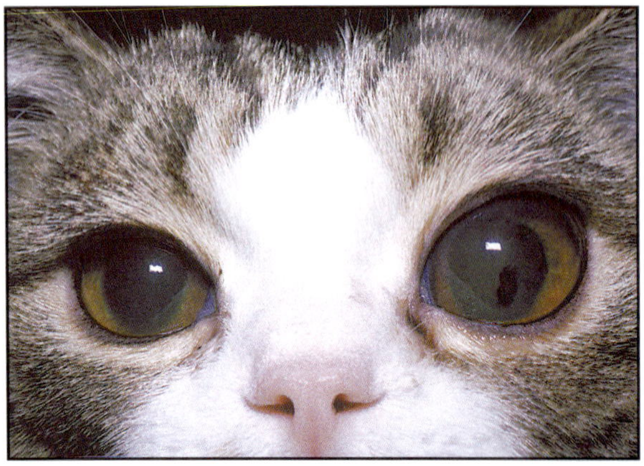

Figure 11.44 A 1-year-old domestic short-haired cat with bilateral glaucoma secondary to uveitis caused by feline infectious peritonitis. The left eye is grossly enlarged and shows signs of a haemorrhagic inflammatory deposit on the corneal endothelium.

Therapy

The treatment of glaucoma in cats is similar to that in dogs, although, due to late presentation and the high incidence of secondary causes, the outcome is often disappointing. The primary aim is to treat the underlying cause of the glaucoma, and in cases with uveitis this may be sufficient to reduce IOP to within normal limits. However, in some instances the underlying uveitis may be low-grade and poorly responsive to medical therapy; in these circumstances a relentless progression of the secondary glaucoma may occur, leading to blindness and end-stage disease.

Cats appear to tolerate topical treatment with dorzolamide and brinzolamide very well, and these drugs can give good control of IOP when used two or three times daily. Cats tolerate systemic carbonic anhydrase inhibitors poorly, and the use of acetazolamide in this species is not recommended. There is no published evidence regarding the use of latanoprost in cats, although it does cause marked miosis.

All too often, medical treatment may ultimately prove to be ineffective in controlling glaucoma in cats. In some instances, there may be side-effects, particularly of systemic therapy, which are not warranted, particularly if vision has already been lost. Should the eye be irreversibly blind and if the pressure cannot readily be kept below a level of around 40 mmHg, then enucleation may be the best policy. Intravitreal gentamicin injections should not be used, as chronically damaged feline eyes are at risk of developing intraocular sarcoma.

The surgical therapies described for dogs can be applied to cats. They are rarely performed, however, as a result of the late presentation and secondary nature of a large proportion of feline cases.

References and further reading

Barnett KC (1990) Glaucoma. In: *A Colour Atlas of Veterinary Ophthalmology*, ed. KC Barnett, pp. 70–74. Wolfe Publishing, London

Barnett KC and Crispin SM (1998) Aqueous and glaucoma. In: *Feline Ophthalmology*, ed. KC Barnett and SM Crispin, pp. 104–111. W B Saunders, London

Bedford PGC (1977) The surgical treatment of canine glaucoma. *Journal of Small Animal Practice* **18**, 713–730

Bedford PGC (1980) The aetiology of canine glaucoma. *Veterinary Record* **107**, 76–82

Bedford PGC (1989) A clinical evaluation of a one-piece drainage system in the treatment of canine glaucoma. *Journal of Small Animal Practice* **30**, 68–75

Bentley E, Miller PE, Murphy CJ and Schoster JV (1999) Combined cycloablation and gonioimplantation for treatment of glaucoma in dogs: 18 cases (1992–1998). *Journal of the American Veterinary Medical Association* **215**, 1469–1472

Blocker T and Van der Woerdt (2001) The feline glaucomas (1995–1999). *Veterinary Ophthalmology* **4**, 81–85

Brooks DE (1990) Glaucoma in the dog and cat. *Veterinary Clinics of North America: Small Animal Practice* **20**, 775–797

Brooks DE, Komaromy AM and Kallberg ME (1999) Comparative optic nerve physiology: implications for glaucoma, neuroprotection and neuroregeneration. *Veterinary Ophthalmology* **2**, 13–25

Cook CS (1997) Surgery for glaucoma. *Veterinary Clinics of North America* **27**, 1109–1129

Cook CS, Davidson M, Brinkmann M, Priehs D, Abrams K and Nasisse M (1997) Diode laser transscleral cyclophotocoagulation for the treatment of glaucoma in dogs: results of six and twelve month follow-up. *Veterinary and Comparative Ophthalmology* **7**, 148–154

Cottrell BD and Barnett KC (1988) Primary glaucoma in the Welsh Springer Spaniel. *Journal of Small Animal Practice* **29**, 185–199

Deehr AJ and Dubielzig RR (1997) Glaucoma in Golden Retrievers. *Proceedings of the American College of Veterinary Ophthalmologists* **28**, 5

Dubielzig RR, Everitt J and Shadduck JA (1990) Clinical and morphological features of post-traumatic ocular sarcomas in cats. *Veterinary Pathology* **27**, 62–65

Ekesten B (1993) Correlation of intraocular distances to the iridocorneal angle in Samoyeds with special reference to angle-closure glaucoma. *Progress in Veterinary and Comparative Ophthalmology* **3**, 67–73

Garcia GA, Brooks DE, Gelatt KN, Kubilis PS, Gil F and Whitley RD (1998) Evaluation of valved and non-valved implants in 83 eyes of 65 dogs with glaucoma. *Animal Eye Research* **17**, 9–16

Gelatt KN and Brooks DE (1999) The canine glaucomas. In: *Veterinary Ophthalmology*, 3rd edn, ed. KN Gelatt, pp. 701–754. Lippincott, Williams & Wilkins, Philadelphia

Gelatt KN, Brooks DE, Miller TR, Smith PJ, Sapienza JS and Pellicane CP (1992). Issues in ophthalmic therapy: the development of anterior chamber shunts for the clinical management of canine glaucomas. *Progress in Veterinary Ophthalmology* **2**, 59–64

Gelatt KN, Gum GG, Samuelson DA, Mandelkorn RM, Olander KW and Zimmerman TJ (1987) Evaluation of the Krupin–Denver valve implant in normotensive and glaucomatous beagles. *Journal of the American Veterinary Medical Association* **191**, 1404–1409

Gelatt KN, Peiffer RL, Gum GG and Gwin RM (1977) Evaluation of applanation tonometers for the dog eye. *Investigative Ophthalmology and Visual Science* **16**, 963–968

Gum GG, Gelatt KN and Knepper PA (1993) Histochemical localisation of glycosaminoglycans in the aqueous outflow pathways in normal Beagles and Beagles with inherited glaucoma. *Veterinary and Comparative Ophthalmology* **3**, 52–57

Gum GG, Larocca RD, Gelatt KN, Mead JP and Gelatt JK (1991) The effect of topical timolol maleate on IOP in normal beagles and beagles with inherited glaucoma. *Progress in Veterinary and Comparative Ophthalmology* **1**, 141–149

Lazarus JA, Pickett JP and Champagne ES (1998) Primary lens luxation in the Chinese Shar Pei: clinical and hereditary characteristics. *Veterinary Ophthalmology* **1**, 101–107

Martin CL (1975) Scanning electron microscopic examination of selected canine iridocorneal angle abnormalities. *Journal of the American Animal Hospital Association* **11**, 300–306

Miller PE and Pickett JP (1992a) Comparison of the human and canine Schiøtz tonometry conversion tables in clinically normal dogs. *Journal of the American Veterinary Medical Association* **201**, 1021–1025

Miller PE and Pickett JP (1992b) Comparison of the human and canine Schiøtz tonometry conversion tables in clinically normal cats. *Journal of the American Veterinary Medical Association* **201**, 1017–1020

Moller I, Cook CS, Peiffer RL, Nasisse MP and Harling DE (1986) Indications for and complications of pharmacological ablation of the ciliary body for the treatment of chronic glaucoma in the dog. *Journal of the American Veterinary Medical Association* **22**, 319–326

Olivero DK, Riis RC, Dutton AG, Murphy CJ, Nasisse MP and Davidson MG (1991) Feline lens displacement. A retrospective analysis of 345 cases. *Progress in Veterinary and Comparative Ophthalmology* **1**, 239–244

Peiffer RL (1981) Feline glaucoma. In: *Veterinary Ophthalmology*, 1st edn, ed. KN Gelatt, p. 547. Lea & Febiger, Philadelphia

Peiffer RL, Wilcock BP and Yin H (1990) The pathogenesis and significance of pre-iridal fibrovascular membrane in domestic animals. *Veterinary Pathology* **27**, 41–45

Petersen-Jones SM (1991) Abnormal ocular pigment deposition associated with glaucoma in the Cairn terrier. *Journal of Small Animal Practice* **32**, 19–22

Read RA, Wood JLN and Lakhani KH (1998) Pectinate ligament dysplasia in Flat Coated Retrievers. I. Objectives, techniques and results of a PLD survey. *Veterinary Ophthalmology* **1**, 85–90

Ridgway MD and Brightman AH (1989) Feline glaucoma: a retrospective study of 29 clinical cases. *Journal of the American Animal Hospital Association* **25**, 485–490

Regnier A (1999) Ocular pharmacology and therapeutics. Part 2. Antimicrobial, anti-inflammatory agents and antiglaucoma drugs. In: *Veterinary Ophthalmology*, 3rd edn, ed. KN Gelatt. pp. 336. Lippincott, Williams & Wilkins, Philadelphia

Wilcock B, Peiffer RL and Davidson MG (1990) The causes of glaucoma in cats. *Veterinary Pathology* **27**, 35–40

Zhan GL, Miranda OC and Bito LZ (1992) Steroid glaucoma: corticosteroid-induced ocular hypertension in cats. *Experimental Eye Research* **54**, 211–218

12

The lens

Simon Petersen-Jones

Embryology, anatomy and physiology

Formation of the lens vesicle
The lens is formed from surface ectoderm of the developing embryo. An outbudding of neurectoderm from the presumptive forebrain forms the optic vesicle. This will give rise to the neurosensory retina, retinal pigment epithelium, ciliary and iridal epithelium and a portion of the iris musculature. As the optic vesicle approaches the surface ectoderm, it induces a thickening of the ectoderm, known as the lens placode. As the optic vesicle invaginates to form the double-layered optic cup, the overlying lens placode also invaginates to become a spherical, hollow monolayer of cells positioned in the mouth of the optic vesicle.

This process is shown in Figure 12.1.

Formation of primary lens fibres
The posterior cells of the lens vesicle elongate to form primary lens fibres which obliterate the cavity within the developing lens. These fibres remain in the adult lens at the very centre of the nucleus. The anterior cells lining the lens vesicle persist as the anterior lens epithelium.

Formation of secondary lens fibres
The remaining anterior lens epithelial cells remain active and form the secondary lens fibres throughout life. Epithelial cells at the equator of the lens elongate such that a single fibre extends into the anterior and posterior cortex. The secondary fibres are hexagonal in cross-section and form a regular arrangement with adjacent fibres, conferring transparency to the adult lens. Where the tips of lens fibres from different regions of the lens equator meet, they form a pattern known as the lens suture lines. In their simplest pattern, the suture lines in the anterior cortex

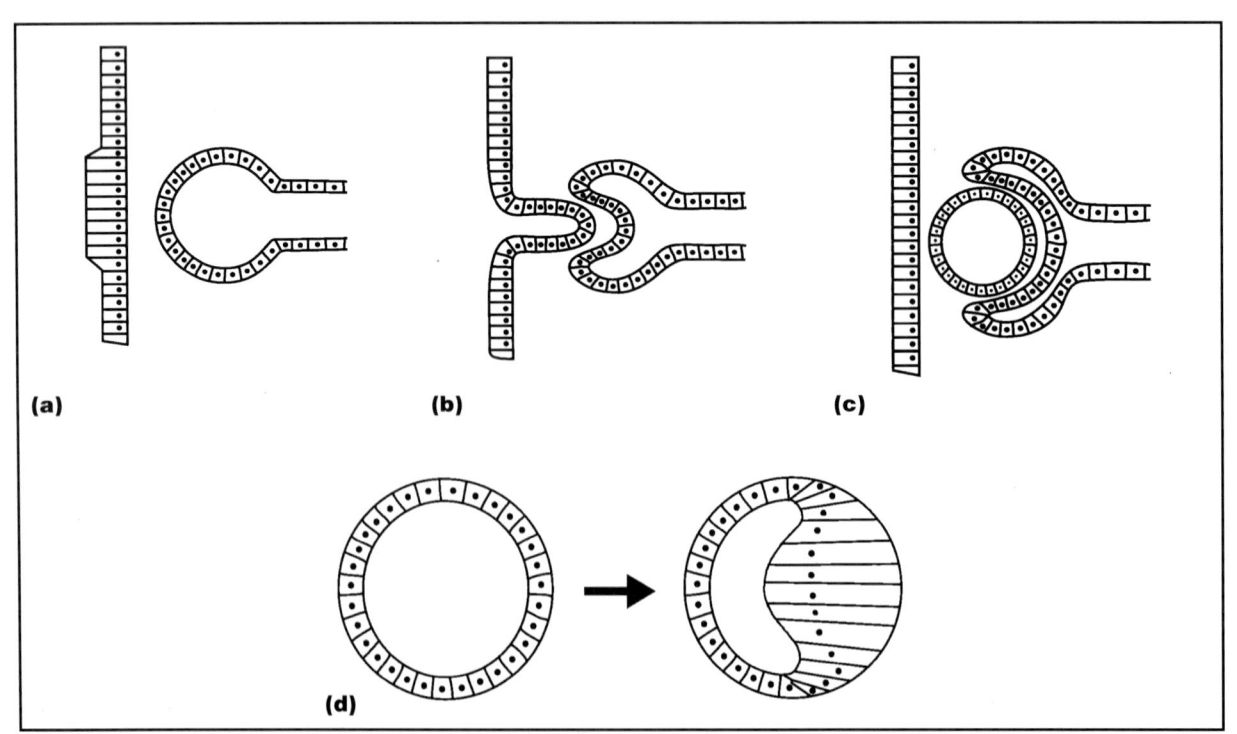

Figure 12.1 Embryology of the lens. (a) The optic vesicle develops as an outbudding of neurectoderm in the region of the developing forebrain. It induces a thickening of the overlying surface ectoderm to form the lens placode. (b) As the optic vesicle invaginates to form the optic cup, the lens placode invaginates from the surface ectoderm. (c) The lens vesicle consists of a hollow sphere with a single layer of cells. (d) The posterior cells of the lens vesicle elongate to form primary lens fibres which obliterate the cavity, forming the lens vesicle.

form an upright Y, while those in the posterior cortex form an inverted Y shape (Figure 12.2). The suture lines may be faintly visible in the adult lens and can become more apparent in some forms of cataract.

Histologically, the nuclei of the epithelial cells are seen to form a line that curves into the lens at the equatorial region; this is known as the lens bow. The constant formation of new secondary lens fibres compresses the more central portions of the lens and is ultimately responsible for the hardening of the lens nucleus that develops in elderly animals. This is known as nuclear sclerosis.

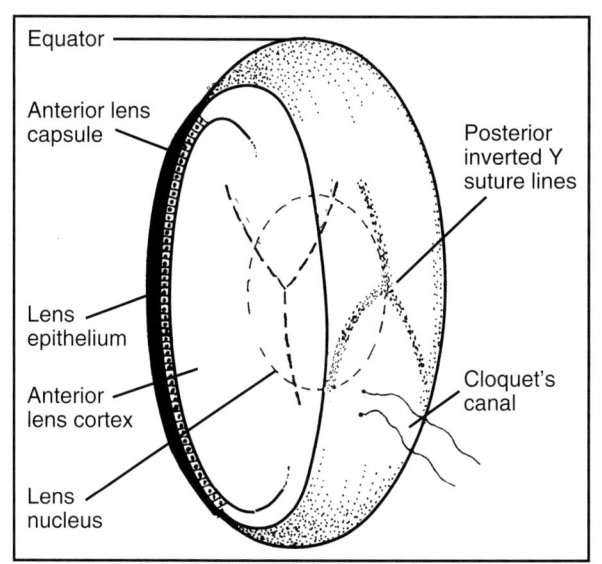

Figure 12.2 Diagram showing different areas of the adult lens and the lens sutures. The anterior lens suture lines are in the form of an upright Y, while the posterior ones are an inverted Y. Cloquet's canal can often be seen arising from the posterior lens surface.

Formation of the lens capsule

An elastic acellular capsule surrounds the lens and is the basement membrane of the lens epithelial cells. Posterior lens epithelial cells are only present during the early development of the lens, so the capsule they form is considerably thinner than the anterior capsule, which continues to be produced throughout life. The anterior capsule, therefore, thickens with age.

Blood supply to the developing lens

During embryological development, the lens is nourished by an extensive blood supply. The hyaloid vasculature enters the optic cup through the ventral optic fissure and traverses the future vitreal cavity to reach the posterior surface of the lens and ramify across its surface as the tunica vasculosa lentis. The hyaloid vasculature and supporting structures are known as the primary vitreous.

Vascular supply is also derived from an annular vessel at the anterior edge of the optic cup. This supplies the pupillary membrane, a network of vessels which is present over the anterior surface of the lens. As the eye matures, this vasculature regresses, with little evidence of its previous presence being visible in the adult eye. Sometimes, developmental anomalies associated with persistence of the embryonic vasculature are encountered, and these include persistent pupillary membrane and persistent hyperplastic tunica vasculosa lentis / persistent hyperplastic primary vitreous.

The adult lens

In the adult animal, the lens is a transparent biconvex structure consisting of a central nucleus, surrounding cortical lens fibres and an elastic acellular capsule (Figure 12.3). It is positioned in the patella fossa of the anterior face of the vitreous and is held in position by numerous bundles of transparent fibres known as zonules or suspensory ligaments. The zonules originate on and between the ciliary processes of the ciliary body and insert on to the lens capsule both anterior and posterior to the lens equator (Figure 12.4). It is possible to see the insertions of the zonular fibres on the lens capsule in the live animal by examining the lens periphery with the aid of magnification.

Muscular action within the ciliary body alters the tension on the zonules and thus alters the lens shape and, therefore, its optical power. This process is known as dynamic accommodation and only occurs to a limited degree in dogs and cats. There is a firm attachment of the vitreous to the mid-periphery of the posterior lens capsule at the hyaloideocapsular ligament. Anteriorly, the posterior surface of the pupillary zone of the iris slides across the surface of the lens as the pupillary diameter alters. The iris bows anteriorly due to the convex shape of the anterior lens surface on which it rests. This can be seen by looking obliquely across the anterior chamber of the eye.

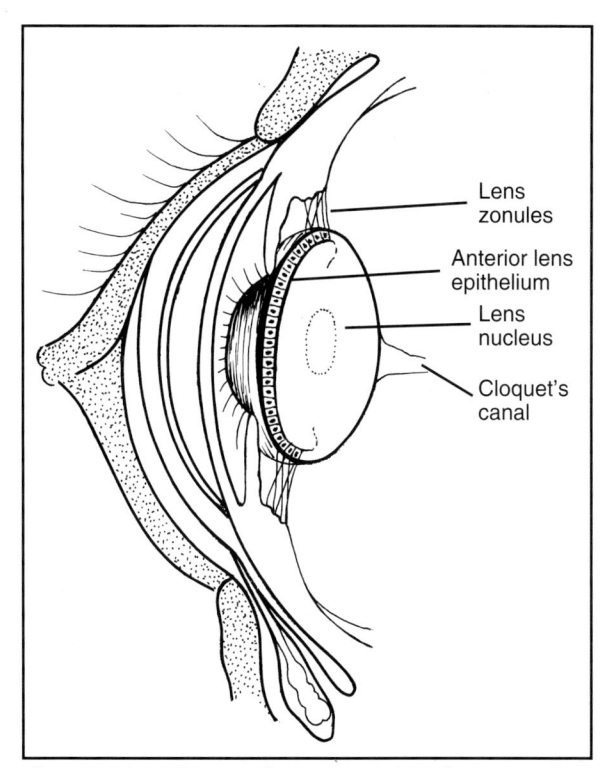

Figure 12.3 Diagram of a cross-section of an eye showing the normal lens position in the patella fossa of the anterior vitreous face. Zonular fibres attach the lens to the ciliary body, holding the lens firmly in place and allowing accommodation. The iris rests on the anterior lens surface.

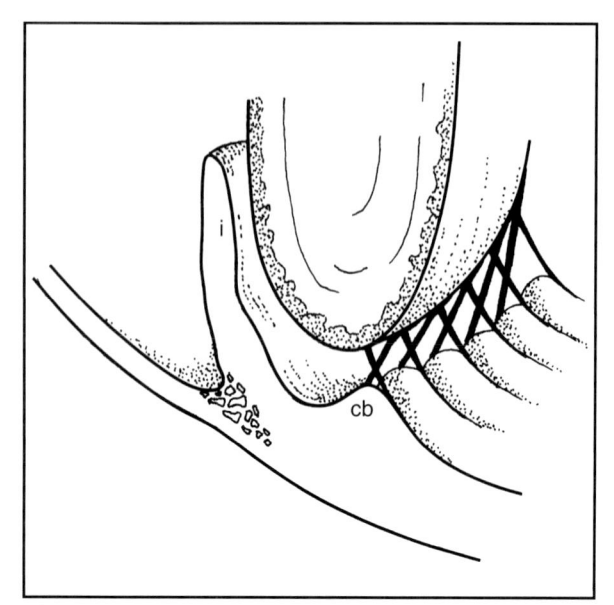

Figure 12.4 Diagram showing the zonular attachments to the lens. Note that zonular fibres arising from the peaks of the ciliary processes insert posterior to the lens equator, while those arising from the valleys between the processes insert anterior to the lens equator. cb=ciliary body; i = iris; l = lens.

Since the adult lens does not have a blood supply, it must rely on the aqueous to supply oxygen and nutrients and to remove waste products. Pathological changes within the lens can result in an increase in the amount of insoluble lens protein, an alteration in the proportions of different lens crystallins and a breakdown in the normal metabolic pathways of the lens, accompanied by increased lens hydration. These changes result in deposition of lens protein, disruption of lens fibres due to vacuole formation and, hence, a loss of lens transparency, known as cataract.

Examination of the lens

This is also discussed in Chapter 1a.

Pupillary dilation
The pupillary light reflex should be assessed prior to the application of a mydriatic.

Dilation of the pupil is required to examine the more peripheral (equatorial) regions of the lens. Tropicamide is the most frequently used mydriatic agent, because of its rapid action (about 20 minutes to dilate the pupil). A mydriatic should be avoided in animals with, or suspected of having, glaucoma, and used with care in those with lens instability.

Examination with a transilluminator
A transilluminator or, if this is not available, a bright penlight should be used to examine the lens.

Initially, the light should be shone along the visual axis of the eye and the lens examined by looking directly along the beam of light. Lens opacities will be highlighted against the tapetal reflection.

Following this, the light is kept shining along the visual axis and the observer moves to examine the eye obliquely, to judge the depth of the anterior chamber. Within the pupil of the normal eye, the convex anterior face of the lens can be seen with the iris resting on the surface. Oblique examination is useful in judging the position of opacities within the lens.

Following this examination, the light is shone into the eye from different directions and the lens is also viewed from different directions. This should enable the examiner to detect any opacity within the lens and see any evidence of lens instability. With experience, the localization of cataracts within the lens can be described accurately.

Inexperienced observers may find parallax helpful in deciding the depth of an opacity in the lens. While continuing to look at the opacity along the beam of the examining light, the examiner moves sideways, looking to see the apparent direction of movement of the opacity:

- Anterior lens opacities will appear to move in the same direction as the examiner
- Posterior lens opacities will appear to move in the opposite direction to the examiner
- At the posterior border of the nucleus, opacities will appear to remain stationary.

Wobbling of the lens or iris with eye movements (phacodonesis and iridodonesis, respectively) are indicators of lens instability. The equatorially attached lens zonules may be seen to be stretched if there is some lens instability with resulting subluxation, or an abnormally small lens.

Distant direct ophthalmoscopy
Careful examination using a transilluminator should enable the examiner to detect lens opacities and to distinguish cataract from nuclear sclerosis. However, distant direct ophthalmoscopy can be used as an additional check for opacities and to help distinguish nuclear sclerosis from cataract. The eye is viewed at arm's length through the direct ophthalmoscope. A zero or +1 dioptre lens is usually selected to bring the eye into focus. The tapetal reflection will highlight any opacity present on the transparent structures from the cornea to the anterior vitreous (including the lens). Actual lens opacities will appear as black shadows against the tapetal reflection, while a sclerotic nucleus appears as an obvious but transparent sphere within the lens.

Magnification to examine the lens
A direct ophthalmoscope can be used to examine opacities of the lens in more detail. A +12 dioptre setting is required for the anterior of the lens and +8 for the posterior of the lens. A slit-lamp biomicroscope provides superior magnification and illumination. With the use of an obliquely directed slit beam of light, lens opacities can be very accurately localized and examined in great detail.

Conditions of the canine lens

Congenital conditions

Aphakia
Aphakia means a lack of lens. Congenital aphakia is extremely rare and only occurs in severely malformed and cystic eyes.

Microphakia
Microphakia means an abnormally small lens. This may occur in dogs with multiple congenital ocular defects, including microphthalmos and cataracts. It may also be a feature of more severe forms of persistent hyperplastic primary vitreous/ persistent tunica vasculosa lentis (see below).

Lens coloboma
A lens coloboma is a rare condition in which an area of the lens, usually at the equator, has not formed, resulting in a notch in the affected region (Figure 12.5).

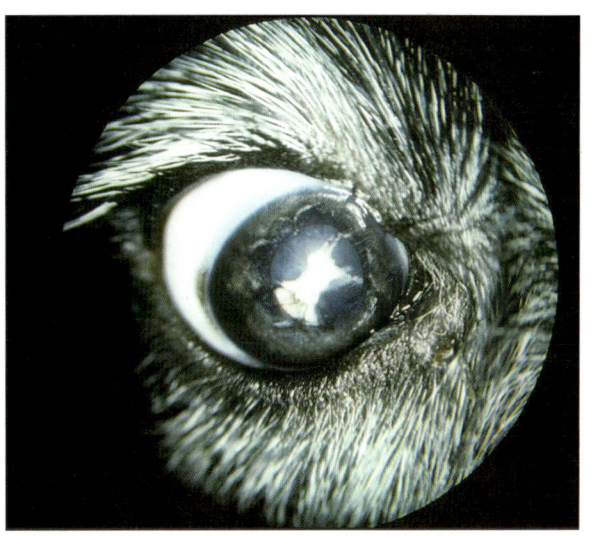

Figure 12.6 An English Cocker Spaniel puppy with microphthalmos, persistent pupillary membrane and cataract. There is a dense white capsular plaque that protrudes into the anterior chamber.

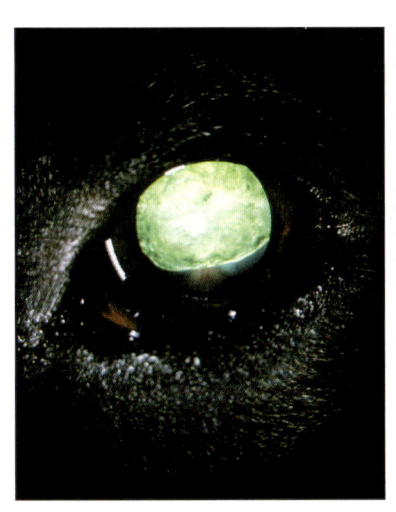

Figure 12.5 An abnormally shaped lens in a young dog. The ventral portion of the lens has not formed (coloboma). Note the gap between the pupil edge and the lens equator ventrally. The lens is also developing a cataract.

Capsular cataracts associated with persistent pupillary membrane (PPM)
PPM represents abnormal remnants of the embryonic vasculature of the anterior chamber. Typically, strands of iris-coloured tissue arise from the iris collarette, approximately one third of the distance from the pupil edge to the iris root. They may insert at a variety of sites (see Chapter 10), including the anterior lens capsule. There is usually a focal capsular and subcapsular cataract at the insertion point. PPM remnants may occur in eyes with microphthalmos and multiple ocular abnormalities (Figure 12.6). Persistent pupillary membrane remnants attaching to the lens capsule should not be confused with posterior synechiae, which are post-inflammatory iris to lens adhesions (see Chapter 10).

Other mesodermal remnants
The mildest form of anterior chamber mesodermal remnants are collections of small circular pigment spots seen axially on the anterior capsule of some dogs (Figure 12.7). English Cocker Spaniels in particular are affected. The pigment spots may be so small that they are difficult to see without magnification.

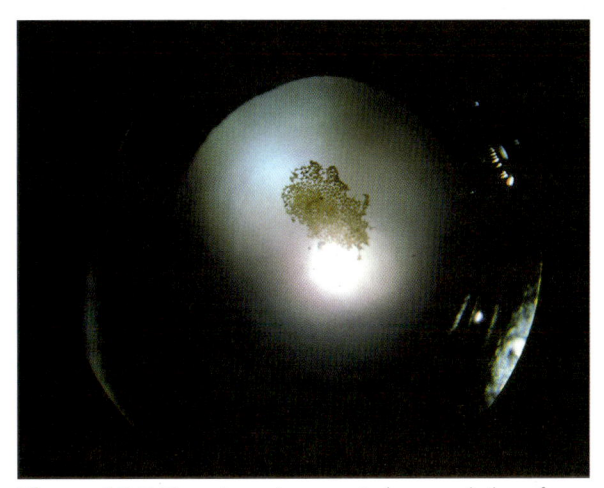

Figure 12.7 Mesodermal remnants (accumulation of pigmented 'spots') on the anterior lens capsule.

Persistent hyperplastic primary vitreous/persistent hyperplastic tunica vasculosa lentis (PHPV/PHTVL)
As described earlier in this chapter, the embryonic lens is supplied by a ramifying network of blood vessels with supporting tissue. In PHPV/PHTVL, variable proportions of this vascular network persist and proliferate into adult life. The severity of the resulting lesions varies considerably between affected dogs. Typically, a fibrovascular plaque is present on the posterior lens surface and involves the lens capsule (Figure 12.8). The lens itself may be abnormally shaped and cataractous. Persistent hyaloid vasculature may also be present. Intravitreal or intralenticular haemorrhage can also occur.

PHPV/PHTVL is variable in its severity, with more severe cases resulting in blindness. Clinically, the presence of blood vessels and sometimes pigment within a plaque on the posterior lens capsule allows the condition to be differentiated from uncomplicated cataract.

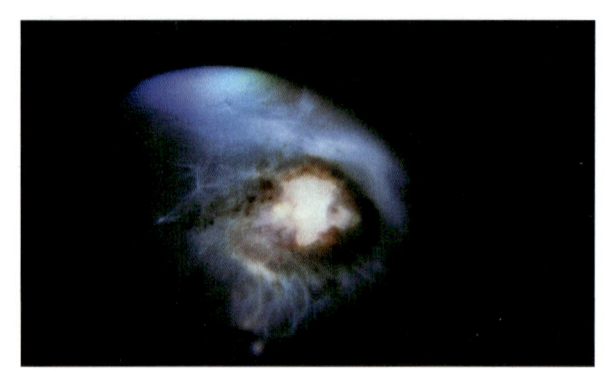

Figure 12.8 PHPV/PHTVL in a young Whippet. The photograph is focused on the fibrovascular plaque on the posterior capsule of the lens.

Surgery on eyes with PHPV/PHTVL to remove the cataract and posterior capsular fibrovascular plaque is possible, but the success rate is lower than that of conventional cataract surgery, because of the risk of complications, such as haemorrhage from patent vessels supplying the fibrovascular plaque. Further discussion of this condition can be found in Chapter 13.

Congenital cataract

Congenital cataracts can occur in otherwise normal eyes. They are considered in the section on cataracts below.

Acquired conditions

Nuclear sclerosis

Nuclear sclerosis is a hardening of the nucleus of the lens that occurs in all older dogs due to the compression of the more central portions of the lens. The difference in refractive index between the compressed nucleus and surrounding cortex gives the lens a bluish-grey appearance that is often mistaken for cataract. Examination of the lens as described previously should allow nuclear sclerosis to be distinguished from cataract.

Cataract

A cataract is an opacity of the lens or its capsule. Cataract formation is common in dogs. Detailed examination of the lens, allowing a description of the extent of the cataract, its position in the lens and the appearance of the opacity, helps in the classification of a cataract.

The position of the opacity in the lens may be capsular, subcapsular, nuclear or cortical. It may involve the visual axis and lie at the anterior or posterior poles of the lens, or involve the equatorial region of the lens. Accurate localization and recording is important in monitoring the progress of cataracts and in deciding whether a cataract is typical of inherited cataracts seen in that particular breed.

Lens opacities vary in appearance. Lens vacuoles may be present: these appear like bubbles of fluid within the lens, or some opacities may manifest as dense white condensations. Sometimes, the cataract involves just a few lens fibres, which can be seen highlighted within the lens; in other cases, the lens suture lines may be involved or the entire lens may be cataractous.

Cataracts may be classified by age at onset, stage of development or aetiology.

Classification by age of onset: Cataracts may be present as a congenital abnormality (congenital cataract), develop in the young animal (juvenile cataract) or develop in old age (senile cataract).

Congenital cataracts: These are often associated with other ocular abnormalities such as microphthalmos, PPM, PHPV/PHTVL and retinal dysplasia. When multiple ocular abnormalities are present, there may also be abnormal eye movements, ranging from a fine oscillatory nystagmus to a more rotatory type of movement. This is described as a searching nystagmus. Congenital cataracts are quite often stationary and may actually decrease in size relative to the entire lens if clear lens fibres are produced as the lens grows. In many instances, cataract surgery is not required.

Congenital cataract associated with microphthalmos is breed related and shown to be inherited in the Miniature Schnauzer. Other breeds in which the condition is common include the English Cocker Spaniel, Golden Retriever, Old English Sheepdog and West Highland White Terrier. In these breeds, the defect, although breed related, does not appear to follow a simple Mendelian mode of inheritance, and environmental factors may play a major role in the aetiology (Strande *et al.*, 1988).

The severity of the condition varies between affected puppies, even within the same litter. Some members of a litter may have marked microphthalmos, whereas others may have eyes which appear grossly to be of normal size and only have small cataracts. The region of the lens involved usually includes the nucleus, but in some eyes there is cortical involvement and the presence of dense white capsular plaques that protrude into the anterior chamber. When the cataracts are axial in position, the dog's vision may be improved by keeping the pupil dilated by the use of topical atropine drops although, sometimes, the pupils will only partially dilate.

The Y suture lines are often clearly visible in puppies' eyes, and this should not be confused with congenital or early-onset cataract. Temporary developmental lens opacities are sometimes seen in puppies of a few weeks of age (Figure 12.9). These are arrow-tip-shaped opacities situated at the equatorial end of one or more of the lens suture lines. These transient opacities disappear within a few weeks.

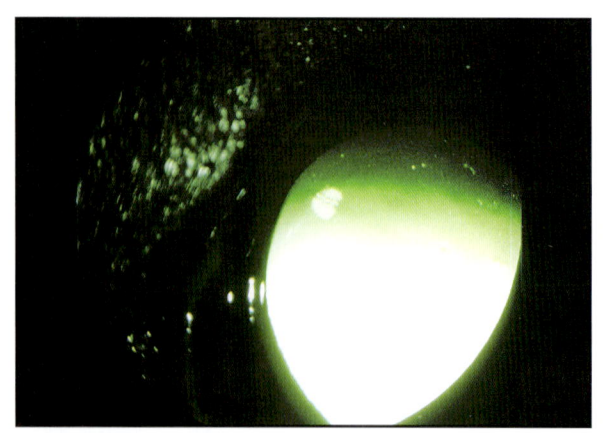

Figure 12.9 Temporary lens opacity at the tip of a lens suture line in a puppy. The three tips of the suture lines were affected. This type of opacity is only temporary.

Juvenile cataracts: Primary cataracts that develop in juvenile animals are inherited in some breeds and may progress to involve the entire lens.

Senile cataracts: These are common in dogs, and most animals presenting for cataract surgery are middle aged and older.

Classification by stage of development

Incipient cataracts: These are very early lens changes (Figure 12.10). These may involve just a few lens fibres or a small area of the lens. The presence of vacuoles suggests that the cataract may progress. Incipient cataracts have little or no effect on vision.

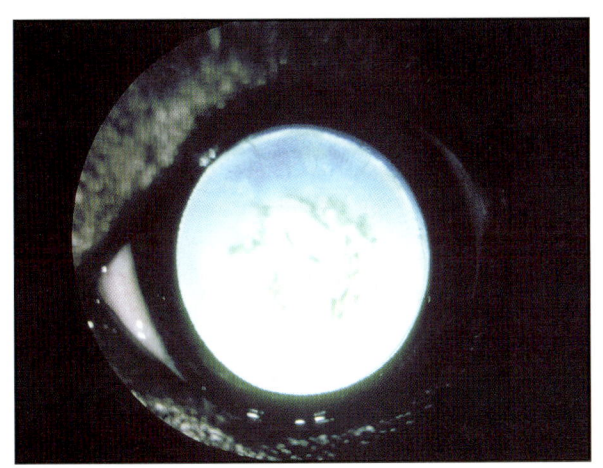

Figure 12.10 Incipient cataract in a young Staffordshire Bull Terrier; the lens opacity can be seen silhouetted against the tapetal reflex.

Immature cataracts: The entire lens is not yet involved and a fundic reflex can still be seen (Figure 12.11). This reflex can be used to highlight lens changes, making them more readily detected. The fundus may still be examinable by indirect ophthalmoscopy.

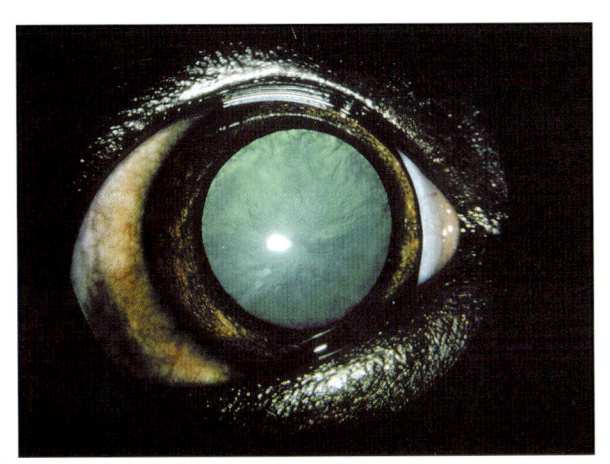

Figure 12.11 A late immature cataract in a dog; the tapetal reflex is still visible.

Mature cataracts: With these, the entire lens is opaque, and a tapetal reflex cannot be seen (Figure 12.12). The affected eye will be blind. The cataract may take up fluid and swell (intumescence), thus becoming

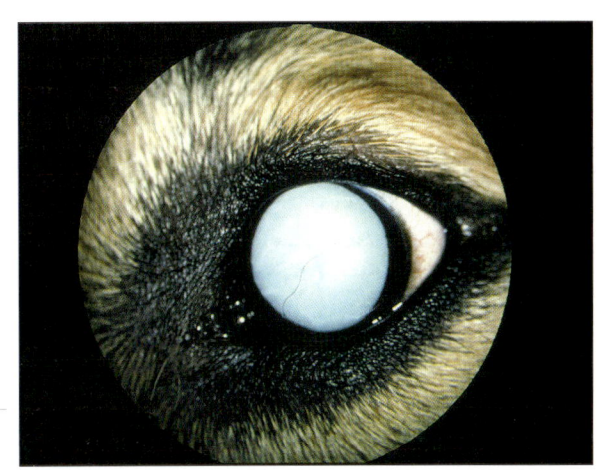

Figure 12.12 A mature cataract in a dog; the tapetal reflex can no longer be seen.

hypermature. Intumescence is commonest in rapidly developing cataracts secondary to diabetes mellitus; it results in a shallow anterior chamber. In some cases, compromise of aqueous drainage and increased intraocular pressure can result. The increase in size of the lens in such cases, which is sometimes dramatic, can be fully appreciated on ocular ultrasonography.

Hypermature cataracts: There are varying degrees of hypermaturity of the cataract. Fluid accumulation may lead to separation of the lens along the suture lines, resulting in a Y-shaped cleft within the lens. Liquefied lens proteins may leak out through the lens capsule. Exposure of the uvea to these proteins, which are considered 'foreign' by the immune system, induces an anterior uveitis. Some degree of lens-induced, or phacolytic, uveitis can be detected in most eyes with mature to hypermature cataracts. Signs include mild episcleral congestion, lowered intraocular pressure and a darkening of the iris. The pupil may be resistant to the effects of mydriatics. Sometimes a more severe uveitis results, leading to the formation of iris rests (pigment deposited from the iris on the anterior lens capsule), posterior synechiae (iris to lens adhesions – Figure 12.13), keratic precipitates and even secondary glaucoma.

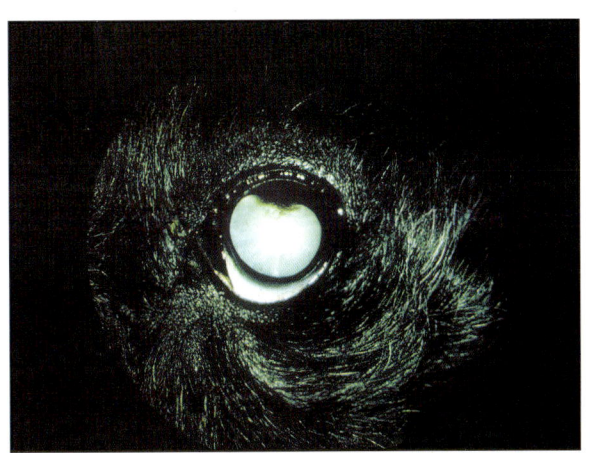

Figure 12.13 A hypermature cataract with lens-induced uveitis. The inflammation has resulted in posterior synechiae, leading to an abnormally shaped pupil.

Secondary changes in the vitreous may also develop; these may eventually cause retinal detachment. In some instances, the cataractous lens may luxate.

Loss of liquefied lens material results in a wrinkled lens capsule (best detected when the anterior surface of the lens is viewed obliquely). If sufficient lens material is lost, the anterior chamber will appear deeper and the face of the iris will appear flatter (the iris is normally bowed anteriorly by the convex shape of the anterior lens surface). Liquefied lens material may be present, swirling in the lens capsule with eye movements. Refractile condensations of lens proteins are common, appearing as shiny flecks of cataractous material.

Some dogs may have significant clearing of the visual axis as a result of lens resorption. This tends to occur more frequently in young animals with rapidly developing cataracts. If the more severe secondary ocular changes (uveitis, glaucoma and retinal detachment) do not develop, useful sight may be restored (Figure 12.14).

Category	Examples
Congenital	Inherited *In utero* insult
Inherited	Seen in certain breeds (see Figure 12.16)
Secondary to other ocular disease	Glaucoma Uveitis Generalized progressive retinal atrophy Chronic lens luxation Persistent hyperplastic primary vitreous Retinal dysplasia
Trauma	Penetrating wounds which damage the lens capsule Blunt trauma
Metabolic	Diabetes mellitus Hypocalcaemia
Toxic or dietary	Orphaned puppies fed inappropriate milk substitutes Various drugs and toxins
Senile	Quite common in older dogs; cause unknown
Radiation	Following treatment for nasal tumours
Electrocution	

Figure 12.15 The aetiology of cataracts.

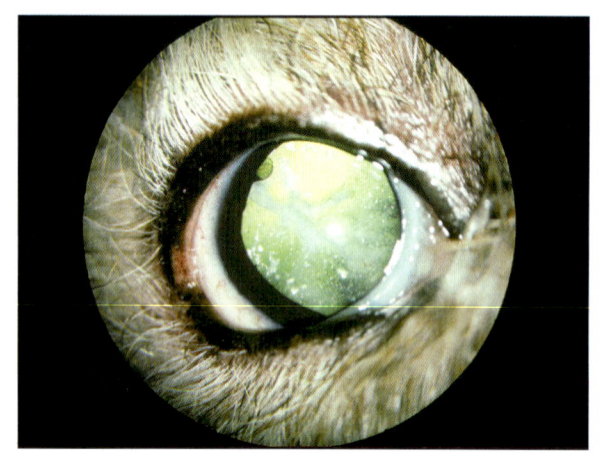

Figure 12.14 A hypermature cataract. There has been liquefaction of the lens proteins that have leaked out of the lens capsule, leaving a few small white condensations of lens proteins. The resulting lens-induced uveitis has resulted in a darkened iris and the development of an anterior uveal cyst (visible at the 11 o'clock position).

Morgagnian cataracts: Morgagnian cataracts are those in which a dense remnant of cataractous nucleus and the capsule is all that remains of the lens. The nuclear remnant sinks ventrally in the collapsed capsular bag.

Classification by aetiology: The causes of cataract formation are shown in Figure 12.15 and discussed below.

Hereditary cataracts: There are many breeds of dog worldwide that have, or are suspected to have, inherited cataracts (Rubin, 1989). Only those which are listed on the British Veterinary Association/Kennel Club/International Sheepdog Society (BVA/KC/ISDS) eye examination scheme are included here. For information of the breeds affected in other countries, see the literature of the appropriate eye screening scheme (e.g. CERF scheme in the USA).

Most inherited cataracts follow a characteristic pattern in age of onset, part of the lens affected and progression. Before condemning a dog as having inherited cataracts and, thus, implicating related dogs, it is important to ascertain that the cataract follows the characteristics for that particular breed. Figure 12.16 shows details of the cataracts listed by the BVA/KC/ISDS eye scheme as being inherited and Figure 12.17 lists breeds that have been noted to have cataracts, but inheritance has not been proven in the UK.

Early developing and progressive inherited cataracts are recognized in a number of breeds. They are classically described in the Boston Terrier and Staffordshire Bull Terrier. Selective breeding and eye screening means that the incidence of these cataracts is now low.

Posterior polar subcapsular cataracts (PPC) are the commonest form of inherited cataract encountered in adult dogs. They were initially described in the Golden and Labrador Retriever breeds. The opacity develops at the confluence of the posterior suture lines, is subcapsular in position and is typically triangular, pyramidal or of an inverted Y shape. Generally both eyes are affected, although the opacity may develop in one eye before the other. Most PPCs do not appear to have a major impact upon vision, although some may involve a larger area of the posterior subcapsular region. Occasionally, affected dogs are reported to develop a progressive cataract, which starts as vacuolation at the lens equator and may spread to involve the entire lens. This second form of cataract can have a marked effect on vision.

The insertion of the remnant of the hyaloid vasculature on the posterior lens capsule is often associated with a small capsular opacity (Mittendorf's dot) which is ventromedial to the confluence of the suture lines and should not be confused with a PPC. Some retrievers are seen with a faint perinuclear 'ring'; this does not appear to be a true opacity and should not be confused with the inherited cataract.

Type of cataract	Breeds affected	Features	Mode of inheritance	Reference(s)
Congenital with microphthalmos and rotatory nystagmus	Miniature Schnauzer	Mainly nuclear, sometimes cortical; rarely progressive. Some have posterior lenticonus and microphakia.	Autosomal recessive	Gelatt et al., 1983; Barnett, 1985
Early onset and progressive	Boston Terrier (1st form)	Bilateral, spreads from nucleus and suture lines, leads to total cataract. Starts 8–10 weeks	Autosomal recessive	Barnett, 1978
	Cavalier King Charles Spaniel	Progressive, bilateral and symmetrical. Becomes total in young adult	Unknown	Barnett, 1985
	German Shepherd Dog	Bilateral, slowly progressive. Starts as vacuoles at suture lines at 8 weeks	Autosomal recessive	Barnett, 1986
	Miniature Schnauzer	Similar to Boston Terrier	Autosomal recessive	Barnett, 1978
	Old English Sheepdog	Bilateral, asymmetrical, progressive. Starts at 7 months–2 years	Unknown	Barnett, 1978
	Staffordshire Bull Terrier	Similar to Boston Terrier	Autosomal recessive	Barnett, 1978
	Standard Poodle	Bilateral, symmetrical, progressive, cortical. Starts from 5 months	Autosomal recessive	Rubin and Flowers, 1972; Barnett and Startup, 1985
	Welsh Springer Spaniel	Bilateral, symmetrical, progressive, cortical vacuolation. Starts from 8 weeks	Autosomal recessive	Barnett, 1980
Posterior polar cataracts – affect confluence of suture lines. Inverted Y shaped, triangular or pyramidal	Chesapeake Bay Retriever	Posterior polar cataract; may involve suture lines and equatorial area of lens as well; may progress	? Dominant with incomplete penetrance	Gelatt et al., 1979
	Golden Retriever	Typical posterior polar subcapsular cataract at confluence of suture lines. A second progressive form exists which is believed to be due to same gene	? Dominant with incomplete penetrance	Curtis and Barnett, 1989
	Labrador Retriever	Similar to Golden Retriever	? Dominant with incomplete penetrance	Curtis and Barnett, 1989
	Large Munsterlander	Similar to Golden Retriever	Unknown	Barnett, 1985
	Siberian Husky	Inverted Y shape	? Autosomal recessive	Peiffer, 1982a
	Belgian Shepherd Dog	Posterior polar cataract	Unknown	BVA/KC/ISDS, 2001
	Norwegian Buhund	Onset from 3–4 months. Posterior polar cataract with extensions around the suture lines. Anterior cortex may be involved	Unknown	Barnett, 1988
Other forms of cataract	American Cocker Spaniel	Onset 2 months–6 years. Variable appearance, non-symmetrical, stationary or progressive	Autosomal recessive	Yakely, 1978
	Boston Terrier (2nd form)	Onset from 3–10 years. Subcapsular, anterior radial wedges (spokes) from equator	Unknown	Curtis, 1984

Figure 12.16 Inherited cataracts in dogs as recorded by the BVA/KC/ISDS eye examination scheme.

A cataract initially affecting the posterior suture lines occurs in the Siberian Husky (Figure 12.18; Gelatt, 1979), Alaskan Malamute and Norwegian Elkhound. However, this differs from that typical for the retriever breeds and can be more progressive. PPC is also recorded in the Rottweiler (Bjerkås and Bergsjø, 1991).

Inherited cataract in the American Cocker Spaniel is the most pleomorphic of the described inherited cataracts. It has a variable age of onset, may be progressive or stationary and may be unilateral or bilateral.

A so-called 'pulverulent' cataract has been described in the Norwegian Buhund as a potentially dominant trait with a high degree of penetrance (Bjerkås and Haaland, 1995). A similarly appearing cataract is also seen in German Shepherd Dogs. In the Buhund, the opacity starts as a series of parallel dots along the posterior suture lines. The central part of the nucleus then becomes involved with fine lines of opacity, which resemble candyfloss. The opacity does not progress to have a significant effect on vision.

212 The lens

Types of cataract	Breeds	References
Congenital	Bloodhound	BVA/KC/ISDS, 2001
	Cavalier King Charles Spaniel	Narfström and Dubielzig, 1984
	Dobermann	Lewis *et al.*, 1986
	English Cocker Spaniel	Olesen *et al.*, 1974
	Golden Retriever	Gelatt, 1972; Barnett and Grimes, 1975; quoted by Barnett, 1978
	Old English Sheepdog	Barrie *et al.*, 1979; Barnett, 1985
	Rottweiler	BVA/KC/ISDS, 2001
	Rough Collie	BVA/KC/ISDS, 2001
	Standard Poodle	Barnett and Startup, 1985
	West Highland White Terrier	Barnett, 1985
	Golden Retriever	Gelatt, 1972
	Old English Sheepdog	Koch, 1972
	West Highland White Terrier	Narfström, 1981
Early developing	Alaskan Malamute	BVA/KC/ISDS, 2001
	Australian Shepherd Dog	BVA/KC/ISDS, 2001
	Bichon Frisé	BVA/KC/ISDS, 2001
	Border Collie	BVA/KC/ISDS, 2001
	Field Spaniel	BVA/KC/ISDS, 2001
	French Bulldog	BVA/KC/ISDS, 2001
	Giant Schnauzer	BVA/KC/ISDS, 2001
	Greenland Dog	BVA/KC/ISDS, 2001
	Griffon Bruxellois	BVA/KC/ISDS, 2001
	Lancashire Heeler	BVA/KC/ISDS, 2001
	Tibetan Terrier	BVA/KC/ISDS, 2001
Variable age of onset	Leonberger	BVA/KC/ISDS, 2001
Late onset	Border Terrier	BVA/KC/ISDS, 2001
	Yorkshire Terrier	BVA/KC/ISDS, 2001

Figure 12.17 Breed-related cataracts which may be inherited ('under investigation' in the BVA/KC/ISDS eye scheme).

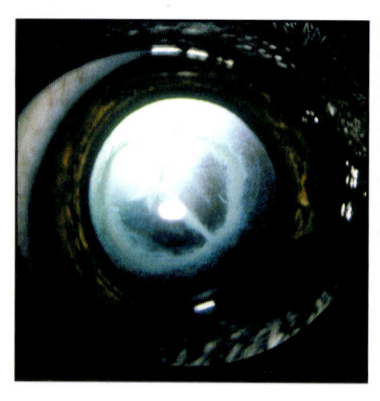

Figure 12.18 Hereditary cataract in a Siberian Husky. This is a posterior polar subcapsular Y-shaped cataract with an additional cortical ring of cataract.

Cataracts secondary to other ocular disorders: Cataracts may develop secondarily to any disease that alters the environment around the lens or directly damages it.

An important cause of secondary cataracts is generalized progressive retinal atrophy (gPRA). Hence, bilateral mature cataracts in dogs of the breed and age known to be at risk of developing gPRA should be investigated fully for the possibility of concurrent gPRA before lensectomy is advocated. Cataract formation is often the presenting sign in middle-aged Miniature Poodles and English Cocker Spaniels with gPRA; the owners wrongly attribute the vision loss to the cataracts. Labrador Retrievers with gPRA also develop secondary cataracts, but these appear to progress at a slower rate than the cataracts in the breeds already mentioned. Careful questioning of the owners may suggest that there was a deterioration in vision, particularly under poor lighting conditions, prior to the development of the cataract. Although the extent and briskness of the pupillary light reflex may give an indication of retinal function, it is highly unreliable. Affected dogs may also still have a dazzle reflex because of residual retinal function. When the fundus of these breeds cannot be viewed by indirect ophthalmoscopy, electroretinography should be performed to assess retinal function before considering cataract surgery. The reason that cataracts develop secondary to gPRA is unknown, but it is suggested that toxic products released by the degenerating retina may be responsible. Other disorders that cause degeneration of widespread areas of the retina may also be associated with cataract formation.

Conditions such as anterior uveitis and glaucoma alter the composition and characteristics of the aqueous on which the lens relies for nutrition and for the removal of waste products. Not surprisingly, both of these conditions can induce cataract formation. Hypermature cataracts and rapidly developing cataracts are often associated with signs of low-grade anterior uveitis. With some chronic inflammations, it is difficult to decide whether the cataract or the uveitis developed first. Chronically luxated lenses often become cataractous, regardless of whether they induce glaucoma or not.

Traumatic cataracts: Trauma to the globe may result in cataract formation (see also Chapter 10). The lens may be damaged directly or as a result of a trauma-induced uveitis. Blunt trauma may result in a more slowly developing cataract secondary to the resulting uveitis or as a result of disruption of lens material, allowing the influx of fluid and the release of lens proteins which will exacerbate the traumatic uveitis. Penetrating wounds that damage the lens capsule will result in rapid cataract formation. Small capsular injuries may heal, leaving a focal opacity, while slightly larger defects will usually result in a rapidly progressing cataract associated with a more severe inflammatory reaction. Larger tears, or ruptures, of the lens capsule will result in a severe purulent uveitis that leads to loss of the eye, often due to secondary glaucoma.

Medication with topical and systemic anti-inflammatory drugs and topical mydriatics is required. Lens extraction by phacoemulsification is indicated if there is release of a large amount of lens material, but the prognosis is guarded.

Metabolic cataracts: Diabetes mellitus is a common cause of cataracts (Basher and Roberts, 1995). Increased blood glucose levels lead to increased lens and aqueous glucose levels, causing the normal metabolic pathways for glucose metabolism in the lens to be saturated. Glucose is then converted by aldose reductase to sorbitol. This is a larger molecule than glucose and cannot diffuse out of lens fibres; its accumulation creates an osmotic gradient. The resulting uptake of fluid into the lens disrupts lens fibres, causing vacuolation and cataract formation. Diabetic cataracts frequently develop rapidly and progress to maturity. Early surgical removal of diabetic cataracts usually carries a similar success rate to that of non-diabetic cataracts (Bagley and Lavach, 1994), so long as the medical complications due to diabetes are controlled and the animal is well stabilized on insulin prior to surgery.

Hypocalcaemia, for example due to hypoparathyroidism, can result in characteristic bilateral lens changes in which there are numerous punctate anterior and posterior subcapsular opacities (Figure 12.19) (Bruyette and Feldman, 1988).

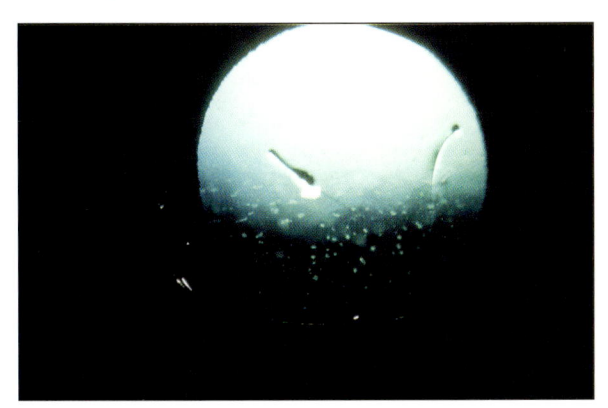

Figure 12.19 Multiple punctate subcapsular lens opacities in a dog with hypocalcaemia due to hypoparathyroidism.

Toxic or dietary cataracts: Cataract formation in orphaned puppies fed inappropriate milk substitutes has been reported (Martin and Chambreau, 1982; Glaze and Blanchard, 1983). Various drugs and toxins are cataractogenic (da Costa *et al.*, 1996; Davidson and Nelms, 1999), and exposure to radiation for the treatment of malignancies can induce cataract formation.

Senile cataracts: There is a higher incidence of cataracts in older animals. The majority of dogs presented for cataract extraction are middle to old aged, often with no apparent cause for their cataracts.

Treatment of cataracts: This is discussed by Nasisse *et al.* (1991); Glover and Constantinescu (1997) and Nasisse and Davidson (1999).

The only current treatment for cataracts is surgical removal. Occasional dogs are encountered with lens opacities that resolve spontaneously, the commonest of which are the temporary opacities seen in puppies at the tips of the suture lines. However, most cataracts will not spontaneously resolve, and there is no proof that medical therapy is effective in resolving cataracts.

It has long been accepted that extracapsular techniques, in which the lens capsule is opened and the contents of the capsule are removed, are preferable to intracapsular techniques, in which the entire lens is removed. The strong zonular attachments to the lens equator and the vitreal attachments to the posterior lens capsule mean that intracapsular techniques are difficult to perform without inducing intraocular bleeding, vitreal loss and an increased risk of retinal detachment. There are exceptions to this: some cataracts do luxate or subluxate due to loss of zonular attachments, and, in such cases, intracapsular extraction may be preferred.

Phacoemulsification is accepted as the preferred technique of cataract removal. This involves the use of a phacoemulsification needle, which is vibrated by ultrasound and breaks up the cataractous material; this is then aspirated from the eye through the needle. Irrigating fluid is used to replace that which is aspirated, thereby keeping the globe formed. A circular defect is created in the anterior lens capsule (typically by careful and controlled tearing); this allows the phacoemulsification needle access to the lens material. Once the cataractous portions of the lens have been emulsified and aspirated, an irrigation/aspiration handpiece is used to remove all residual lens fibres. This entire procedure is performed through an incision just large enough to allow the introduction of the phacoemulsification needle and surrounding irrigating sheath (typically 3.2 mm). The incision is then enlarged if an intraocular lens is to be implanted. Intraocular lens implantation following cataract removal is routine, and, although aphakic dogs can usually cope well, implantation of an intraocular lens that corrects the visual deficit will obviously improve vision. Intraocular lenses following phacoemulsification are positioned within the remaining capsular bag. This holds the lens in position within the eye (Figure 12.20).

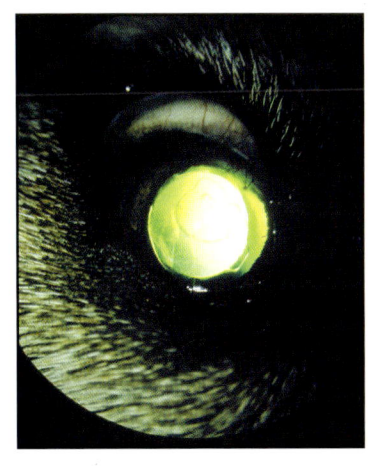

Figure 12.20 A canine eye following phacoemulsification and intraocular lens (IOL) implantation. The IOL can be seen positioned in the remaining capsular bag. The capsulorrhexis can also be seen overlying the IOL.

Cataract surgery is a skilled procedure that should always be performed with the aid of an operating microscope. Those undertaking it should have received considerable training, as well as possessing all the required equipment. Nevertheless, it is important that the practitioner is aware of what is involved, the selection criteria and the possible complications. A detailed description of the surgical procedure is beyond the scope of this manual.

Selection criteria for cataract surgery: The ideal stage of cataract development for extraction is the immature stage (Davidson *et al.*, 1991). Secondary changes present in eyes with mature and hypermature cataracts typically result in a more severe postoperative inflammatory reaction, increased risk of retinal detachment and other complications that reduce the likely success rate.

With careful patient selection, typical success rates will be over 90% in the short term. However, the success rate will be lower if the patients are followed for extended periods, because of slowly developing complications, such as those resulting from proliferation of residual lens epithelial cells. The success rate for eyes with more advanced cataracts and pre-existing lens-induced uveitis can be considerably lower, particularly when the longer term outcome is considered (Paulsen *et al.*, 1986; van der Woerdt *et al.*, 1992).

Before performing cataract surgery, it is essential to show that either the cataract is having a significant effect on vision or that it is progressive and, therefore, very likely to lead to blindness if it is not treated.

With older dogs, it is particularly important to differentiate between nuclear sclerosis and cataract. Veterinary ophthalmologists commonly receive referrals for cataract evaluation, only to find that the dog has nuclear sclerosis.

Many dogs that develop cataracts are either older or have systemic disease such as diabetes mellitus. It is essential that dogs with cataracts are fully evaluated for systemic disease problems before surgery is considered. A detailed evaluation of the eye for accompanying abnormalities is essential. This dictates that the eyes are fully evaluated and this typically includes the following:

- Schirmer tear test – to ensure that tear production is normal
- Intraocular pressure measurement – to examine for secondary glaucoma and active uveitis
- Gonioscopy – to evaluate the predisposition to primary narrow angle/goniodysgenesis forms of glaucoma
- Detailed slit-lamp examination – to check for lens-induced uveitis and other changes that may complicate surgery
- Indirect ophthalmoscopy – to evaluate the posterior segment through an immature cataract
- Ocular ultrasonography – particularly to look for evidence of retinal detachment
- Evaluation of retinal function – to rule out generalized retinal dysfunction, such as that caused by gPRA. Although the pupillary light reflex and dazzle reflex can give an indication that the retina is functional, they are not completely reliable and many veterinary ophthalmologists will perform electroretinography before cataract extraction.

Figure 12.21 summarizes the ocular conditions that particularly need to be considered prior to cataract surgery.

- **Globe**
Microphthalmos may make intraocular manipulations difficult
- **Eyelids**
Infections of the eyelids are a potential source of post-operative intraocular infection
- **Ocular surface**
Pre-existing ocular surface inflammation or infection should be treated prior to surgery. Particularly, consider tear film dysfunction
- **Corneal endothelium**
Pre-existing corneal endothelial disease will be worsened by intraocular surgery. This may result in permanent corneal opacity
- **Aqueous drainage**
Glaucoma or a predisposition to glaucoma due to an abnormal iridocorneal drainage angle are contraindications
- **Uveitis**
A pre-existing uveitis will be exacerbated by surgical intervention. However, a mild previous uveitis which has been successfully suppressed is not a contraindication
- **Pupil**
Persistent pupillary membrane and posterior synechiae may interfere with cataract extraction and may be contraindications
- **Lens**
The cataract should significantly affect vision before considering surgery (perform an obstacle course test; do not rely on the owner's assessment of vision). Lens instability due to zonule breakdown may mean that an intracapsular rather than an extracapsular extraction is indicated
- **Posterior segment**
Abnormalities of the vitreous and fundus may not be visible due to the cataract. The pupillary light reflex is a guide as to retinal function, but is unreliable. Ultrasonography will detect abnormalities such as retinal detachments, and electroretinography can be used to assess overall retinal function and diagnose primary disorders such as generalized progressive retinal atrophy

Figure 12.21 Ocular assessment prior to cataract surgery.

There are many possible complications associated with cataract surgery, including:

- Those that arise during the surgery, often related to surgical technique
- The occurrence of rises in intraocular pressure within a few hours of the end of surgery (Smith *et al.*, 1996; Miller *et al.*, 1997)
- Those associated with inflammation as a result of the release of lens proteins into the eye during surgery
- Those seen in the longer term as a result of attempts by the residual lens epithelial cells to produce new lens fibres. This can occur, leading to opacification of the posterior lens capsule. This is particularly a problem in younger dogs and may impede vision and cause a lens-induced uveitis. The presence of an intraocular lens may limit the space for lens epithelial proliferation (Nasisse *et al.*, 1995).

Complications, such as glaucoma (Biros *et al.*, 2000; Lannek and Miller, 2001), damage from uncontrolled uveitis, retinal detachment and permanent corneal oedema, are among the more serious complications that can result in failure of the surgery.

Lens luxation

Dislocation of the lens from its normal position results from a breakdown of the zonules which should firmly attach the lens to the ciliary body. This may occur as a primary or secondary condition.

Primary lens luxation: This disease is discussed by Curtis *et al.* (1983) and Curtis (1990).

This is an inherited condition that affects the terrier breeds (Jack Russell Terrier, Fox Terrier, Tibetan Terrier, Sealyham Terrier, Miniature Bull Terrier), the Border Collie (Foster *et al.*, 1986) and Shar Pei (Lazarus *et al.*, 1998), and is a relatively common cause of secondary glaucoma. It occurs occasionally in other breeds and crossbreeds. Studies in the Tibetan Terrier suggest that it is inherited in an autosomal recessive manner (Willis *et al.*, 1979).

Affected terriers are typically 3 to 6 years of age. Gradual zonular breakdown allows the lens to move relative to the rest of the globe under the effects of inertia. Lens instability (phacodonesis) and iridodonesis ('iris wobble') are early signs that are best detected when closely viewing the anterior chamber from an oblique angle just after an eye movement. Zonular breakdown allows strands of vitreous to pass anteriorly to appear through the pupil as faint wisps of slightly translucent material (see Figure 13.14). Following dilation of the pupil, evidence of early lens subluxation is more readily observed. The lens equator may be seen and an aphakic crescent (a gap between the pupil edge and the lens equator) may be present (Figure 12.22). Eventually the lens will luxate fully. Most luxate anteriorly through the pupil (Figure 12.23) and, in the majority of cases, cause a 'pupil block' and secondary glaucoma.

It can be difficult to measure the intraocular pressure reliably of an eye with an anteriorly luxated lens. An applanation tonometer, such as a Tonopen, can be used. It should be pressed on the peripheral cornea, which does not have the luxated lens lying against its posterior surface. Measurement of intraocular pressure with an indentation tonometer, such as the Schiøtz

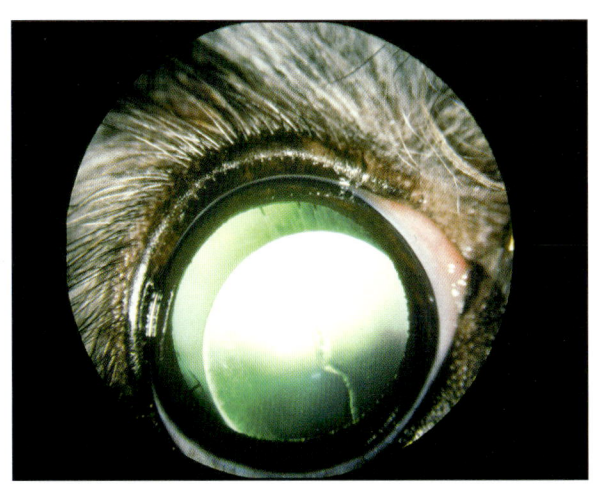

Figure 12.22 Primary lens luxation in a Tibetan Terrier. The lens in this photograph was subluxated, whereas the lens in the other eye had already luxated into the anterior chamber. An aphakic crescent is visible, and stretched zonular fibres can be seen dorsally, stretching from the lens equator to the ciliary processes.

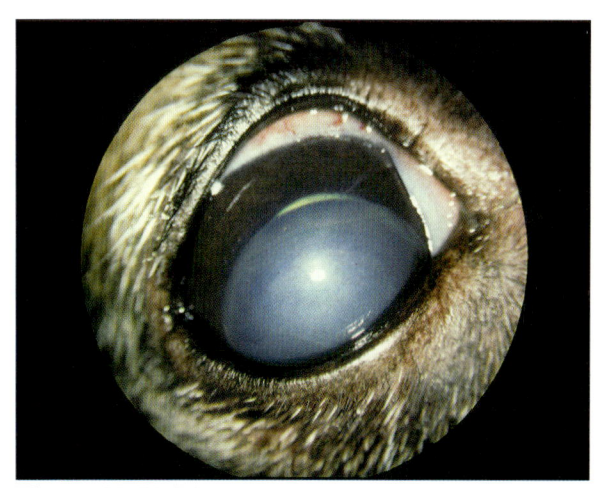

Figure 12.23 Primary anterior lens luxation in a Jack Russell Terrier. The lens is clearly visible in the anterior chamber.

tonometer, will not give an accurate result in such cases. Contact between the luxated lens and the corneal endothelium will result in the development of an area of corneal oedema just ventral to the centre of the cornea. Sometimes the anteriorly luxated lens will spontaneously move into the vitreous, at which time the intraocular pressure often returns to normal and, therefore, the eye becomes more comfortable. In such cases, a characteristic patch of corneal oedema usually remains and acts as an indicator of the previous presence of the lens in the anterior chamber. Such lenses often luxate anteriorly again. However, while they remain in the vitreous, they generally causes few problems. In long-standing luxations, the lens often becomes cataractous.

Treatment: This is discussed by Nasisse *et al.* (1995) and Nasisse and Glover (1997).

Emergency treatment to reduce intraocular pressure is indicated prior to surgical removal. The osmotic diuretic, mannitol, is most commonly used for this purpose (see Chapter 11).

Referral to a veterinary ophthalmologist equipped for intraocular surgery is recommended. The lens and its capsule can be removed through a small incision by phacoemulsification of the lens nucleus and cortex and manual extraction of the remaining capsule. More commonly, the luxated lens is removed in one piece through a corneal incision that approaches 180 degrees. It is possible to suture in an intraocular lens following intracapsular lens extraction.

Primary lens luxation is a bilateral condition, so the lens of the second eye is very likely to luxate at some stage. The eye should be examined for signs of impending luxation. Many veterinary ophthalmologists will elect to remove the lens from the second eye if it shows signs of instability. This saves the eye from possibly suffering glaucoma, with consequent irreversible damage, in the future. If the decision is made not to remove the unstable but not luxated lens at the same time as the luxated lens, the owners should be warned to seek veterinary help immediately if the second eye shows signs of having developed an anterior luxation.

Posteriorly luxated lenses can also be associated with the development of a secondary glaucoma (Glover *et al.,* 1995); the risk of this should be weighed against the potential difficulties of removal and the possible risk of complications due to the surgery, such as retinal detachment.

Secondary lens luxation: Lens luxation may occur secondary to glaucoma, cataract formation or trauma, or it may be associated with uveitis. The globe enlargement due to glaucoma does not often result in complete lens luxation. A few zonular fibres usually remain intact and attach the lens to one area of the ciliary processes. An aphakic crescent is seen between the edge of the pupil and the equator of the subluxated lens. Removal of a lens that has been subluxated secondarily to glaucoma is not indicated.

Conditions of the feline lens

Lens abnormalities occur less commonly in cats than in dogs. There are few reports of inherited lens diseases, and most lens pathology is secondary to injury or other ocular disorders.

Congenital conditions

Aphakia (Peiffer,1982b) and microphakia (Molleda *et al.,* 1995) have been reported, but are very rare. Lens defects may be seen in kittens born with multiple congenital defects. Focal capsular and subcapsular opacities are associated with the insertion of persistent pupillary membrane remnants on to the anterior lens capsule, but this is an uncommon condition in cats. Congenital cataracts have been reported in related Himalayan kittens, leading to suggestions of inheritance (Rubin, 1986).

Acquired conditions

Cataract

Primary cataracts are very rare in cats (Figure 12.24). Cataracts usually develop secondary to injury or other ocular disease, but cataracts secondary to other ocular disease are not as common in cats as in dogs.

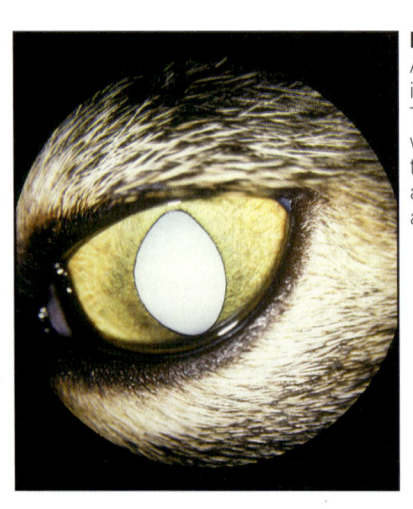

Figure 12.24 A mature cataract in a young cat. The condition was bilateral and there was no apparent aetiology.

Blunt trauma can injure the lens, leading to a slowly progressive cataract. Penetrating wounds, such as those caused by cat claws, may involve the lens and may lead to cataract formation. Development of cataracts secondary to diabetes mellitus is uncommon in cats (Salgado *et al.,* 2000). Metabolic cataracts resulting from hypocalcaemia due to hypoparathyroidism have been reported (Parker, 1991; Bassett, 1998). Cataracts are common sequelae to chronic anterior uveitis in cats. The cataracts tend to be slowly progressive, but may eventually cause blindness. Chronically luxated lenses may become cataractous. Furthermore, cataracts may develop secondary to chronic glaucoma.

Cataract extraction: Although less frequently indicated in the cat than in the dog, cataract surgery generally has a good prognosis, and the cat's eye tends to be much less reactive than that of the dog. Removal of cataracts that develop secondary to anterior uveitis can give good results, although the anterior uveitis must be suppressed prior to surgery, and the possibility of it being associated with a serious systemic disease must be considered and fully investigated. Persistence of inflammation with continued formation of pre-iridal fibrovascular membranes may lead to secondary glaucoma.

Lens luxation

This has been studied by Olivero *et al.* (1991).

Lens luxation or subluxation in the cat most commonly occurs secondary to trauma, glaucoma, anterior uveitis or cataract formation. Glaucoma usually results in tearing of part of the zonules due to globe enlargement, resulting in an aphakic crescent and lens subluxation. Cats with anterior lens luxation secondary to anterior uveitis (Figure 12.25) are sometimes presented because of the change in appearance due to the lens luxation. The owners may not have noticed the signs of the preceding anterior uveitis. Close examination of such eyes reveals evidence of previous anterior uveitis (see Chapter 10).

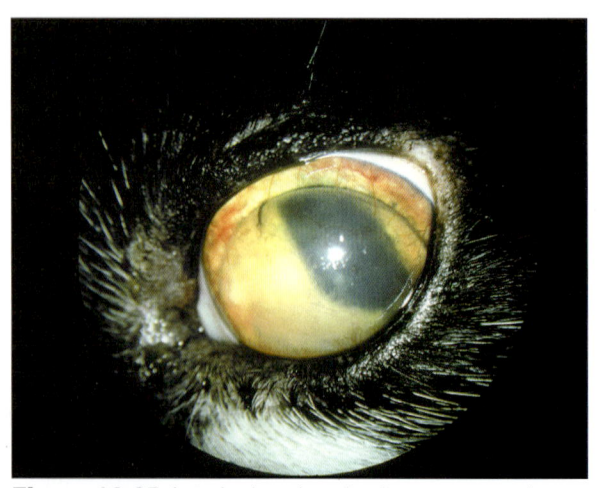

Figure 12.25 Anterior lens luxation in a cat secondary to chronic anterior uveitis. The lens is clearly visible in the anterior chamber. Iris neovascularization is present as an indicator of chronic anterior uveitis.

Inherited primary lens luxation is not recognized in the cat, but an apparently spontaneous luxation is occasionally encountered in older cats with no evidence of an accompanying anterior uveitis.

Removal of anteriorly luxated lenses is advisable. They do not cause a secondary glaucoma as frequently as anterior lens luxations do in dogs, but they may result in corneal oedema due to endothelial damage, and the lens may become cataractous. The outcome of removal of anterior lens luxations in cats is generally good. If lens luxation is secondary to anterior uveitis, the possible aetiologies of the uveitis should be fully investigated and appropriately treated.

References and further reading

Bagley LH II and Lavach JD (1994) Comparison of postoperative phacoemulsification results in dogs with and without diabetes mellitus: 153 cases (1991–1992). *Journal of the American Veterinary Medical Association* **205**, 1165–1169

Barnett KC (1978) Hereditary cataract in the dog. *Journal of Small Animal Practice* **19**, 109–120

Barnett KC (1980) Hereditary cataract in the Welsh Springer Spaniel. *Journal of Small Animal Practice* **21**, 621–625

Barnett KC (1985) The diagnosis and differential diagnosis of cataract in the dog. *Journal of Small Animal Practice* **26**, 305–316

Barnett KC (1986) Hereditary cataract in the German Shepherd Dog. *Journal of Small Animal Practice* **27**, 387–395

Barnett KC (1988) Inherited eye disease in the dog and cat. *Journal of Small Animal Practice* **29**, 462–475

Barnett KC and Startup FG (1985) Hereditary cataract in the Standard Poodle. *Veterinary Record* **117**, 15–16

Barrie KP, Peiffer RL, Gelatt KN and Williams LW (1979) Posterior lenticonus, microphthalmia, congenital cataracts, and retinal folds in an Old English Sheepdog. *Journal of the American Animal Hospital Association* **15**, 715–717

Basher AW and Roberts SM (1995) Ocular manifestations of diabetes mellitus: diabetic cataracts in dogs. *Veterinary Clinics of North America: Small Animal Practice* **25**, 661–676

Bassett JR (1998) Hypocalcemia and hyperphosphatemia due to primary hypoparathyroidism in a six-month-old kitten. *Journal of the American Animal Hospital Association* **34**, 503–507

Biros DJ, Gelatt KN, Brooks DE, Kubilis PS, Andrew SE, Strubbe DT and Whigham HM (2000) Development of glaucoma after cataract surgery in dogs: 220 cases (1987–1998). *Journal of the American Veterinary Medical Association* **216**, 1780–1786

Bjerkås E and Bergsjø T (1991) Hereditary cataract in the Rottweiler dog. *Progress in Veterinary and Comparative Ophthalmology* **1**, 7–10

Bjerkås E and Haaland MB (1995) Pulverulent nuclear cataract in the Norwegian Buhund. *Journal of Small Animal Practice* **36**, 471–474

British Veterinary Association/Kennel Club/International Sheepdog Society eye examination scheme (2001) *Inherited ocular disease: breeds affected and type of condition*

Bruyette DS and Feldman EC (1988) Primary hypoparathyroidism in the dog: report of 15 cases and review of 13 previously reported cases. *Journal of Veterinary Internal Medicine* **2**, 7–14

da Costa PD, Merideth RE and Sigler RL (1996) Cataracts after long-term ketoconazole therapy. *Progress in Veterinary and Comparative Ophthalmology* **6**, 176–180

Curtis R (1984) Late-onset cataract in the Boston Terrier. *Veterinary Record* **115**, 577–578

Curtis R (1990) Lens luxation in the dog and cat. *Veterinary Clinics of North America: Small Animal Practice* **20**, 755–773

Curtis R, Barnett KC and Lewis SJ (1983) Clinical and pathological observations concerning the aetiology of primary lens luxation in the dog. *Veterinary Record* **112**, 238–246

Curtis R and Barnett KC (1989) A survey of cataracts in Golden and Labrador Retrievers. *Journal of Small Animal Practice* **30**, 277–286

Davidson MG and Nelms S (1999) Disease of the lens and cataract formation. In: *Veterinary Ophthalmology, 3rd edn*, ed. KN Gelatt, pp. 797–825. Lippincott, Williams and Wilkins, Philadelphia

Davidson MG, Nasisse MP, Jamieson VE, English RV and Olivero DK (1991) Phacoemulsification and intraocular lens implantation: a study of surgical results in 182 dogs. *Progress in Veterinary and Comparative Ophthalmology* **1**, 233–238

Foster SJ, Curtis R and Barnett KC (1986) Primary lens luxation in the Border Collie. *Journal of Small Animal Practice* **27**, 1–6

Gelatt KN (1972) Cataracts in the Golden Retriever dog. *Veterinary Medicine/Small Animal Clinician* **67**, 1113–1115

Gelatt KN (1979) Lens and cataract formation in the dog. *Compendium of Continuing Education for the Practicing Veterinarian* **1**, 75–80

Gelatt KN, Whitley D, Lavach JD, Barrie KP and Williams LW (1979) Cataracts in Chesapeake Bay Retrievers. *Journal of the American Veterinary Medical Association* **175**, 1176–1178

Gelatt KN, Samuelsen DA, Barrie KP, Das ND, Wolf ED, Bauer JE and Andersen TL (1983) Biometry and clinical characteristics of congenital cataracts in the Miniature Schnauzer. *Journal of the American Veterinary Medical Association* **183**, 99–102

Glaze M and Blanchard G (1983) Nutritional cataracts in a Samoyed litter. *Journal of the American Animal Hospital Association* **19**, 951–954

Glover TD and Constantinescu GM (1997) Surgery for cataracts. *Veterinary Clinics of North America: Small Animal Practice* **27**, 1143–1173

Glover TL, Davidson MG, Nasisse MP and Olivero DK (1995) The intracapsular extraction of displaced lenses in dogs: a retrospective study of 57 cases (1984–1990). *Journal of the American Animal Hospital Association* **31**, 77–81

Koch SA (1972) Cataracts in interrelated Old English Sheepdogs. *Journal of the American Veterinary Medical Association* **160**, 299–301

Lannek EB and Miller PE (2001) Development of glaucoma after phacoemulsification for removal of cataracts in dogs: 22 cases (1987–1997). *Journal of the American Veterinary Medical Association* **218**, 70–76

Lazarus JA, Pickett JP and Champagne ES (1998) Primary lens luxation in the Chinese Shar Pei: clinical and hereditary characteristics. *Veterinary Ophthalmology* **1**, 101–107

Lewis DG, Kelly DF and Sansom J (1986) Congenital microphthalmia and other developmental ocular abnormalities in the Dobermann. *Journal of Small Animal Practice* **27**, 559–566

Martin CL and Chambreau T (1982) Cataract production in experimentally orphaned puppies fed a commercial replacement for bitch's milk. *Journal of the American Animal Hospital Association* **18**, 115–119

Molleda JM, Martin E, Ginel PJ, Novales M, Moreno P and Lopez R (1995) Microphakia associated with lens luxation in the cat. *Journal of the American Animal Hospital Association* **31**, 209–212

Miller PE, Stanz KM, Dubielzig RR and Murphy CJ (1997) Mechanisms of acute intraocular pressure increases after phacoemulsification lens extraction in dogs. *American Journal of Veterinary Research* **58**, 1159–1165

Narfström K (1981) Cataract in the West Highland White Terrier. *Journal of Small Animal Practice* **22**, 467–471

Narfström K and Dubielzig R (1984) Posterior lenticonus, cataracts and microphthalmia: congenital ocular defects in the Cavalier King Charles Spaniel. *Journal of Small Animal Practice* **25**, 669–677

Nasisse MP, Davidson MG, Jamieson VE, English RV and Olivero DK (1991) Phacoemulsification and intraocular lens implantation: a study of technique in 182 dogs. *Progress in Veterinary and Comparative Ophthalmology* **1**, 225–232

Nasisse MP, Dykstra MJ and Cobo LM (1995) Lens capsule opacification in aphakic and pseudophakic eyes. *Graefe's Archive for Clinical and Experimental Ophthalmology* **233**, 63–70

Nasisse MP, Glover TL, Davidson MG, Nelms S and Sullivan T (1995) Technique for suture fixation of intraocular lenses in dogs. *Progress in Veterinary and Comparative Ophthalmology* **5**, 146–150

Nasisse MP and Glover TL (1997) Surgery for lens instability. *Veterinary Clinics of North America: Small Animal Practice* **27**, 1175–1192

Nasisse MP and Davidson MG (1999) Surgery of the lens. In: *Veterinary Ophthalmology, 3rd edn*, ed. KN Gelatt, pp. 827–856. Lippincott, Williams and Wilkins, Philadelphia

Olesen HP, Jensen OA and Norn MS (1974) Congenital hereditary cataract in Cocker Spaniels. *Journal of Small Animal Practice* **15**, 741–750

Olivero DK, Riis RC, Dutton AG, Murphy CJ, Nasisse MP and Davidson MG (1991) Feline lens displacement: a retrospective analysis of 345 cases. *Progress in Veterinary and Comparative Ophthalmology* **1**, 239–244

Parker JSL (1991) A probable case of hypoparathyroidism in a cat. *Journal of Small Animal Practice* **32**, 470–473

Paulsen M, Lavach J, Severin G and Eichenbaum J (1986) The effect of lens-induced uveitis on the success of extracapsular cataract extraction: a retrospective study of 65 lens removals in the dog. *Journal of the American Animal Hospital Association* **22**, 49–56

Peiffer RL (1982a) Inherited ocular disease of the dog and cat. *Compendium of Continuing Education for the Practicing Veterinarian* **4**, 152–166

Peiffer RL (1982b) Bilateral congenital aphakia and retinal detachment in a cat. *Journal of the American Animal Hospital Association* **18**, 128–130

Roberts SR and Helper LC (1972) Cataracts in Afghan Hounds. *Journal of the American Veterinary Medical Association* **160**, 427–432

Rubin LF (1986) Hereditary cataract in Himalayan cats. *Feline Practice* **16**, 14–15

Rubin LF (1989) *Inherited Eye Disease in Purebred Dogs*. Williams and Wilkins, Baltimore

Rubin LF and Flowers RD (1972) Inherited cataract in a family of Standard Poodles. *Journal of the American Veterinary Medical Association* **161**, 207–208

Salgado D, Reusch C and Spiess B (2000) Diabetic cataracts: different incidence between dogs and cats. *Schweizer Archiv für Tierheilkunde* **142**, 349–353

Smith PJ, Brooks DE, Lazarus JA, Kubilis PS and Gelatt KN (1996) Ocular hypertension following cataract surgery in dogs: 139 cases (1992–1993). *Journal of the American Veterinary Medical Association* **209**, 105–111

Strande A, Nicolaissen B and Bjerkås I (1988) Persistent pupillary membrane and congenital cataract in a litter of English Cocker Spaniels. *Journal of Small Animal Practice* **29**, 257–260

van der Woerdt A, Nasisse MP and Davidson MG (1992) Lens-induced uveitis in dogs: 151 cases (1985–1990). *Journal of the American Veterinary Medical Association* **201**, 921–926

Willis MB, Curtis R, Barnett KC and Tempest WM (1979) Genetic aspects of lens luxation in the Tibetan Terrier. *Veterinary Record* **104**, 409–412

Yakely WL (1978) A study of heritability of cataracts in the American Cocker Spaniel. *Journal of the American Veterinary Medical Association* **172**, 814–817

13

The vitreous

Christine Heinrich

Introduction

The vitreous humour is a transparent hydrogel that occupies the posterior segment of the globe. Its function is not only to act as a clear medium for transmission of light between lens and retina, but its viscoelastic properties also provide mechanical support and protection for the internal structures of the eye during movement and deformation of the globe. The vitreous takes part in intraocular metabolism and acts as a nutrient reservoir and metabolic waste repository for the retina and neighbouring tissues.

Embryology

The development of the vitreous has traditionally been divided into three stages.

In the first stage, the relatively small retrolental space is filled by the primary vitreous, which consists of the hyaloid artery and its branches, and provides nutrition to the developing lens via the tunica vasculosa lentis. The primary vitreous is thought to be of a mixed ectodermal and mesenchymal origin. Not only the vascular mesenchyme of the primitive ophthalmic artery but also surface ectoderm-derived elements which surround the lens during invagination contribute to its formation. Vitrosin (see below) may be of neuroectodermal origin. With the development of the iris and ciliary body, a need for a direct vascular supply is lost, so the hyaloid vasculature regresses. This begins at day 45 of gestation and is completed at around 2–4 weeks post partum in the dog.

In the second phase, secondary or adult vitreous fills the increasing space of the posterior optic cavity. The atrophying primary vitreous becomes condensed in the centre of the posterior segment and forms Cloquet's canal, which runs between the optic disc and lens.

The area of previous hyaloid artery attachment to the posterior lens capsule remains visible in the adult dog as Mittendorf's dot. This mark can be seen ventromedial to the confluence of the posterior suture line; a fine remnant of the atrophied vessel is usually visible on slit lamp examination within the anterior vitreous.

The posterior remnant of the hyaloid artery, Bergmeister's papilla, is not usually visible on examination of the adult dog, but the area where the hyaloid artery has originated from the posterior pole can be seen easily on ophthalmoscopic examination as the physiological pit on the surface of the optic nerve head.

The origin of the secondary or adult vitreous remains unclear, but hyalocytes, ciliary epithelium, mesenchymal cells at the rim of the optic cup, hyaloid vessels during fetal development and retinal glial cells (Müller cells) are thought to contribute to its development (Forrester et al., 1996).

In the third stage of vitreal development, the collagen condensations of the vitreal base and the zonular fibres are formed. As with the secondary vitreous, the exact origin of the tertiary vitreous is unclear, but it is suspected that the non-pigmented ciliary epithelium is involved in its formation.

The development and regression of the structures of the primary vitreous are of the utmost importance for normal ocular development; failure of the normal regression of these embryological structures gives rise to several congenital vitreal abnormalities.

Anatomy, physiology and biochemistry

The vitreous is bound anteriorly by the lens, its zonules and the ciliary body, and posteriorly by the retinal cup (Figure 13.1). Filling most of the posterior cavity of the globe, the vitreous is almost spherical in shape with a

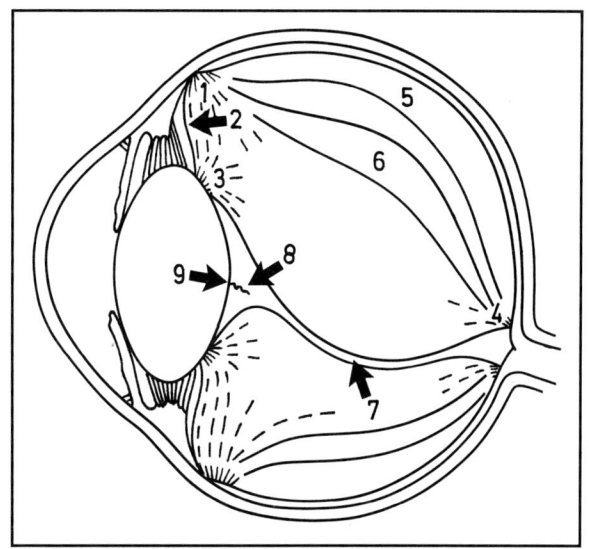

Figure 13.1 Globe and vitreous. 1. Vitreous base; 2. anterior hyaloid face; 3. hyaloideocapsular ligament; 4. attachment to margin of optic disc; 5. cortical vitreous; 6. lamellae and tracts; 7. Cloquet's canal; 8. hyaloid vessel remnant; 9. Mittendorf's dot.

depression on its anterior face – the fossa hyaloidea, which offers a resting space for the lens. The vitreous can be divided into a cortical zone and a central zone. A further, geographical, description divides the vitreous into an anterior, an intermediate and a posterior zone.

The vitreous consists of approximately 99% water, with the remaining 1% comprising collagen, vitreal cells (hyalocytes), soluble protein and hyaluronic acid.

The vitreous gel is approximately 2–4 times more viscous than water, the viscosity being largely dependent on the concentration of sodium hyaluronate. During ageing or pathological processes, this structure is lost and the vitreous becomes liquefied – a process known as syneresis. The hyaluronic acid molecules degrade and the collagen fibrils clump together, to form vitreal 'floaters' (see below).

The cortical vitreous is attached by the condensation of the fine collagen fibrils to the peripheral retina and the pars plana (vitreous base), the posterior lens capsule (hyaloideocapsular ligament), the margins of the optic nerve head at the base of the hyaloid canal and the inner limiting membrane of the retina. Breakdown and disruption of the vitreous base is found during diseases such as primary lens luxation, although detachment of the vitreal face from the internal limiting membrane, where it has its weakest attachments, is more common. This condition, described as posterior vitreal detachment, can easily be demonstrated on ultrasonographic examination of the posterior segment and may predispose the eye to the development of a retinal detachment.

Cellular elements

Although the vitreous is essentially acellular and avascular, a small number of macrophage-derived cells named hyalocytes are found in it, with their highest number in the cortical zone. The function of these cells is not clear but their high numbers of phagolysosomes indicates that they may be active phagocytes. It has also been shown that hyalocytes are able to produce hyaluronate in vitro, and it is suspected that hyalocytes contribute to the synthesis of vitreous humour.

Matrix

The vitreous contains vitrosin, a unique fibrous protein, which is most similar to type 2 collagen, but differs from normal collagen in being inseparably linked with complex polysaccharides. Unlike type 1 collagen, which has weak interactions with only small amounts of proteoglycans and therefore presents as a compact fibril, vitrosin, in common with type 2 collagen, appears in extracellular matrices that are rich in proteoglycans and have a strong collagen–proteoglycan interaction. Vitrosin fibrils form a skeleton for the vitreal gel by entrapping large coiled hyaluronic acid molecules, which, in turn, keep the collagen fibrils widely spaced. Electronegative charges of the hyaluronic acid triple helix are responsible for the hydrophilic character of the molecule.

Hyaluronic acid, a glycosaminoglycan molecule, is present in the gel and affects the flow of fluid within the vitreous. The transvitreal movement of substances is influenced by a number of mechanisms, such as diffusion, hydrostatic and osmotic pressure, convection and active transport. The strong electrostatic charges within the gel also affect electrolyte transport through the vitreous.

Glucose and other sugars are also present, suggesting that the vitreous could temporarily supply nutrients to the retina. Waste products of retinal and lenticular metabolism can accumulate within the vitreous, and increased intravitreal glutamate levels are thought to be an indicator for retinal and optic nerve fibre injury in glaucoma.

Light transmission

Light transmission in the vitreous occurs according to the same principles as in the cornea, i.e. vitreal collagen fibrils are thinner than half the wavelength of light, and the distribution of glycosaminoglycans between the fibrils reduces the effects of diffraction.

Congenital and developmental anomalies in the dog

Persistent primary vitreous

Persistent hyaloid artery (PHA)

Failure of the normal regression of the hyaloid vascular system is a relatively rare and sporadic congenital ocular anomaly in the dog. Clinical signs vary in accordance with the part of the hyaloid artery structure that has persisted. The most common form is a small vascular remnant that protrudes from the posterior lens capsule into the anterior vitreous (Figure 13.2). A localized capsular opacity may be seen at the point of insertion of the vessel remnant on the posterior lens capsule, but the opacity is rarely progressive. The remnant does not usually carry blood, but a patent hyaloid artery may persist in rare cases and haemorrhage from this vessel into the lens or vitreous may occur. Extensive cataract formation may ensue, and persistent hyperplastic tunica vasculosa lentis/persistent hyperplastic primary vitreous (PHTVL/PHPV) should be considered as a differential diagnosis (see later).

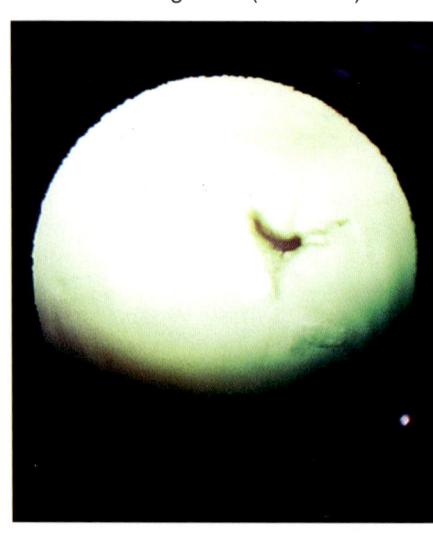

Figure 13.2 Small hyaloid remnant on posterior lens capsule.

Persistence of the posterior part of the hyaloid artery is sometimes seen in collies affected with collie eye anomaly. The remnant of the glial sheath of the primitive hyaloid artery, Bergmeister's papilla, may in these cases give rise to a patent blood vessel, with resulting vitreal haemorrhage.

Persistent tunica vasculosa lentis

Persistence of the posterior tunica vasculosa lentis in isolation is rare, but does occasionally present on ophthalmoscopic examination as a fine filamentous web or punctate or pigmented opacities on the posterior lens capsule. It is rarely of any clinical significance, may be unilateral or bilateral and has a similar clinical presentation to mild degrees of PHTVL/PHPV.

PHTVL/PHPV

In this condition, the hyaloid system and the tunica vasculosa lentis become hyperplastic during relatively early embryological development and continue to proliferate following birth. The extent of the lesions varies between affected animals. The degree of visual impairment that results depends on the degree of proliferation of the hyaloid system and the presence of complications, such as cataract formation and haemorrhage.

Clinically visible lesions vary in severity from fine pigment spots on the posterior lens capsule (Figure 13.3) to large fibrovascular plaques involving the posterior lens capsule and may be accompanied by other abnormalities, including abnormal lens shape (lenticonus or lentiglobus), cataract, intralenticular haemorrhage (Figures 13.4 and 13.5), elongated ciliary processes, persistent hyaloid artery, persistent pupillary membrane and capsulopupillary vessels. These last vessels appear in the form of pigmented strands or even patent vessels that originate from the retrolental plaque, course over the lens equator and, in most cases, insert on the anterior surface of the iris.

PHTVL/PHPV has been reported as a bilateral inherited trait in the Staffordshire Bull Terrier (Leon *et al.*, 1986) and the Dobermann (Stades, 1980). It has been studied extensively in the latter breed, where an incomplete dominant mode of inheritance has been suggested (Stades, 1983a). A grading system has been applied for the condition in the Dobermann, to allow clinical classification of the lesions:

1. Very minor posterior capsular cataract and retrolental pigment dots
2. More intense central posterior capsular cataract, with yellow/brown retrolental fibrous tissue and peripheral retrolental pigment dots. Persistent pupillary membrane is also commonly seen
3. Persistent tunica vasculosa lentis–hyaloid system visible as retrolental meshwork and abnormalities as in Grade 2
4. Lenticonus and abnormalities as Grade 2
5. Combination of Grade 3 and Grade 4 abnormalities
6. Combination of former grades associated with lens coloboma, microphakia and accumulations of pigment and blood.

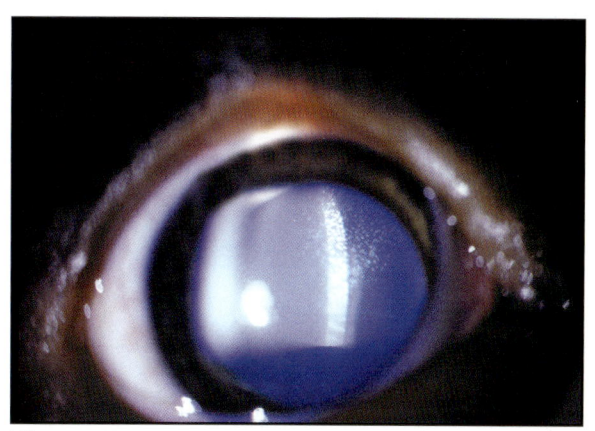

Figure 13.3 Fine opacities on posterior lens capsule: Grade 1 PHTVL/PHPV.

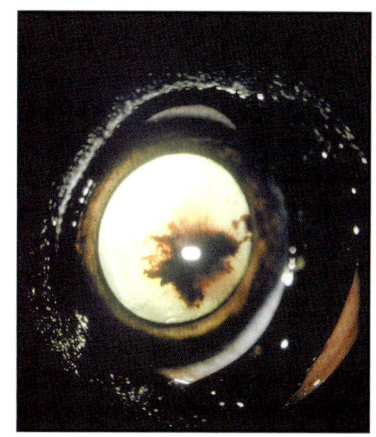

Figure 13.4 PHTVL/PHPV showing intralenticular haemorrhage and early cataract formation. (Courtesy of SM Crispin.)

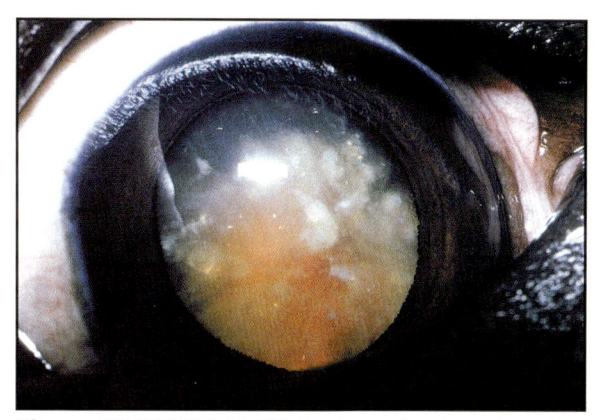

Figure 13.5 PHTVL/PHPV showing extensive cataract formation following intralenticular haemorrhage. (Courtesy of P Renwick.)

Preventive measures, in the form of selective breeding (excluding severely affected dogs classed as Grade 2–6 from breeding programmes), have been successful in reducing the incidence of PHTVL/PHPV in the Dobermann in the Netherlands (Stades *et al.*, 1991). Unlike the Dobermann, where dogs with anomalies from Grade 2 to 6 will develop progressive cataract and blindness, extensive cataracts are uncommon in association with the typical fibrovascular plaque on the posterior lens capsule seen in the Staffordshire Bull Terrier (Figure 13.6).

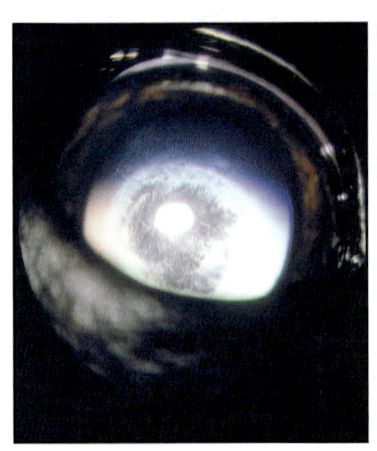

Figure 13.6 Typical fibrovascular plaque on posterior lens capsule in PHTVL/PHPV in the Staffordshire Bull Terrier. (Courtesy of D Gould.)

PHTVL/PHPV can occasionally occur in any breed of dog, and may be unilateral. When vision is severely impaired but retinal morphology and function are unaffected, phacoemulsification with posterior capsulectomy and anterior vitrectomy can be considered. The overall success rate in dogs with this condition is much lower than for uncomplicated cataracts, due to the risks associated with vitrectomy and the potential for haemorrhage from a patent hyaloid artery (Stades, 1983b). Wet field cautery may be required to cauterize any patent hyaloid vessels, but is not without hazard.

Vitreoretinal dysplasia

Vitreoretinal dysplasia describes an abnormal development of vitreous and neurosensory retina. Affected puppies either have retinal non-attachment, seen as a funnel-shaped abnormally formed retina in the vitreal cavity, or develop an early-onset detachment of an abnormally formed retina. Vitreal non-development is thought to be an important factor in the aetiopathogenesis of vitreoretinal dysplasia in the Bedlington Terrier and Sealyham Terrier. Vitreoretinal dysplasia due to non-allelic gene defects has been described in the Labrador Retriever and Samoyed. Animals homozygous for the gene defect have skeletal dysplasia in addition to the vitreoretinal dysplasia. Heterozygotes have a multifocal retinal dysplasia (see Chapter 14a).

Acquired conditions in the dog

Degeneration

Syneresis
As a result of ageing, or due to concurrent ocular disease, such as vitreal haemorrhage or glaucoma, the vitreal collagen framework can break down, leading to vitreal liquefaction. Collagen fibrils that are clumped together are easily visible ophthalmoscopically as 'floaters' in the liquefied vitreous. This process is irreversible and can predispose the eye to the development of a retinal detachment.

Asteroid hyalosis
Asteroid hyalosis is a form of endogenous vitreal degeneration in which, in contrast to synchysis scintillans (see below), the vitreous does not become liquefied. Although the aetiopathogenesis of asteroid hyalosis remains unclear, it is thought that the dispersed particles consist of a lipid and calcium complex. Clinical diagnosis is straightforward, as the presence of small refractile particles suspended throughout the vitreal framework is pathognomonic (Figures 13.7 and 13.8). The diagnosis can be made with pen light examination alone in the majority of cases, and the condition is not thought to affect vision or give rise to other ocular disease.

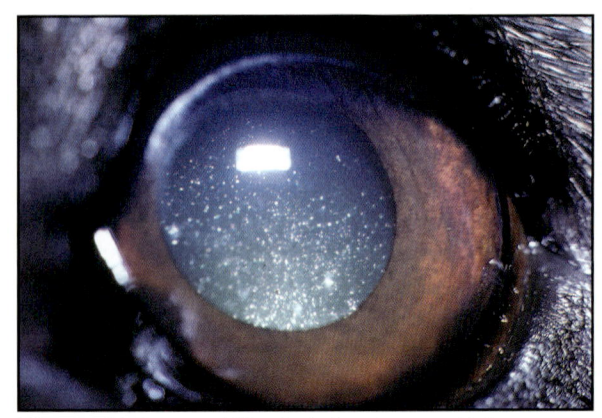

Figure 13.7 Asteroid hyalosis in a 3-year-old German Shepherd Dog. (Courtesy of P Renwick.)

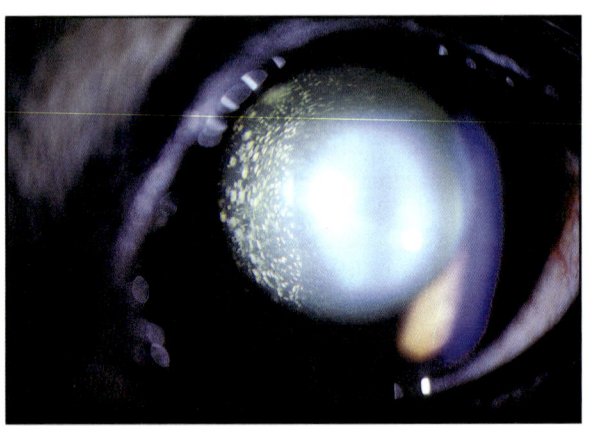

Figure 13.8 Asteroid hyalosis shown by slit lamp photography in an 11-year-old crossbreed dog.

Synchysis scintillans
In synchysis scintillans (also named cholesterolosis bulbi), fine scintillating particles containing cholesterol are found in the liquefied vitreous. The particles settle out ventrally if the eye is kept still, but following rapid ocular movement the particles become dispersed throughout the vitreous (Figure 13.9). This condition is not thought to interfere with vision, but as it is commonly the result of concurrent ocular disease, other abnormalities may be present. In humans, synchysis scintillans is usually the result of a previous intravitreal haemorrhage, and, in such cases, the particles may be darker in colour.

Vitreal haemorrhage
As the vitreous is primarily avascular, vitreal haemorrhage is always the result of a pathological process of a neighbouring ocular tissue or associated with a

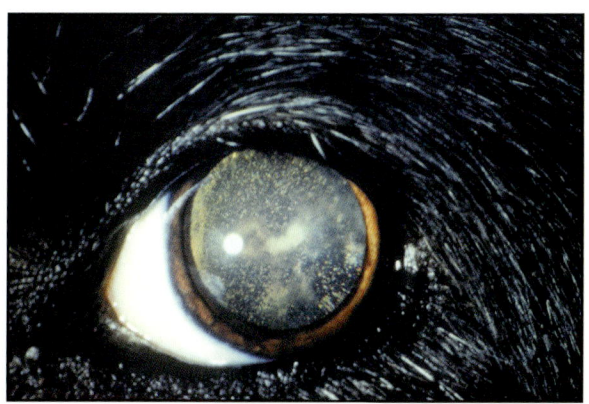

Figure 13.9 Synchysis scintillans in a crossbreed dog. (Courtesy of SM Crispin.)

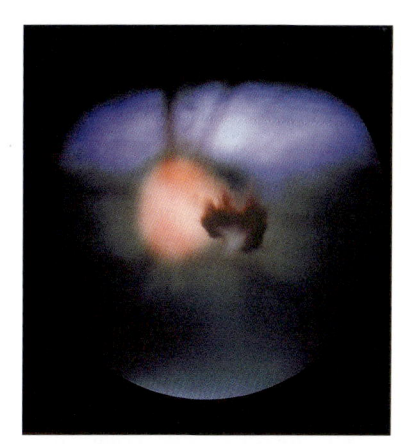

Figure 13.11 Small intravitreal haemorrhage in a 6-week-old Border Collie. (Courtesy of P Renwick.)

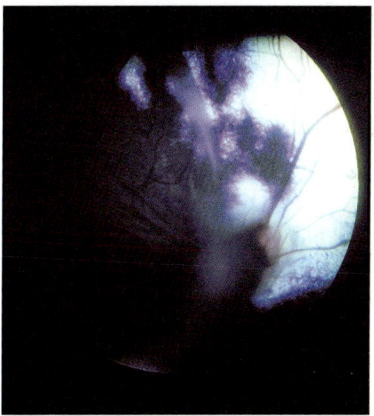

Figure 13.12 Vitreal haemorrhage and vitreoretinal traction band formation with persistent hyaloid artery in a 1-year-old Welsh Terrier.

congenital anomaly involving abnormal persistence of blood vessels (see above). It is commonly seen in cases of trauma and hypertensive retinopathy; other causes include retinal detachment, neoplasia, coagulopathies, severe uveitis, glaucoma and optic neuritis. Vitreal haemorrhage can be severe and prevent detailed ophthalmoscopic examination of the posterior segment. However, as many cases of vitreal haemorrhage are the result of an underlying systemic disease, careful examination of the other eye may suggest an aetiology.

Vitreal haemorrhage can be divided into pre-retinal (between the posterior vitreal face and the internal limiting membrane) and intravitreal. Whereas pre-retinal haemorrhages are usually keel-boat shaped (Figure 13.10) and resorb rapidly, haemorrhage into the vitreal body is often diffuse (Figure 13.11) and will clear only very slowly over weeks and months. Liquefaction of the vitreal gel is common following haemorrhage, and condensations of vitreal collagen around the clot with pseudocapsule and vitreal membrane formation can occur. Severe vitreal haemorrhage can be deleterious to the retina due to toxic effects from blood breakdown products or the formation of pre-retinal fibrous membranes and vitreoretinal traction band formation (Figure 13.12). This may lead to rhegmatogenous retinal detachment, i.e. a retinal detachment arising from a tear.

The treatment of vitreal haemorrhage is aimed at correcting any underlying disease. In human patients, where vitreal haemorrhage is often associated with diabetic retinopathy, vitrectomy has become an established mode of treatment. Vitrectomy is not, as yet, a commonly applied treatment for vitreal haemorrhage in veterinary medicine.

Vitritis

Being almost acellular, the vitreous is unlikely to mount an inflammatory response. However, involvement of the vitreous in inflammatory processes of surrounding tissues is common and described as vitritis or hyalitis. With intraocular inflammation, breakdown of the blood–ocular barrier occurs, allowing inflammatory cells and proteins, together with blood, to leak into the vitreous and destroy the gel structure. Vitritis presents clinically as a generalized 'blurring' of fundic detail on ophthalmoscopy, and severe vitritis may render fundic examination impossible. The most severe form of vitritis is seen in endophthalmitis resulting from infections caused by penetrating injuries, intraocular surgery or spread from systemic disease. Potential bacterial and fungal aetiologies must be considered.

Although rare in the UK, granulomatous endophthalmitis is commonly seen in other parts of the world as the result of ocular mycoses, such as blastomycosis, cryptococcosis and histoplasmosis.

Foreign bodies

Vitreal foreign bodies are generally associated with severe ocular trauma. The most common intraocular foreign bodies in dogs and cats are airgun pellets and

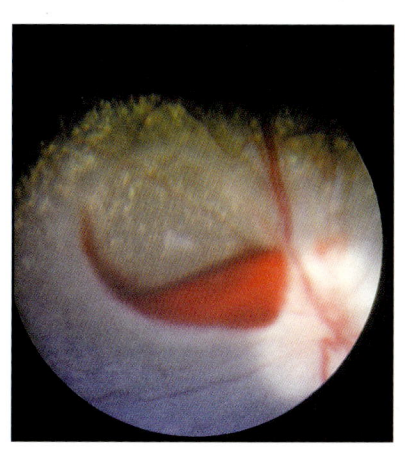

Figure 13.10 Keel-boat shaped pre-retinal haemorrhage.

lead shot. A gunshot injury must therefore be considered in every case of sudden-onset ocular pain. Signs of ocular penetration, in the form of corneal or scleral wounds, should raise suspicion of the possible presence of a foreign body within the vitreal space. Ocular ultrasonography must be carried out if vitreal haemorrhage or opacification of the anterior segment prevents ophthalmoscopic assessment.

Although both lead shot and pellets are visible on radiographic examination, it is usually not possible to determine on radiographs alone whether the foreign body is situated within the vitreous or within the orbit. The use of ocular ultrasonography can aid in the exact location of the foreign body. Vegetable material that has penetrated the outer ocular coats is usually contaminated with organisms; thus, endophthalmitis is likely to result if a piece of vegetable material remains in the vitreous.

The prognosis for salvage of the eye is dependent on the extent of trauma at the time of entry of the foreign body, especially on the involvement of the lens. Whether removal of a vitreal foreign body is attempted depends on whether the particle is surgically accessible and also on the type of material and its interactions with intraocular tissues. Whereas high-quality glass, stone, high-quality plastics, stainless steel and other high-quality alloys are considered to be relatively inert and are probably best left *in situ,* others, such as organic matter, iron, copper, low-grade alloys and low-grade glass and plastics are known to be poorly tolerated (Belin, 1992). However, if, following an ocular perforation, a foreign body is retained intravitreally, referral for a specialist assessment is advised.

Neoplasia

Primary vitreal neoplasia has not been reported, but involvement of the vitreous is seen in neoplasia of the adjacent tissues, both by infiltration with neoplastic cells and by displacement of the vitreous by solid tumours. Possibly the most common type of neoplastic vitreal involvement is seen in lymphoma, where neoplastic cells originating from the uveal tract infiltrate the vitreous. Exudate and haemorrhage from leaky new blood vessels that often accompany intraocular neoplasia commonly lead to vitreal degeneration.

Clinically, vitritis, retinal detachment or masses within the vitreal cavity may be seen; further diagnostic aids, such as ocular ultrasonography and vitreocentesis, should be considered. Cytology of a vitreal aspirate may aid in the diagnosis of systemic metastasis, especially if the primary tumour site has not been identified. However, the procedure is not without risk and, in sighted eyes, should be left to those experienced in the technique. The treatment will depend on the type of tumour present, but most eyes with solid neoplasms within the vitreal space will require enucleation.

Cysts

Uveal cysts can sometimes be found on examination of the vitreous and present as variably pigmented semitransparent spherical structures floating in the vitreous body. They can vary in size and usually have no impact on vision (Figure 13.13).

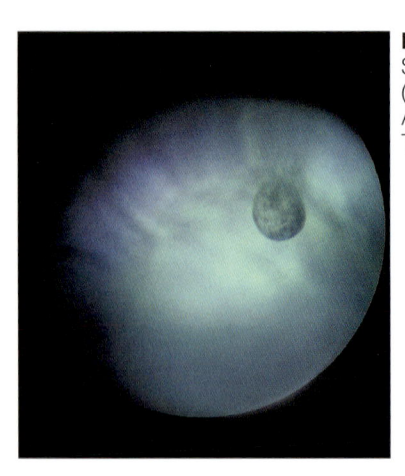

Figure 13.13 Small vitreal cyst. (Courtesy of the Animal Health Trust.)

Parasites

Occasionally, aberrant parasites can be found in the vitreous on ocular examination. Reported parasites include *Toxocara canis, Dirofilaria immitis, Angiostrongylus vasorum* and *Echinococcus* spp. Species of Diptera have also been seen, associated with ophthalmomyiasis interna. Although some parasites can be killed by the use of systemic medication, surgical removal of larger parasites is indicated to avoid deleterious inflammatory reactions following parasitic death. However, surgical intervention is a skilled procedure and should only be performed by those with experience of posterior segment surgery.

Vitreal prolapse and herniation

Extraocular prolapse of vitreous can be seen in traumatic ocular injuries with scleral or corneal lacerations or during some types of intraocular surgery. Herniation of degenerate vitreous through the pupil into the anterior chamber (Figure 13.14) is often the first sign of lens instability. As a result of zonular breakdown, the anchoring collagen fibril arrangements at the capsulohyaloid ligament weaken and the anterior vitreous undergoes syneresis. In severe cases, the herniated vitreous can obstruct the iridocorneal angle, leading to an increase in the intraocular pressure. Herniated vitreous is often present on first incision into the anterior chamber in cases of lens luxation; closure of the corneal incision should not be carried out until the prolapsed vitreous has been removed.

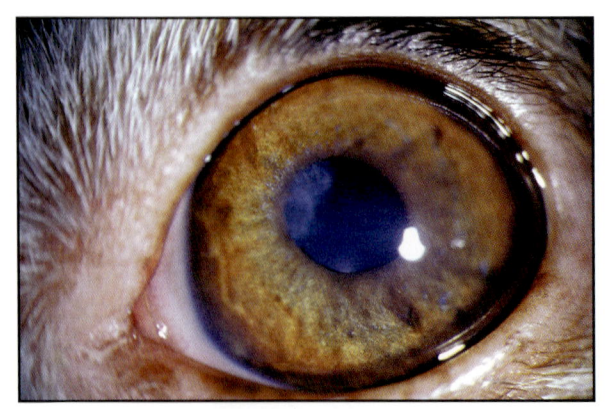

Figure 13.14 Vitreal material in the pupil of a 5-year-old Jack Russell Terrier caused by lens zonule breakdown.

Vitreal interventions

Vitrectomy

As mentioned previously, herniation of vitreous into the anterior chamber is a common presentation in lens luxation. Vitreal prolapse through accidental tears in the posterior lens capsule is a major complication during phacoemulsification. Vitreous that prolapses into the anterior chamber as a result of posterior capsular defects or zonular breakdown during lens surgery should be removed. The prolapsed vitreous can impair aqueous drainage, potentially leading to glaucoma. If it is incarcerated into a corneal wound, it can lead to surface epithelial cell downgrowth into the anterior chamber, which may result in additional complications. If vitreous is left touching the corneal endothelium, it may lead to corneal endothelial dysfunction and corneal oedema.

Surgical removal of herniated or prolapsed vitreous (vitrectomy) can be carried out manually, with cellulose sponges and scissors, or mechanically, with automated vitreous cutting devices. These instruments are usually an integral part of phacoemulsification equipment and can be used through a small corneal incision (approximately 2–3 mm).

If removal is carried out manually, great care must be taken not to exert excessive traction on the adherent vitreal gel, to avoid retinal detachment.

Vitrectomy can also be carried out as a diagnostic procedure in cases of endophthalmitis, and vitreous samples are forwarded for microscopic examination, bacterial and fungal culture. It must be emphasized that vitrectomy is a challenging procedure with severe potential complications and should only be carried out by experienced veterinary ophthalmologists.

Therapeutic intravitreal injection

Adequate treatment with antibiotics and anti-inflammatory drugs is of utmost importance for the outcome in cases of hyalitis or endophthalmitis. Topical application of any drug is rarely able to achieve therapeutic levels in the vitreous, especially in cases of bacterial endophthalmitis. As the vitreous is avascular, systemic delivery of drugs is limited by the blood–ocular barrier, and only lipid-soluble drugs, such as chloramphenicol, are likely to reach a significant concentration after systemic administration. With the breakdown of the blood–ocular barrier in uveitis, adequate levels of other drugs may also be achieved within the vitreous following systemic medication.

The most efficient way, however, to achieve adequate levels of medication in the vitreous is by intravitreal injection. Drugs used for intravitreal injection are usually antibiotics or steroids, and recommended doses of intravitreal antibiotics have been extrapolated from use in rabbits, primates or humans. It must be remembered that intravitreal injection is associated with risks, such as lens injury, haemorrhage, infection and retinal detachment, and that the drug itself can have a deleterious effect on vitreous gel structure and other intraocular tissues. For this reason, intravitreal injections should only be carried out by experienced veterinary ophthalmologists.

Vitreal conditions in the cat

The anatomy, embryology and biochemistry of the feline vitreous are very similar to those of the canine vitreous, but there are minor differences: the cortical vitreous in the cat is more liquid and the central vitreous has a more solid nature.

Congenital conditions

Congenital conditions of the vitreous are extremely rare in the cat and published reports are limited to the presence of a persistent hyaloid artery (Ketring and Glaze, 1994; Barnett and Crispin, 1998). Persistent tunica vasculosa lentis posterioris has not been reported in the cat.

Acquired conditions

Chronic feline uveitis

Involvement of the vitreous in chronic feline uveitis is common; the extent of vitreal involvement is dependent on the location of the uveitis (anterior, intermediate or posterior). An interesting phenomenon is the accumulation of inflammatory cells within the anterior vitreous in pars planitis (Figure 13.15). The clinical appearance of this change has led to the use of the descriptive term 'snowbanking'. It is thought frequently to be associated with feline immunodeficiency virus infection. Snowbanking is also occasionally seen in uveitis as the result of toxoplasmal infection (see Chapter 10).

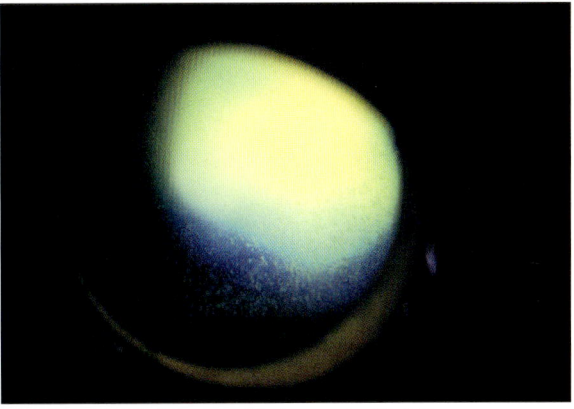

Figure 13.15 Pars planitis in a cat with feline immunodeficiency virus infection. (Courtesy of SM Crispin.)

Vitreal haemorrhage

Vitreal haemorrhages (Figure 13.16) are possibly more commonly noted in the cat than in the dog and should alert the observer to the possible presence of an underlying hypertensive retinopathy (Barnett and Crispin, 1998, and see Chapter 14). Vitreal haemorrhage can also be the result of head trauma and may be an indicator of the severity of the trauma, considering how well the feline globe is protected by the deep orbit.

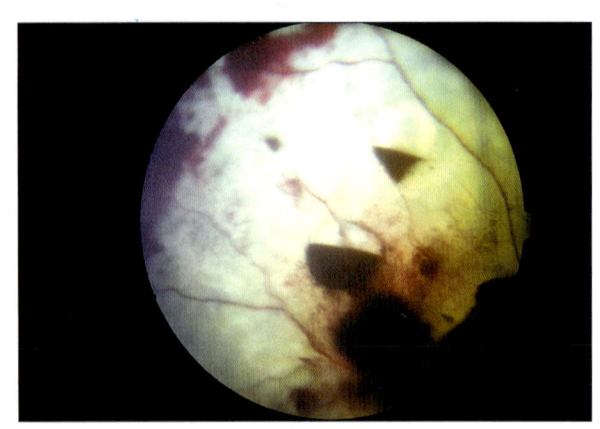

Figure 13.16 Retinal and vitreal haemorrhage in a cat with systemic hypertensive disease. (Courtesy of SM Crispin.)

References and further reading

Barnett KC (1990) *A Colour Atlas of Veterinary Ophthalmology*. Wolfe, London
Barnett KC and Crispin SM (1998) Vitreous. In: *Feline Ophthalmology: An Atlas and Text*, pp. 144–145. WB Saunders, Philadelphia
Belin NW (1992) Foreign bodies and penetrating injuries to the eye. In: *Ocular Emergencies*, ed. RA Catalano, pp. 197–213. WB Saunders, Philadelphia
Forrester JV, Dick AD, McMenamin P and Lee WR (1996) *The Eye – Basic Sciences in Practice*. WB Saunders, Philadelphia
Ketring KL and Glaze MB (1994) Vitreous. In: *Atlas of Feline Ophthalmology*, pp. 201–207. Veterinary Learning Systems, Trenton, NJ
Leon A, Curtis R and Barnett KC (1986) Hereditary persistent hyperplastic primary vitreous in the Staffordshire Bull Terrier. *Journal of the American Animal Hospital Association* **22**, 765–774
Stades F C (1980) Persistent hyperplastic tunica vasculosa lentis and persistent hyperplastic primary vitreous (PHTVL/PHPV) in 90 closely related Doberman Pinschers: clinical aspects. *Journal of the American Animal Hospital Association* **16**, 739–751
Stades FC (1983a) Persistent hyperplastic tunica vasculosa lentis and persistent hyperplastic primary vitreous in Doberman Pinschers: genetic aspects. *Journal of the American Animal Hospital Association* **19**, 957–964
Stades FC (1983b) Persistent hyperplastic tunica vasculosa lentis and persistent hyperplastic primary vitreous in Doberman Pinschers: techniques and results of surgery. *Journal of the American Animal Hospital Association* **19**, 393–402
Stades FC, Boeve MH, van der Brom WE and van der Linde-Sipman JS (1991) The incidence of PHTVL/PHPV in the Doberman and the results of breeding rules. *Veterinary Quarterly* **13**, 24–29

14a

The canine fundus

Gillian McLellan

Introduction

The term 'fundus' describes the part of the posterior segment of the eye that is viewed with the ophthalmoscope. Structures that contribute to the ophthalmoscopic appearance of the fundus include the optic disc (also known as the optic nerve head (ONH) or optic papilla), the neurosensory retina and the retinal pigment epithelium, the underlying choroid and, in some instances, the sclera.

The neurosensory retina is continuous anteriorly with the non-pigmented epithelium of the ciliary body at the ora ciliaris retinae. The retinal pigment epithelium (RPE) is continuous with the pigmented epithelium of the ciliary body. The optic disc represents the commencement of myelination of the retinal ganglion cell axons, as they converge to form the optic nerve and leave the globe through the lamina cribrosa of the sclera.

Anatomy and physiology of the retina and choroid

Retina

The retina develops from the two layers of neuroectoderm that constitute the optic cup. The optic cup develops from an evagination of the primitive forebrain, known as the optic vesicle; therefore, the retina may be regarded as an extension of the forebrain via the optic nerve. The neurosensory layer of the retina forms from the inner, non-pigmented layer and the RPE forms from the outer pigmented layer of the optic cup (Figure 14.1).

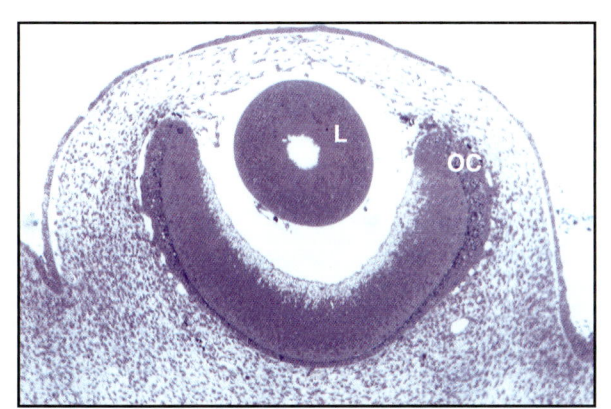

Figure 14.1 Photomicrograph that demonstrates both the inner (neurosensory) and the outer retinal pigment epithelial layers of the optic cup (OC) in a canine embryo. The developing lens (L) is also shown.

In the dog, development of photoreceptor cells occurs in the first 2–3 weeks postnatally, and organization of retinal layers may not be completed for up to 6–8 weeks postnatally (Gum et al., 1984).

Histologically, the retina may be described in terms of layers (Figure 14.2).

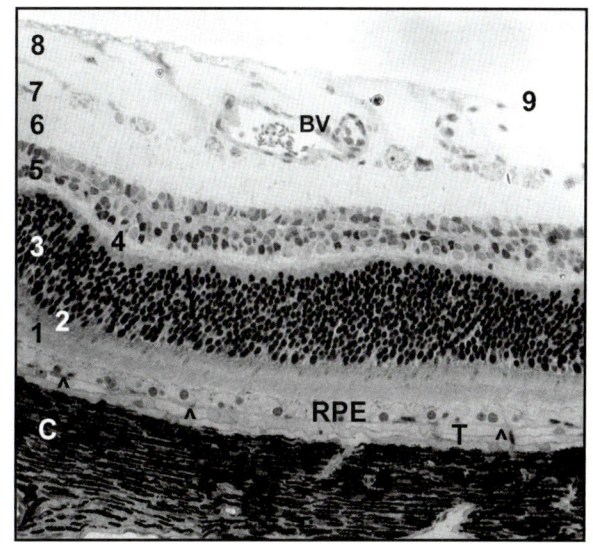

Figure 14.2 Histological section of the retina and choroid of a normal dog, illustrating the tapetum (T) and choriocapillaris (^) within the choroid (C), the retinal pigment epithelium (RPE) and the neurosensory retina. The neurosensory retina consists of the visual cell/photoreceptor layer (1), the outer limiting membrane (2), the outer nuclear layer (3), the outer plexiform layer (4), the inner nuclear layer (5), the inner plexiform layer (6), the ganglion cell layer (7), the nerve fibre layer (8), and the inner limiting membrane (9). Retinal blood vessels are also shown (BV).

The outermost layer of the neurosensory retina, the *photoreceptor layer*, contains the outer segments of the rod and cone photoreceptor cells. In dogs, the photoreceptor layer consists mainly of rod photoreceptors.

An area of greater cone density (known as the area centralis) exists as an oval area extending horizontally, dorsally and laterally to the optic disc. Rod photoreceptors are slender and cylindrical in profile, and function more effectively in dim light than cones, and are thus more suited to night vision. However, the visual acuity produced by rod photoreceptors is lower than that of cones.

Photoreceptor outer segments consist of stacks of membranous discs which undergo constant shedding and renewal. Photoreceptor inner segments contain large numbers of mitochondria and other organelles. The photoreceptor inner segments are separated from their nuclei, within the *outer nuclear layer,* by a very thin *outer limiting membrane.*

Progressing inwards, the *outer plexiform layer* consists of the terminal branches of the photoreceptor cell axons and their synapses with the horizontal and bipolar cells. The cell bodies of the horizontal and bipolar cells, the amacrine cells and those of the Müller cells, which serve as supportive cells extending through the neurosensory retina, are located in the *inner nuclear layer.* The horizontal, bipolar and amacrine cells, which maintain a connection between the photoreceptors and ganglion cells, are involved in the modification and integration of stimuli.

The *inner plexiform layer,* which is thicker than the outer plexiform layer, represents a region of synapses between the bipolar and amacrine cells and the ganglion cells. Functionally, this layer accentuates contrast in the retinal image and enhances detection of motion.

The *ganglion cell layer* contains retinal ganglion cell bodies, the axons of which gather in the *nerve fibre layer.* These axons pass centripetally, without branching, to form the optic nerve. To maintain retinal transparency, the nerve fibres are typically not myelinated until they reach the optic disc. The nerve fibre layer also contains some neuroglial cells and the innermost tips of the Müller cells. Retinal blood vessels occupy the nerve fibre, ganglion cell, and inner plexiform layers.

The *inner limiting membrane* is formed by the fused terminations of the Müller cells.

The outermost layer of the retina, the RPE, consists of a single layer of cells which play a vital role in the maintenance of the overlying neurosensory retinal tissue. The RPE is responsible for the control of metabolite movement to and from the outer retina, and it phagocytoses spent photoreceptor outer segment debris. The RPE also plays an important role in the metabolism of vitamin A, which is vital to normal photoreceptor function. Although elsewhere normally densely pigmented, the RPE cells that overlie the tapetum lack melanin granules. Numerous microvilli extend from the inner surface of the RPE cells and surround the photoreceptor outer segments. These microvillus processes increase the surface area available for metabolite exchange and transport, facilitate phagocytosis of photoreceptor material and promote adhesion between the RPE and neurosensory retina.

Choroid

The choroid is external to the RPE; it is a highly vascular, pigmented tissue. The choroid also consists of a number of distinct layers.

Immediately underlying the RPE is a thin capillary layer, the *choriocapillaris,* beneath which, in the dorsal portion of the fundus, lies the highly reflective *tapetum.* The presence of a tapetum increases visual sensitivity in dim light by reflecting incident light back through the photoreceptors.

In dogs, the cellular tapetum consists of layers of polyhedral cells that contain reflective crystals within a regular array of membrane-bound rodlets. Beneath the tapetum lie *medium-sized and large vessel layers* and, in turn, the elastic pigmented connective tissue of the *suprachoroidea,* which represents a transition between the choroid and sclera (Samuelson, 1999). Small blood vessels penetrate the tapetum to connect the medium vessel and choriocapillaris layers.

Investigation of disorders of the fundus

Behavioural tests

The ability to 'follow' moving objects (e.g. cotton balls) and negotiate obstacles and stairs should be tested in both photopic (bright) and scotopic (dim) lighting conditions.

Reflexes

Pupillary light reflexes, menace response and dazzle reflexes may allow a crude assessment of visual capability. The pupillary light reflex and dazzle reflex are, however, subcortical reflexes that do not require conscious perception of visual stimuli. Therefore, as discussed in Chapter 15, these neuro-ophthalmological tests have significant limitations as a means of assessing retinal function and vision.

Ophthalmoscopy

Indirect and direct ophthalmoscopy (previously described in detail in Chapter 1a) are central to any investigation of retinal disease. Usually, both techniques are employed to facilitate thorough evaluation of the fundus; the former provides an overview and the latter allows a more detailed, magnified image of specific regions. Normal ophthalmoscopic features and commonly recognized abnormalities of the canine fundus are considered in later sections of this chapter.

Ultrasonography

As described in Chapter 1b, this is particularly useful in those cases in which opacification of the ocular media precludes ophthalmoscopic examination of the fundus. Total, infundibular retinal detachment appears as a 'gull wing' shape, with its apex at the site of attachment of the retina at the optic nerve (Figure 14.3).

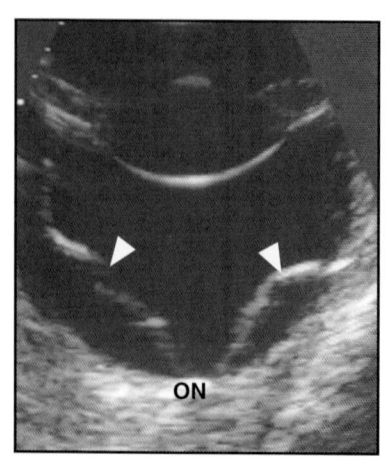

Figure 14.3 Ultrasonographic appearance of a total bullous retinal detachment. White arrowheads indicate the detached retina; ON = optic nerve. (Courtesy of CR Lamb.)

Fluorescein angiography

This is used infrequently in the clinical investigation of fundic disorders in dogs, due to the requirement for specialist instrumentation.

Fluorescein angiography is particularly helpful in the investigation of retinal vascular disease, although tapetal autofluorescence combined with an absence of RPE melanin within the tapetal fundus may mask visualization of capillaries in this region.

Electroretinogram

The electroretinogram (ERG) measures the electrical response of the retina to a light flash or pattern stimulus and is dependent on photoreceptor activity. Measurement of visually evoked potentials (VEPs) allows the evaluation of gross electrical activity elicited in the occipital cortex in response to a light stimulus. This electrophysiological technique gives a more accurate indication of visual perception. However, this technique is rarely used in the clinical investigation of disorders of the ocular fundus in dogs.

Electroretinography is considered further in the following section.

Understanding the ERG – Basic retinal electrophysiology

A basic understanding of photoreceptor electrophysiology and the process of phototransduction, which is responsible for the generation of electrical impulses in response to a light stimulus, is required before considering the principles of electroretinography.

The visual pigment of rods is rhodopsin, which contains a derivative of vitamin A. Rhodopsin is localized within the disc membranes of rod photoreceptor outer segments. The initial event in the process of phototransduction within the photoreceptor outer segment is the light-triggered isomerization of the 11-cis retinal component of rhodopsin. The 'activated' form of rhodopsin which results from the isomerization process is then able to interact with the protein transducin. Activated transducin molecules, in turn, interact with the phosphodiesterase (PDE) enzyme complex, causing a marked increase in PDE activity and consequent drop in the level of cyclic guanosine monophosphate (cGMP). High levels of cGMP in darkness interact with cGMP-gated ion channels in the photoreceptor outer segment plasma membrane, allowing an influx of cations and resulting in membrane depolarization. Thus, the fall in cGMP levels associated with phototransduction interrupts this 'dark current', leading to photoreceptor hyperpolarization. This hyperpolarization, in turn, leads to a modulation in the rate of secretion of a synaptic transmitter by the photoreceptor synaptic terminal, issuing a message to the retinal bipolar and horizontal cells.

The ERG gathers information on the electrophysiological function of the neuroretinal tissues, including photoreceptors, bipolar and ganglion cells, associated glia (Müller cells) and, if appropriately modified recording protocols are utilized, the RPE.

Recording the ERG

A consistent, bright light source is required to generate the light flashes which stimulate photoreceptor hyperpolarization. The subject's pupils should be widely dilated in order to allow optimum retinal illumination. Recording equipment generally consists of reference and earthed subdermal electrodes and an active recording electrode, most commonly a corneal contact lens electrode. The subdermal electrodes are typically positioned near the lateral canthus and at the nuchal crest. The signal generated is then amplified and averaged over a number of flashes. For complex, sensitive protocols, such as those employed in the early diagnosis of inherited photoreceptor dystrophies and degenerations, patients must be anaesthetized. In contrast, simple, scotopic ERG protocols (conducted after a period of dark adaptation) may be performed in conscious or lightly sedated patients. Scotopic ERG protocols are frequently used in veterinary patients to assess retinal function prior to proceeding with cataract surgery, and are invaluable in the diagnosis of sudden acquired retinal degeneration (see below).

An example of a typical, scotopic ERG trace is shown in Figure 14.4.

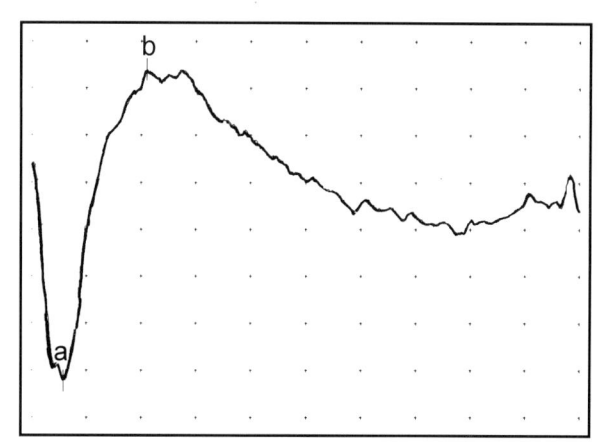

Figure 14.4 Scotopic ERG trace (normal adult dog). Horizontal divisions represent 300 milliseconds and vertical divisions represent 20 microvolts.

The ERG trace may be described in simple terms:

- The *a wave* mainly reflects photoreceptor electrical activity, as they hyperpolarize in response to a bright flash of light which interrupts the 'dark current'
- The *b wave* reflects bipolar cell activity and associated changes in the electrical potential of glial cells. Oscillatory potentials on the b wave provide information on the electrical activity within the inner retina
- The *c wave* reflects mainly RPE activity; however, this component is not usually detected using routine ERG protocols, as brighter stimuli of longer duration are required, together with alterations to the standard recording equipment (Acland, 1988).

Molecular genetic tests for inherited retinal disease

Current research leading to the development of DNA-based tests will increasingly offer the means of eradicating a number of inherited canine retinal disorders. Molecular genetic tests offer considerable advantages over traditional methods of inherited disease control, such as costly and time-consuming test-mating procedures.

DNA-based tests are of particular value in those disorders which are of late onset (e.g. progressive rod–cone degeneration (prcd) and late-onset generalized progressive retinal atrophy (gPRA)). They can be useful in predicting which animals will be clinically affected, and in predicting those that are carriers of recessively inherited traits, early in life, before they reach breeding age.

For diseases, such as collie eye anomaly, which have a very high incidence within specific breeds, and, in particular, for those diseases which are inherited as autosomal recessive traits, the development of a specific molecular genetic test would allow the identification of carrier animals. This would allow for their inclusion in the breeding programme if they display highly desirable traits, provided that matings involve genotypically unaffected animals. Thus, use of the available gene pool could be maximized, reducing the likelihood of promoting the emergence of other recessively inherited traits, while allowing the inherited retinal disorder to be eliminated from the breed population gradually, over a number of generations (Petersen-Jones, 1999).

It should, however, be borne in mind that DNA-based tests are specific for individual gene mutations that may be specific for a single breed. They should therefore be considered to represent an adjunct, rather than an alternative, to traditional clinical screening schemes in the control of inherited ocular disease.

Molecular genetic tests which are presently available for inherited canine retinal dystrophies and degenerations are discussed in greater detail later in this chapter.

Normal ophthalmoscopic features of the canine fundus

Marked variation in the ophthalmoscopic appearance of the fundus exists both within and between species; the degree to which fundic appearance may vary between normal dogs is striking. It is imperative that the clinician is familiar with the spectrum of normal variation if incorrect diagnosis is to be avoided.

Tapetal fundus

In most dogs, a bright shiny sweep of colour, roughly triangular in shape, occupies the dorsal area of the fundus (Figure 14.5). In this region, the RPE lacks pigment and there are tapetal cells present within the choroid, beneath the choriocapillaris. Although the normal thickness of the retina does attenuate light reflected from the underlying tapetum, the retina is essentially transparent, so the ophthalmoscopic appearance is of retinal blood vessels against a background of tapetum. The small blood vessels connecting the medium-vessel and choriocapillaris layers, may be observed end-on as they penetrate the tapetum as multiple dark spots known as 'stars of Winslow'; however, this ophthalmoscopic feature is less obvious in dogs than in certain other species, such as horses.

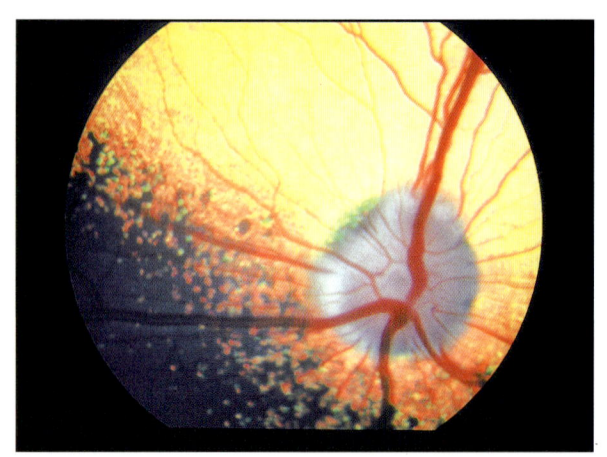

Figure 14.5 Normal adult canine fundus in a Cocker Spaniel.

Tapetal fundus coloration differs greatly between individuals, although in dogs it is generally yellow, orange, green or blue. The tapetal colour often differs slightly at its margins, e.g. a yellow tapetum may have a blue or green border. The margins of the tapetum may be clearly demarcated or irregular and broken up (the latter appearance being particularly prevalent in long-haired breeds). Islands of pigment may be visible within the tapetal fundus, and islands of tapetum may be visible within the non-tapetal fundus. Typically, the tapetum extends to the level of the optic disc; however, the extent of the tapetum may also vary, tending to be small in small dogs (Figure 14.6) and larger in large dogs. The tapetum may be absent, particularly in subalbinotic dogs.

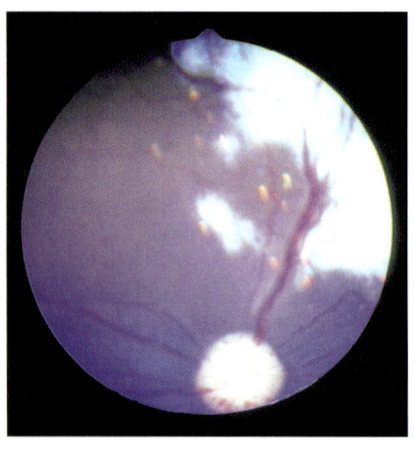

Figure 14.6 Normal adult canine fundus in a Chihuahua.

It should be borne in mind that tapetal development is incomplete in puppies up to 12–14 weeks of age. In very young puppies, the future tapetal region first appears dark grey, changing to violet or lilac (Figure 14.7) and then bright blue, before achieving its definitive adult coloration.

Non-tapetal fundus

The non-tapetal fundus, ventral to the optic disc and peripheral to the tapetum, typically appears dark grey, brown or black in colour (Figure 14.8). This appearance is due to the presence of melanin within the RPE cells beneath the neurosensory retina, with retinal

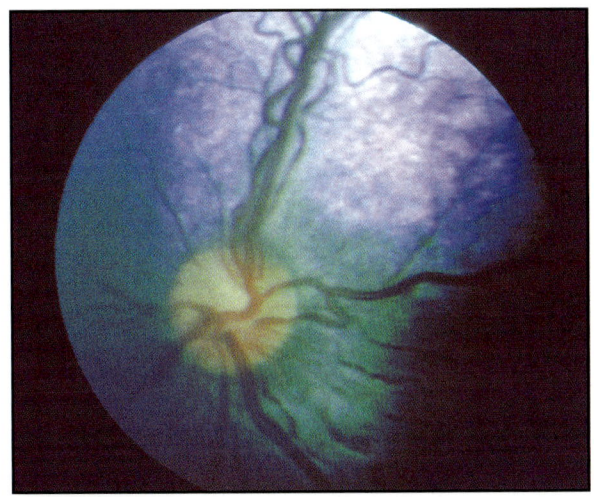

Figure 14.7 Normal canine fundus in a 7-week-old puppy.

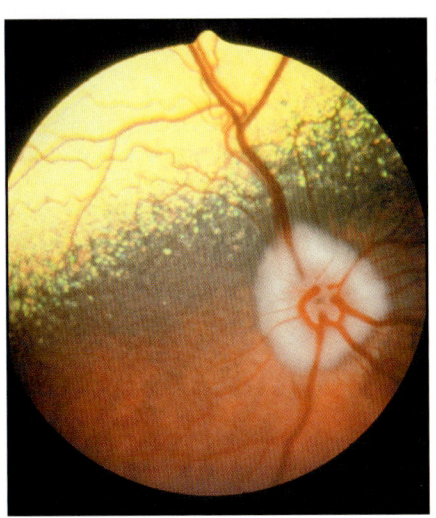

Figure 14.8 Normal adult canine fundus in an Old English Sheepdog (left eye with pale brown iris). (Courtesy of SM Crispin.)

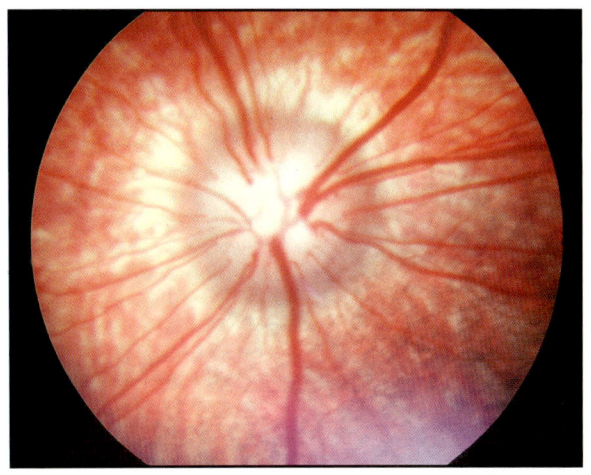

Figure 14.9 Normal adult canine fundus in an Old English Sheepdog (right eye with blue iris).

blood vessels observed against a background of RPE and choroidal pigment. However, degrees of pigment dilution lead to variations ranging from a reddish tan to a striped appearance, which is characteristic of subalbinotic dogs (Figure 14.9). This appearance is due to an absence of pigment in the RPE, exposing the underlying choroidal blood vessels, which are thus observed against a background of choroidal pigmentation. Choroidal vessels have a more orange appearance than the retinal vasculature and are orientated approximately radially. The 'tigroid' striped appearance is accentuated in animals that lack choroidal pigmentation, where the choroidal vessels are viewed against the white background of the underlying sclera. The latter appearance is most commonly associated with a merle coat colour, and with blue and heterochromic irides.

Optic disc

The normal canine optic disc appears white or pink, due to myelination of nerve fibres as they converge to form the optic nerve. Although the optic nerve is circular in cross-section, the shape of the optic disc may vary as a result of myelin extending into the nerve fibre layer of the retina beyond the margins of the optic nerve head. In puppies the optic disc is round, as myelination is a postnatal phenomenon. It is not uncommon for the optic disc to have an oval, triangular or irregular outline in adult dogs. This excessive myelination is frequently exaggerated in Golden Retrievers and German Shepherd Dogs and is termed 'pseudopapilloedema' (Figure 14.10). This may be distinguished from pathological swelling of the optic nerve head by observing the course of retinal blood vessels (which should not be deviated over the optic disc) and by identification of the normal physiological pit (a small grey spot at the centre of the optic disc). Occasionally, a small glial remnant of the hyaloid vasculature ('Bergmeister's papilla') may be observed at the centre of the optic disc. Some dogs have a hyperreflective crescent around the disc, known as conus: this is the only instance of 'normal' hyperreflectivity. Others have a ring of pigment around the disc.

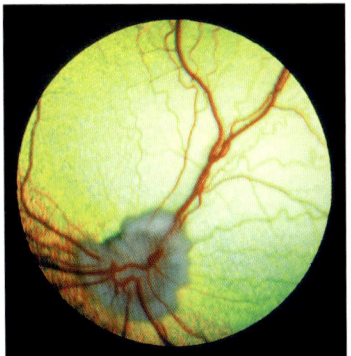

Figure 14.10 Normal adult canine fundus demonstrating 'pseudopapilloedema' due to extensive myelination of the optic disc.

Retinal vasculature

Dogs possess a holangiotic retina, in which the inner neurosensory retina receives a direct blood supply. Typically, 3–5 major veins are visible, which converge at the optic disc and may anastomose on its surface to a variable degree. The number of major retinal blood vessels may vary, as may the extent of their anastomoses on the surface of the optic disc. Slightly narrower diameter major retinal arterioles emerge at the optic disc and follow the course of the retinal veins. These major retinal blood vessels branch as smaller venules and arterioles throughout the fundus. Vasculature tends

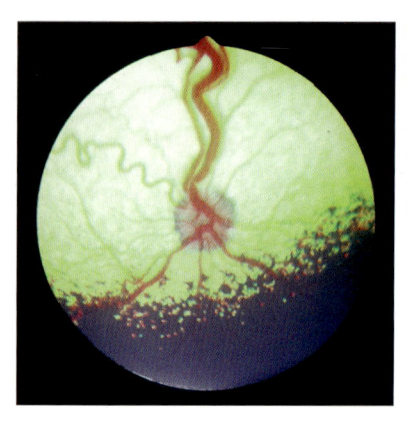

Figure 14.11 Normal adult canine fundus demonstrating tortuous retinal vasculature and a small optic disc/micropapilla.

to curve around, rather than traverse, the area centralis, dorsolateral to the optic disc. Tortuosity of the retinal vasculature may be a normal feature in some individuals (Figure 14.11).

General ophthalmoscopic abnormalities

Altered tapetal reflectivity
Tapetal hyperreflectivity signifies a thinning of the neurosensory retina, e.g. due to atrophy or degeneration. The tapetum is viewed through a thinner layer of retinal tissue than normal and, consequently, appears brighter, due to a reduction in the degree of attenuation of reflected light (see Figures 14.20, 14.23 and 14.29).

Tapetal reflectivity may be reduced by disease processes that are associated with thickening of the retina, e.g. due to folding, detachment, oedema or cellular infiltration of the neurosensory retina (see Figures 14.16, 14.25 and 14.27).

Altered pigmentation
Lesions within the pigmented region of the fundus which result in thickening, oedema, or exudates within the neurosensory retina will appear as paler areas against the background of RPE pigment (see Figure 14.17).

Proliferation, migration and aggregation of melanocytes and RPE cells within either the tapetal or non-tapetal fundus are non-specific responses to insult, such as inflammation, injury and degenerative processes (see Figure 14.29). Black or dark brown melanin pigment should be distinguished from the lighter brown or tan-coloured lipopigment which accumulates within the RPE of animals affected by retinal pigment epithelial dystrophy (see below, and Figure 14.23).

Vascular changes
Attenuation of retinal vasculature occurs secondarily to retinal degeneration and is most readily observed in the peripheral fundus, affecting the smaller arterioles around the optic disc. The major venules 'disappear' only in very advanced retinal degeneration (see Figure 14.20), although their calibre may be reduced earlier in the degenerative process.

Perivascular cuffing with inflammatory cell infiltrates may be observed in chorioretinitis.

Changes may be observed in the retinal vasculature in response to systemic disease processes, such as anaemia, hyperviscosity syndrome, systemic hypertension and hyperlipoproteinaemia (see below).

Haemorrhage
The appearance of retinal haemorrhages depends on their relative depth within the retina. Subretinal haemorrhages generally appear very dark red and are often diffuse and ill-defined; intraretinal haemorrhages appear as small dark round spots (Figure 14.12); superficial retinal haemorrhages appear as radial, flame-like streaks, reflecting the course of axons within the nerve fibre layer (see Figure 14.34); preretinal haemorrhages may assume a 'keel-boat' shape (Figure 14.12).

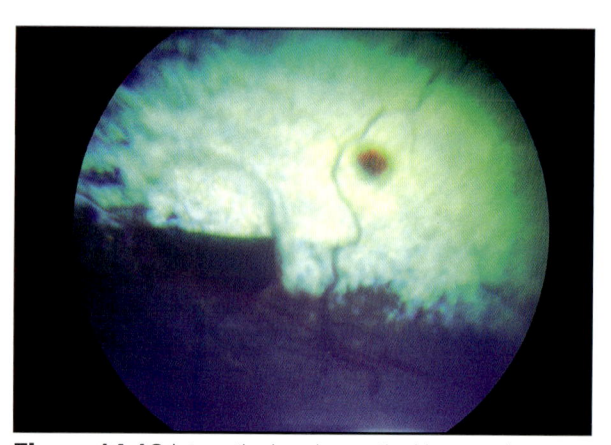

Figure 14.12 Intraretinal and preretinal haemorrhages associated with vascular disease and coagulopathy due to multiple myeloma in an adult dog.

Developmental lesions of the retina and choroid

Collie eye anomaly
As its name suggests, this congenital disorder is most prevalent in the Collie breeds, in particular the Rough and Smooth Collie and the Shetland Sheepdog. The clinical incidence of this disorder in Collie breeds is high, with the reported percentage of affected dogs of these breeds ranging from approximately 40% to more than 75% depending on geographic location, the age group examined and criteria employed in the interpretation of disease status (Roberts, 1969; Bedford, 1982b; Bjerkås, 1991; Wallin-Håkanson et al., 2000 a and b). However, the incidence of the disease in the Border Collie appears to be much lower (Bedford, 1982a). A similar syndrome has been described in other breeds, most notably the Lancashire Heeler (Bedford, 1998) and the Australian Shepherd Dog (Rubin et al., 1991).

Clinical and pathological features
The characteristic lesion of collie eye anomaly (CEA) is an area of choroidal hypoplasia (also termed chorioretinal dysplasia) lateral to the optic disc. Choroidal hypoplasia appears, on ophthalmoscopy, as a pale patch lateral to the optic disc, within which abnormal

choroidal vessels may be observed against a white scleral background (Figures 14.13 and 14.14). Abnormal choroidal vessels may be recognized by their altered diameter and irregular distribution, which departs from the normal, approximately radial, pattern of the choroidal vasculature. Within this region, the choroid is attenuated, has a poorly developed vascular bed and lacks pigment (Roberts, 1969).

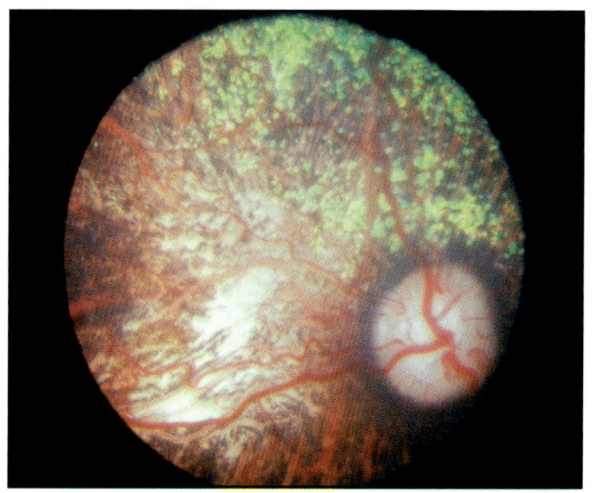

Figure 14.13 Choroidal hypoplasia in the right eye of a Rough Collie. (Courtesy of SR Hollingsworth.)

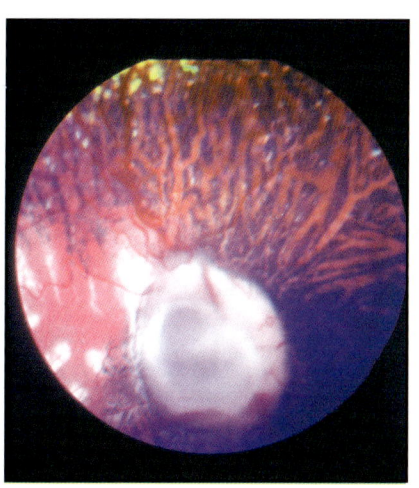

Figure 14.14 Choroidal hypoplasia and optic disc coloboma in the right eye of a Shetland Sheepdog. (Courtesy of PGC Bedford.)

Embryological studies have implicated faulty obliteration of the optic vesicle and abnormal differentiation of the RPE in the process of impaired differentiation of mesodermal, i.e. choroidal and scleral, tissues (Latshaw et al., 1969).

Choroidal hypoplasia may be accompanied by other ocular abnormalities, including optic nerve, or peripapillary, coloboma (Figures 14.14 and 14.15) (see below) and, as secondary complications, retinal detachment and intraocular haemorrhage. In a study of the incidence of CEA in Collies in the UK, 34% of dogs with choroidal hypoplasia, the essential lesion of CEA, had concurrent colobomas; 6% had retinal detachment, and approximately 1% had intraocular haemorrhage (Bedford, 1982b). Retinal detachment and intraocular haemorrhage generally occur within the first few years of life.

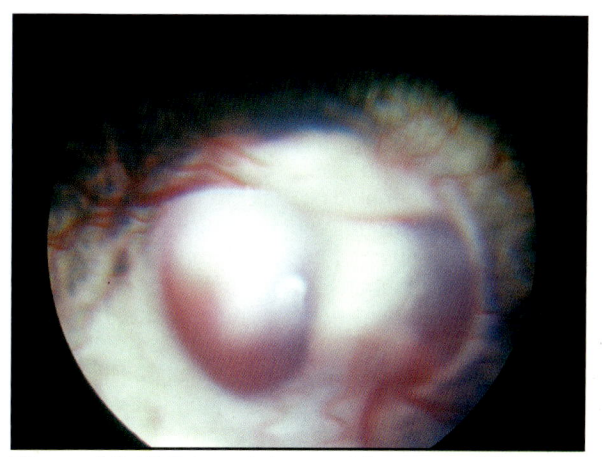

Figure 14.15 Extremely large colobomatous defect involving the optic disc in a Border Collie with collie eye anomaly. (Courtesy of R Elks.)

CEA is usually a bilateral condition, but the severity of the ocular lesions can differ greatly between the two eyes of affected individuals. Minor lesions of choroidal hypoplasia have little effect on vision, but very large colobomatous defects, extensive areas of retinal detachment or intraocular haemorrhage may lead to blindness. Fortunately, bilateral blindness as a result of CEA is not common.

Heritability and disease control

CEA has been suggested to be a pleomorphic trait with simple autosomal recessive inheritance (Yakely et al., 1968; Bedford, 1982b). The findings of recently published studies from Scandinavia suggest, however, that the colobomatous defect may not be inherited directly along with choroidal hypoplasia. On the basis of their findings, these authors suggested a polygenic inheritance of CEA (Wallin-Håkanson et al., 2000a and b).

Control of CEA by selective breeding has proved difficult for several reasons. Ophthalmoscopic diagnosis in mature dogs may be confounded by the 'go-normal' phenomenon, in which regions of choroidal hypoplasia are obscured by postnatal tapetal maturation in a proportion of affected dogs. For this reason, screening of litters of puppies at approximately 6–7 weeks of age, prior to tapetal development, is advised. Ophthalmoscopic diagnosis of small areas of choroidal hypoplasia may prove challenging in dogs with a subalbinotic fundus, particularly in merle animals. Very small optic nerve colobomas may prove difficult to distinguish from the normal physiological pit, particularly in very young puppies.

Nonetheless, clinically affected dogs, regardless of how mildly they may be affected, should not be included in breeding programmes. Unfortunately, the prevalence of this disease in the Rough and Smooth Collie and Shetland Sheepdog breeds means that an extremely large proportion of the breeding stock are genetically affected.

In future, the development of a molecular genetic test may enable carrier animals to be identified. However, at present, efforts to reduce the incidence of CEA must rely on the identification of affected animals by ophthalmoscopic screening.

Retinal dysplasia

Retinal dysplasia may be defined as abnormal retinal differentiation with disorderly proliferation and disorganization of retinal layers. The condition is characterized histopathologically by folding and rosette formation within the neurosensory retina (O'Toole et al.,1983). Retinal dysplasia in dogs may arise spontaneously, or may be acquired as a result of external insults to the developing retina, such as systemic infections (e.g. canine herpesvirus); X-irradiation; vitamin A deficiency; and a range of intrauterine insults (Percy et al., 1971; Narfström and Ekesten, 1999). The lesions of retinal dysplasia may occur in isolation, or in conjunction with other congenital ocular defects, such as microphthalmos, or in association with systemic abnormalities, such as skeletal dysplasia, as reported in Labrador Retrievers and Samoyeds with short-limbed dwarfism (Carrig et al., 1977; Meyers et al., 1983). In dogs, retinal dysplasia occurs most frequently as a primary genetic disorder.

Clinical features

Three major forms of retinal dysplasia are recognized clinically:

- In the mildest form, focal or multifocal retinal dysplasia, dysplastic lesions appear as single or multiple greyish vermiform linear streaks and small circular lesions which are most frequently observed as regions of reduced reflectivity within the tapetal fundus dorsal to the optic disc (Figure 14.16). Lesions of retinal dysplasia are generally observed in the region of the dorsal retinal blood vessels, although, occasionally, dysplastic lesions may be visible within the pigmented non-tapetal fundus (Figure 14.17). The lesions of focal or multifocal retinal dysplasia generally remain static, although, occasionally, they may become less obvious with time, or they may become more clearly demarcated by the development of adjacent hyperreflective or hyperpigmented areas.
- In geographic retinal dysplasia, larger, circumscribed horseshoe-shaped or approximately circular areas are typically observed within the tapetal fundus, generally in close association with the dorsal retinal vasculature. The abnormal, dysplastic areas may include regions of retinal detachment, and there may be tapetal hyperreflectivity and hyperpigmentation (Figure 14.18). As with multifocal retinal dysplasia, the appearance of these lesions may alter throughout life. Generally, geographic lesions become more obvious with the passage of time. This may be due to increased tapetal hyperreflectivity, and greater distinction between the dysplastic region and the adjacent, normally differentiated, retina related to altered pigmentation within, and at the margins of, the lesion. In addition, focal or total retinal detachment or intravitreal haemorrhage may occur as infrequent complications of retinal dysplasia in affected dogs, within the first few years of life (Lavach et al., 1978).
- In the most severe form, total retinal dysplasia, there is congenital infundibular detachment, or non-attachment, of the retina, which is seen as greyish folds floating behind the lens.

In its mildest form, retinal dysplasia usually does not affect vision. However, geographic retinal dysplasia may lead to significant visual impairment. The lesions of retinal dysplasia may be unilateral or bilateral. Total retinal dysplasia invariably results in blindness, and is frequently associated with a 'searching' nystagmus. Secondary complications associated with retinal dysplasia include intraocular haemorrhage, cataract and secondary glaucoma.

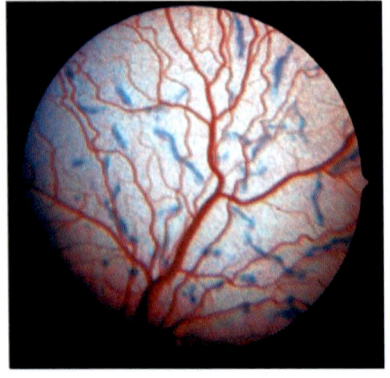

Figure 14.16 Multiple retinal folds within the tapetal fundus of an American Cocker Spaniel with multifocal retinal dysplasia. (Courtesy of NC Buyukmihci.)

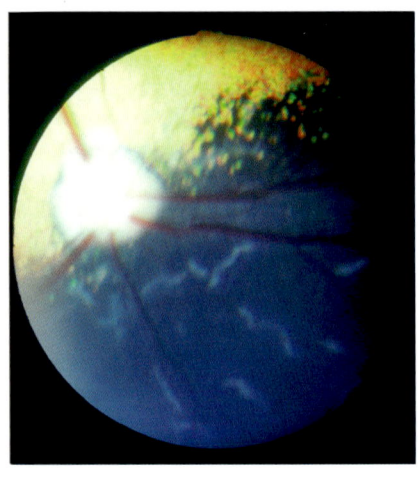

Figure 14.17 Multiple retinal folds within the non-tapetal fundus associated with multifocal retinal dysplasia.

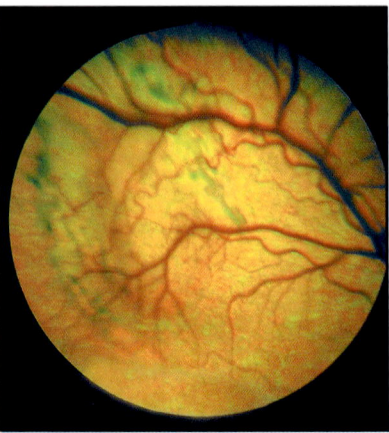

Figure 14.18 Area of geographic retinal dysplasia within the tapetal fundus of an adult English Springer Spaniel.

Heritability and disease control

Primary retinal dysplasia may occur sporadically in any breed; however, those breeds which are presently considered by the British Veterinary Association/Kennel Club/International Sheepdog Society eye scheme to be affected by inherited retinal dysplasia in the UK are listed in Figure 14.19. A dominant mode of inheritance, with incomplete penetrance, has been suggested for both the multifocal form of retinal dysplasia identified in field trial Labrador Retrievers in the USA (Nelson and MacMillan, 1983) and the more severe retinal dysplasia associated with short-limbed dwarfism in Labrador Retrievers (Carrig et al.,1988). With these exceptions, a simple autosomal recessive mode of inheritance has been proposed for retinal dysplasia in all affected breeds that have been adequately studied (Rubin, 1968; MacMillan and Lipton, 1978; Schmidt et al., 1979; Meyers et al., 1983; Long and Crispin, 1999).

Form of retinal dysplasia	Breeds affected
Multifocal/focal	American Cocker Spaniel Cavalier King Charles Spaniel English Springer Spaniel Golden Retriever Hungarian Puli Labrador Retriever Rottweiler
Geographic	Cavalier King Charles Spaniel English Springer Spaniel Golden Retriever Labrador Retriever
Total	Bedlington Terrier English Springer Spaniel Labrador Retriever Sealyham Terrier

Figure 14.19 Breeds considered to be affected by inherited retinal dysplasia in the UK.

Diagnostic problems

As with many forms of retinal disease, problems exist in the interpretation of ophthalmoscopic findings. In particular, areas of focal, multifocal or geographic retinal dysplasia associated with tapetal reflectivity and hyperpigmentation may prove difficult to distinguish from postinflammatory lesions. In breeds which are known to be affected by inherited forms of retinal dysplasia, e.g. the English Springer Spaniel, lesions of this type should be viewed with suspicion, especially if bilateral and closely associated with the dorsal retinal vasculature.

Transient retinal folds may be observed in immature dogs of any breed, possibly as a result of disparity between the rates of growth of the tissues of the neurosensory retina and outer layer of the optic cup. However, these disappear with age. Results of an investigation conducted in a number of affected breeds in the USA suggested that lesions of retinal dysplasia, in particular the geographic form, may not be ophthalmoscopically visible until animals are 6–18 months old (Holle et al., 1999). However, as previously described, multifocal forms may become less obvious as animals mature. The screening of puppies has, therefore, been recommended at 4–6 and 10–12 weeks of age (Crispin et al., 1999), together with later examination which may help in distinguishing mismatched growth from genuine dysplasia and may help to ensure that lesions of geographic retinal dysplasia do not go undetected.

Acquired disease of the retina

Inherited retinal dystrophies and degenerations

Generalized progressive retinal atrophy

Generalized progressive retinal atrophy (gPRA) is an important inherited cause of blindness in pedigree dogs. gPRA is a general term encompassing a range of different diseases in which rod and/or cone photoreceptors either fail to develop normally (photoreceptor dysplasia) or degenerate prematurely following normal postnatal photoreceptor maturation (photoreceptor degenerations). These genotypically and phenotypically heterogeneous disorders are all characterized by a bilateral degeneration of the neurosensory retina, with gradual loss of vision that invariably leads to complete blindness. With the exception of X-linked PRA, which has been described in a strain of Siberian Huskies in the US (Zeiss et al., 1999), most forms of gPRA demonstrate a simple autosomal recessive mode of inheritance.

Clinical features: Typically, gPRA is first recognized as night blindness (nyctalopia), with subsequent progression to complete blindness, even under bright lighting conditions. Both the age of onset of clinical signs and the rate of progression of loss of vision differ between breeds and between affected individuals. Specific breed-related differences in clinical presentation have been reviewed in detail elsewhere (Curtis, 1988; Millichamp, 1990; Clements et al., 1996; Narfström and Ekesten, 1999).

Characteristic ophthalmoscopic findings, irrespective of the form of gPRA, include retinal vascular attenuation and tapetal hyperreflectivity (Figure 14.20). Progressive attenuation of the superficial retinal vasculature, initially recognized as a reduction in the number of, and narrowing of, the retinal arterioles, proceeds to a loss of retinal venules in the later stages of the disease process.

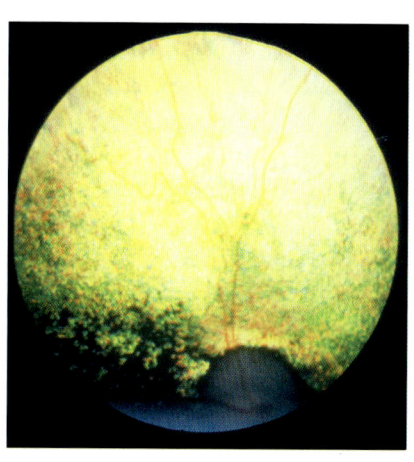

Figure 14.20 Generalized progressive retinal atrophy in a Miniature Poodle with pronounced attenuation of the retinal vasculature.

In the early stages of the degenerative process, altered granularity or coloration, often in a radial, or striate, pattern, may be noted within the peripheral tapetal fundus. Subsequently, tapetal hyperreflectivity develops as a result of thinning of the neurosensory retina. Although the primary defect in gPRA lies within the photoreceptors, RPE atrophy or hypertrophy with intraretinal migration of RPE cells may be observed in very advanced stages of the disease. This leads to a mottled appearance of the non-tapetal fundus (Figure 14.21), which has been described as 'pavementing' (Narfström and Ekesten, 1999).

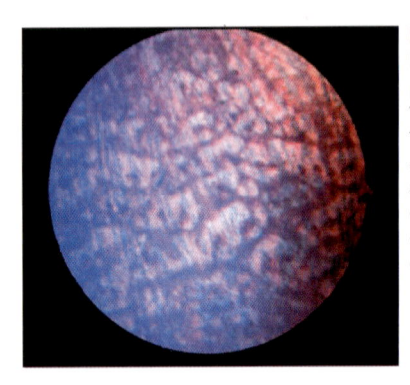

Figure 14.21 Mottled pigmentation within the non-tapetal fundus of a dog with advanced generalized retinal degeneration. (Courtesy of NC Buyukmihci.)

Ultimately, secondary optic nerve atrophy may also be observed. Pupillary light responses may be reduced, and the pupils of affected dogs frequently appear relatively dilated under normal lighting conditions. However, it should be borne in mind that pupillary light reflexes may be retained long after functional vision has been lost.

Secondary cataract formation is a common finding in advanced cases of gPRA, hence the importance of evaluating retinal function, particularly in 'at risk' breeds, prior to embarking on cataract surgery (Millichamp, 1990; Narfström and Ekesten, 1999).

Breed incidence and disease control: Figure 14.22 shows those breeds that are currently listed in the UK as being affected by gPRA, by the British Veterinary Association/Kennel Club/International Sheepdog Society eye examination scheme. It should, however, be noted that the incidence of gPRA in a large number of other breeds of dog is presently under investigation by veterinary ophthalmologists, both in the UK and worldwide. In addition to the breeds listed in Figure 14.22, the incidence of gPRA in the Australian Cattle Dog, the Miniature Smooth-haired Dachshund, the Irish Wolfhound, the Japanese Akita, the Papillon and the Golden Retriever remains under investigation by the BVA/KC/ISDS eye scheme in the UK. Information on breeds affected by inherited retinal degenerations in other countries can be obtained by consulting the literature of the appropriate eye disease screening scheme (e.g. 'Ocular Disorders Presumed to be Inherited in Purebred Dogs', published in the US by the Genetics Committee of the American College of Veterinary Ophthalmologists). In the UK, gPRA is most commonly encountered in the Toy and Miniature Poodle, the Labrador Retriever and the English Cocker Spaniel.

Early diagnosis: In those canine breeds in which electrophysiological changes associated with photoreceptor degeneration have been adequately charac-

Breed	Disease/Gene symbol	Approximate age at which ophthalmoscopic changes are generally first visible	Approximate age at which nyctalopia is first apparent	References
Briard *	Hereditary retinal dystrophy (csnb)	> 3 years	From 5 weeks	Narfström et al., 1994; Narfström, 1999; Veske et al., 1999
Rough Collie	rcd2	4 months	6 weeks	Wolf et al., 1978
Cardigan Welsh Corgi*	rcd3	4–5 months	6–8 weeks	Keep, 1972
Miniature Longhaired Dachshund	gPRA	6–9 months	6 months	Curtis and Barnett, 1993
Norwegian Elkhound	erd	6–12 months	6 weeks	Acland and Aguirre, 1987
Irish Setter*	rcd1	4–6 months	6–8 weeks	Parry, 1953; Clements et al., 1993
Miniature Schnauzer	pd	12 months–5 years	6 months–2 years	Parshall et al., 1991
Miniature and Toy Poodle*	prcd	3–5 years	4–5 years	Barnett, 1965a
Labrador and Chesapeake Bay Retrievers*	prcd	3–5 years	4–6 years	Narfström and Ekesten, 1999
English and American Cocker Spaniel*	prcd	4–8 years	4–8 years	Aguirre and Acland, 1988
English Springer Spaniel	gPRA	12 months		Barnett, 1965b
Tibetan Spaniel	gPRA	3–5 years	3–5 years	Bjerkås and Narfström, 1994
Tibetan Terrier	gPRA	12–18 months	11–15 months	Millichamp et al., 1988

Figure 14.22 Breeds considered to be affected by progressive retinal degeneration related to primary inherited retinal disease in the UK. (csnb = congenital stationary night blindness; rcd = rod–cone dysplasia; erd= early retinal degeneration; rd = rod dysplasia; pd = photoreceptor dysplasia; prcd = progressive rod–cone degeneration). Molecular genetic DNA-based tests are currently available commercially in those breeds which are marked by an asterisk.

terized, early diagnosis of gPRA may be made in advance of the development of ophthalmoscopically visible fundic changes by means of electroretinography (Acland, 1988).

This diagnostic modality is of particular value in those breeds which are affected by the later-onset photoreceptor degenerations. For example, prcd-affected Miniature and Toy Poodles may not demonstrate clinical signs of retinal degeneration until they reach middle age, by which time they may have produced both affected and carrier offspring.

On the other hand, specialist ERG studies can detect affected dogs at 18 months of age. However, the complex, time-consuming protocol required means that ERG diagnosis of gPRA is not commonly performed and has not been widely adopted as a means of control of gPRA in the UK.

Molecular genetics: In recent years, significant advances have been made in the understanding of the molecular genetics of canine gPRA (Petersen-Jones, 1998; Petersen-Jones, 1999). A mutation in the gene which encodes the β-subunit of cyclic guanosine monophosphate phosphodiesterase (cGMP-PDE) has been identified in gPRA-affected Irish Setters, which has allowed the development of a DNA-based diagnostic test for the disease in this breed (Clements et al., 1993). Recently, a mutation in the α-subunit of cGMP-PDE has been identified and characterized as a cause of gPRA in Cardigan Welsh Corgis (Petersen-Jones et al., 1999; Petersen-Jones and Zhu, 2000), and a further mutation in the β-subunit of cGMP-PDE has been identified as a cause of gPRA in the Sloughi breed (Dekomien et al., 2000).

Breeding studies involving Toy and Miniature Poodles, Labrador Retrievers and English Cocker Spaniels have demonstrated that the later-onset form of gPRA observed in these breeds, known as progressive rod–cone degeneration (prcd), is inherited at a common genetic locus. Linkage analysis studies have mapped the gene responsible for prcd – paving the way for a DNA-based diagnostic test for gPRA in the Labrador Retriever, English and American Cocker Spaniel and Portuguese Water Dog, although the specific genetic mutation responsible for gPRA in these breeds has not yet been identified (Acland et al., 1998).

In addition, many candidate genes (canine homologues for many of the genes known to be associated with retinal degenerations in other species) have been excluded as causal genes for gPRA in a number of other dog breeds.

Retinal pigment epithelial dystrophy

Retinal pigment epithelial dystrophy (RPED) is a progressive retinal degeneration, previously known as central progressive retinal atrophy (CPRA), that has been described in several breeds of dog in the UK. These are the Cocker Spaniel, the Border Collie, the Golden and the Labrador Retriever, the Smooth and the Rough Collie, the Briard (Barnett, 1969, 1976; Bedford, 1984) and the Polish Lowland Sheepdog or Nizzini (Watson et al., 1993). Although this breed predisposition implies an inherited basis for the disease, a specific mode of inheritance has not yet been elucidated.

Pathological features: Characteristic histopathological findings in this disease include an accumulation of autofluorescent lipopigment within the cells of the RPE (Lightfoot et al., 1996). It is thought that auto-oxidative processes may play a role in the accumulation of this lipopigment. The pronounced clinical and pathological similarities which exist between canine RPED and the retinopathy associated with deficiency of the important antioxidant, vitamin E, are consistent with this hypothesis. RPED-affected Cocker Spaniels have been found to have extremely low plasma levels of vitamin E. A characteristic neurological syndrome, including ataxia and proprioceptive deficits particularly affecting the hind limbs, has been demonstrated in a number of these dogs (McLellan et al., 2000).

Clinical features: Typically, RPED-affected animals suffer a slowly progressive loss of central vision. The age of onset and rate of progression of this disease are variable, and complete blindness may or may not result. Clinical signs are generally not apparent until affected animals are 2 to 6 years of age. However, as the early stages of RPED are not associated with significant visual impairment, it is likely that the disease is frequently overlooked until later in its course (Parry, 1954).

The loss of central vision, which is a characteristic feature of RPED, means that affected animals, although still able to see moving objects, may not be able to locate quite large stationary objects directly in front of them. In some cases, the disease may stabilize, with no progression from mid-stage for several years, while in others, complete blindness may result within 12 months.

RPED is characterized ophthalmoscopically by the appearance of light brown pigment spots and patches within the lateral tapetal fundus that progressively increase in number, coalesce and become associated with patchy areas of tapetal hyperreflectivity and vascular attenuation (Figure 14.23). Lesions are initially more severe within the central region of the tapetal fundus, becoming more widespread across the whole tapetal fundus as the disease progresses. Optic nerve atrophy, pigmentary disturbances within the non-tapetal fundus and the development of secondary cortical cataract are inconsistent findings in RPED and, if they occur, are generally only recognized in advanced stages of the disease process.

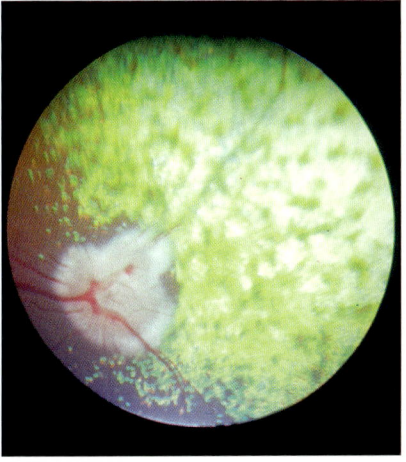

Figure 14.23 Retinal pigment epithelial dystrophy in a Cocker Spaniel.

Management: An ophthalmoscopic diagnosis of RPED thus warrants the measurement of plasma vitamin E values. Should a diagnosis of vitamin E deficiency be made, then high dose oral supplementation is recommended, with 600–900 IU of natural source vitamin E, administered twice daily with food. Although supplementation may arrest the progression of retinal and neurological lesions in clinically affected animals, this is unlikely to be accompanied by an improvement in vision.

Retinal dystrophy in Briard dogs

Congenital hereditary retinal dystrophy, characterized by night blindness and variable day blindness, has been described in Scandinavian Briard dogs (Narfström *et al.*, 1994), with sporadic reports of the disease in Briards in the USA, France and the UK. Low amplitude or non-recordable ERGs are diagnostic for this disease in 5-week-old puppies (Narfström *et al.*, 1994). However, no distinctive fundoscopic changes are observed in this disease until animals are at least 2–3 years old. Often, a subtle alteration in the tapetal colour (or 'sheen') is observed, which may be followed by the development of focal yellow-white spots throughout the fundus (Narfström, 1999).

Although there generally appears to be no evidence for continuing deterioration in vision in affected animals, histological changes have been shown to be progressive.

Results of a breeding programme conducted in Sweden were consistent with a simple autosomal recessive mode of inheritance but with varying expression, possibly due to the effect of modifying genes on the clinical manifestation of the disease. Recently, molecular genetic studies have identified a mutation in the RPE65 gene, which codes for a protein involved in RPE retinoid metabolism, in dogs affected by this form of retinal dystrophy (Veske *et al.*, 1999).

Other acquired retinal disorders

Sudden acquired retinal degeneration

Sudden acquired retinal degeneration (SARD) refers to a syndrome recognized in dogs, in which an acute onset of blindness is associated with a complete absence of photoreceptor activity on ERG. In SARD-affected dogs, vision is usually lost within days or, at most, within a few weeks of the owner first observing that their pet is visually impaired. Most affected dogs demonstrate moderately or widely dilated pupils, with decreased or absent pupillary light reflexes. In the early stages of the disease process, the fundus appears normal on ophthalmoscopy, although, over a period of several weeks to months, vascular attenuation and alteration of tapetal reflectivity become apparent. Ultimately, in SARD-affected dogs, degeneration of the neurosensory retina leads to an ophthalmoscopic appearance that becomes indistinguishable from advanced retinal degeneration associated with other disorders, such as gPRA.

In its early stages, prior to the development of fundoscopic changes, SARD may be distinguished from other causes of acute onset blindness in which there are no fundoscopic abnormalities, i.e. retrobulbar optic neuritis or CNS disease, by electroretinography. In SARD, as the photoreceptors are no longer functioning, the ERG trace is extinguished.

It has been demonstrated that initial retinal morphological abnormalities in SARD are restricted to the photoreceptor layer, with subsequent degeneration of other layers of the neurosensory retina. However, the aetiopathogenesis of the photoreceptor loss observed in SARD remains unclear.

Clinical features: The disorder typically affects middle-aged or older dogs (van der Woerdt *et al.*, 1991). Dogs of any breed or sex may be affected; however, affected animals are often obese, or have a recent history of weight gain. In addition, many SARD-affected dogs have a history of polyuria and polydipsia. It is not uncommon for affected dogs to demonstrate haematological or serum biochemical abnormalities, such as a neutrophilia, lymphopenia and elevations in serum liver enzyme values. A proportion of dogs also show abnormal responses to ACTH stimulation or dexamethasone suppression tests, suggesting an association between SARD and hyperadrenocorticism (Holt *et al.*, 1999).

Unfortunately, there is no treatment for this disorder, with affected animals remaining permanently blind.

Retinal detachment

Pathological features: The neurosensory retina is only firmly attached to the underlying tissue at the optic disc and the ora ciliaris retinae; between these points the attachment is relatively weak, relying on its close apposition to the underlying RPE and the support of the vitreous. Thus, detachment almost always reflects separation of the neurosensory retina from the RPE. In cases with total detachment of the retina, the neurosensory retina may become disinserted from the ora ciliaris retinae peripherally, remaining attached only at the optic disc (Figure 14.24).

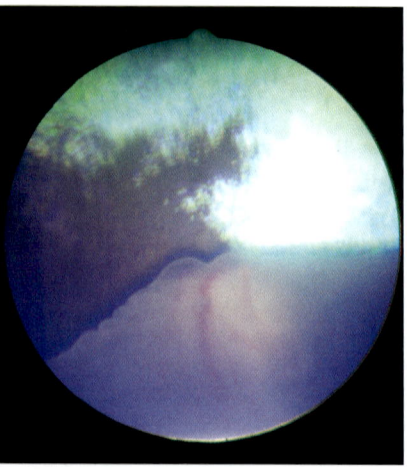

Figure 14.24 Total retinal detachment of unknown cause, with disinsertion from the ora ciliaris retinae, in a Jack Russell Terrier.

Congenital retinal detachment (or non-attachment) may be recognized in association with disorders such as retinal dysplasia or collie eye anomaly (see above).

Clinical features: On ophthalmoscopy, areas of detachment may appear as focal greyish areas within the tapetal fundus (with local reduction in tapetal reflectivity) (Figure 14.25) or non-tapetal fundus (where they appear paler than the surrounding area). More extensive retinal detachments will no longer be observed within the normal plane of the retina and will appear as greyish billowing folds, with surface blood vessels appearing progressively out of focus as they billow towards the observer. In tapetal regions of the fundus where the neurosensory retina is absent due to tearing or disinsertion, hyperreflectivity may be noted.

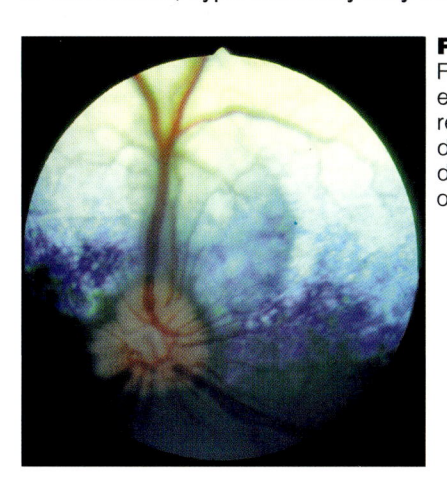

Figure 14.25 Focal area of exudative retinal detachment dorsal to the optic disc.

Classification: Retinal detachment in dogs may be classified according to the extent of retinal involvement as focal, multifocal or total. Focal areas of detachment may not be associated with clinically appreciable visual impairment in dogs, but total detachment is inevitably associated with blindness and reduced or absent pupillary light reflex in the affected eye. Potential secondary complications of retinal detachment include intraocular haemorrhage, cataract and glaucoma.

Acquired retinal detachments may also be classified in terms of the pathophysiology of the detachment:

- *Exudative* or *serous* detachments occur as a result of the accumulation of fluid or cellular infiltrates within the potential 'subretinal space' which exists between the neurosensory retina and the RPE, thereby separating the two layers. This may occur as a result of choroidal inflammatory and vascular disease, and is the most common form of retinal detachment encountered in small animal patients. Causes of exudative, or serous, retinal detachments include chorioretinitis, vascular disease related to hypertension, hyperviscosity syndrome, diabetes mellitus, coagulopathies (see below), neoplasia and idiopathic retinal detachment.

   Provided that the underlying cause of detachment is addressed, and that retinal tears have not occurred, areas of serous detachment may reattach and this may be accompanied by improvement in vision. However, a variable degree of degeneration of the neurosensory retina is to be expected when photoreceptors are separated from the underlying RPE.

   Idiopathic serous retinal detachments are generally bilateral and appear to occur more commonly in German Shepherd Dogs and their crossbreeds than in other canine breeds. This form of serous retinal detachment often responds favourably to immunosuppressive therapy. Provided that no specific local or systemic disorder can be identified as a cause of retinal detachment, oral prednisolone therapy may be instituted at an immunosuppressive dose (2 mg/kg/day, divided into twice daily doses). Perhaps surprisingly, although the time which elapses prior to reattachment of the neurosensory retina may be prolonged, useful vision is often regained in dogs, regardless of the subsequent development of ophthalmoscopic signs of multifocal or diffuse retinal degeneration (Andrew *et al.*, 1997)
- Occasionally, *solid* detachments are observed, due to elevation of the retina by solid infiltration, particularly by neoplastic cells, of the choroid or retrobulbar space
- *Traction* retinal detachment occurs when bands composed of inflammatory and/or fibrotic tissue form within the vitreous and subsequently exert anterior traction forces on the neurosensory retina. Traction retinal detachments are less common in small animal patients, although they may ensue following trauma, intraocular haemorrhage or posterior segment inflammation, as a result of the organization of inflammatory infiltrates within the vitreous. Unfortunately, this form of retinal detachment is rarely amenable to medical or surgical therapy in dogs
- *Rhegmatogenous* detachments are caused by tears in the neurosensory retina which allow fluid, e.g. liquefied vitreous, to enter the potential 'subretinal space'. Subretinal fluid is then responsible for dissecting the neurosensory retina from the underlying RPE. Rhegmatogenous detachment is relatively common in dogs (Hendrix *et al.*, 1993), and may occur as a result of trauma, or of tearing of the thinned neurosensory retina in cases of advanced retinal degeneration. Displacement, movement or fibroblastic changes within the vitreous body may contribute to the formation of rhegmatogenous retinal detachments. Rhegmatogenous retinal detachment is not uncommon in dogs with hypermature cataract or lens luxation and may occur as an unfortunate postoperative complication following cataract surgery.

Tears in the neurosensory retina may occur in dogs with colobomatous lesions of the fundus, and these have been implicated in the development of retinal detachment in cases of collie eye anomaly (Vainisi *et al.*,1989). Giant retinal tears (i.e. those which involve more than 25% of the circumference of the ora ciliaris retinae) have also been reported to occur in Shih Tzus, in conjunction with vitreous degeneration and liquefaction (Vainisi and Packo, 1995). Intraretinal cystic degeneration, which is a common finding within the peripheral retina of elderly dogs, may lead to the formation of splits within the neurosensory retina, with separation occurring between retinal layers (retinoschisis).

Surgical repair of rhegmatogenous retinal detachment is possible, but is rarely undertaken in veterinary patients at present, due to the requirement for specialist skills and instrumentation (Sullivan, 1997). However, an increasing number of veterinary ophthalmologists have the facility to perform laser retinopexy at the margins of retinal tears, in order to prevent the propagation of retinal detachment.

Chorioretinitis

Due to the intimate anatomical relationship between the retina and underlying choroid, inflammatory disease processes rarely affect either structure in isolation. Generally, inflammation affects both the choroid and retina concurrently and, often, the inflammatory process within the choroid is predominant, as reflected in the term chorioretinitis. As the choroid is also continuous with the structures of the anterior uveal tract, chorioretinitis is often recognized in association with a degree of anterior uveitis, and has a similar range of causes (see Chapter 10).

Causes: Causes of chorioretinitis in dogs include many systemic infectious diseases, which are summarized in Figure 14.26; trauma; foreign bodies; immune-mediated disorders, such as uveodermatological syndrome, discussed in Chapter 10; and neoplasia. Specific disorders associated with canine chorioretinitis have previously been reviewed in greater detail by Narfström and Ekesten (1999).

Viral
Canine distemper virus
Canine herpesvirus
Infectious rhinotonsillitis
Bacterial
Generalized bacteraemia/septicaemia
Protozoal
Toxoplasmosis
Neosporosis
Leishmaniasis
Parasitic
Toxocariasis
Angiostrongylosis
Ophthalmomyiasis interna posterior (dipteran larvae)
Rickettsial
Ehrlichiosis
Rocky Mountain spotted fever
Mycotic
Aspergillosis
Blastomycosis
Histoplasmosis
Cryptococcosis
Coccidioidomycosis
Geotrichosis
Algal
Protothecosis

Figure 14.26 Infectious causes of chorioretinitis in dogs.

Clinical and pathological features: Chorioretinitis may be unilateral or, as is usually the case in systemic infectious disorders, bilateral. However, the lesions of chorioretinitis are rarely bilaterally symmetrical. In the acute stages of chorioretinitis, ophthalmoscopic findings may include irregular greyish ill-defined areas of inflammatory cell infiltrates. These lesions may be focal, multifocal or perivascular in location. Cellular infiltrates and more diffuse areas of retinal oedema may be recognized as areas of reduced reflectivity within the tapetal fundus and as pale greyish areas within the non-tapetal fundus (Figure 14.27).

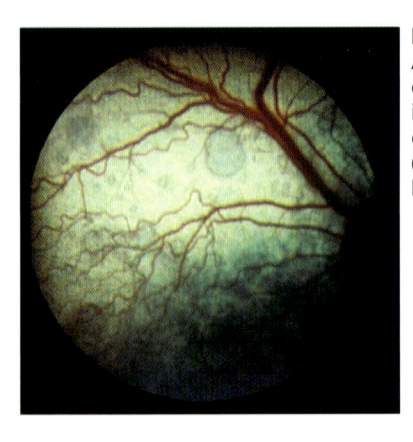

Figure 14.27 Active chorioretinitis in a dog with distemper. (Courtesy of NC Buyukmihci.)

A variable degree of detachment of the neurosensory retina may occur where inflammation and exudation are severe (as discussed in the previous section), leading to impairment of vision. Severe inflammation may also lead to retinal or intravitreal haemorrhage (see Figure 14.34) and secondary vitreal involvement may lead to vitreous haze or the accumulation of inflammatory material within the vitreous, with subsequent vitreous syneresis.

Particularly in mycotic disease, well demarcated raised subretinal granulomas, with deviation of overlying retinal vasculature, may be observed (Figure 14.28), although such disorders are rarely encountered in dogs in the UK. Chorioretinitis may also be associated with inflammation of the optic nerve (see below).

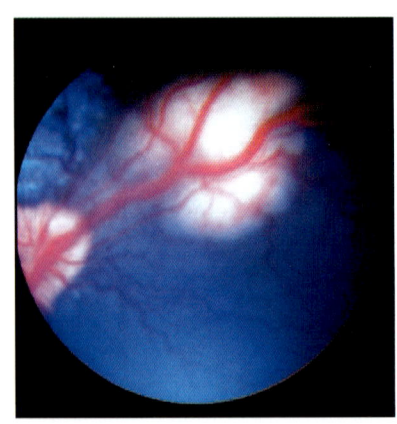

Figure 14.28 Subretinal granuloma in a dog with ocular and systemic blastomycosis. (Courtesy of NC Buyukmihci.)

In later stages of chorioretinitis, degeneration of the neurosensory retina may lead to regions of tapetal hyperreflectivity, often associated with well demarcated hyperpigmented foci due to hypertrophy and migration of RPE cells (Figure 14.29). Within the nontapetal fundus, areas of depigmentation may be observed. Small localized focal postinflammatory lesions in dogs are rarely associated with clinically appreciable impairment of vision, and may be observed as an incidental finding in dogs with no history of prior ocular or systemic disease. However, widespread degeneration of the neurosensory retina in more severely affected patients can lead to permanent severe visual impairment, or even total blindness.

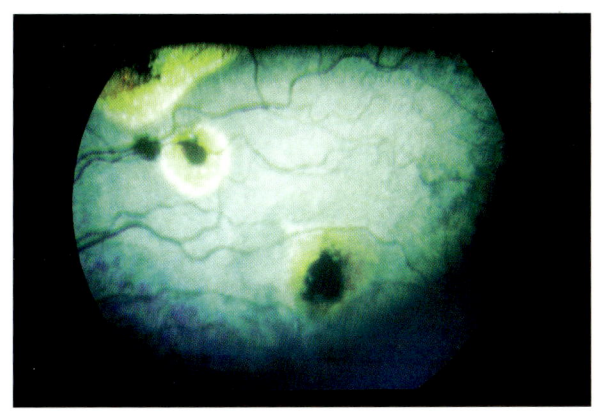

Figure 14.29 Postinflammatory chorioretinopathy in a Jack Russell Terrier.

Management: As chorioretinitis frequently represents an ocular manifestation of a systemic disease process, affected animals should be subjected to a thorough general clinical examination. The presence of further ocular, neurological or other disease signs may arouse a high degree of clinical suspicion for a particular disorder, e.g. in cases of distemper virus infection. Where possible, every effort should be made to investigate, identify and address any underlying systemic disorder. In those rare cases in which mycotic disease is suspected, vitreous paracentesis may allow identification of the fungal organism involved.

Treatment: Although systemic anti-inflammatory therapy is generally warranted, systemic corticosteroids are contraindicated in the management of chorioretinitis associated with infectious disease processes; they should, therefore, be used with great caution. Systemic therapy with non-steroidal anti-inflammatory drugs may be of benefit.

Retinal vascular disease

The transparency of the ocular media affords the clinician an unparalleled opportunity to directly visualize abnormalities of the vascular system, non-invasively. Retinal vascular distension, tortuosity and haemorrhage are examples of relatively commonly observed abnormalities that may be noted on ophthalmoscopic examination of the fundus and that may indicate severe underlying systemic vascular disease (Lane *et al.*, 1993).

Coagulopathies: Quantitative and qualitative disorders affecting platelet function and disorders of the intrinsic and extrinsic coagulation pathways, including inherited and immune-mediated coagulopathies and toxicities, may lead to retinal haemorrhage. The ophthalmoscopic appearance of retinal haemorrhage has been described above. In some instances, intraocular haemorrhage can be the major presenting sign of potentially life-threatening systemic bleeding disorders.

Systemic hypertension: Systemic arterial hypertension, which is generally secondary to other disorders in the dog, such as renal or endocrine disease, but which may be primary or idiopathic, may lead to disease of the retina, choroid and optic nerve. Associated ocular abnormalities, such as visual impairment or intraocular haemorrhage, may be initial presenting signs in affected dogs (Sansom and Bodey, 1997). Fundic lesions that may be observed in hypertensive dogs include narrowing of retinal arterioles; retinal, subretinal and vitreal haemorrhages (Figure 14.30); retinal oedema and serous detachment; and papilloedema. These lesions are consistent with the angiographic abnormalities which have been demonstrated in hypertensive dogs, which include choroidal, particularly choriocapillary, ischaemia, arteriolar vasoconstriction and subretinal oedema. The response of ocular lesions to appropriate antihypertensive therapy varies considerably, and to some extent it is likely to be influenced by the duration and aetiopathogenesis of hypertension in individual patients (Villagrasa and Cascales, 2000).

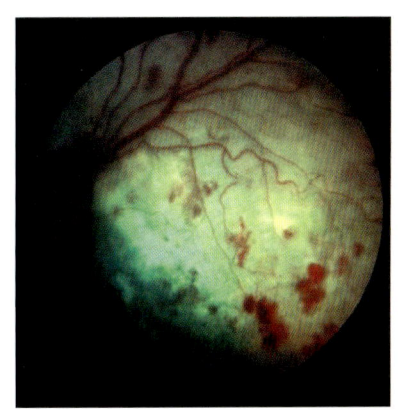

Figure 14.30 Retinal haemorrhage and detachment in a 9-year-old Labrador Retriever with systemic hypertension. (Courtesy of NC Buyukmihci.)

Hyperviscosity syndrome: Blood or serum hyperviscosity may occur as a result of polycythaemia, or hyperproteinaemia (e.g. monoclonal gammopathy related to multiple myeloma). In such cases, the retinal blood vessels may appear tortuous and distended and may demonstrate a characteristic 'sausage' or 'boxcar' appearance, with multiple sacculations due to 'sludging' of blood. Retinal haemorrhage and detachment may also be recognized (Figure 14.31, and see Figure 14.12).

Diabetic retinopathy: In contrast to human diabetic patients, in whom retinal vascular disease is a major cause of blindness, the most common ocular complication of diabetes mellitus in dogs is cataract formation. However, retinal vascular changes have been described in canine patients with long-standing diabetes and it would appear that the difference in the reported incidence of diabetic retinopathy between the species reflects differences in longevity

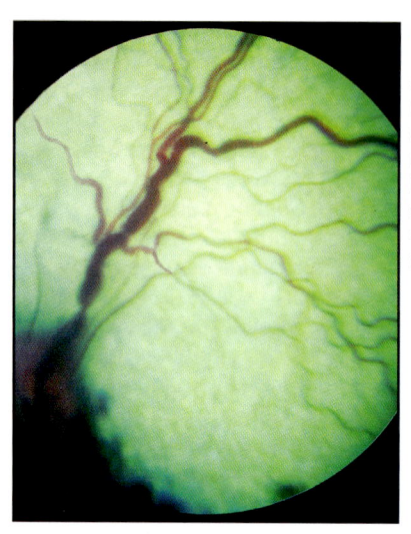

Figure 14.31 Retinal vascular changes, haemorrhage and detachment related to hyperviscosity syndrome in a dog with multiple myeloma.

and duration of diabetes. Retinal lesions that have been described in diabetic dogs include microaneurysms with irregular variations in the calibre of retinal blood vessels and multifocal retinal haemorrhages. Ultimately, areas of retinal degeneration with associated tapetal hyperreflectivity may become apparent (Barnett, 1981; Muñana, 1995).

Lipaemia retinalis: Raised serum triglycerides, in particular due to chylomicronaemia, may result in the retinal vessels appearing white to pale pink, which is most readily appreciated within the peripheral blood vessels of the pigmented non-tapetal fundus (Wyman and McKissick, 1973; Crispin, 1993). Lipaemia retinalis is not associated with impairment of vision, unless sustained or severe; however, this fundic abnormality should prompt investigation and characterization of the underlying disorder affecting systemic lipid metabolism.

Neuronal ceroid-lipofuscinoses

The neuronal ceroid-lipofuscinoses (NCL) are a group of inherited storage diseases which are well recognized in animals and in man, in which NCL is often referred to as Batten's disease (Jolly *et al.*, 1992). These diseases are characterized by an intracellular accumulation of autofluorescent lipopigment within many tissues throughout the body, in particular in the nervous system and retina. Within this heterogeneous group of related disorders, various clinical syndromes with differing age of onset and clinical course are recognized.

Clinical manifestations of NCL include multifocal nervous signs, such as tremors and seizures (due to brain atrophy), and loss of vision (due to retinal changes as well as degenerative changes within the central nervous system). Ophthalmoscopic evidence of retinal degeneration is not a consistent or prominent feature of NCL in dogs. The disease has been described in certain breeds, such as the English Setter, the Border Collie, the Tibetan Terrier and the Dalmatian, but in none of these have marked fundoscopic changes been described. Severe retinal degeneration associated with canine NCL has been described in the Miniature Schnauzer (Smith *et al.*, 1996). It is important to distinguish NCL from gPRA-affected Tibetan Terriers, particularly as the neurological signs associated with NCL may be relatively mild in this breed, with nyctalopia being a prominent clinical sign (Cummings *et al.*, 1990; Riis *et al.*, 1992).

Vitamin E deficiency

The long-term feeding of vitamin E-deficient diets to dogs leads to the development of a pigmentary retinopathy which is clinically and pathologically indistinguishable from RPED (Riis *et al.*, 1981). A relative deficiency of vitamin E may be encountered in dogs which are fed poor quality, high fat diets (Davidson *et al.*, 1998), particularly those diets which have a high content of polyunsaturated fatty acids.

Photic retinopathy

Retinal damage resulting from exposure to intense light has been well documented in a number of species and should be a consideration in patients that may be exposed to the light of an indirect ophthalmoscope or operating microscope for prolonged periods of time. Ophthalmoscopic and histopathological evidence of degeneration of the outer retina has been described in the tapetal region of dogs that were subjected to illumination from the light source of an indirect ophthalmoscope for 1 hour (Buyukmihci, 1981). Use of a yellow-tinted, rather than clear glass, condensing lens to focus light on the retina prevented the development of retinal lesions.

Neoplasia

Primary tumours rarely affect the canine posterior segment, with choroidal melanoma (Figure 14.32) being the most frequently reported primary neoplasm of the canine fundus. In contrast to the situation in man, canine choroidal melanoma appears to be relatively benign, with most reported cases being considered melanocytomas (Collinson and Peiffer, 1993).

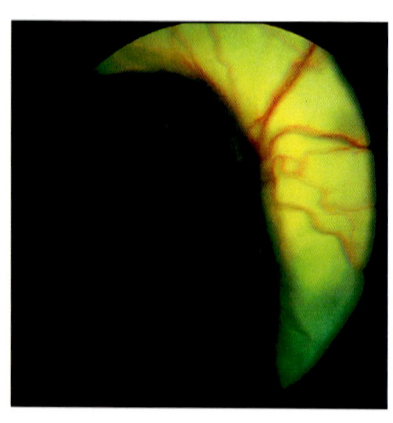

Figure 14.32 Choroidal melanoma in an adult dog. (Courtesy of N Wallin-Håkanson.)

Secondary neoplastic involvement of the posterior segment, specifically the choroid, is less common than that of the anterior uvea. Generalized and metastatic neoplasms, such as lymphoma, carcinoma, melanoma and haemangiosarcoma have, however, all been reported at this site.

Congenital abnormalities of the optic nerve

Optic nerve hypoplasia
Optic nerve hypoplasia refers to a marked reduction in the number of optic nerve axons, because of reduced numbers of retinal ganglion cells. Characteristically there is an abnormally small, dark optic nerve head, within an otherwise relatively normal fundus (Figure 14.33). Optic nerve hypoplasia is associated with impaired vision in the affected eye and reduced pupillary light reflex, with pupillary dilation (Kern and Riis, 1981). Patients with bilateral optic nerve hypoplasia may be totally blind. The condition has been reported in a number of breeds, and may be inherited in the Miniature and Toy Poodle. Optic nerve hypoplasia should be differentiated from micropapilla, in which a small optic disc is also observed on ophthalmoscopy, but which is associated with normal pupillary light reflexes and apparently normal, functional vision.

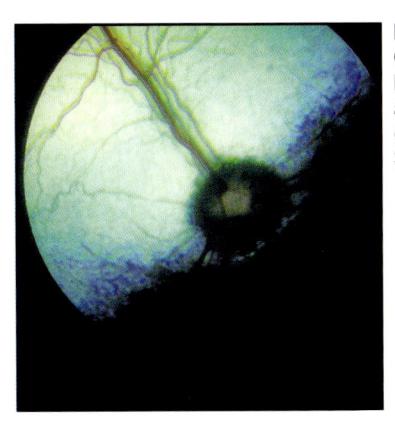

Figure 14.33 Optic nerve hypoplasia in an adult crossbred dog. (Courtesy of SR Hollingsworth.)

Optic nerve coloboma
Optic nerve colobomas represent focal absence of ocular tissue in the region of the optic nerve that may be related to failure, or incomplete, closure of the ventral foetal fissure during ocular development. Although colobomas may be observed sporadically as congenital lesions in any breed, they are most commonly recognized in dogs affected by collie eye anomaly (see earlier), in which they are invariably seen in conjunction with lesions of choroidal hypoplasia. Optic nerve coloboma is also considered to be inherited in the Basenji (Rubin, 1989).

Colobomas of the optic nerve head range in ophthalmoscopic appearance from small greyish pits to deep excavations within the optic disc, into which vessels may be seen to plunge at the margins of the lesion (see Figures 14.14 and 14.15). 'Typical' colobomas are located in a ventral midline position (i.e. in the location of the foetal fissure) and 'atypical' colobomas are located at, or near, the temporal or nasal margins of the disc. Colobomas frequently have little or no appreciable effect on vision, although large defects may be associated with severe visual impairment. The presence of optic nerve coloboma has been implicated in the development of retinal detachment as a complication of collie eye anomaly (Vainisi et al., 1989).

Acquired diseases of the optic disc and optic nerve

Papilloedema
Papilloedema is a term which refers to an abnormal swelling of the optic disc. This may be the result of elevated intracranial/cerebrospinal fluid pressure. Oedema of the optic disc may also reflect primary optic nerve neoplasia (see below); it may result from compression of the retrobulbar optic nerve by orbital space-occupying lesions, or it may accompany systemic hypertension, acute glaucoma or uveitis. The affected optic disc appears 'fluffy' and swollen, with deviation of the retinal blood vessels as they cross the margins of the disc. Papilloedema recognized on ophthalmoscopy may or may not be directly associated with PLR deficits or loss of vision (Palmer et al., 1974).

Optic neuritis
Optic neuritis (inflammation of the optic nerve) in dogs may be due to viral, bacterial, parasitic or fungal infectious disease processes, such as canine distemper, toxoplasmosis, cryptococcosis or blastomycosis. Alternatively, it may result from extension of local disease processes, such as orbital cellulitis, or may reflect granulomatous or neoplastic infiltration, for example, in cases of granulomatous meningoencephalitis (GME) or lymphoma. However, in many dogs affected by optic neuritis, the inflammatory process is deemed to be idiopathic, and is assumed to be immune-mediated on the basis of clinical response to immunosuppression.

Clinical features
Inflammation of the optic nerve usually leads to a sudden loss of pupillary light reflexes in association with visual impairment, or blindness. Optic neuritis, with involvement of the ONH, may lead to ophthalmoscopically visible changes, such as optic disc congestion and swelling, which is recognized by:

- The absence of a normal physiological pit in the optic disc
- Cellular infiltrates within the posterior vitreous
- Haemorrhages within or surrounding the disc
- Peripapillary retinal oedema or detachment (Figures 14.34 and 14.35). However, inflammation of the retrobulbar portion of the optic nerve may lead to pupillary light reflex deficits and visual impairment in the absence of fundoscopic abnormalities. Bilateral retrobulbar optic neuritis should therefore be considered as an important differential diagnosis, together with SARD (see earlier) and central nervous system disorders, in those patients that present with a history of blindness of acute onset and widely dilated pupils, and that have a normal fundic appearance on ophthalmoscopy.

Diagnosis: Normal ERG responses are maintained in patients with retrobulbar optic neuritis, a feature which distinguishes this condition from SARD. A thorough

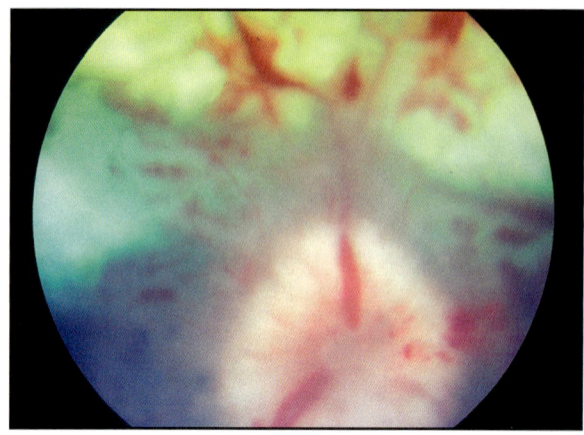

Figure 14.34 Optic neuritis and chorioretinitis of undetermined cause in an adult dog. Note flame-like haemorrhages within the nerve fibre layer of the retina.

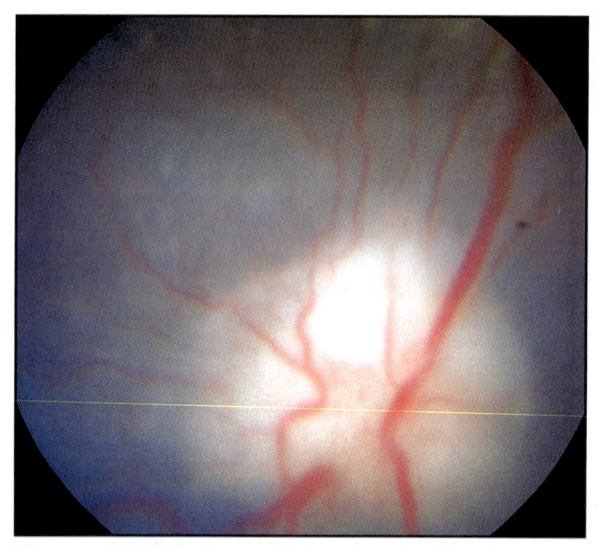

Figure 14.35 Optic neuritis in a Cavalier King Charles Spaniel with granulomatous meningoencephalitis.

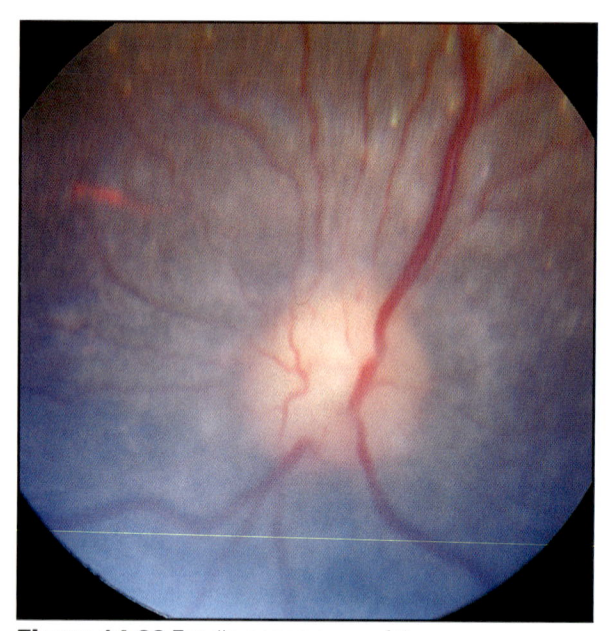

Figure 14.36 Fundic appearance of the same eye as shown in Figure 14.35 following immunosuppressive therapy with oral corticosteroid.

doses of corticosteroids may be encouraging in the early stages, but the long-term prognosis for restoration and maintenance of vision is generally poor, as optic atrophy frequently ensues. Prednisolone should be administered orally at 2mg/kg/day (divided into twice daily doses) for 10–14 days, with the dosage being gradually reduced by half at two-weekly intervals until an alternate day maintenance dosage is reached. Patients should be monitored throughout the treatment period to ensure that signs of improvement, such as resolution of optic disc swelling and/or restoration of vision and PLRs, are achieved and maintained (Figure 14.36) (Nafe and Carter, 1981).

neurological examination is warranted, in order to detect other neurological abnormalities consistent with the presence of CNS disease.

Orbital ultrasonography is particularly useful in those cases of optic disc swelling that are accompanied by exophthalmos, in which optic nerve neoplasia or optic nerve involvement in other orbital disease processes is suspected.

Advanced imaging techniques, such as magnetic resonance imaging or computed tomography, may detect lesions, such as CNS neoplasia, and may demonstrate optic nerve swelling.

Cerebrospinal fluid (CSF) analysis may be valuable, particularly in those cases in which optic neuritis is a manifestation of more diffuse CNS inflammatory disease, such as GME, in which the CSF typically displays a mononuclear pleocytosis and elevation in protein concentration (Thomas and Eger, 1989). CSF samples may also be subjected to tests for canine distemper, toxoplasmosis or cryptococcosis.

Management

In cases of idiopathic optic neuritis, or of suspected GME, the response to systemic, immunosuppressive

The prognosis in those cases of optic neuritis related to GME is extremely guarded, as ultimately other manifestations of CNS disease occur. However, remission may be achieved in response to systemic, immunosuppressive doses of corticosteroids (Thomas and Eger, 1989).

Optic nerve neoplasia

Optic nerve tumours are uncommon in the dog, with meningioma being the most frequently reported. The optic nerve may be involved secondarily, by local extension or by metastasis of neoplasia from other sites. Meningioma may involve the optic nerve by secondary extension of intracranial neoplasia, or by primary neoplastic transformation of cells within the optic nerve sheath (Mauldin et al., 2000). Affected dogs may present with slowly progressive exophthalmos, accompanied by loss of vision and pupillary light reflex deficits. Orbital exenteration may be curative, although intracranial and chiasmal extension and pulmonary metastasis of primary optic nerve meningiomas have been reported (Barnett and Singleton, 1967; Paulsen et al., 1989; Dugan et al., 1993; Mauldin et al., 2000).

Optic atrophy

Optic atrophy may occur as a result of a previous episode of optic nerve inflammation; a traumatic incident (particularly as a common sequel to prolapse or proptosis of the globe); previous optic nerve compression (e.g. by space-occupying lesions within the orbit); or as a result of an elevation in the intraocular pressure associated with glaucoma (which leads to optic disc 'cupping'). The atrophic ONH appears grey and dark, with loss of myelin leading to an irregular, crenated appearance, and loss of blood vessels (Figure 14.37).

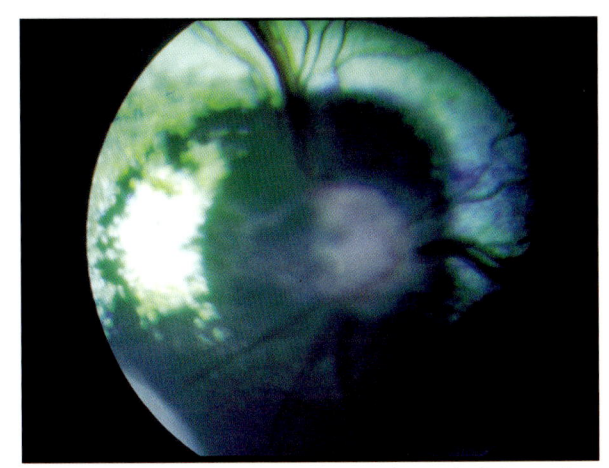

Figure 14.37 Advanced optic atrophy and glial scarring following optic nerve trauma.

References and further reading

Acland GM (1988) Diagnosis and differentiation of retinal diseases in small animals by electroretinography. *Seminars in Veterinary Medicine and Surgery (Small Animal)* **3**, 15–27

Acland GM and Aguirre GD (1987) Retinal degenerations in the dog: IV. Early retinal degeneration (erd) in Norwegian elkhounds. *Experimental Eye Research* **44**, 491–521

Acland GM, Ray K, Mellersh CS, Gu W, Langston AA, Rine J, Ostrander EA and Aguirre GD (1998) Linkage analysis and comparative mapping of canine progressive rod-cone degeneration (prcd) establishes potential locus homology with retinitis pigmentosa (RP17) in humans. *Proceedings of the National Academy of Sciences USA* **95**, 3048–3053

Aguirre GD and Acland GM (1988) Variation in retinal degeneration phenotype inherited at the prcd locus. *Experimental Eye Research* **46**, 663–687

Andrew SE, Abrams K L, Brooks DE and Kubilis PS (1997) Clinical features of steroid responsive retinal detachments in twenty-two dogs. *Veterinary and Comparative Ophthalmology* **7**, 82–87

Barnett KC (1965a) Canine retinopathies – II. The Miniature and Toy poodle. *Journal of Small Animal Practice* **6**, 93–109

Barnett KC (1965b) Canine retinopathies – III. The other breeds. *Journal of Small Animal Practice* **6**, 185-196

Barnett KC (1969) Primary retinal dystrophies in the dog. *Journal of the American Veterinary Medical Association* **154**, 804–808

Barnett KC (1976) Central progressive retinal atrophy in the labrador retriever. *Veterinary Annual* **17**, 142–144

Barnett KC (1981) Diabetic retinopathy in the dog. *British Journal of Ophthalmology* **65**, 312–314

Barnett KC and Singleton WB (1967) Retrobulbar and chiasmal meningioma in a dog. *Journal of Small Animal Practice* **8**, 391–394

Bedford PGC (1982a) Collie eye anomaly in the Border collie. *Veterinary Record* **111**, 34–35

Bedford PGC (1982b) Collie eye anomaly in the United Kingdom. *Veterinary Record* **111**, 263–270

Bedford PGC (1984) Retinal pigment epithelial dystrophy (CPRA): a study of the disease in the Briard. *Journal of Small Animal Practice* **25**, 129–138

Bedford PGC (1998) Collie eye anomaly in the Lancashire heeler. *The Veterinary Record* **143**, 354–356

Bjerkås E (1991) Collie eye anomaly in the rough collie in Norway. *Journal of Small Animal Practice* **32**, 89–92

Bjerkås E and Narfström K (1994) Progressive retinal atrophy in the Tibetan spaniel in Norway and Sweden. *Veterinary Record* **134**, 377–379

Buyukmihci N (1981) Photic retinopathy in the dog. *Experimental Eye Research* **33**, 95–109

Carrig CB, MacMillan A, Brundage S, Pool RR, Morgan JP (1977) Retinal dysplasia associated with skeletal abnormalities in Labrador retrievers. *Journal of the American Veterinary Medical Association* **170**, 49–57

Carrig CB, Sponenberg DP, Schmidt GM, Tvedten HW (1988) Inheritance of associated ocular and skeletal dysplasia in Labrador retrievers. *Journal of the American Veterinary Medical Association* **193**, 1269–1272

Clements PJ, Gregory CY, Peterson-Jones SM, Sargan DR and Bhattacharya SS (1993) Confirmation of the rod cGMP phosphodiesterase subunit b (PDEB) nonsense mutation in affected rcd-1 Irish setters in the UK and development of a diagnostic test. *Current Eye Research* **12**, 861–866

Clements PJM, Sargan DR, Gould DJ and Petersen-Jones SM (1996) Recent advances in understanding the spectrum of canine generalised progressive retinal atrophy. *Journal of Small Animal Practice* **37**, 155–162

Collinson PN and Peiffer RL (1993) Clinical presentation, morphology, and behavior of primary choroidal melanomas in eight dogs. *Progress in Veterinary and Comparative Ophthalmology* **3**, 158–164

Crispin SM (1993) Ocular manifestations of hyperlipoproteinaemia. *Journal of Small Animal Practice* **34**, 500–506

Crispin SM, Long SE and Wheeler CA (1999) Incidence and ocular manifestations of multifocal retinal dysplasia in the golden retriever in the UK. *Veterinary Record* **145**, 669–672

Cummings JF, De Lahunta A, Riis RC and Loew ER (1990) Neuropathologic changes in a young adult tibetan terrier with subclinical neuronal ceroid-lipofuscinosis. *Progress in Veterinary Neurology* **1**, 301–309

Curtis R (1988) Retinal diseases in the dog and cat: an overview and update. *Journal of Small Animal Practice* **29**, 397–415

Curtis R and Barnett KC (1993) Progressive retinal atrophy in miniature longhaired dachshund dogs. *British Veterinary Journal* **149**, 71–85

Davidson MG, Geoly FJ, McLellan GJ, Gilger BC and Whitley W (1998) Retinal degeneration associated with vitamin E deficiency in a group of hunting dogs. *Journal of the American Veterinary Medical Association* **213**, 645–651

Dekomien G, Runte M, Gödde R and Epplen JT (2000) Generalized progressive retinal atrophy of Sloughi dogs is due to an 8-bp insertion in exon 21 of the PDE6B gene. *Cytogenetics and Cell Genetics* **90**, 261–267

Dugan SJ, Schwarz PD, Roberts SM and Ching SV (1993) Primary optic nerve meningioma and pulmonary metastasis in a dog. *Journal of the American Animal Hospital Association* **29**, 11–16

Gum GG, Gelatt KN and Samuelson DA (1984) Maturation of the retina of the canine neonate as determined by electroretinography and histology. *American Journal of Veterinary Research* **45**, 1166–1171

Hendrix DV, Nasisse MP, Cowen P and Davidson MG (1993) Clinical signs, concurrent diseases, and risk factors associated with retinal detachment in dogs. *Progess in Veterinary and Comparative Ophthalmology* **3**, 87–91

Holle DM, Stankovics ME, Sarna CS and Aguirre GD (1999) The geographic form of retinal dysplasia in dogs is not always a congenital abnormality. *Veterinary Ophthalmology* **2**, 61–66

Holt E, Feldman EC and Buyukmihci N (1999) The prevalence of hyperadrenocorticism (Cushing's syndrome) in dogs with sudden acquired retinal degeneration (SARD). *Proceedings of the 30th Annual Meeting of the American College of Veterinary Ophthalmologists*, p.35. Chicago

Jolly RD, Martinus RD and Palmer DN (1992) Sheep and other animals with ceroid-lipofuscinoses: their relevance to Batten disease. *American Journal of Medical Genetics* **42**, 609–614

Keep JM (1972) Clinical aspects of progressive retinal atrophy in the Cardigan Welsh corgi. *Australian Veterinary Journal* **48**, 197–199

Kern TJ and Riis RC (1981) Optic nerve hypoplasia in three miniature poodles. *Journal of the American Veterinary Medical Association* **178**, 49–54

Lane IF, Roberts SM and Lappin MR (1993) Ocular manifestations of vascular disease: hypertension, hyperviscosity and hyperlipidemia. *Journal of the American Animal Hospital Association* **29**, 28–36

Latshaw WK, Wyman M and Venzke WG (1969) Embryologic development of an anomaly of ocular fundus in the collie dog. *American Journal of Veterinary Research* **30**, 211–217

Lavach JD, Murphy JJ and Severin GA (1978) Retinal dysplasia in the English springer spaniel. *Journal of the American Animal Hospital Association* **14**, 192–199

Lightfoot RM, Cabral L, Gooch L, Bedford PGC and Boulton ME (1996) Retinal pigment epithelial dystrophy in Briard dogs. *Research in Veterinary Science* **60**, 17–23

Long SE and Crispin SM (1999) Inheritance of multifocal retinal dysplasia in the golden retriever in the UK. *Veterinary Record* **145**, 702–704

MacMillan AD and Lipton DE (1978) Heritability of multifocal retinal dysplasia in American cocker spaniels. *Journal of the American Veterinary Medical Association* **172**, 568–572

Mauldin EA, Deehr AJ, Hertzke D and Dubielzig RR (2000) Canine orbital meningiomas: a review of 22 cases *Veterinary Ophthalmology* **3**, 11–16

McLellan GJ, Cappello R, Mayhew IG, Elks, R, Lybaert P, Watté C, Moore DL and Bedford PGC (2000) Systemic manifestations of vitamin E deficiency in canine RPED (CPRA). *Proceedings of the 31st Annual Meeting of the American College of Veterinary Ophthalmologists*, p.41. Montreal

Meyers VN, Jezyk PF, Aguirre GD and Patterson DF (1983) Short-limbed dwarfism and ocular defects in the Samoyed dog. *Journal of the American Veterinary Medical Association* **183**, 975–979

Millichamp NJ (1990) Retinal degeneration in the dog and cat. *Veterinary Clinics of North America: Small Animal Practice* **20**, 799–835

Millichamp NJ, Curtis R and Barnett KC (1988) Progressive retinal atrophy in Tibetan terriers. *Journal of the American Veterinary Medical Association* **192**, 769–776

Muñana KR (1995) Long-term complications of diabetes mellitus, part 1: retinopathy, nephropathy, neuropathy. *Veterinary Clinics of North America: Small Animal Practice* **25**, 715–730

Nafe LA and Carter JD (1981) Canine optic neuritis. *Compendium on Continuing Education for the Practising Veterinarian* **3**, 978–981

Narfström K (1999) Retinal dystrophy or "congenital stationary night blindness" in the Briard dog. *Veterinary Ophthalmology* **2**, 75–76

Narfström K and Ekesten B (1999) Diseases of the canine ocular fundus. In: *Veterinary Ophthalmology 3rd edn*, ed. KN Gelatt, pp. 869–933. Lippincott, Williams and Wilkins, Philadelphia

Narfström K, Wrigstad A, Ekesten B and Nilsson SEG (1994) Hereditary retinal dystrophy in the briard dog: clinical and hereditary characteristics. *Veterinary & Comparative Ophthalmology* **4**, 85–92

Nelson DL and MacMillan AD (1983) Multifocal retinal dysplasia in field trial labrador retrievers. *Journal of the American Animal Hospital Association* **19**, 388–392

O'Toole D, Young S, Severin GA and Neuman S (1983) Retinal dysplasia of English springer spaniel dogs: light microscopy of the postnatal lesions. *Veterinary Pathology* **20**, 298–311

Palmer AC, Malinowski W and Barnett KC (1974) Clinical signs including papilloedema associated with brain tumours in twenty-one dogs. *Journal of Small Animal Practice* **15**, 359–386

Parry HB (1953) Degenerations of the dog retina. II. Generalized progressive retinal atrophy of hereditary origin. *British Journal of Ophthalmology* **37**, 487–502

Parry HB (1954) Degenerations of the dog retina VI. Central progressive atrophy with pigment epithelial dystrophy. *British Journal of Ophthalmology* **38**, 653–668

Parshall CJ, Wyman M, Nitroy S, Acland G and Aguirre G (1991) Photoreceptor dysplasia: an inherited progressive retinal atrophy of Miniature schnauzer dogs. *Progress in Veterinary and Comparative Ophthalmology* **1**, 187–203

Paulsen ME, Severin GA, Lecouteur, RA and Young S (1989) Primary optic nerve meningioma in a dog. *Journal of the American Animal Hospital Association* **25**, 147–152

Percy DH, Carmichael LE, Albert DM, King JM and Jonas AM (1971) Lesions in puppies surviving infection with canine herpesvirus. *Veterinary Pathology* **8**, 37–53

Petersen-Jones SM (1998) A review of research to elucidate the causes of the generalized progressive retinal atrophies. *The Veterinary Journal* **155**, 5–18

Petersen-Jones SM (1999) Clinical and molecular genetics. In: *Veterinary Ophthalmology, 3rd edn*, ed. KN Gelatt, pp. 219–238. Lippincott, Williams and Wilkins, Philadelphia

Petersen-Jones SM, Entz DD and Sargan DR (1999) cGMP phosphodiesterase-a mutation causes progressive retinal atrophy in the Cardigan Welsh corgi dog. *Investigative Ophthalmology and Visual Science* **40**, 1637–1644

Petersen-Jones SM and Zhu FX (2000) Development and use of a polymerase chain reaction-based diagnostic test for the causal mutation of progressive retinal atrophy in Cardigan Welsh corgis. *American Journal of Veterinary Research* **61**, 844–846

Riis RC, Cummings JF, Loew ER and De Lahunta A (1992) A Tibetan terrier model of canine ceroid lipofuscinosis. *American Journal of Medical Genetics* **42**, 615–621

Riis RC, Sheffy BE, Loew E, Kern TJ and Smith JS (1981) Vitamin E deficiency retinopathy in dogs. *American Journal of Veterinary Research* **42**, 74–86

Roberts SM (1969) The collie eye anomaly. *Journal of the American Veterinary Medical Association* **155**, 859–878

Rubin LF (1968) Heredity of retinal dysplasia in Bedlington terriers. *Journal of the American Veterinary Medical Association* **152**, 260–262

Rubin LF (1989) *Inherited Eye Diseases in Purebred Dogs*. Williams and Wilkins, Baltimore

Rubin LF, Nelson EJ and Sharp CA (1991) Collie eye anomaly in Australian shepherd dogs. *Progress in Veterinary and Comparative Ophthalmology* **1**, 105–108

Samuelson DA (1999) Ophthalmic anatomy. In: *Veterinary Ophthalmology, 3rd edn*, ed. KN Gelatt, pp. 31–150. Lippincott, Williams and Wilkins, Philadelphia

Sansom J and Bodey A (1997) Ocular signs in four dogs with hypertension. *Veterinary Record* **140**, 593–598

Schmidt GM, Ellersieck MR, Wheeler CA, Blanchard GL and Keller WF (1979) Inheritance of retinal dysplasia in the English springer spaniel. *Journal of the American Veterinary Medical Association* **174**, 1089–1090

Smith RIE, Sutton RH, Jolly RD and Smith KR (1996) A retinal degeneration associated with ceroid-lipofuscinosis in adult miniature schnauzers. *Veterinary and Comparative Ophthalmology* **6**, 187–191

Sullivan TC (1997) Surgery for retinal detachment. *Veterinary Clinics of North America: Small Animal Practice* **27**, 1193–1214

Thomas JB and Eger C (1989) Granulomatous meningo-encephalomyelitis in 21 dogs. *Journal of Small Animal Practice* **30**, 287–293

Vainisi SJ and Packo KH (1995) Management of giant retinal tears in dogs. *Journal of the American Veterinary Medical Association* **206**, 491–495

Vainisi SJ, Peyman GA, Wolf ED and West CS (1989) Treatment of serous retinal detachments associated with optic disk pits in dogs. *Journal of the American Veterinary Medical Association* **195**, 1233–1236

Van der Woerdt A, Nasisse MP and Davidson MG (1991) Sudden acquired retinal degeneration in the dog: clinical and laboratory findings in 36 cases. *Progress in Veterinary and Comparative Ophthalmology* **1**, 11–18

Veske A, Nilsson SE, Narfström K and Gal A (1999) Retinal dystrophy of Swedish Briard / Briard-beagle dogs is due to a 4-bp deletion in RPE65. *Genomics* **57**, 57–61

Villagrasa M and Cascales MJ (2000) Arterial hypertension: angiographic aspects of the ocular fundus in dogs. A study of 24 cases *The European Journal of Companion Animal Practice*, **10**, 177–190

Wallin-Håkanson B, Wallin-Håkanson N and Hedhammar Å (2000a) Influence of selective breeding on the prevalence of chorioretinal dysplasia and coloboma in the rough collie in Sweden. *Journal of Small Animal Practice* **41**, 56–59

Wallin-Håkanson B, Wallin-Håkanson N and Hedhammar Å (2000b) Collie eye anomaly in the rough collie in Sweden: genetic transmission and influence on offspring vitality. *Journal of Small Animal Practice* **41**, 254–258

Watson P, Narfström K and Bedford PGC (1993) Retinal Pigment Epithelial Dystrophy (RPED) in Polish Lowland Sheepdogs. *Proceedings of the British Small Animal Veterinary Association Congress*, p.231. Birmingham

Wolf ED, Vainisi SJ and Santos-Anderson R (1978) Rod-cone dysplasia in the collie. *Journal of the American Veterinary Medical Association* **173**, 1331–1333

Wyman M and McKissick GE (1973) Lipemia retinalis in a dog and cat: case reports. *Journal of the American Animal Hospital Association* **9**, 288–291

Yakely WL, Wyman M, Donovan EF and Fechheimer NS (1968) Genetic transmission of an ocular fundus anomaly in Collies. *Journal of the American Veterinary Medical Association* **152**, 457–461

Zeiss CJ, Acland GM and Aguirre GD (1999) Retinal pathology of canine X-linked progressive retinal atrophy the locus homologue of RP3. *Investigative Ophthalmology and Visual Science* **40**, 3292–3304.

14b

The feline fundus

Joan Dziezyc and Nicholas J. Millichamp

Anatomy and physiology

The anatomy of the feline posterior segment is similar to that of the other domestic species, but the normal feline fundus shows less variation than the normal canine fundus. The sensory (neural) retina is found closest to the vitreous, with the ganglion cell layer nearest the vitreous and the layer of rods and cones (photoreceptors) nearest to the sclera. Adjacent to the photoreceptors is the one-cell layer of the retinal pigment epithelium (RPE). In the non-tapetal fundus, this layer normally contains melanin granules. In the tapetal fundus, the RPE is non-pigmented.

The next layer is the choroid, which consists of choriocapillaris, tapetum, and large blood vessels. The tapetum is only found in the dorsal fundus. It is a reflective structure, consisting of stacks of riboflavin-rich tapetal cells – the iridocytes; its purpose is to enhance light gathering by reflecting light back to the photoreceptors. The majority of the choroid consists of numerous large vessels which radiate from the optic nerve and which may be seen in some fundi as a striped pattern on the white background of the sclera. The choroid is usually pigmented, except in blue-eyed cats.

The most external layer is the sclera. This is a fibrous layer to which the extraocular muscles of the eye are attached and is continuous with the cornea anteriorly.

The optic nerve head (optic disc) is found in the tapetal fundus. It is unmyelinated and therefore circular, smaller than the canine disc, and greyish in colour. Three paired major retinal arterioles and veins extend into the retina from the periphery of the optic disc. One vessel pair runs dorsally and the other two run ventrally: one medially and one laterally. Small arterioles also extend from the disc between the three major vessels.

The area around the optic nerve may be darker or more reflective than the rest of the tapetal fundus (Figure 14.38). The tapetum itself is usually yellow-green, with less variation in size than in dogs. The non-tapetal fundus is dark brown. In blue-eyed cats with the Siamese coat colour pattern (e.g. Siamese, Himalayan) there is often a yellow-green tapetum but the RPE in the non-tapetal fundus is not pigmented and the normal 'tiger-striping' of the choroidal vessels is seen against the white of the sclera. In other blue-eyed cats there is no tapetum and no RPE pigment and the entire fundus shows the 'tiger-striping' of the choroidal vessels against the white sclera (Figure 14.39). These two fundic variations are known as subalbinotic fundi. Cats with chocolate coats (e.g. Burmese) may have a tigroid fundic pattern in the non-tapetal fundus, with choroidal blood vessels seen against a background of brown choroidal pigment (Rubin, 1974; Barnett and Crispin, 1998; Glaze and Gelatt, 1999).

The area centralis is the cat's equivalent of the human macula. It is located dorsolateral to the disc and contains the highest concentration of cones in the retina. Sometimes the normal tapetum in this area may look slightly more granular or greener than the rest of the tapetum.

The ora ciliaris retinae and ciliary processes can often be visualized when performing feline fundoscopy through a dilated pupil.

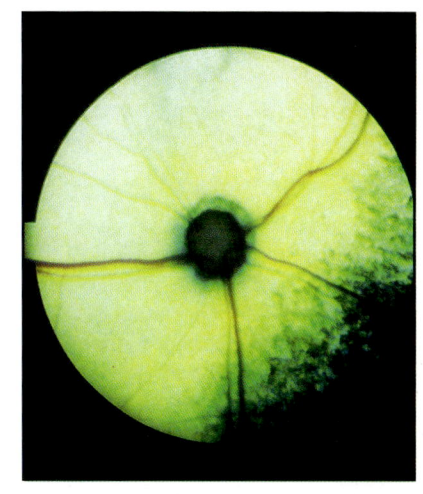

Figure 14.38 A normal fundus in a cat.

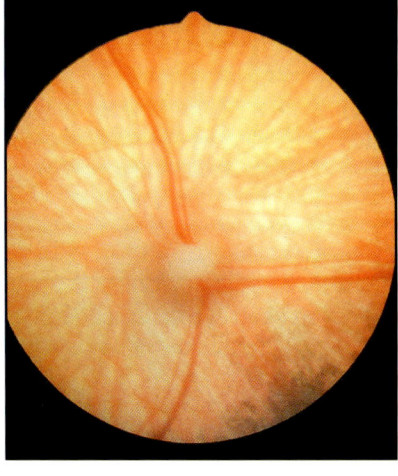

Figure 14.39 A normal subalbinotic fundus in a Siamese cat. (Courtesy of SM Crispin.)

Developmental diseases

Developmental diseases of the posterior segment of cats are rare, but several have been described. Persistent hyaloid artery is rare in cats (Ketring and Glaze, 1994; Barnett and Crispin, 1998; Glaze and Gelatt, 1999). Persistent hyperplastic tunica vasculosa lentis/persistent hyperplastic primary vitreous (PHTLV/PHPV) has been rarely reported; it is associated with persistent pupillary membrane remnants and corneal and lens opacities (Allgoewer and Pfefferkorn, 2001).

Coloboma

A coloboma is a congenital defect in which tissue is missing. Congenital defects in the optic nerve head have been reported, and are seen as pits (single or multiple) affecting varying percentages of the optic nerve head (Bellhorn et al., 1971). Optic nerve head colobomas do not usually affect vision unless they are very extensive.

Retinal dysplasia

Retinal dysplasia is the abnormal development of the retina that produces the characteristic pathology of retinal folds, rosettes or areas of degeneration. It is very uncommon in the cat and has only been described in association with perinatal infection with feline panleukopenia virus or experimental infection with feline leukaemia virus (FeLV) (Percy et al., 1975; Albert et al., 1977). In the non-tapetal fundus, dysplasia is seen as depigmented areas. In the tapetal fundus, the dysplastic areas can look darker than the surrounding fundus or can be hyper-reflective in regions of degeneration.

Optic nerve aplasia

Optic nerve aplasia has been reported in a cat in which there was no evidence of optic nerve or retinal vessels on fundic examination (Barnett and Grimes, 1974).

Acquired diseases

Most of the retinal disease seen in cats is acquired. It can be divided into three categories depending on the clinical signs:

- *Non-inflammatory degenerative disease:* Lesions are seen as bilateral symmetrical changes in the fundus. Degenerations may be hereditary or associated with nutritional deficiencies or toxicity to the retina. In their final stages, all of these cause diffuse changes throughout the fundus. In the early stages, changes may be localized or best seen in only one part of the fundus
- *Inflammatory disease:* Lesions are usually multifocal, asymmetrical and of varying size, and can be found anywhere in the tapetal or non-tapetal fundus.
  - Active inflammatory lesions in the tapetal fundus are seen as hyporeflective areas, which are dull green, white, or grey; the edges appear fuzzy. In the non-tapetal area, lesions are hypopigmented, either white or greyish. Retinal detachments are seen as elevated areas. Perivascular cuffing may be seen as fuzzy white opacities surrounding or running alongside retinal vessels. This is best appreciated in the non-tapetal fundus, especially with smaller-calibre vessels. Active lesions are hyporeflective or hypopigmented because cells and fluid are infiltrating the retina or are collecting between sensory retina and RPE. The retina becomes thickened and oedematous, and therefore absorbs and scatters more light. Thus the reflection from the tapetum is dulled and the RPE in the non-tapetal fundus is obscured.
  - Chronic, inactive inflammatory lesions in the tapetal fundus are seen as hyper-reflective areas with sharp edges. Hyper-reflectivity is seen as an area that looks bright – often like a mirror – when seen at certain angles. However, when the light is coming from a different angle, the lesion will look dark or greyish. This is a feature of the appearance of focal retinal degeneration that is especially evident in cats. Inactive lesions are hyper-reflective because retinal thinning occurs after the active pathology ceases. With retinal thinning, there is less scatter of light by the retina and more light is reflected back from the tapetum to the observer.

    Pigment may be seen within the areas of hyper-reflectivity in the tapetal fundus. Inactive lesions in the non-tapetal fundus can be either depigmented (whitish) or hyperpigmented (very dark brown), or, often, a combination of both. The edges of the lesion are sharply demarcated and the lesions look flat. Colour changes are a result of RPE changes (loss of pigment and/or increased pigmentation due to RPE hyperplasia or hypertrophy). Whatever the cause of the lesion, it is no longer active and there is usually no way of determining the aetiological agent.

    If the lesion is chronic and inactive, no further time need be spent on the problem. On the other hand, if the lesion is active, an attempt should be made to determine the aetiology. If a diagnosis is made, the underlying disease process, which is frequently a systemic problem, should be treated whenever possible. If no diagnosis is made, then non-specific anti-inflammatory drugs can be used to suppress the inflammation.
- *Retinal detachment:* This occurs between the neural retina and the RPE, with attachment usually remaining at the optic nerve and the ora ciliaris retinae. The retina can often be seen as a billowing grey sheet with blood vessels just behind the lens. Total retinal detachments can usually be diagnosed with a penlight. Indirect ophthalmoscopy will, however, give a better view of the detachment, and haemorrhage or inflammatory exudates can be seen more readily.

Non-inflammatory fundic diseases

Taurine deficiency/Feline central retinal degeneration

The cat has an essential requirement for the amino acid taurine. Taurine deficiency has been associated with a well described syndrome of retinal degeneration (Aguirre, 1978) as well as, more recently, cardiomyopathy (Pion et al., 1992).

Clinically, the earliest obvious lesion of taurine deficiency is an elliptical area of hyper-reflectivity at the area centralis (dorsolateral to the disc) in both eyes (Figure 14.40). With continued taurine deficiency, this area increases in size. Then a similar lesion begins to appear in the medial tapetal fundus, dorsal to the disc. As the two lesions grow, they become confluent and extend horizontally across the fundus above the disc (Figure 14.41) (Bellhorn et al., 1974). This area increases in size until the entire tapetum becomes hyper-reflective, retinal vessels become markedly attenuated, and the optic disc appears dark (Barnett and Burger, 1980).

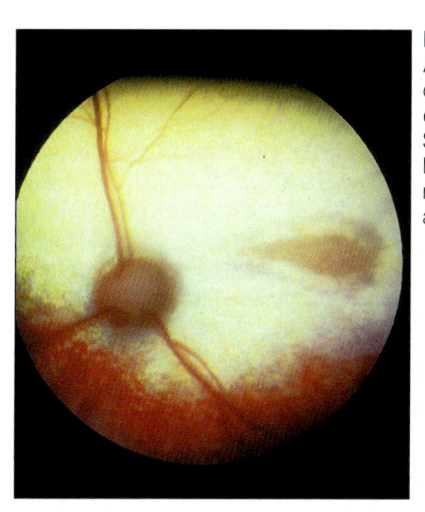

Figure 14.40 An early lesion of taurine deficiency in a Siamese cat. Note the hyper-reflectivity in the area centralis.

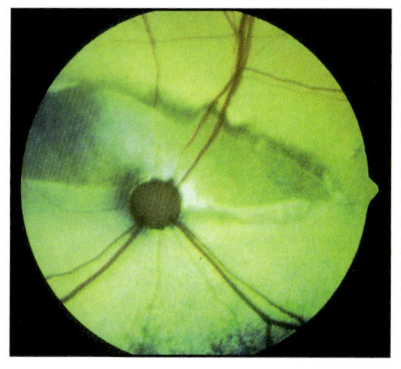

Figure 14.41 A later lesion of taurine deficiency in a domestic shorthair. There is a horizontal area of hyper-reflectivity extending dorsal to the optic disc. (Courtesy of SM Crispin.)

Cats with early taurine deficiency lesions do not appear to have any decrease in vision clinically, although electroretinograms (ERGs) performed at this time show a marked decrease in cone function. Later, a marked decrease in rod responses is also seen (Rabin et al., 1973; Glaze and Gelatt, 1999). The electrophysiological data suggest that the cones are initially more involved in the disease. However, there is evidence that the distribution of lesions histologically, which progresses from the central area of retina to a circumferential band of degeneration around the periphery of the retina, cannot be entirely explained by the distribution of cones in the feline retina (Leon et al., 1995).

Taurine deficiency retinopathy has been seen most commonly in cats exclusively fed dog food (Schmidt et al., 1976; Aguirre, 1978). Dog food may have very low levels of taurine, as it is not an essential amino acid for the dog. If taurine is supplemented at any point in the course of the disease, no further progression will be seen. Although ophthalmoscopic lesions do not change, there is an improvement in retinal function as assessed by the ERG.

Under experimental conditions, it takes 4–12 months for cats fed taurine-deficient diets to develop ophthalmoscopically detectable signs of retinal degeneration. Changes in the ERG are apparent after about 10 weeks (Rubin and Lipton, 1973). Normal retinal taurine levels are maintained until liver reserves are near zero. Differences in onset of disease may be correlated with differences in liver taurine reserves or difference in sensitivity to a dietary deficiency of taurine.

Feline central retinal degeneration (FCRD) is a clinical entity described as a bilateral elliptical area of hyper-reflectivity at the area centralis. It is clear that taurine deficiency is a cause of FCRD. However, cats with a good dietary history can also be seen with FCRD. It is possible that these cats also have taurine-deficiency retinopathy. They may be particularly sensitive to taurine deficiency, have had an episode of dietary taurine deficiency in the past, have impaired gut absorption of taurine, or it may be that cat foods that were presumed to have adequate taurine levels did not. In the USA, recommended minimum levels for dietary taurine have been raised and, consequently, cat food manufacturers have raised the level of taurine in cat foods. A cardiologist should examine cats diagnosed with FCRD because of the known association with dilated cardiomyopathy.

Progressive retinal degeneration

In photoreceptor dysplasia, photoreceptors begin to form in the developing retina, but never attain normal configuration and, subsequently, they degenerate. The retina normally completes its development in the cat during the first 3 months after birth (Hamasaki and Maguire, 1985; Jacobson et al., 1987) and clinical signs can be detected during this period in affected cats.

Progressive retinal degenerations have been described in both purebred and mixed breed cats. It is assumed (and proven in the Abyssinian) to be a hereditary problem. In cats (as in dogs), these inherited diseases (which may comprise several genetic forms) are collectively referred to as progressive retinal atrophy (PRA).

Abyssinian cats: The Abyssinian suffers from two well described forms of inherited PRA. One is an early-onset photoreceptor dysplasia. Affected kittens begin to develop pupillary dilation at 2–3 weeks, nystagmus at 4–5 weeks and ophthalmoscopically detectable retinal degeneration at 8 weeks. The tapetal fundus becomes increasingly hyper-reflective, with vessel attenuation. The disease is inherited as an autosomal dominant trait and has been described in a closed colony of cats in the UK (Voaden et al., 1982; Curtis et al., 1987). The second form of PRA in the Abyssinian is a later-onset disease that is inherited recessively and is common in Scandinavia (Narfström, 1983, 1985). Definitive clinical signs are first seen at 18 months to 2 years; a grey tapetal discoloration is seen in the midperipheral and peripheral fundus. This progresses to hyper-reflectivity and within 3–4 years the retinas are severely degenerate, with blood vessel attenuation. This form of PRA is a degeneration which affects rod and then cone photoreceptors, starting in the midperipheral fundus. Abnormally immature rod photoreceptors are present in the retina as early as 5 weeks of age, with considerable degeneration evident in the rods at 5 months of age. The cones may remain largely normal until 2–3 years of age (Narfström and Nilsson, 1986, 1989).

Siamese cats: A generalized retinal degeneration is seen in older Siamese cats in the UK (Figure 14.42). The affected animals typically present with visual impairment at approximately 10 years of age, at which time advanced retinal degeneration is present. Inheritance in these cases has not been proven (Barnett, 1965).

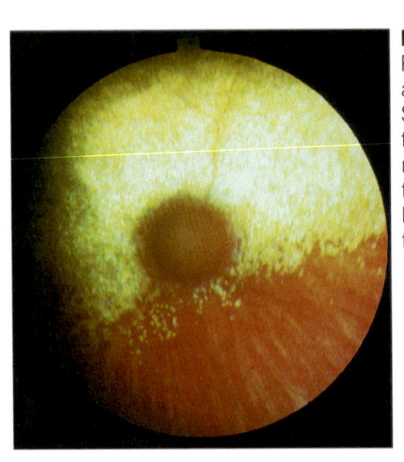

Figure 14.42 Progressive retinal atrophy in a Siamese cat. Note the attenuated retina vessels and the diffusely hyper-reflective tapetum.

Persian cats: In Persians in the USA, early- and late-onset forms of suspected inherited PRA have been reported (Rubin and Lipton, 1973; West-Hyde and Buyukmihci, 1982).

End-stage degeneration: A number of diseases may progress to end-stage degeneration and any breed can be affected (Figure 14.43). Clinically, the cat has impaired vision. However, because blind cats can function remarkably well in their own surroundings, owners often do not realize that the cat is blind. It can also be difficult to determine visual function by using a maze test.

On ocular examination, the pupillary light response is usually present, but slow and incomplete. The tapetal fundus is diffusely hyper-reflective, vessels are attenuated to the point where they are almost invisible and the optic nerve head looks darker than normal. This appearance is identical to end-stage taurine deficiency.

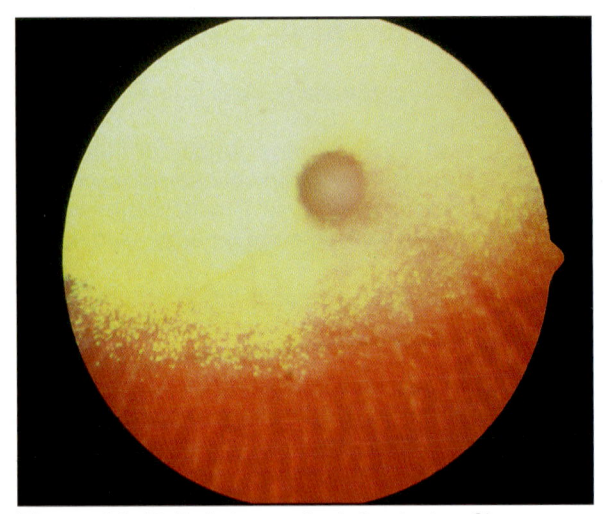

Figure 14.43 End-stage retinal atrophy in a Siamese cat with complete lack of retinal vessels and optic atrophy. This might be seen in advanced progressive retinal atrophy, at a late stage of taurine deficiency or resulting from enrofloxacin-associated retinal degeneration. (Courtesy of SM Crispin.)

Quinolone-associated retinopathy

An apparent toxic retinal degeneration has been reported in cats, associated with the use of the antimicrobial drug enrofloxacin (Gelatt et al., 2001) This is a sporadic toxicity which occurs in cats given enrofloxacin near or above the recommended dose of 5mg/kg per day, and is particularly associated with parenteral administration of the drug.

Clinical signs include a decrease in vision and an acute onset of mydriasis, which is often the first sign noticed by owners. Pupillary light reflexes may still be present although sluggish and incomplete. The fundus may appear normal on examination initially, although signs of retinal degeneration can develop within a few days of enrofloxacin administration. Signs include increased tapetal hyper-reflectivity, vascular attenuation, the presence of rust- to gold-coloured spots throughout the tapetal fundus, and variable pigmentary changes in the non-tapetal fundus. The ERG in affected cats is extinguished. Although some cats may regain some vision if the drug is discontinued immediately, others will remain blind. Similar changes have been reported experimentally in cats given the quinolone orbifloxacin (Kay-Mugford, 2001).

Anaemic retinopathy

Anaemia has been reported to be the cause of retinal haemorrhages in cats, when blood haemoglobin levels are less than 50 g/l (Figure 14.44) (Fischer, 1970). Concurrent diseases in these cats included thrombocytopenia, lymphoma, septicaemia, uraemia and panleucopenia. Blood pressure measurements were not performed. It is certainly possible that other factors or underlying disease processes, rather than the anaemia *per se*, were the cause of the retinal haemorrhages.

Inherited enzyme deficiencies

There have been occasional reports of hereditary enzyme deficiency or lysosomal storage disease that

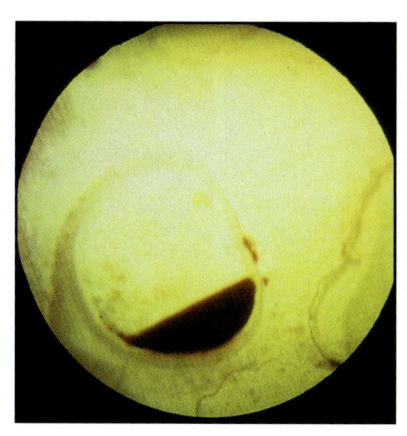

Figure 14.44 Preretinal haemorrhage in the fundus of a cat with both a blood clotting defect and anaemia. Note that the red blood cells settle ventrally in the areas of haemorrhage.

affect the retina as well as other body systems. These include: alpha-mannosidosis (Blakemore, 1986), which is manifested as a dull grey, granular appearance to the area centralis; GM_1-gangliosidosis (Murray et al., 1977), which is associated with focal fundic lesions; gyrate atrophy (ornithinase deficiency) resulting in generalized retinal atrophy (Valle et al., 1983); and Chédiak–Higashi syndrome, manifested as a lack of tapetum and decreased pigmentation, allowing choroidal vessels to be seen (Collier et al., 1985).

Inflammatory fundic diseases

Active inflammatory posterior segment disease is described clinically as a chorioretinitis because often both layers are involved and, clinically, it is difficult to distinguish between choroiditis and retinitis. The same disease entities that cause anterior uveitis (see Chapter 10) cause posterior uveitis (choroiditis). Certain differences in clinical signs between disease entities will be mentioned, but none is pathognomonic for a particular disease (with the possible exception of ophthalmomyiasis interna).

Diagnosis

Cases of active inflammatory chorioretinitis should be investigated further to determine aetiology. The work-up of a cat with active chorioretinitis should include a complete blood count and differential white cell count, biochemistry, urinalysis, feline leukaemia virus (FeLV) and feline immunodeficiency virus (FIV) tests, and IgG and IgM antibody titres for toxoplasmosis.

Other diseases to consider are feline infectious peritonitis (FIP) and, at least in tropical and subtropical zones, systemic fungal infections. Unfortunately, there are no reliable serological tests for FIP or systemic mycotic infection.

The cat should always be screened for other systemic illness – there are cases where the diagnosis of the cause of chorioretinitis can be made based on lesions elsewhere in the body that are more accessible than the retina and choroid. For instance, aspirates can be taken from enlarged lymph nodes and skin lesions; CSF paracentesis is also indicated if neurological signs are present. Thoracic radiography, abdominal ultrasonography and computerized tomography (CT) or magnetic resonance imaging (MRI) may be indicated in cases of systemic illness (with respiratory, alimentary or genitourinary or central nervous system signs). In rare cases, anterior chamber, vitreous or subretinal aspirates may be indicated for serology, although collecting subretinal aspirates carries a significant risk of complications and should not be attempted by non-specialists.

Treatment

If a cause is determined, this should be treated with appropriate systemic drugs (see Chapter 10). If all the titres are negative and no other evidence of systemic illness is present, and this will be true in a large percentage of cases, then systemic corticosteroids (prednisolone 1–2 mg/kg orally, divided into two daily doses) are the treatment of choice. Only systemic drugs, not topical preparations, will reach the posterior segment, and the long-term use of non-steroidal anti-inflammatory drugs is probably unsafe in cats. When the clinical signs of inflammation have subsided, the dosage of corticosteroids can be gradually reduced. In some animals, the inflammatory signs will disappear. However, in other animals, inflammation will recur and the cat will need to stay on long-term reduced levels of corticosteroids to keep the inflammation under control.

Cats with inflammatory chorioretinitis should be re-examined periodically to monitor any recrudescence of disease. The possibility of a systemic disease that can be worsened by the use of systemic corticosteroids must also be kept in mind. If chorioretinitis is accompanied by anterior uveitis, the latter should also be treated with topical drugs (see Chapter 10).

Viral diseases

Feline infectious peritonitis (FIP) causes a pyogranulomatous inflammation, especially of blood vessels (vasculitis). In the posterior segment, this presents as retinal perivascular exudates, retinal haemorrhage, choroidal exudation (hyporeflective tapetum), focal retinal detachments and optic neuritis (FIP also affects the central nervous system) (Figures 14.45 and 14.46) (Vianisi and Campbell, 1969; Campbell and Reed, 1975; Campbell and Schiessl, 1978; Andrew, 2000).

Feline leukaemia virus (FeLV) is described as a cause of anterior and posterior uveitis, although little has been published on the ocular signs associated with this infection (Brightman et al., 1991; Corcoran et al., 1995). Abnormal lymphocytes can invade the posterior segment, causing perivascular cuffing, chorioretinal infiltrates, retinal detachment and optic neuritis (Figure 14.47).

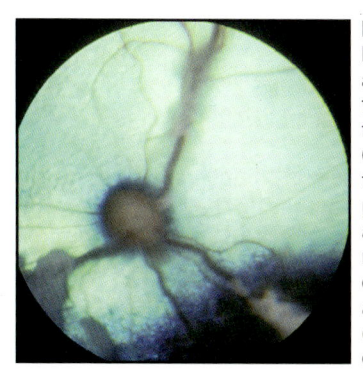

Figure 14.45 Perivascular exudates are the most obvious feature in the fundus of this 14-month-old Chinchilla cat with feline infectious peritonitis. There are also some acquired retinal folds, indicative of subretinal effusion and early retinal detachment. (Courtesy of SM Crispin.)

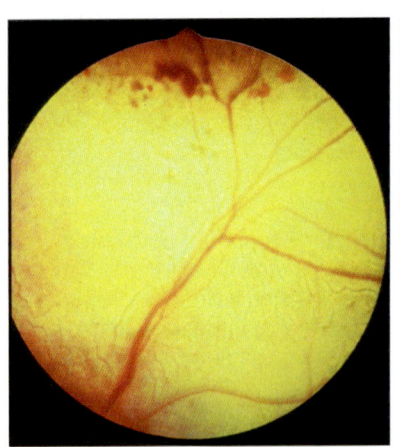

Figure 14.46 Multifocal retinal haemorrhages are present in the dorsal tapetum of this Siamese cat with feline infectious peritonitis.

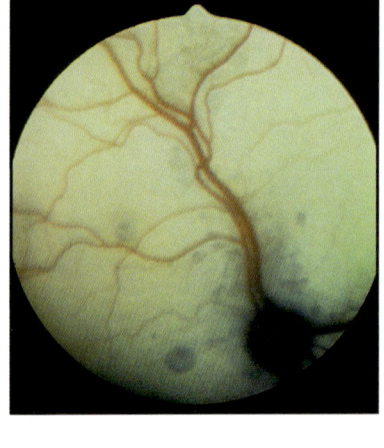

Figure 14.48 Focal inflammatory lesions and retinal folds in a domestic shorthair with toxoplasmosis. The retinal folds are indicative of subretinal effusion and early retinal detachment. The cat also had mild vitritis. (Courtesy of SM Crispin.)

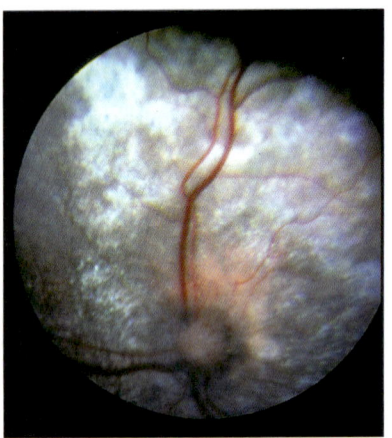

Figure 14.47 The fundus of a cat infected with feline leukaemia virus. There is evidence of chorioretinitis with cellular (neoplastic) infiltrates, especially dorsal to the optic disc.

FIV seropositivity has been associated with the development of posterior segment signs, including retinal perivasculitis and white punctate infiltrates in the anterior vitreous, most noticeable peripherally. These are interpreted as signs of pars planitis (English et al., 1990). FIV can cause ocular signs by direct damage to the uveal tract, by causing immune reactions and thus secondary damage, or by allowing opportunistic organisms such as *Toxoplasma gondii* to invade the eye (Davidson et al., 1993; Lappin et al., 1993).

Parasitic diseases

Toxoplasmosis: *Toxoplasma gondii* has been shown to produce retinitis and choroiditis (Figure 14.48), as well as anterior uveitis (Vianisi and Campbell, 1969). The retina has been reported as the primary site of inflammation, but inflammation and organisms can also be found in the choroid (Dubey and Carpenter, 1993; Davidson and English, 1998). The organism is transmitted through the ingestion of infected tissues, ingestion of oocytes (passed in infected cats' faeces), or transplacentally.

The inflammatory lesions produced by *T. gondii* are not, however, pathognomonic. In the past, it was difficult to reach a specific diagnosis of toxoplasmosis. IgG antibody titres do not accurately reflect recent disease because IgG levels may not become positive until a month after infection. Once positive, they can remain very highly positive for a least a year. IgM antibody titres have been used to diagnose recent infection with *T. gondii* more accurately. IgM antibodies are produced within 2 weeks post-infection and become negative by 16 weeks. IgM titres of >1:256 indicate recent infection (Lappin et al., 1989a,b). In most cases, cats only become sick with recent infection, although clinical relapse can occur in immunosuppressed animals.

Clindamycin (12.5–25 mg/kg orally twice a day for 2 weeks) has been suggested as the treatment of choice for toxoplasmosis, although it may not control ocular signs, and recent work has indicated that it may exacerbate the disease (Chavkin et al., 1992; Davidson and English, 1998). Corticosteroids should not be used to treat cases of chorioretinitis in cats with toxoplasmosis, in view of the risk of exacerbating generalized disease that often accompanies chorioretinal involvement in the disease (Davidson and English, 1998).

Animals with toxoplasmosis should have their FIV status tested. FIV, being an immunosuppressive agent, may reactivate latent *T. gondii* infections. A strong association between FIV-positive status and positive *T. gondii* titres has been demonstrated. However, FIV-positive animals may have an impaired antibody response, making diagnosis of toxoplasmosis difficult. Animals that are FIV-positive may also respond poorly to treatment for toxoplasmosis (Davidson and English, 1998).

Ophthalmomyiasis interna posterior: Aberrant migration of parasites in the posterior segment has been described in several cats. The lesions, which are considered pathognomonic, consist of curvilinear tracks of uniform width, resembling a road map. In the tapetal fundus, the tracks can be darker than, or more reflective than, the rest of the tapetal area. In the non-tapetal fundus, they appear lighter than the surrounding fundus, with pigment clumping possible. In addition to the tracks, there can be large areas of chorioretinal scarring. While the parasite is not usually present in the eye at the time of examination, the problem is assumed to be caused by botfly larvae, such as *Hypoderma* spp., which are capable of invading living tissue (Brooks et al., 1984; Harris et al., 2000).

Systemic fungal diseases

In tropical and subtropical zones, systemic fungal disease is a cause of chorioretinitis. These organisms are opportunistic, often enter the body through the respiratory tract, and are usually spread haematogenously to the eye. Organisms reported as causing disease include *Histoplasma capsulatum*, *Blastomyces dermatitidis*, *Cryptococcus neoformans* (Figure 14.49), *Coccidioides immitis* and *Candida albicans*.

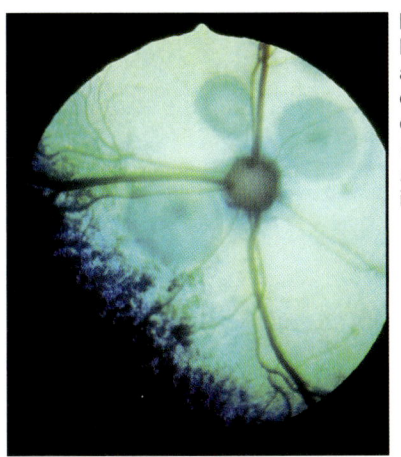

Figure 14.49 Multifocal areas of active chorioretinitis in a cat with active *Cryptococcus neoformans* infection.

Of these fungal diseases, the ones most likely to present with posterior segment inflammation in the cat are cryptococcosis (chorioretinitis and optic neuritis) (Blouin and Cello, 1980), blastomycosis (chorioretinitis with subretinal and intraretinal pyogranulomas and retinal detachment) (Gionfriddo, 2000) and histoplasmosis. Diagnosis needs to be confirmed by finding the organisms in infected tissues, because serology in cats often results in false negatives.

Various therapies have been proposed for intraocular inflammation caused by mycoses in cats (Gionfriddo, 2000, and see Chapter 3).

Retinal detachments

Animals with retinal detachments are usually presented when the retina in the second eye also detaches, at which point the owner notices that the animal has suddenly gone blind. On examination, pupillary light reflexes are present, but are usually slow and incomplete. Retinal vessels and folds of retina can often be seen behind the lens when examining the eye with a penlight.

Serous retinal detachments are the commonest type reported in cats. They are caused by choroidal exudates or transudates forming subretinal fluid which detaches sensory retina from RPE. They are not associated with retinal tears or vitreal traction bands. They can be divided into two categories: inflammatory and non-inflammatory.

Inflammatory retinal detachments

Because inflammatory disease is usually multifocal, there will be areas of retina that remain attached and normal. In abnormal areas, there will be cellular thickening of the retina or choroid, which can look white or yellow. Haemorrhage may be present (Figure 14.50). In cases of inflammatory disease, the differential diagnosis is as for inflammatory chorioretinitis.

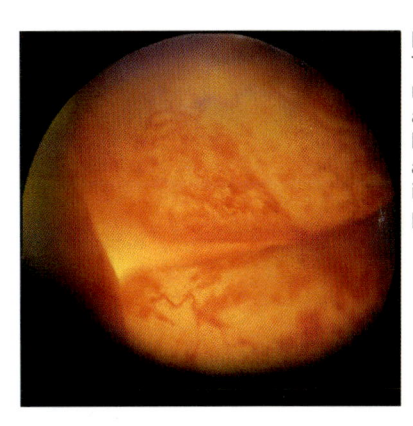

Figure 14.50 Total bullous retinal detachment and retinal haemorrhages in a cat with feline infectious peritonitis.

Non-inflammatory retinal detachments

Non-inflammatory retinal detachments are usually bilateral. The neural retina separates from the RPE and choroid throughout the posterior segment, but remains attached at the optic nerve and ora ciliaris retinae. The retina is usually uniformly greyish-white and may undulate with eye movement. These are described as 'morning glory' detachments because their appearance is similar to that of the flower. Haemorrhage can also be seen either in the retina, vitreous, subretinal space, or choroid.

Causes of non-inflammatory bullous retinal detachments in the cat include systemic hypertension, hyperviscosity syndromes and neoplasia. If the underlying cause of the retinal detachment can be controlled, the retina may spontaneously reattach. Unfortunately, in most instances, the reattached retina will not regenerate and the cat remains blind.

Degeneration of the feline retina begins within 1 hour of detachment. The degenerative changes in the neural retina and retinal pigment epithelium continue with time, and many are irreversible (Anderson *et al.*, 1981; Anderson *et al.*, 1983). The time between detachment and reattachment is critical for the regeneration of the retina (Anderson *et al.*, 1986). While no precise critical time period has been reported, it would appear that this period is shorter in the cat than it is in the dog.

Systemic hypertension: Although there have been few reports of hypertension-induced retinal detachments, this is not an uncommon problem (Morgan, 1986; Stiles *et al.*, 1994; Sansom *et al.*, 1994; Maggio *et al.*, 2000).

The most obvious lesions are bullous retinal detachments, which can be partial or total (Figures 14.51 and 14.52). Retinal and optic nerve oedema can be marked and vitreal haemorrhages are also seen, as well as hyphaema (Figure 14.52). In the early stages of the disease, retinal oedema may give the impression of narrowing of the retinal arterioles (retinal venules are largely unaffected). In more chronic stages of the disease, the arterioles are definitely narrowed and, histopathologically, reveal arteriosclerosis. These vessels may appear white and, occasionally, more tortuous than usual. Retinal detachment is probably largely due to subretinal oedema (transudate) from terminal choroidal arterioles and capillaries, and breakdown of the blood–retinal barrier that allows this fluid access to the subretinal space (Crispin and Mould, 2001). In chronic cases, retinal and optic nerve atrophy will ensue.

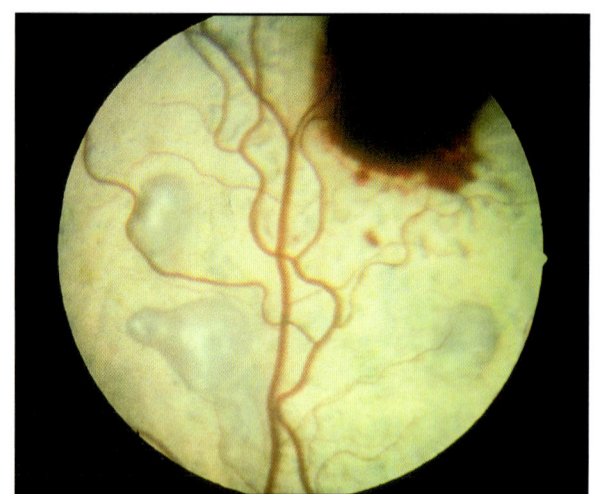

Figure 14.51 There is a large pre-retinal haemorrhage (top of picture) in this domestic shorthair (approximately 10 years old) with systemic hypertensive disease (mean systolic blood pressure 280 mmHg). The retinal arterioles also show some variation in calibre, especially ventral to the haemorrhage. Multiple bullous detachments are also present. Whereas the haemorrhage originated from retinal vessels, the bullous detachments are indicative of effusion from choroidal vessels. (Courtesy of SM Crispin.)

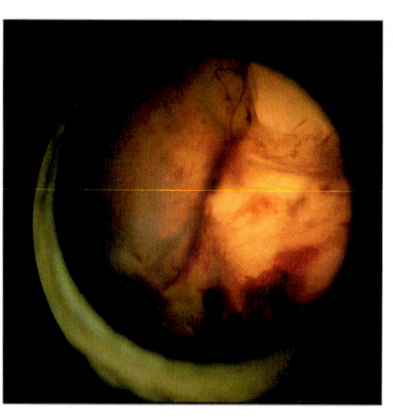

Figure 14.52 Total bullous retinal detachment with large areas of retinal and vitreal haemorrhage.

Hypertension in the cat is defined as sustained systolic pressure >170 mmHg and sustained diastolic pressure >100 mmHg. It is associated with chronic renal disease, hyperthyroidism, left ventricular hypertrophy and diabetes mellitus. Primary hypertension should be considered where these associated diseases can be ruled out. Although direct blood pressure measurements are more accurate, indirect blood pressure measurements can be used to confirm the diagnosis (Labotto and Ross, 1991).

Treatment consists of treating the underlying condition, as well as specific medical antihypertensive therapy. Reduction of peripheral vascular resistance with angiotensin-converting enzyme inhibitors (such as enalapril maleate) or calcium channel blockers (such as amlodipine besylate) will usually result in retinal reattachment, with some restoration of vision. Amlodipine besylate appears to be the treatment of choice (Maggio *et al.*, 2000). Retinal degeneration may, however, occur after the retina is reattached, causing further deterioration of vision. This possibly reflects the severity of retinal and choroidal vasculopathy resulting from systemic hypertension (Crispin and Mould, 2001).

Serum hyperviscosity: Serum hyperviscosity syndromes are rare, but have been described in the cat associated with multiple myeloma and tetralogy of Fallot. Serum hyperproteinaemia or polycythaemia (Figure 14.53) cause hyperviscosity which can cause retinal and vitreal haemorrhages and retinal detachments (Williams, 1981; Glaze and Gelatt, 1999).

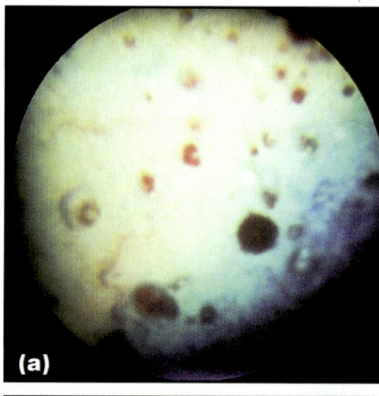

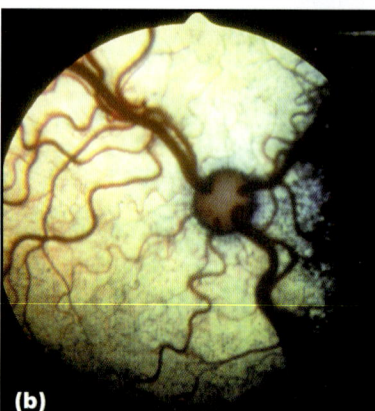

Figure 14.53 Retinal haemorrhage. (a) A cat with hyperviscosity syndrome. There are multiple areas of retinal haemorrhage, as well as small multifocal areas of tapetal hyper-reflectivity, which probably mark areas where there have been previous haemorrhages. (b) Secondary polycythaemia associated with tetralogy of Fallot in a 10-month-old domestic shorthair. The retinal vessels are dark, congested and tortuous. (Courtesy of SM Crispin.)

Neoplasia: Primary or secondary neoplasia can invade the posterior segment, causing retinal detachments and haemorrhage. Sometimes the tumour can be seen ophthalmoscopically. Tumours reported include retinal astrocytoma, metastatic squamous cell carcinoma, metastatic adenocarcinoma, metastatic haemangiosarcoma and lymphoma (Figure 14.54) (Glaze and Gelatt, 1999). Primary bronchogenic carcinoma is associated with ischaemic chorioretinopathy and necrosis of the extremities and appears to be a unique neoplastic syndrome in the cat (Cassotis *et al.*, 1999).

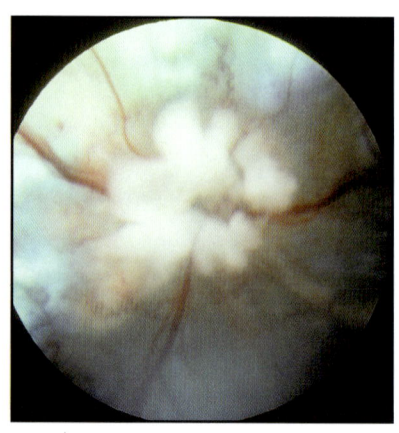

Figure 14.54 Multicentric lymphoma in a 7-year-old domestic shorthair. There is neovascularization and possible neoplastic infiltration in the papillary and peripapillary region. (Courtesy of SM Crispin.)

Other conditions of the feline fundus

Lipaemia retinalis

Lipaemia can cause retinal vessels to look creamy or pale (Figure 14.55). This condition is usually of diagnostic significance only and, in cats, is most frequently associated with an inherited form of primary chylomicronaemia due to mutation of the lipoprotein lipase gene (Ginzinger et al., 1996) but secondary associations also occur (Gunn-Moore et al., 1997).

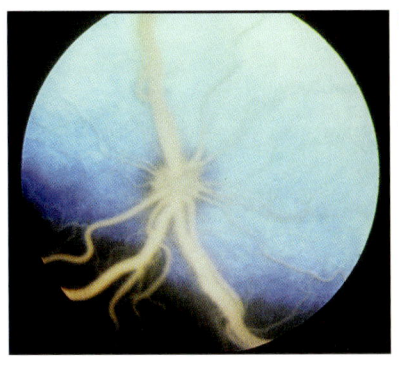

Figure 14.55 Lipaemia retinalis in a kitten with primary chylomicronaemia.

Optic nerve lesions

Oedema of the optic nerve head may be seen in cases of systemic hypertension and, possibly, be associated with central nervous system neoplasia and inflammation. Optic neuritis can be associated with CNS inflammation or chorioretinitis, and is not infrequently seen in cats with systemic fungal disease (see above). Atrophy of the optic nerve occurs secondary to neuritis and retinal degenerations. Cupping of the optic nerve in glaucoma, which is commonly seen in chronic disease in the dog, is difficult to appreciate in the cat (Barnett and Crispin, 1998; Glaze and Gelatt, 1999).

References

Aguirre GD (1978) Retinal degeneration associated with the feeding of dog foods to cats. *Journal of the American Veterinary Medical Association* **172**, 791–796

Albert DM, Lahav M, Colby ED, Shadduck J A and Sang DN (1977) Retinal neoplasia and dysplasia. I. Induction by feline leukemia virus. *Investigative Ophthalmology and Visual Science* **16**, 325–337

Allgoewer I and Pfefferkorn B (2001) Persistent hyperplastic tunica vasculosa lentis and persistent hyperplastic primary vitreous (PHTVL/PHPV) in two cats. *Veterinary Ophthalmology* **4**, 161–164

Anderson DH, Guerin CJ, Erickson PA, Stern WH and Fisher SK (1986) Morphological recovery in the reattached retina. *Investigative Ophthalmology and Visual Science* **27**, 168–183

Anderson DH, Stern WH, Fisher SK, Erickson PA and Borgula GA (1981) The onset of pigment epithelial proliferation after retinal detachment. *Investigative Ophthalmology and Visual Science* **21**, 10–16

Anderson DH, Stern WH, Fisher SK, Erickson PA and Borgula GA (1983) Retinal detachment in the cat: the pigment epithelial-photoreceptor interface. *Investigative Ophthalmology and Visual Science* **24**, 906–926

Andrew SE (2000) Feline infectious peritonitis. *Veterinary Clinics of North America: Small Animal Practice* **30**, 987–1000

Barnett KC (1965) Retinal atrophy. *Veterinary Record* **77**, 1543–1559

Barnett KC and Burger IH (1980) Taurine deficiency retinopathy in the cat. *Journal of Small Animal Practice* **21**, 521–534

Barnett KC and Crispin SM (1998) *Feline Ophthalmology. An Atlas and Text.* WB Saunders, Philadelphia

Barnett KC and Grimes TD (1974) Bilateral aplasia of the optic nerve in a cat. *British Journal of Ophthalmology* **58**, 663–667

Bellhorn RW, Aguirre GD and Bellhorn MB (1974) Feline central retinal degeneration. *Investigative Ophthalmology* **13**, 608–616

Bellhorn RW, Barnett KC and Henkind P (1971) Ocular colobomas in domestic cats. *Journal of the American Veterinary Medical Association* **159**, 1015–1021

Blakemore, C. (1986) A case of mannosidosis in the cat: Clinical and histopathological findings. *Journal of Small Animal Practice* **27**, 447–455

Blouin P and Cello RM (1980) Experimental ocular cryptococcosis. Preliminary studies in cats and mice. *Investigative Ophthalmology and Visual Science* **19**, 21–30

Brightman AH, Ogilvie Gk and Tomkins M (1991) Ocular disease in FeLV positive cats. *Journal of the American Animal Hospital Association* **27**, 1049–1051

Brooks DE, Wolf ED and Meredith R (1984) Ophthalmomyiasis interna in two cats. *Journal of the American Animal Hospital Association* **20**, 157–160

Campbell H and Reed C (1975) Ocular signs associated with feline infectious peritonitis in two cats. *Feline Practice* **5**, 32–34

Campbell H and Schiessel MM (1978) Ocular manifestation of toxoplasmosis, infectious peritonitis and lymphosarcoma in cats. *Modern Veterinary Practice* **59**, 761–765

Cassotis NJ, Dubielzig RR, Gilger BC and Davidson MG (1999) Angioinvasive pulmonary carcinoma with posterior segment metastasis in four cats. *Veterinary Ophthalmology* **2**, 125–131

Chavkin MJ, Lappin MR, Powell CC, Roberts SM, Parshall CJ and Reif JS (1992) Seroepidemiologic and clinical observations of 93 cases of uveitis in cats. *Veterinary and Comparative Ophthalmology* **2**, 29–36

Collier LL, King EJ and Prieur DJ (1985) Tapetal degeneration in cats with Chédiak-Higashi syndrome. *Current Eye Research* **4**, 767–773

Corcoran KA, Peiffer RL and Kock SA (1995) Histopathologic features of feline ocular lymphosarcoma. *Veterinary and Comparative Ophthalmology* **5**, 35–41

Crispin SM and Mould JR (2001) Systemic hypertensive disease and the feline fundus. *Veterinary Ophthalmology* **4**, 131–140

Curtis R, Barnett KC and Leon A (1987) An early-onset retinal dystrophy with dominant inheritance in the Abyssinian cat. *Investigative Ophthalmology and Visual Science* **28**, 131–139

Davidson MG and English RV (1998) Feline ocular toxoplasmosis. *Veterinary Ophthalmology* **1**, 71–80

Davidson MG, Rottman JB, English RV, Lappin MR and Tompkins MB (1993) Feline immunodeficiency virus predisposes cats to acute generalized toxoplasmosis. *American Journal of Pathology* **143**, 1486–1497

Dubey JP and Carpenter JL (1993) Histologically confirmed clinical toxoplasmosis in cats: 100 cases (1952–1990). *Journal of the American Veterinary Medical Association* **23**, 1556–1566

English RV, Davidson MG, Nasisse MP, Jamieson VE and Lappin MR (1990) Intraocular diseases associated with feline immunodeficiency virus infection in cats. *Journal of the American Veterinary Medical Association* **196**, 1116–1119

Fischer CA (1970) Retinopathy in anemic cats. *Journal of the American Veterinary Medical Association* **156**, 1415–1427

Gelatt KN, van der Woerdt A, Ketring KL, Andrew SE, Brooks DE, Biros DJ, Denis HM and Cutler TJ (2001) Enrofloxacin-associated retinal degeneration in cats. *Veterinary Ophthalmology* **4**, 99–100

Ginzinger DG, Lewis ME, Ma Y, Jones BR, Liu G and Jones SD (1996) A mutation in the lipoprotein lipase gene is the molecular basis of chylomicronemia in a colony of domestic cats. *Journal of Clinical Investigation* **97**, 1257–1266

Gionfriddo JR (2000) Feline systemic fungal infections. *Veterinary Clinics of North America: Small Animal Practice* **30**, 1029–1050

Glaze MB and Gelatt KN (1999) Feline Ophthalmology. In: *Veterinary Ophthalmology*, ed. KN Gelatt, pp. 997–1052. Lippincott, Williams & Wilkins, Philadelphia

Gunn-Moore DA, Watson TD, Dodkin SJ, Blaxter AC, Crispin SM and Gruffydd-Jones TJ (1997) Transient hyperlipidaemia and anaemia in kittens. *Veterinary Record* **140**, 355–359

Hamasaki DI and Maguire GW (1985) Physiological development of the kitten's retina: an ERG study. *Vision Research* **25**, 1537–1543

Harris BP, Miller PE, Bloss JR and Pellitteri PJ (2000) Ophthalmomyiasis interna anterior associated with *Cuterebra* spp in a cat. *Journal of the American Veterinary Medical Association* **216**, 352–355

Jacobson SG, Ikeda H and Ruddock KH (1987) Cone-mediated retinal function in cats during development. *Documenta Ophthalmologica* **65**, 7–14

Kay-Mugford PA (2001) Ocular effects of orally administered orbifloxacin in cats. In: *Proceedings, Conference of the American College of Veterinary Ophthalmologists*. Sarasota

Ketring K and Glaze MB (1994) *Atlas of Feline Ophthalmology.* Veterinary Learning Systems, Trenton, NJ

Labotto MA and Ross LA (1991) Diagnosis and management of hypertension. In: *Consultations in Feline Internal Medicine,* ed. JR August, pp. 301–308. WB Saunders, Philadelphia

Lappin MR, Greene CE, Prestwood AK, Dawe DL and Tarleton RL (1989a) Diagnosis of recent *Toxoplasma gondii* infection in cats by use of an enzyme-linked immunosorbent assay for immunoglobulin M. A*merican Journal of Veterinary Research* **50**, 1580–1590

Lappin MR, Greene CE, Winston S, Toll SL and Epstein ME (1989b) Clinical feline toxoplasmosis. Serologic diagnosis and therapeutic management of 15 cases. *Journal of Veterinary Internal Medicine* **3**, 139–143

Lappin MR, Marks A, Greene CE, Rose BJ, Gasper PW, Powell CC and Reif JS (1993) Effect of feline immunodeficiency virus infection on *Toxoplasma gondii*-specific humoral and cell-mediated immune responses of cats with serologic evidence of toxoplasmosis. *Journal of Veterinary Internal Medicine* **7**, 95–100

Leon A, Levick WR and Sarossy MG (1995) Lesion topography and new histological features in feline taurine deficiency retinopathy. *Experimental Eye Research* **61**, 731–741

Maggio F, DeFrancesco TC, Atkins CE, Pizzirani S, Gilger BC and Davidson MG (2000) Ocular lesions associated with systemic hypertension in cats: 69 cases (1985–1998). *Journal of the American Veterinary Medical Association* **217**, 695–702

Morgan RV (1986) Systemic hypertension in four cats: ocular and medical findings. *Journal of the American Animal Hospital Association* **22**, 615–621.

Murray JA, Blakemore C and Barnett KC (1977) Ocular lesions in cats with GM1-gangliosidosis with visceral involvement. *Journal of Small Animal Practice* **18**, 1–10

Narfström K (1983) Hereditary progressive retinal atrophy in the Abyssinian cat. *Journal of Heredity* **74**, 273–276

Narfström K (1985) Progressive retinal atrophy in the Abyssinian cat: clinical characteristics. *Investigative Ophthalmology and Visual Science* **26**, 193–200

Narfström K and Nilsson SE (1986) Progressive retinal atrophy in the Abyssinian cat. Electron microscopy. *Investigative Ophthalmology and Visual Science* **27**, 1569–1576

Narfström K and Nilsson SE (1989) Morphological findings during retinal development and maturation in hereditary rod–cone degeneration in Abyssinian cats. *Experimental Eye Research* **49**, 611–628

Percy DH, Scott FW and Albert DM (1975) Retinal dysplasia due to feline panleukopenia virus infection. *Journal of the American Veterinary Medical Association* **167**, 935–937

Pion PD, Kittleson MD, Thomas WP, Skiles ML and Rogers QR (1992) Clinical findings in cats with dilated cardiomyopathy and relationship of findings to taurine deficiency. *Journal of the American Veterinary Medical Association* **201**, 267–274

Rabin AR, Hayes KC and Berson EL (1973) Cone and rod responses in nutritionally induced retinal degeneration in the cat. *Investigative Ophthalmology* **12**, 694–704

Rubin LF (1974) *Atlas of Veterinary Ophthalmoscopy.* Lea & Febiger, Philadelphia

Rubin LF and Lipton DE (1973) Retinal degeneration in kittens. *Journal of the American Veterinary Medical Association* **162**, 467–469

Sansom J, Barnett KC, Dunn KA, Smith KC and Dennis R (1994) Ocular disease associated with hypertension in 16 cats. *Journal of Small Animal Practice* **35**, 604–611

Schmidt SY, Berson EL and Hayes KC (1976) Retinal degeneration in cats fed casein. I. Taurine deficiency. *Investigative Ophthalmology* **15**, 47–52

Stiles J, Polzin DJ and Bistner SJ (1994) The prevalence of retinopathy in cats with systemic hypertension and chronic renal failure or hyperthyroidism. *Journal of the American Animal Hospital Association* **30**, 564–572

Valle D, Jezyk PF and Aguirre GD (1983) Gyrate atrophy of the choroid and retina. *Comparative Pathology Bulletin* **15**, 2–4

Vianisi SJ and Campbell LH (1969) Ocular toxoplasmosis in cats. *Journal of the American Veterinary Medical Association* **154**, 141–152

Voaden MJ, Curtis R, Barnett KC, Leon A, Doshi M and Hussain AA

West-Hyde L and Buyukmihci NC (1982) Photoreceptor degeneration in a family of cats. *Journal of the American Veterinary Medical Association* **181**, 243–246

Williams DA (1981) Gammopathies. *Compendium on Continuing Education for the Practicing Veterinarian* **3**, 815–822

15

Neuro-ophthalmology

Fabiano Montiani Ferreira and Simon Petersen-Jones

The basic rationale for the practice of neuro-ophthalmology is very objective, almost mathematical, and relies heavily on our current knowledge of neuroanatomical circuitry. Neuro-ophthalmology combines apparently disparate specialties, including neuroanatomy, internal medicine, neurology, neurosurgery, radiology and ophthalmology, in a fascinating way.

Clinical tests

Clinical evaluation of animals suspected of having disease involving neuro-ophthalmic pathways requires a good knowledge of neuroanatomy. Clinical history data and several tests can be used. The objective of the clinical examination is to detect the presence of a neuro-ophthalmic disease and establish the location of the lesion in the nervous system. The diagnostic procedures and clinical tests, as well as the order in which they are performed, vary among specialists but it is important for every clinician to understand the basic principles and to establish their own method and sequence of tests, so as to be consistent in every examination. The cranial nerves influencing the globe and adnexa, their actions and the clinical tests used in their evaluation, are listed in Figure 15.1.

A brief description of the most commonly used clinical tests is presented here. Further details can be found in neurology textbooks (de Lahunta, 1983; King, 1987; Bagley, 1996; Hanson et al., 2001).

Tests of vision

Vision requires transparent ocular media (a clear cornea, aqueous humour, lens and vitreous) and functional retina, optic nerve (II) and central projection pathways to the visual (occipital) cortex. Tests of vision also require cortical association and projection pathways, and motor neurons necessary to complete the responses to visual stimuli. Several neurological tests rely on the optic nerve as the afferent arm.

Maze test
The animal should be watched as it negotiates a maze or strange environment (see Figure 1.3). This should be performed in both bright and dim light.

Visual tracking
This can be tested by dropping cotton wool balls about 30 cm in front of the animal's face (see Figure 1.2). Most sighted animals will follow the ball to the floor, although stressed animals may not respond, and some cats are indifferent. This is also called a fixating response. It can be used to evaluate not only visual fields but also eye movements.

Type of nerve supply	Nerves involved	Function	Clinical evaluation
Sensory (afferent) nerves:			
General somatic afferent	Trigeminal (V) (ophthalmic branch and part of maxillary branch)	Globe and adnexa (e.g. touch, pain, reflex tearing, temperature)	Corneal and/or palpebral reflex Use of the Cochet–Bonnet aesthesiometer
Special somatic afferent	Optic (II)	Vision and afferent arm to subcortical reflexes	Check pupillary size and anisocoria Pupillary light reflex Menace response Dazzle reflex Visual placing (postural reaction) Fundoscopy (optic disc)
	Vestibulocochlear (VIII)	Fibres from vestibular nuclei course in the medial longitudinal fasciculus, reticular formation and cerebellum to influence the nuclei of cranial nerves III, IV and VI (coordinated conjugate eyeball movements associated with changes in head position)	Check presence of nystagmus Gait analysis Oculocephalic reflex Optokinetic nystagmus Post-rotatory nystagmus

Figure 15.1 Cranial nerves influencing the globe and adnexa. (continues) ▶

Type of nerve supply	Nerves involved	Function	Clinical evaluation
Motor (efferent) nerves			
Somatic efferent	Oculomotor (III)	Levator palpebrae superioris and all extraocular muscles except superior oblique, lateral rectus and retractor bulbi	Check presence of strabismus or ptosis of the upper eyelid Check eyeball movements during vestibulo-ocular reflexes
	Trochlear (IV)	Superior oblique muscle	Check presence of strabismus (in the cat) Fundoscopy (check position of dorsal retinal vessels in the dog) Check vestibulo-ocular reflexes
	Abducens (VI)	Lateral rectus muscle and retractor bulbi	Check presence of strabismus Check vestibulo-ocular reflexes (check temporal movement particularly) Globe retraction on corneal or palpebral touch reflex
General visceral efferent: Parasympathetic branch	Within oculomotor (III) (ciliary ganglion)	Pupillary constrictor (sphincter) muscles	Pupillary light reflex (always check consensual) Pilocarpine test
	Within facial (VII) (pterygopalatine ganglion)	Secretory control of lacrimal glands	Schirmer tear test
General visceral efferent: Sympathetic branch	Pass via thoracolumbar outflow (T1–T3) and vagosympathetic trunk (cranial cervical ganglion)	Pupillary dilator (radial) muscles Smooth muscle within orbit and eyelids	Check for signs of Horner's syndrome
Special visceral efferent	Facial (VII)	Muscles of facial expression	Palpebral touch reflex Menace response Dazzle reflex

Figure 15.1 continued Cranial nerves influencing the globe and adnexa.

Menace response

The menace response is a little less subjective than the above. The test consists of making a menacing gesture, using the hand with the fingers spread (Figure 15.2), directed at each eyeball in turn, while the other eyeball is covered. The examiner should not touch the facial hairs of the patient nor produce air turbulence that will be felt by the patient. The response observed is closure of the palpebral fissure – a blink. The menace response tests the optic nerve (II) as the afferent arm and the facial nerve (VII) as the efferent arm (blink). The central interconnecting pathway is shown in Figure 15.2.

This is a learned response and is often absent in animals under 10–12 weeks old. Some normal adult animals do not respond – sometimes due to stress, and sometimes for no obvious reason.

- If the menace response is present and the palpebral or corneal touch reflex is absent, this may indicate reduced sensation, e.g. due to a trigeminal nerve (V) lesion
- If a unilateral cerebellar cortical lesion is present, the menace response is usually lost on the same side
- The menace response is lost with most cerebrocortical lesions.

Dazzle reflex

The dazzle reflex is elicited when a bright light (preferably a halogen light) is shone along the visual axis. The pathway for this reflex involves the optic nerve (II) as the afferent arm, rostral colliculus, subcortical connections and the facial nerve (VII) (Figure 15.3). The expected response is a rapid blink.

It is important to bear in mind that the dazzle reflex is a subcortical reflex. Fibres project directly from several regions near the region of the Edinger–Westphal nucleus to the facial nucleus, resulting in a blink (Takada et al., 1984). This reflex may be more prominent with forebrain disease due to loss of inhibition from the controlling upper motor neuron.

- If the dazzle reflex is present and the menace response is absent, this may indicate the presence of a cerebrocortical lesion, because only the menace response requires a normal visual cortex.

Pupillary light reflex and 'swinging flashlight test'

A bright light (preferably a halogen light) is shone into the eye, causing both pupils to constrict (Figure 15.4). The afferent fibres from the optic nerve (II) cross both in the optic chiasma and in the pretectum to influence oculomotor nuclei bilaterally (consensual reflex). The efferent arm of the reflex is via parasympathetic fibres in the oculomotor nerve (III), causing miosis. Figure 15.4 shows the entire pathway. Part of this pathway also mediates lens accommodation.

It is important to be aware that every time a light is shone into the eye, the normal response is an initial

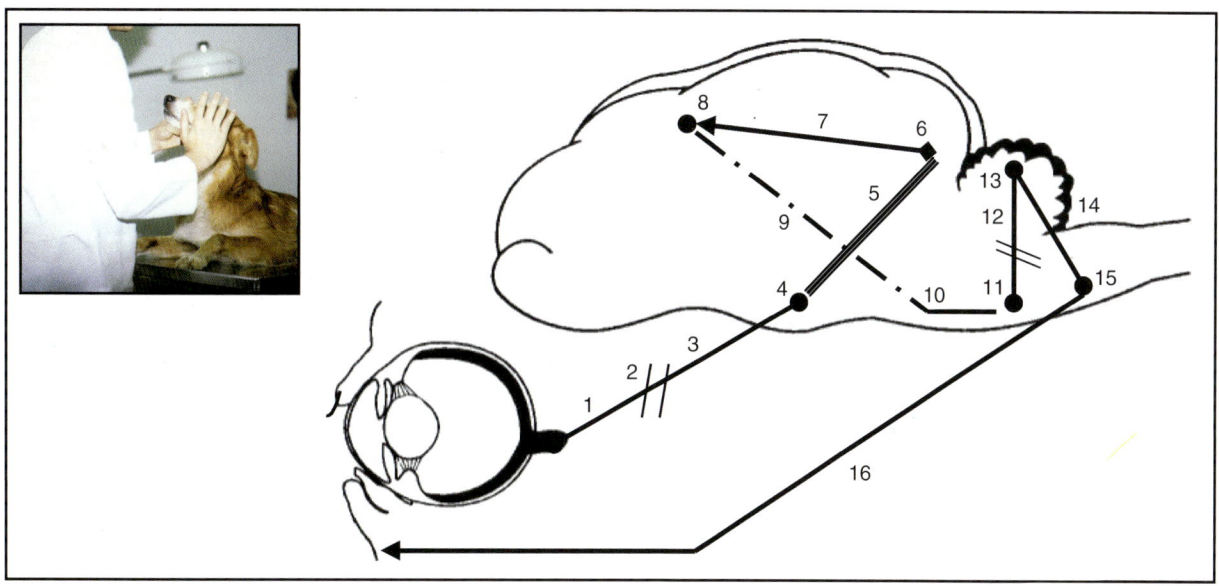

Figure 15.2 Menace response. The afferent and final efferent components of the menace response are illustrated. The photograph shows the test being performed. 1 – Optic nerve (II); 2) – Optic chiasma; 3 – Optic tract; 4 – Lateral geniculate nucleus; 5 – Optic radiation; 6 – Visual cortex; 7 – Internal capsule, association fibres; 8 – Motor cortex; 9 – Internal capsule, projection fibres, crus cerebri; 10 – Longitudinal fibres of pons; 11 – Pontine nuclei; 12 – Transverse fibres of pons and middle cerebellar peduncle; 13 – Cerebellar cortex; 14 – Efferent cerebellar pathway; 15 – Facial nuclei; 16 – Facial nerve; // – indicates axons crossing the midline.

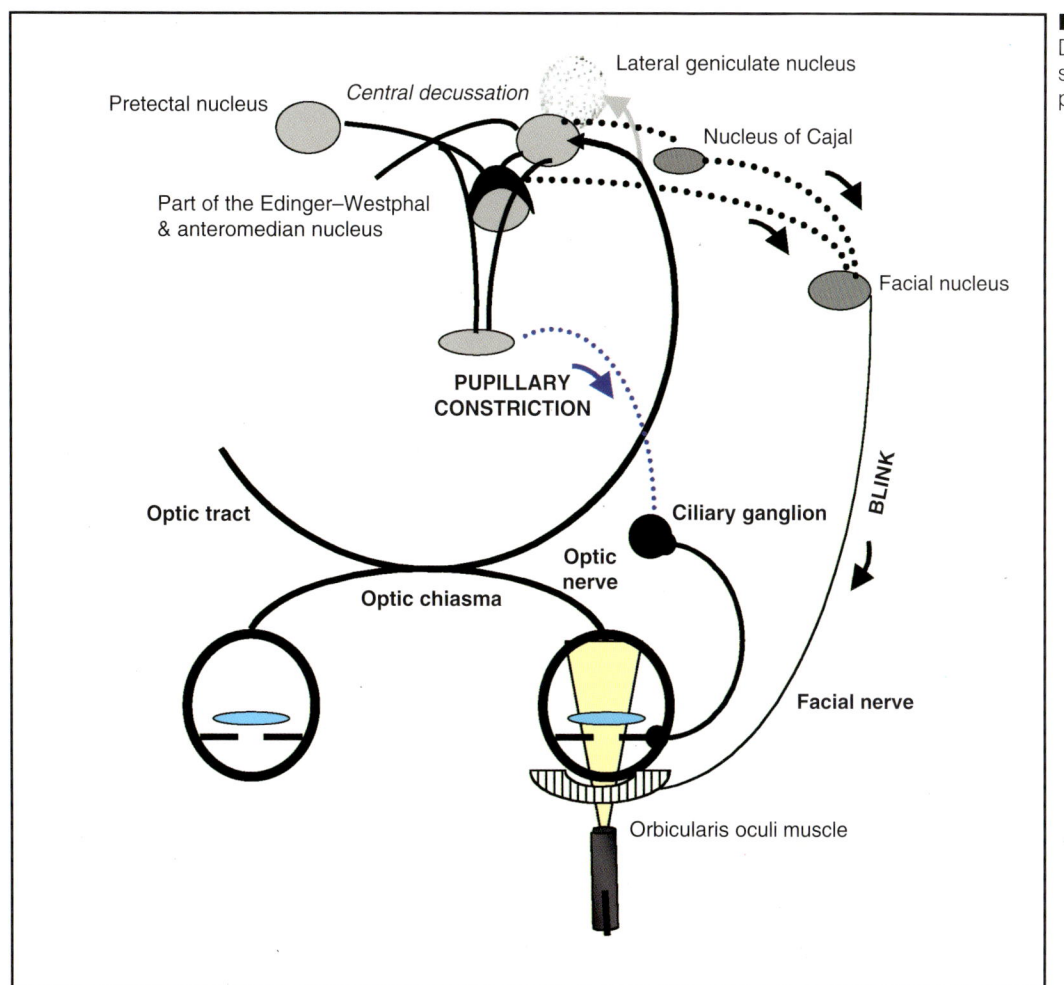

Figure 15.3 Dazzle reflex: subcortical pathway.

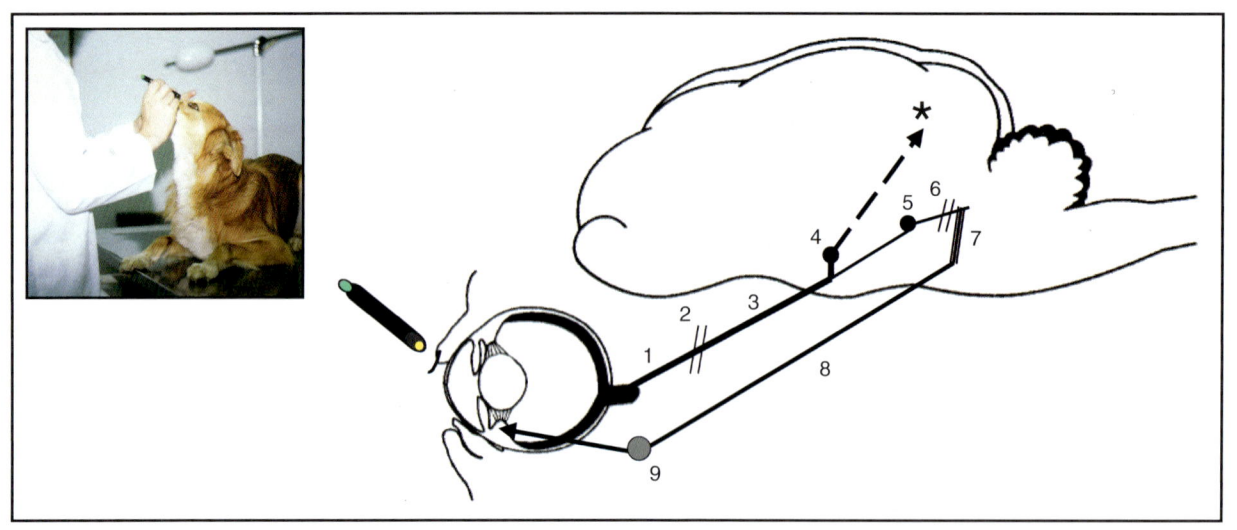

Figure 15.4 Pupillary light reflex. The afferent and efferent components of the reflex are illustrated. The photograph shows the test being performed. 1 – Optic nerve (II); 2 – Optic chiasma; 3 – Optic tract; 4 – Lateral geniculate nucleus; 5 – Pretectal nucleus; 6 – Central decussation; 7 – Ventral tegmental area, anteromedian nucleus, periaqueductal grey and Edinger–Westphal nucleus; 8 – Oculomotor nerve + parasympathetic supply to the iris; 9 – Ciliary ganglion; // – indicates axons crossing the midline; * – Optic radiation to visual cortex.

pupillary constriction followed by a slight redilation. The degree of the latter depends upon the intensity of the light source and the duration of the stimulus. There is a greater degree of redilation with weak light sources or longer time of light exposure. This is due to light adaptation of the photoreceptors, and it is referred to as 'pupillary escape'.

The pupillary light reflex requires fewer functioning optic nerve (II) fibres than does the menace response. Thus, it is not rare to find blind animals that still have a reasonable pupillary light reflex.

The 'swinging flashlight' test is simply a method of observing both direct and consensual pupillary light reflexes. The test involves swinging the penlight from one eye to the other. When it is shining on the first eye, the direct reflex constriction of that pupil is observed; as it is swung to the second eye, the pupil can be seen to be already constricted (the consensual reflex from the first eye) and will remain constricted (the direct reflex from the second eye). The pupil under direct illumination normally constricts slightly more than the contralateral pupil.

Reflex pupillary dilation

Reflex dilation in response to reduced illumination can be obtained by completely covering both eyes or by leaving the animal in a dark room for about 30 seconds. The afferent arm is the optic nerve and the efferent arm is reduced parasympathetic tone to the pupillary constrictor muscle leaving the dilator muscle (under sympathetic innervation) unopposed.

Ophthalmoscopy

Ophthalmoscopy allows direct inspection of the head of the optic nerve (II) for diagnosing, for example, optic neuritis and papilloedema. It also enables inspection of the position of the retinal vessels, useful in detecting rotation of the globe due to trochlear nerve (IV) lesions in dogs (see below).

Corneal and palpebral reflexes

The corneal and palpebral (touch) reflexes are used to test sensory innervation to the cornea, palpebrae and surrounding skin. The afferent arm of the reflex is the trigeminal nerve (V) (ophthalmic branch for the whole eyeball, including medial canthus).

This reflex is triggered by gently touching the cornea or the medial canthus (Figure 15.5), taking care not to induce a menace response.

- Touching the lateral canthus tests the maxillary branch (overlapping with the ophthalmic branch) of the trigeminal nerve (V). The normal response is eyelid closure, mediated by the efferent arm that is the facial nerve (VII) innervating the orbicularis oculi muscle.
- If the examiner touches the cornea, an additional response is seen, which uses a different efferent pathway in addition to the one already mentioned. This response is eyeball retraction via activation of the efferent arm that is the abducens nerve (VI) innervating the retractor bulbi muscle (Figure 15.5). Contraction of the retractor bulbi displaces orbital fat and connective tissue, and this displacement has an indirect mechanical effect on the third eyelid, causing it to sweep across the eye. This is also known as the nictitating reflex.

Sensory deficits are uncommon compared with facial paralysis.

- If the animal blinks with the menace response and dazzle reflex but not with the corneal or palpebral reflex, a trigeminal nerve (V) lesion is suspected
- Corneal sensation can be quantified using an aesthesiometer (see below).

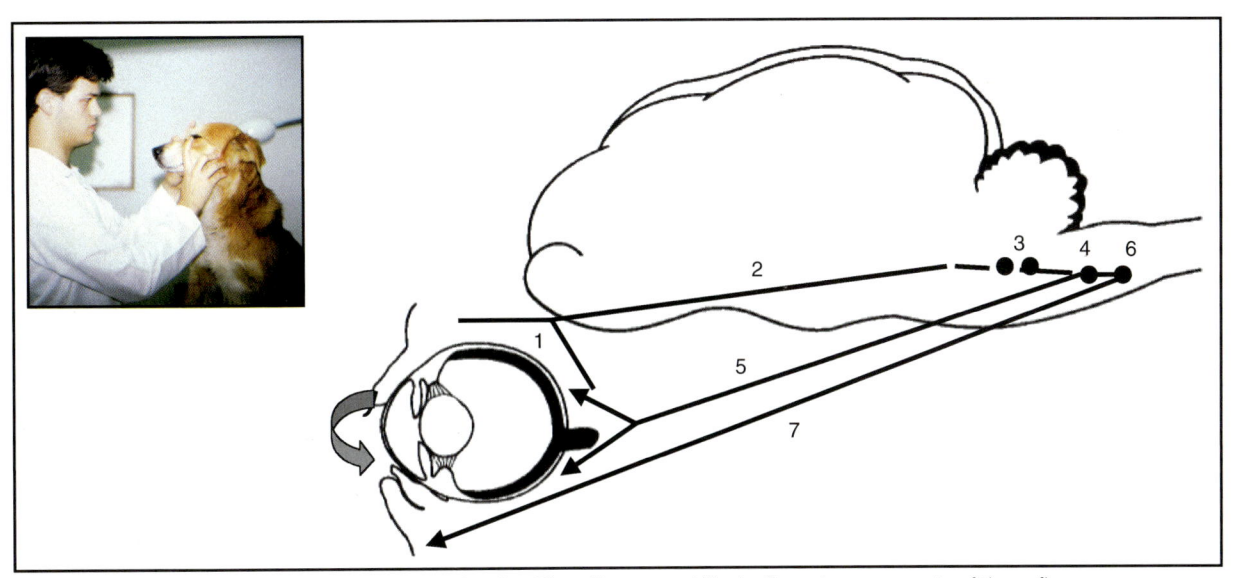

Figure 15.5 Corneal and/or palpebral (blink) reflex. The afferent and final efferent components of the reflex are illustrated. The photograph shows the test being performed. 1 – Corneal and palpebral sensory terminals of the trigeminal nerve; 2 – Trigeminal nerve (V); 3 – Pontine and spinal tract nuclei of the trigeminal nerve (V); 4 – Abducens nucleus ; 5 – Abducens nerve (VI) to retractor bulbi muscle; 6 – Facial nucleus; 7 – Facial nerve (VII) to orbicularis oculi muscle.

Inducing physiological nystagmus to test extraocular muscle innervation and vestibular system

Nystagmus is an involuntary rapid rhythmical eye movement associated with vestibular or visual stimuli, commonly with a slow and fast phase. Less commonly the eye excursions can be equal in extent; this is called pendular nystagmus. Usually the slow phase is a slow movement of the eyes away from their central position; the fast phase then rapidly re-centres the eyes. Physiological nystagmus is said to occur in the direction of the fast phase, i.e. if the animal's head is rotated to the left, nystagmus (fast phase) will occur to the left. Inducing physiological nystagmus serves to test the cranial nerves that innervate the extraocular muscles, i.e. oculomotor (III), trochlear (IV) and abducens (VI) (Figure 15.6 and see Figure 15.17) and the extraocular muscles themselves.

Vestibular nystagmus

The examiner may elicit vestibular eye movements (doll's eye, oculocephalic or oculovestibular reflexes) simply by moving the animal's head from side to side and then up and down. With the head moving, the eye will attempt to maintain eye direction towards the area where the animal was looking initially. This will result in a slow drifting of the eyes in the opposite direction to the movement. As the head continues to be moved, the extraocular muscles influenced by the vestibular system produce a quick deviation of the eyes in the direction of the movement. This slow/quick eye movement is continued as the head movement is being accelerated or decelerated (Bagley, 1996).

- In physiological nystagmus the eyes move in unison. After the head has stopped moving the nystagmus stops; if it continues this is abnormal
- The nystagmus produced by this reflex is due to the vestibular apparatus and will occur in blind dogs (so long as the necessary vestibular apparatus and pathways are normal)
- If the animal's body is rotated rapidly and then stopped, there is normally a post-rotatory nystagmus for a few moments. Vestibular disease is suspected when there is a different response to post-rotatory nystagmus following rotation in one direction compared with that following rotation in the other direction
- The response is depressed when the patient is rotated in a direction opposite to the side of a peripheral receptor lesion (de Lahunta, 1983).

Optokinetic nystagmus

Higher centres also influence the normal nystagmus induced by head movements. The autonomic 'pursuit' eye movements coordinated by the cerebral cortex allow fixation on a moving object in the surroundings or on a stationary object if the head is moving. Nystagmus induced, for instance, when looking out of a moving train, is an example of optokinetic nystagmus. Moving the visual stimuli with the patient's head stationary, or moving the patient's head and body with the visual stimuli stationary, can reproduce this reaction. Clinically this can be achieved by rotating a striped drum (optokinetic device) in front of the animal. The test also is an objective means of detecting vision in animals. It requires an intact central visual pathway. Further discussion on cranial nerves influencing eye movements is found below.

262 Neuro-ophthalmology

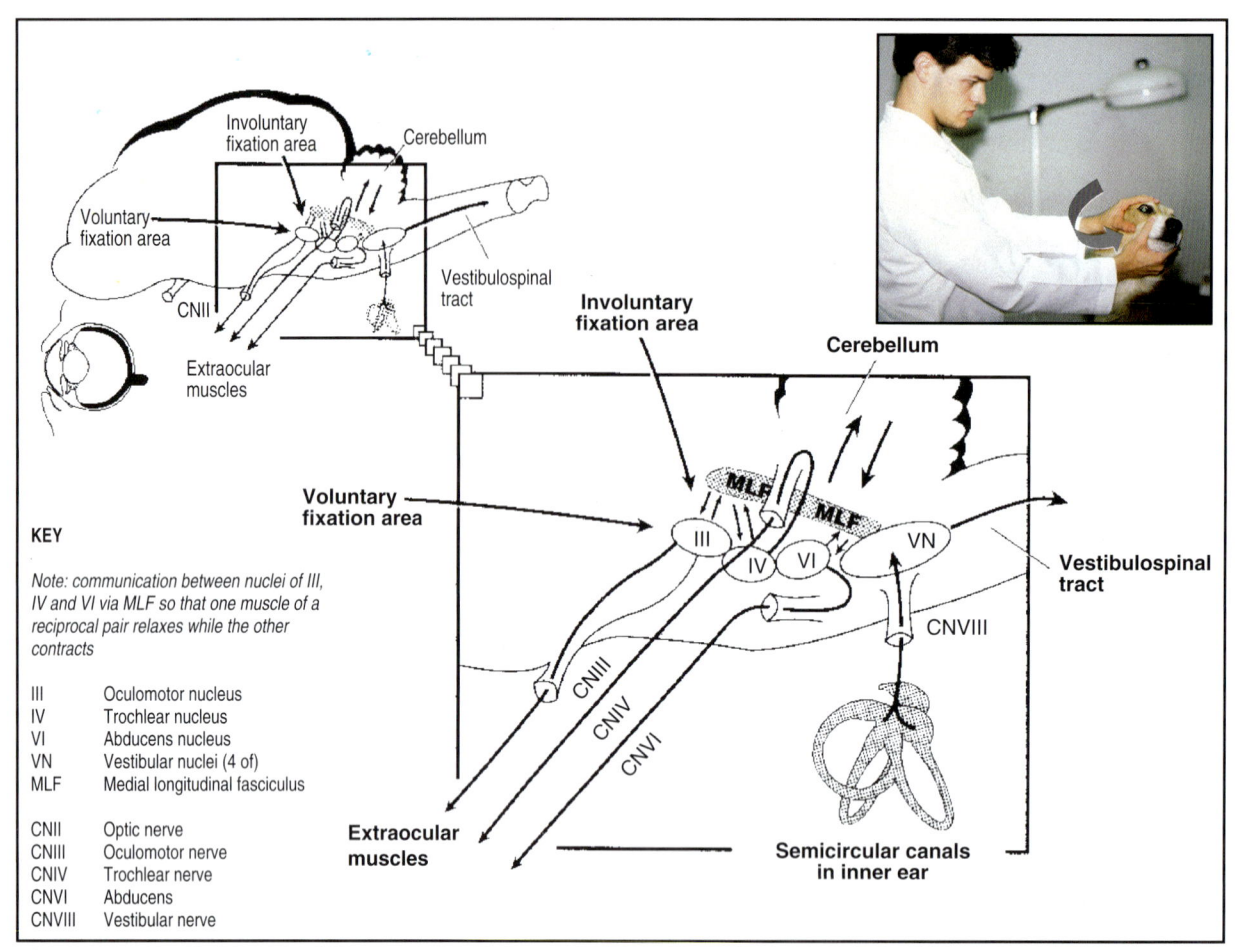

KEY

Note: communication between nuclei of III, IV and VI via MLF so that one muscle of a reciprocal pair relaxes while the other contracts

III	Oculomotor nucleus
IV	Trochlear nucleus
VI	Abducens nucleus
VN	Vestibular nuclei (4 of)
MLF	Medial longitudinal fasciculus
CNII	Optic nerve
CNIII	Oculomotor nerve
CNIV	Trochlear nerve
CNVI	Abducens
CNVIII	Vestibular nerve

Figure 15.6 The neural pathway for vestibular influence of eye movement. The photograph shows testing the oculocephalic reflex (doll's eye reflex) in a dog. (Adapted from the BSAVA Manual of Small Animal Neurology.)

A problem-oriented approach to neuro-ophthalmology

The following neuro-ophthalmic problems are considered together for the dog and cat:

- Central blindness
- Difference in size of pupils – anisocoria
- Abnormalities of eye position and movements
- Disorders of blinking
- Abnormalities of lacrimation.

This is intended as a guide to the investigation of each presenting sign; a fairly detailed anatomical description of important neurological pathways is included. Suggested further reading is included at the end of the chapter.

Central blindness

Visual deficits may result from lesions at any level of the central visual pathways, from the optic nerve to the occipital lobe of the cerebral cortex (optic nerves, optic chiasma, optic tracts and optic radiation).

Causes

Among the most common causes are:

- Trauma
- Feline cerebral infarction
- Congenital defects
- Neoplasia
- Proliferative conditions such as granulomatous meningoencephalitis (GME) and other space-occupying lesions
- Infections (e.g. canine distemper, systemic mycoses, *Toxoplasma gondii*, feline infectious peritonitis)
- Necrotizing vasculitis and inflammatory diseases
- Hydrocephalus
- Metabolic storage diseases
- Ischaemic damage.

Diagnosis

The complete arsenal of techniques for the diagnosis of central blindness may include: laboratory data; physical and neurological examination; cerebrospinal fluid analysis (culture, serology and cytology); and computed tomography (CT) or magnetic resonance imaging (MRI). Although superseded by advanced imaging techniques, optic tecography can be performed by injecting contrast medium into the cerebellomedullary cistern. With the animal's head tilted downward for several minutes, skull radiographs can reveal contrast enhancement of possible optic nerve masses (Moore *et al.*, 1996). Orbital ultrasonography can be used to diagnose optic nerve lesions and retrobulbar masses, although CT or MRI are superior for this task. Ocular ultrasonography is very useful in the identification of retinal detachment or intraocular masses, especially in cases where opacification of ocular media is present. Visual evoked potential (VEP) analysis can evaluate the functional integrity of the post-retinal visual pathways and visual cortex. In the VEP the electrical activity in the visual cortex produced in response to light stimulation of the eye is recorded by scalp electrodes. This technique can be very useful in cases of blindness due to lesions in the optic nerve, visual tracts or visual cortex (Hamilton and McLaughlin, 2000).

Animals with blindness of intracranial origin usually have a normal fundic examination unless there is a retrograde degeneration of the optic nerves. Initially they will also have a normal electroretinogram (ERG) (Hamilton and McLaughlin, 2000). Vision tests, menace response, dazzle and pupillary reflexes can be used to localize lesions. The anatomy of the central visual pathways and the pupillary light reflex pathways must be understood before these tests can be interpreted.

The central visual pathways

It is important to appreciate that visual information from one side of the body projects to the opposite cerebral cortex. This does not mean that the information from the left eye projects to the right cortex, but rather that the information from the *left visual field of each eye* (i.e. objects that are seen to the left of the body) project to the right cerebral cortex and vice versa. Ganglion cell axons in the temporal retina project ipsilaterally, whereas those located nasally project contralaterally. In domestic animals more than half of the optic nerve fibres cross (decussate) at the optic chiasma to the opposite side of the body. In cats, 65% of fibres decussate, whereas in dogs 75% of fibres cross over. This is in contrast with humans, where 50% of the visual fibres decussate.

Optic tract projections

In small animals, as in most mammals, fibres from the optic tracts terminate in one of six destinations (Figure 15.7):

- *Lateral geniculate nucleus* (LGN), a caudodorsolateral protrusion of the thalamus. The LGN is the main retinofugal projection site in the CNS (Hoffmann et al., 1984). From the LGN, there are two basic pathways axons can follow: (1) a pathway for conscious perception of vision (cortical pathway); and (2) a reflex pathway (subcortical pathway). There is a complete retinotopic anatomical relationship maintained throughout the central visual pathway, mainly in the LGN, rostral colliculus and visual cortex (Laties and Sprague, 1966). In other words, there is a map of the retinal visual space maintained in these structures
- *Suprachiasmatic nucleus* of the hypothalamus, via the retinohypothalamic bundle. This is the site of a 'biological clock' (Pu, 2000). The retinal input serves to regulate and reset the clock according to circadian and circannual light cycles. Some of these cycling phenomena are also mediated through the pineal body via a suprachiasmatic–spinal lateral horn–cranial cervical ganglion–pineal sympathetic pathway
- *Accessory optic system* of the midbrain, across the cerebral peduncles to small nuclei in the midbrain tegmentum, which project to the inferior olive and cerebellum. This pathway mediates adjustment in direction of visual gaze correlated with head and neck movements. This system is crucial for the optokinetic response (nystagmus) (Hoffmann and Fischer, 2001).
- *Pretectum (pretectal nucleus)*, situated frontal to the rostral colliculus at the junction of the thalamus and midbrain tectum. Some of these retinofugal fibres help to mediate the pupillary light reflex (PLR), are involved in perception of diffuse light and help coordination of eye movements and visually guided behaviour, as well as maintaining binocularity. It is also the sensorimotor link between the retina and premotor structures in the pathway mediating optokinetic response (Hoffman et al., 1984)
- *Rostral (anterior) colliculus* (Hoffman et al., 1984), called the optic tectum in non-mammalian vertebrates. Output from the colliculus goes to the spinal cord (tectospinal tract), to the pontine cerebellar peduncle, to the midbrain tegmental nuclei and to the thalamic pulvinar and posterolateral nuclei. These last two nuclei project to the associated cortex, which thus completes a route from retina to cortex. Visual acoustically guided activities are mediated via this pathway. Additionally, a population of cells capable of encoding the amplitude and sign of horizontal visual disparity is found in the anterior colliculus. Horizontal disparities are the main cue for stereopsis (Gonzalez and Perez, 1998).

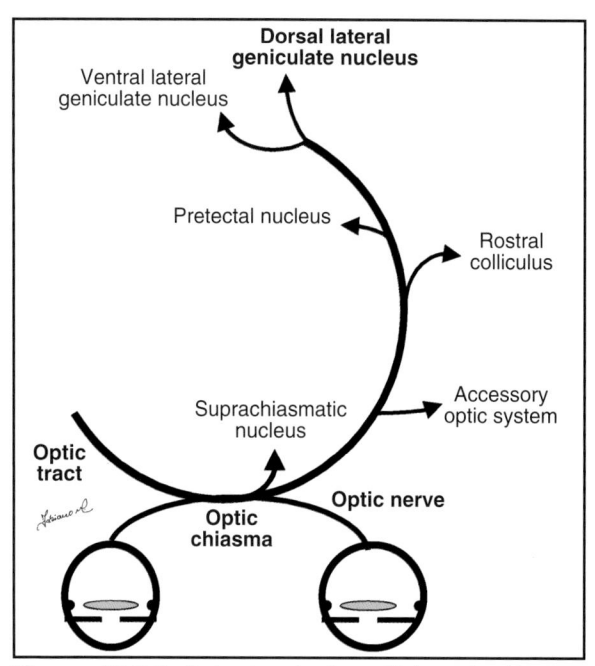

Figure 15.7 Optic tract projections. (Adapted, with permission, from a drawing by Dr John I. Johnson.)

There is also a strong projection from the visual cortex to the rostral colliculus
- *Ventral lateral geniculate nucleus* (VLGN), a major portion of the ventral thalamus. There are projections from the VLGN to each of the other terminals of the retinofugal pathways. Basically, any nucleus receiving retinal input also receives input from VLGN. The significance of these projections is still undetermined.

The neuronal pathway for the pupillary light and accommodation reflexes

Axons from the ganglion cells of the retina that are involved in the PLR accompany those concerned with conscious perception of vision from the retina to the LGN. However, rather than terminating in the LGN, they pass the LGN to project to the pretectal nucleus (PN). From the PN these fibres project to several areas of the midbrain, such as the ventral tegmental area, periaqueductal grey, peripheral part of the Edinger–Westphal nucleus and the anteromedian nuclei (Toyoshima *et al.*, 1980; Takada *et al.*, 1984; Evinger, 1988). Despite detailed studies using retrograde tracers and microstimulation techniques, the exact preganglionic origin of the pupillary light reflex and accommodation reflex of small animals has not been fully determined (Loewy *et al.*, 1978). From electron microscopy studies it seems likely that accommodation-related pre-ganglionic neurons are predominantly located anterior and dorsal to the somatic nuclei of the oculomotor nuclear complex (i.e. the anteromedian and Edinger–Westphal nuclei, and the ventral central grey area), while pupilloconstriction-related oculomotor parasympathetic pre-ganglionic neurons are predominantly located ventral to the somatic nuclei (i.e. the ventral tegmental area) (Ichinohe *et al.*, 1996). Other authors found, using microstimulation, that accommodation-related areas include the posterolateral pretectum, the posteromedial pretectum and the mesencephalic reticular formation, while pupilloconstriction-related areas include the posteromedial pretectum, the nucleus of the posterior commissure and the anterior pretectum around the olivary pretectal nucleus (Konno and Ohtsuka, 1997). These parasympathetic nerve fibres to the iris and ciliary body are initially carried within the oculomotor nerve and then leave to synapse in the ciliary ganglion. This pathway is responsible for the efferent arm of the PLR and accommodation reflex (Figure 15.8).

As with the axons concerned with vision, over 50% of those concerned with the PLR decussate at the chiasma in domestic animals. A similar percentage then cross back to the original side at the central decussation. This means that if a light is shone in one eye the pupil of that eye will constrict slightly more than the contralateral pupil, although in practice this difference can be difficult to appreciate.

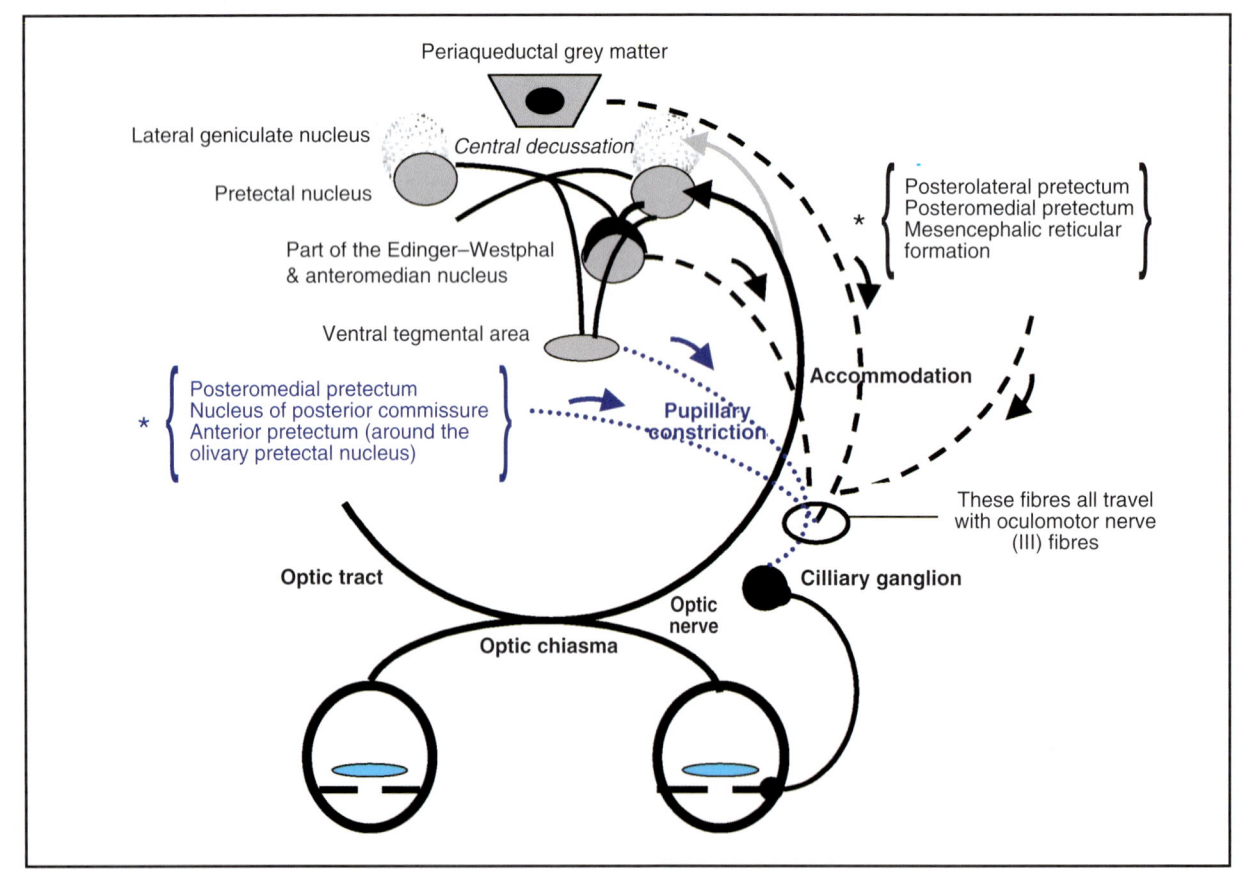

Figure 15.8 Pupillary and lens accommodation reflex pathways. Note the details of the nuclei believed to be involved. * – Microstimulation responsive areas; ••••• – Pupillary constriction-related fibres; ▬ ▬ ▬ – The response is always bilateral even though only one side is depicted in this cartoon.

Linking the results of vision tests with those for pupillary reflexes

Figure 15.9 shows the effect of lesions within the central visual pathways on the visual fields; Figure 15.10 is a flow diagram to help link the results of vision testing with the pupillary responses.

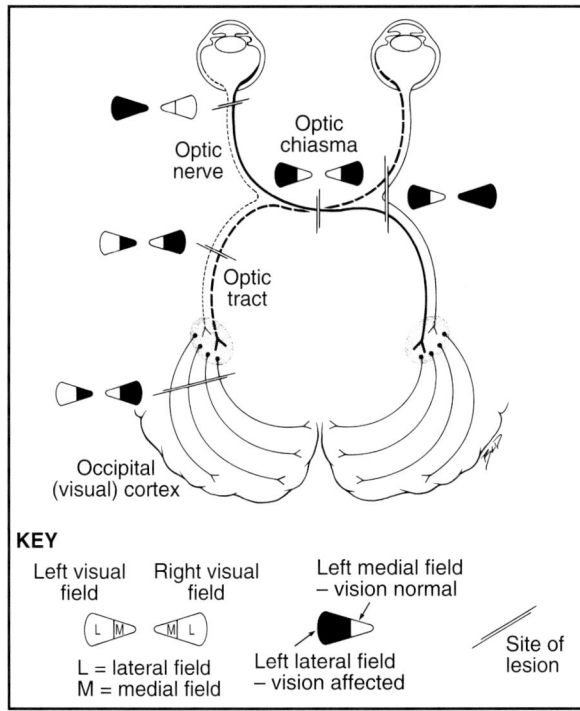

Figure 15.9 Effect on visual fields of lesions at various levels of the central visual pathways. (Reproduced from the *BSAVA Manual of Small Animal Neurology.*)

Optic nerve lesions

Complete lesions affecting the optic nerve will render the eye on the affected side blind. Under normal room lighting a static anisocoria will be present, with the pupil of the affected eye being slightly more dilated than the other pupil. However, in darkness both pupils will dilate evenly. The affected eye will have no direct or consensual PLR and the swinging flashlight test will be abnormal. In other words, if there is a unilateral afferent lesion, when the light is directed into the normal eye both pupils constrict but as the light swings into the affected eye, the pupil slowly dilates from its previous (consensual) constricted position as it does not respond to the direct stimulus. The abnormality detected with this test is an afferent defect, also known as the Marcus–Gunn pupil (Figure 15.11). In normal room light, if the unaffected eye is covered, the abnormal eye's pupil will dilate. This is defined as a 'positive' (abnormal) cover test result. Bilateral lesions result in dilated non-responsive pupils and blindness.

Fundoscopy and, if necessary, electroretinography will help differentiate retinal from pre-chiasmal optic nerve lesions. Retinal disease such as sudden acquired retinal degeneration syndrome (see Chapter 14a) will result in an abnormal ERG, whereas central causes of blindness do not initially affect the ERG. Optic nerve lesions include congenital optic nerve hypoplasia, optic neuritis (Fischer and Jones, 1972), papilloedema, neoplasia (Williams *et al.*, 1961; Barnett *et al.*, 1967), trauma and optic nerve compression. It is suggested that optic nerve hypoplasia may be inherited, but a mode of transmission has not been determined in most breeds, although in the Miniature Poodle it may be an autosomal recessive trait (Ackerman, 1999).

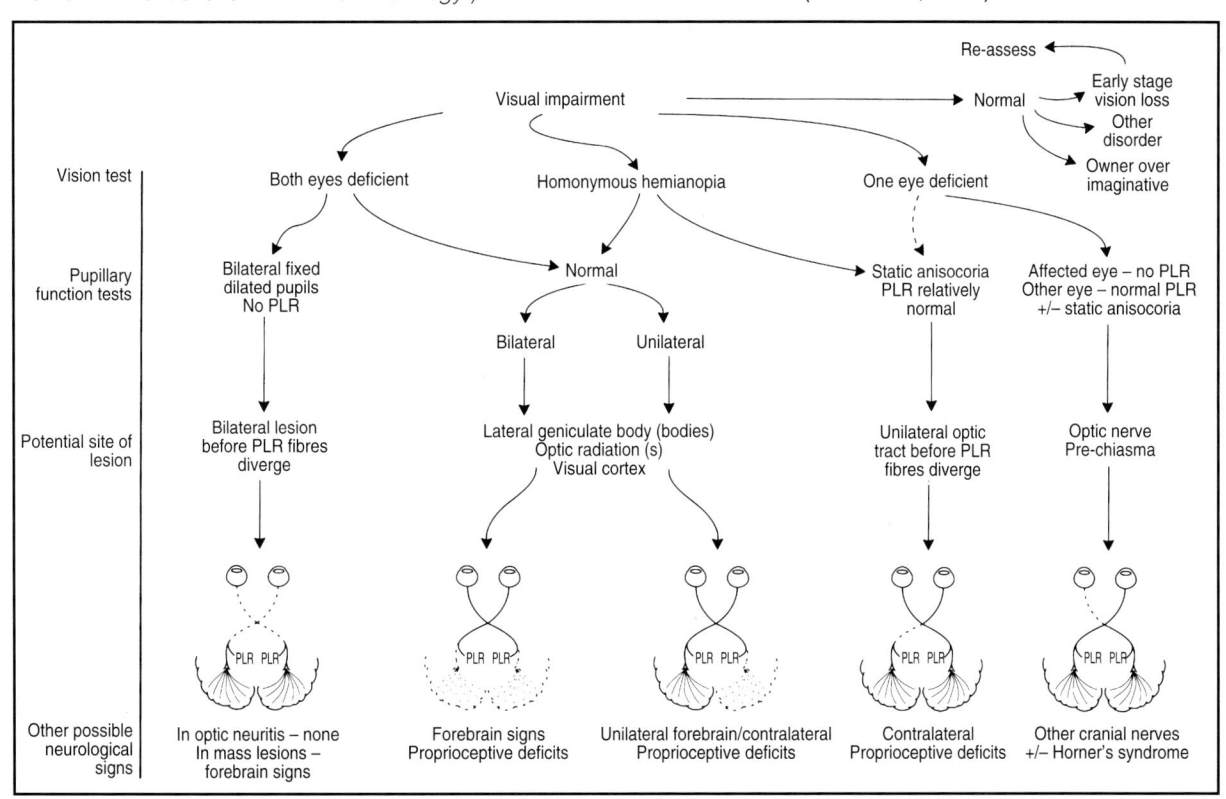

Figure 15.10 Flow diagram to help link the results of vision testing with those of pupillary light reflex testing. (The broken lines on the visual pathway indicate the site of the lesion.) (Reproduced from the *BSAVA Manual of Small Animal Neurology.*)

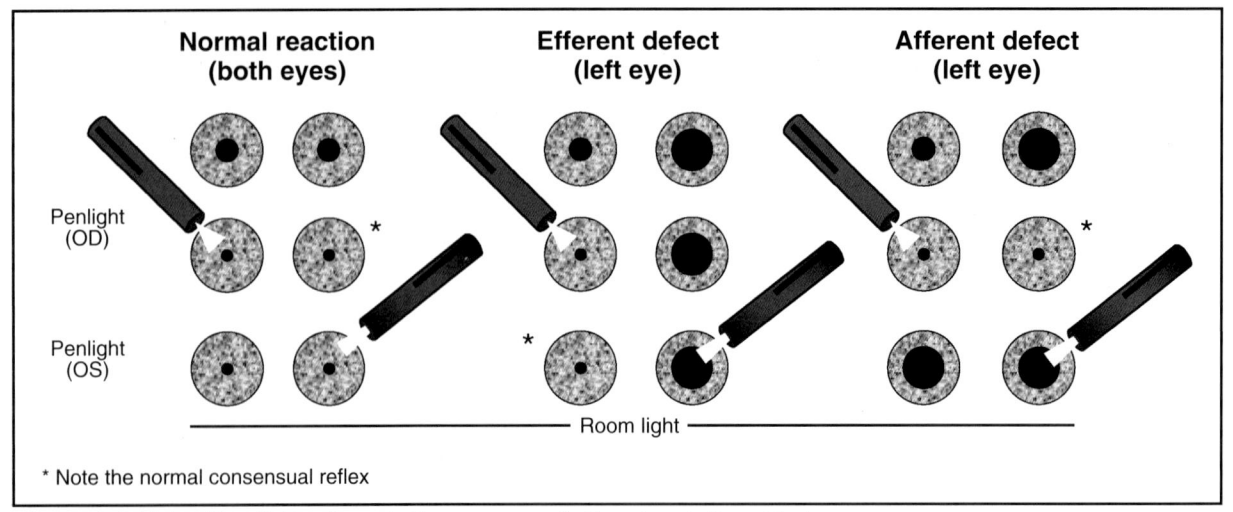

Figure 15.11 Pupillary light reflexes in the presence of afferent and efferent lesions.

* Note the normal consensual reflex

Optic neuritis can be due to infectious agents (canine distemper virus, *Toxoplasma gondii*, *Blastomyces dermatitidis*, *Cryptococcus neoformans*, *Histoplasma capsulatum*), feline infectious peritonitis, GME (in dogs), neoplasia, trauma and idiopathic causes (Hamilton and McLaughlin, 2000). When optic neuritis also involves the initial portion of the optic nerve (papillitis), ophthalmoscopic changes such as a swollen optic disc, often with haemorrhages, is present. Optic neuritis posterior to the globe (retrobulbar optic neuritis) can result in blindness without any ophthalmoscopic changes. Neoplasia of the presphenoid bone or meninges (de Lahunta, 1983) or any kind of neoplasia involving or compressing the optic nerves may result in loss of vision. Papilloedema, a non-inflammatory swelling of the optic nerve head, does not itself cause blindness (presence of vision loss is dependent on the disease process causing the swelling), and should be differentiated from papillitis (inflammation involving the optic nerve head) that is typically associated with vision loss.

Lesions of the optic chiasma

Blindness can be the only neurological deficit of tumours in the optic chiasma (Davidson *et al.*, 1991). Space-occupying lesions such as neoplasia (Braund *et al.*, 1977; Skerritt *et al.*, 1986) and abscesses may affect the optic chiasma; meningiomas can develop between the optic chiasma and pituitary gland, causing compression of both (deLahunta, 1983); and pituitary macroadenomas may grow to compress the chiasma. Cerebral vascular infarction in cats is occasionally reported to cause ischaemic necrosis of the optic chiasma. Complete lesions of the optic chiasma result in blindness with non-responsive pupils.

Post-chiasmal optic tract lesions prior to divergence of the fibres of the PLR

Visual impairment due to unilateral post-chiasmal lesions is more difficult to demonstrate than that due to pre-chiasmal lesions because neither eye is rendered totally blind, although the contralateral eye is more severely affected. Careful use of the menace test may show loss of the medial visual field of one eye and the lateral visual field of the other eye – a defect described as homonymous hemianopia. The swinging flashlight test and cover tests are relatively normal, except that a static anisocoria is present, with the pupil of the eye contralateral to the lesion remaining more dilated.

The internal capsule and rostral crus cerebri are in close association with the optic tracts and may also be affected by lesions involving the optic tracts; a hemisensory deficit affecting the side of the body contralateral to the lesion will result. Unilateral lesions may be caused by space-occupying lesions such as neoplasms (de Lahunta and Cummings, 1967) or abscesses. Ischaemia following vascular occlusions may also occur. Canine distemper virus infection can cause bilateral inflammation of both optic tracts.

Lesions affecting the LGN, optic radiation or occipital cortex

Homonymous hemianopia will be present, as described above for post-chiasmal optic tract lesions. The PLR will be unaffected. An animal with bilateral complete lesions will be blind and yet have a normal PLR. The LGN and initial portion of the optic radiation is situated just lateral to the internal capsule, so lesions may also affect the sensory and motor components within this structure. The posterior part of the optic radiation branches away from the internal capsule towards the occipital cortex, so lesions closer to the cortex may spare the internal capsule fibres.

Unilateral lesions may result from neoplasia, abscessation or trauma; encephalitis and vascular occlusions are additional causes. Trauma resulting in cerebral swelling, or space-occupying lesions such as hydrocephalus and neoplasia which result in brain herniation (pushing of posterior cerebrum under the tentorium towards the cerebellum), and encephalitis may all result in bilateral visual deficits usually accompanied by additional severe neurological abnormalities.

Cerebellar lesions

Although the cerebellum is not directly involved in vision, cerebellar lesions can influence the visual system. In addition to nystagmus due to lesions of the flocular nodular lobe, which is a vestibular nucleus, it is known that the cerebellum positively influences the menace response because animals with exclusively cerebellar lesions lack a menace response ipsilaterally. Affected animals retain normal responses in vision tests (cotton wool ball tests) and have a blink reflex induced by other tests, e.g. by inducing palpebral and dazzle reflexes. The cerebellum in the cat, and probably in the dog, also receives fibres from the Edinger–Westphal nucleus (Roste and Dietrichs, 1988). The physiological significance of this projection is still not completely clear.

Anisocoria

Anisocoria is defined as a resting bilateral inequality in pupil size. It may result not only from interference with the nervous control of the pupils but also from intraocular disease, e.g. glaucoma (ipsilateral mydriasis), uveitis, synechiae and iris atrophy.

Causes
- Anisocoria of neurological origin may result from lesions of the PLR arc, or of the sympathetic nerve supply to the eye, or from cerebellar disease
- Painful conditions of the cornea, such as ulcers, may cause miosis (oculosensory pupillary reflex) via the trigeminal nerve (V)
- Several drugs may interfere with pupillary symmetry (Figure 15.12).

Lesions within the afferent pathway of the PLR

Afferent nerve fibres involved in the PLR diverge from fibres concerned with vision just before the LGN. Lesions affecting the fibres prior to that point also affect vision (see above).

Afferent fibres concerned with the PLR may be damaged as they pass between the optic tracts and the oculomotor nuclei. Lesions at these sites spare vision. The effect on the pupillary responses of lesions prior to the central decussation (via caudal commissure) is the same as caused by lesions of the ipsilateral optic tract prior to the LGN.

Lesions within the efferent pathway for control of pupil size

Parasympathetic control of pupil size and lens accommodation are illustrated in Figures 15.4 and 15.8. Lesions of the oculomotor nerve (III) will affect the parasympathetic nerve supply to the pupillary sphincter muscle. Total lesions result in a dilated unresponsive pupil. The oculomotor supply to the extraocular muscles may also be affected; ptosis and a lateral and ventral strabismus result.

Pharmacological testing may help to localize the site of the lesions within the PLR arc:

- *Direct acting parasympathomimetics* (e.g. pilocarpine): Topically administered pilocarpine can be used to differentiate between upper motor neuron (UMN) (pretectal nucleus to oculomotor nucleus) and lower motor neuron (LMN) (between the oculomotor nucleus and iris) lesions. Pilocarpine 1% ophthalmic solution is diluted to 0.05% with normal saline and 1 drop applied to the ocular surface. Dogs with LMN lesions have a denervation hypersensitivity and the pupil will constrict rapidly. Even at the 0.05% dilution, some normal dogs may show some constriction of the pupils after 45–60 minutes. If no response is seen 90 minutes after instilling the 0.05% solution, the test can be repeated with 1% pilocarpine to show that the pupil is physically capable of constricting
- *Indirect acting parasympathomimetics* (e.g. 0.5% physostigmine drops): These have no effect on pupil size if the lesions are post-ganglionic. They cause a rapid pupillary constriction when either pre-ganglionic lesions or UMN lesions are present. The pupil of the normal eye constricts within 40–60 minutes.

Potential causes of lesions of the PLR arc include those listed as causes of central blindness. Feline dysautonomia may affect the parasympathetic control of the pupils, resulting in fixed dilated pupils, although this condition is less common nowadays. Brain herniation under the tentorium cerebelli, due to displacement by space-occupying lesions, can cause compression of the mid-brain, including the oculomotor nuclei and the oculomotor nerve trunks (Wheeler, 1991). Figure 15.11 shows the influence of afferent and efferent lesions on the pupillary responses.

Clinical condition	Drug	Pupillary response
Normal	Sympathomimetic	Mydriasis
Normal	Parasympathomimetic	Miosis
Normal	Prostaglandin analogue	Miosis
Normal	Opioids (oral or intravenous formulations)	Miosis (dog); mydriasis (cat)
Normal	Beta blocker	Miosis (some cases)
Normal	Alpha-2 agonist	Miosis (cat); mydriasis (some dogs)
Adie's pupil	Pilocarpine 0.05–0.1%	Miosis
Pre-ganglionic Horner's syndrome	Hydroxyamphetamine 1%	Dilation
Post-ganglionic Horner's syndrome	Hydroxyamphetamine 1%	No dilation

Figure 15.12 Effects of pharmacological agents on the pupil in small animals.

Sympathetic innervation of the eye

The sympathetic nervous system supply to the eye is shown in Figure 15.13 (Barlow and Root, 1949). Sympathetic control is initiated in the hypothalamus and diencephalon. The impulse descends through the brainstem and cervical spinal cord in the lateral tectotegmental spinal pathway. This UMN pathway synapses on cell bodies of the pre-ganglionic sympathetic nerves to the eye. The nerve cell bodies are located in the T1–T3 spinal cord segments. Pre-ganglionic fibres exit the spinal cord and course cranially in the cervical sympathetic trunk within the cranial thorax. This pathway continues through the cervical area, with the vagus nerve forming the vagosympathetic trunk. The pre-ganglionic neurons then synapse in the cranial cervical ganglion caudoventral to the ear. The post-ganglionic fibres run through the tympanic bulla and middle ear, and course with the glossopharyngeal nerve (IX), then enter the skull and course in the cavernous sinus with the carotid artery (de Lahunta, 1983; Bagley, 1996). The axons join the ventral surface of the trigeminal ganglion and the ophthalmic nerve. These axons exit the skull through the orbital fissure (de Lahunta, 1983).

In the cat, post-ganglionic sympathetic fibres to the smooth muscle of the third eyelid and to the iris dilator muscle do not pass through the trigeminal ganglion; rather, they unite with the ophthalmic division of the trigeminal nerve beyond the ganglion after first passing through the middle ear (de Lahunta, 1983).

Smooth muscle within the iris (radial or dilator muscle), orbit, upper and lower eyelid (Müller's muscle) and third eyelid is also innervated by the sympathetic nervous system. This musculature serves to keep the eyeball protruded, the palpebral fissure widened and the third eyelid retracted. Additionally, smooth muscle within the walls of blood vessels of the head also have sympathetic innervation.

Sympathetic stimulation of the iris, either via circulating adrenaline or by neuronal pathways, results in a degree of pupillary dilation that can be further increased by, for example, excitement and stress. Note that reduced tone in the pupillary constrictor muscle (parasympathetic supply) is responsible for pupillary dilation in reduced light (reflex dilation) (King, 1987; Bagley, 1996).

The sympathetic nervous system innervates the pupillary dilator muscles, and interruption of its pathway to the iris results in a miotic (constricted) pupil. This occurs as part of Horner's syndrome.

Horner's syndrome

Interference with the sympathetic nerve supply to the head results in a combination of signs collectively referred to as Horner's syndrome (Figure 15.14).

Clinical features

- Miosis: the pupil on the affected side is smaller than the pupil on the normal side (anisocoria)
- Protrusion of the nictitating membrane (third eyelid): due to lack of tone in the smooth muscle retracting it (normally under sympathetic innervation) and also secondary to the enophthalmos
- Upper eyelid ptosis (incomplete elevation): due to reduced tone in Müller's muscle; laxity of the lower eyelid may also be observed. The palpebral fissure may appear narrowed

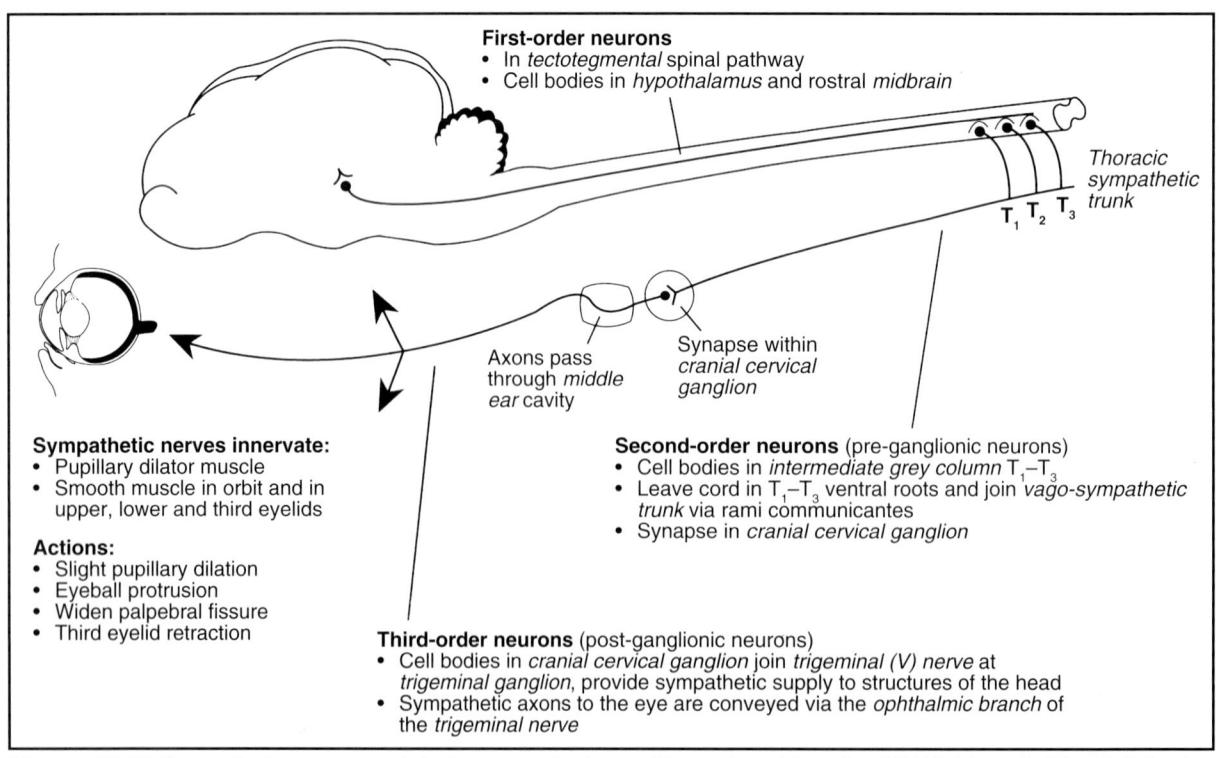

Figure 15.13 Sympathetic nerve supply to the eye and adnexa. (Reproduced from the *BSAVA Manual of Small Animal Neurology*.)

Neuro-ophthalmology 269

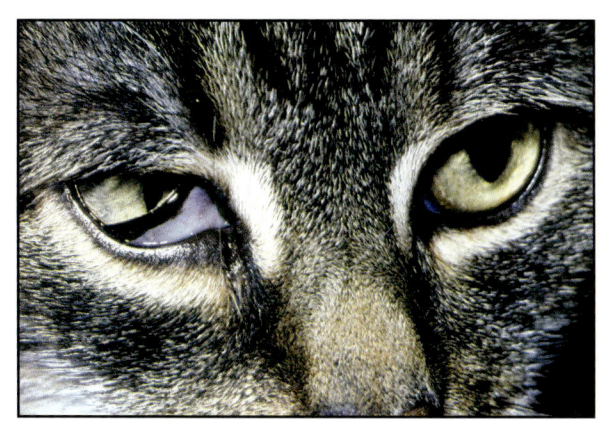

Figure 15.14 Horner's syndrome in a cat. Note the narrowed palpebral fissure, protruded third eyelid and miotic pupil.

- Enophthalmos: resulting from a lack of tone in the orbital smooth muscle, allowing the eye to sink back into the orbit
- The intraocular pressure may be slightly reduced, and increased peripheral vasodilatation causes a warmer pinna and a slight engorgement of conjunctival blood vessels on the affected side.

Causes

Horner's syndrome may result from lesions of the sympathetic supply to the head at one of three anatomical levels, resulting in a first-, second- or third-order Horner's syndrome. These levels and possible aetiologies of lesions are illustrated in Figure 15.15. Special attention should be given to otitis media and its potential to involve the third-order neuron (post-ganglionic sympathetic axons). Other clinical signs and pharmacological differentiation may aid localization of the lesion.

Diagnosis and differentiation

Hydroxyamphetamine: Hydroxyamphetamine 1% (an indirect acting adrenergic amine) can be applied topically to both eyes. This drug will normally displace the noradrenaline vesicles from the nerve terminal to the synaptic cleft, producing mydriasis by constriction of the radial muscle of the iris. This test is useful for differentiation of pre- and post-ganglionic Horner's syndrome. If the patient has pre-ganglionic Horner's syndrome there will be mydriasis. If the lesion is post-ganglionic (third-order neuron) there will be no mydriasis because the disrupted neuron will have lost its amine vesicles.

Phenylephrine: Phenylephrine 10% (a direct acting adrenergic agonist) can be applied topically to both eyes. The pupil of a normal eye or an eye with a first-order Horner's syndrome will dilate in 60–90 minutes; dilation occurs in about 45 minutes in second-order Horner's syndrome and in about 20 minutes in third-order Horner's syndrome. The decreased time and increased sensitivity to phenylephrine in second- and third-order Horner's syndrome is due to denervation hypersensitivity (Bistner *et al.*, 1970). This occurs because in the normally innervated eye the termination of phenylephrine action is due to the pre-synaptic neuronal high affinity re-uptake system. With the second- or third-order lesion the

Site of lesion for first-order Horner's syndrome
Possible causes:
- Cervical spine lesions (usually severe)
- Rostral thoracic spine lesions

Thoracic sympathetic trunk
T_1 T_2 T_3

Site of lesion for second-order Horner's syndrome
Possible causes:
- Brachial plexus root lesions
- Injuries to soft tissue of neck
  - Puncture wounds
  - Infections
  - Iatrogenic

Site of lesion for third-order Horner's syndrome
Possible causes:
- Middle ear lesions (otitis media, neoplasia, etc.)
- Fractures of the skull
- Retrobulbar contusions
- Iatrogenic

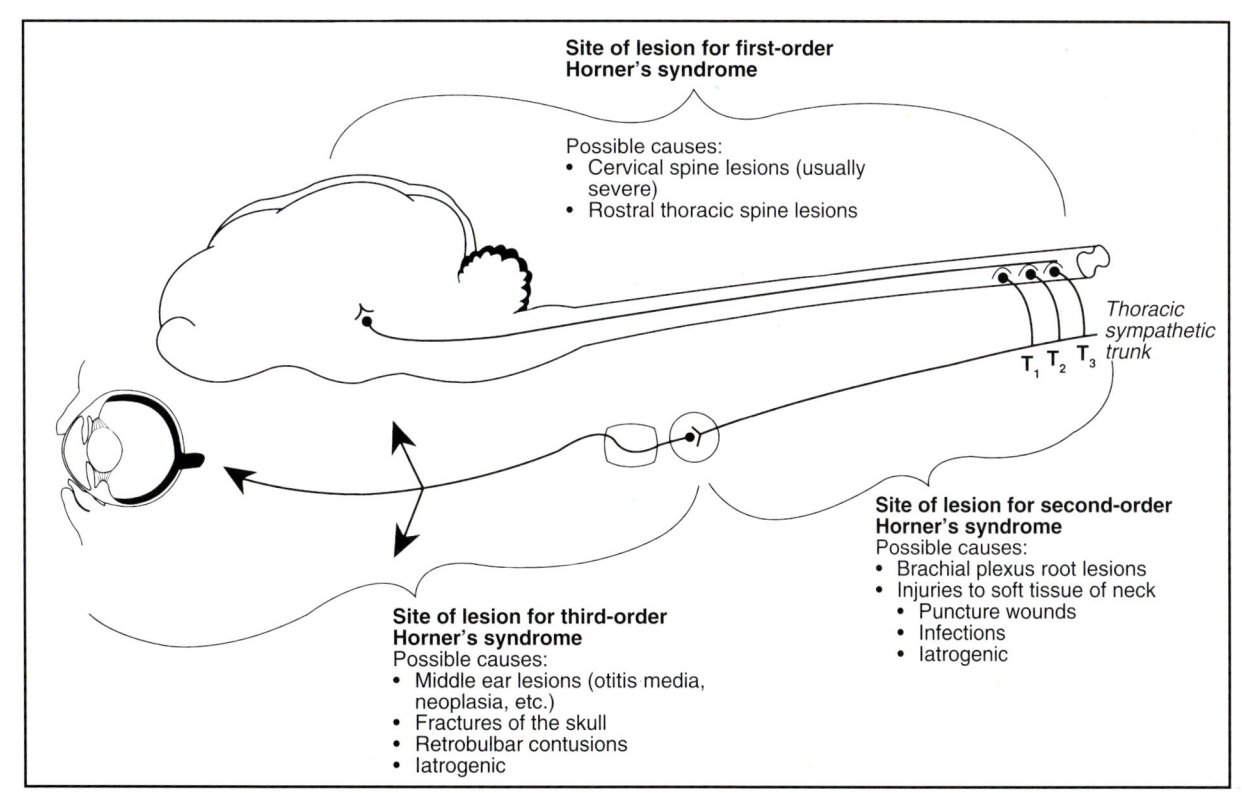

Figure 15.15 Sites of lesions resulting in Horner's syndrome and possible aetiologies. (Reproduced from the *BSAVA Manual of Small Animal Neurology.*)

re-uptake system is disrupted and more drug remains in the synaptic cleft, causing an exaggerated response. Another important contributory factor is the upregulation of receptors in the denervated radial muscle of the iris. In addition to dilating the pupil, other local signs of Horner's syndrome are abolished by topical phenylephrine.

Other diagnostic aids: Radiographs of the anterior thorax, cervicothoracic spine and middle ear may help localize the lesion. Neuropathies, including Horner's syndrome, can be associated with hypothyroidism, and this possibility should be considered. Despite these investigations the aetiology in many cases of Horner's syndrome remains obscure, especially in dogs. Male Golden Retrievers in particular seem predisposed to an apparently idiopathic second-order Horner's syndrome, from which they recover, partly or totally, after several weeks (Boydell, 2000).

Pupil abnormalities accompanying intracranial disease

In severe bilateral cerebrocortical disease, pupils are often miotic. There are two theories that attempt to explain this phenomenon: (a) miosis is caused by the lack of inhibitory response from the UMN; and (b) there is a disruption of the central sympathetic system at the level of the hypothalamus or brainstem. Severe midbrain, or bilateral oculomotor nerve damage results in fixed dilated pupils.

Other pupil abnormalities

- Hippus is a rhythmic contraction and subsequent dilation of the pupil. Its cause is still not well understood, but some believe it indicates CNS disease (Bagley, 1996)
- Spastic pupil syndrome is a static anisocoria of cats that remains unchanged during dark adaptation. It is believed to be associated with feline leukaemia virus (FeLV) infection. Vision is unaffected and other ophthalmic abnormalities are absent. C-type FeLV particles have been identified in the ciliary ganglia and short ciliary nerves of these cats, suggesting viral invasion and damage of these nerve tissues (Bagley, 1996; Stiles, 1999)
- Idiopathic post-ganglionic parasympathetic denervation of the pupil is referred to as Adie's syndrome (Hanson *et al.*, 2001). The disease is rarely seen in domestic animals but has been reported in a dog (Goldfarb and Swann, 1984). In humans it is predominantly seen in young women and is usually unilateral. In ordinary light, the affected pupil is usually larger. Pupillary light reflexes are usually decreased or absent. Instillation of a cholinergic drug (e.g. pilocarpine 1% drops) will cause a more rapid constriction of the affected pupil, indicating denervation hypersensitivity (Bradford, 1999)
- A dysfunction of the autonomic nervous system called dysautonomia can occur in small animals.

In addition to other signs such as urinary tract abnormalities (detrusor atony), regurgitation and constipation, ophthalmic signs such as dilated poorly responsive pupils can be seen (Bagley, 1996; Lane, 2000; Hanson *et al.*, 2001; Jamieson *et al.*, 2002)
- 'D' or 'reverse D' pupil (or hemidilated pupil) can occur in cats when there is impairment in the nasal or temporal parasympathetic innervation, respectively, of the iridal sphincter muscle (Scagliotti, 1999). As with feline spastic pupil syndrome, most affected cats test positive for FeLV.

Abnormalities of eye position and movements

Strabismus

Strabismus (squint) occurs quite commonly. It may be due to a congenital abnormality or result from lesions of the extraocular muscles or their nerve supply. A full knowledge of the actions and innervations of the extraocular muscles (see Figure 15.17) is required to enable the aetiology of a squint to be investigated. Disorders of eye movement can be observed during the oculocephalic reflex (see above). Surgery to correct squints in animals is possible but seldom necessary.

Congenital

Congenital strabismus may be seen in any breed of dog or cat. A common example is the bilateral convergent strabismus (esotropia) of some Siamese, Himalayan and similarly coloured cats. A genetically determined massive misrouting of retinal ganglion cell axons towards the contralateral hemisphere is believed to underlie the extreme paucity of binocular cells in the primary visual cortex. This impairs binocular information (stereopsis) in these cats and causes strabismus as well as an accompanying fine pendular nystagmus (Bacon *et al.*, 1999). These binocular cells normally process spatially coordinated stereopsis input, an ability on which normal ocular alignment depends. Furthermore, in Siamese cats, there is an abnormal degree of decussation of the optic nerve axons originating from the temporal retina (nasal visual field) that normally remain uncrossed. Therefore, esotropia may be a compensatory change in eyeball position in an attempt to place the functional temporal visual field (nasal fundus) to a more frontal position (Scagliotti, 1999).

Strabismus can also occur in non-Siamese non-albino cats. Animals with a congenital convergent squint due to lack of binocularity in the striate cortex were discovered within a colony of Mill Hill cats (von Grunau and Rauschecker, 1983).

Exotropia (divergent strabismus) is commonly seen in animals with congenital hydrocephalus. Both eyes often deviate ventrolaterally. This is thought to result from cranial cavity distortion during early development (Hanson *et al.*, 2001) (Figure 15.16).

Neuro-ophthalmology

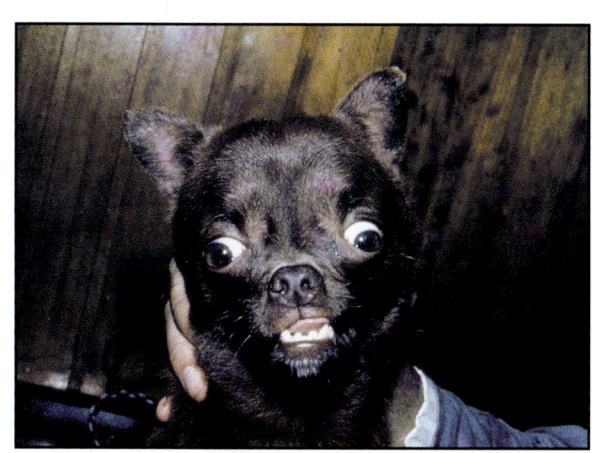

Figure 15.16 Exotropia in a dog with congenital hydrocephalus. (Courtesy of L. Kavinski.)

Other causes

Trauma: Traumatic proptosis of the globe can result in a strabismus due to tearing of the rectus muscles (usually the medial rectus muscle). A divergent strabismus or exotropia results from tearing of the medial rectus muscle. Retrobulbar swelling (due to infection or neoplasia) may cause a deviation of the globe in addition to exophthalmos (see Chapter 4).

Extraocular polymyositis: This is a focal inflammatory myopathy in the extraocular muscles, producing bilateral exophthalmos (see Chapter 4). This disease occurs particularly in young (6–18 months) large-breed dogs, most commonly in Golden Retrievers (Taylor, 2000).

Fibrosing strabismus: Following polymyositis it is possible for fibrosis of the extraocular muscles to occur which, in itself, can be the cause of strabismus. This condition, called fibrosing strabismus, typically occurs in young dogs. Breeds in which the disease has been described include Akita, Dalmatian, Golden Retriever, Shar Pei ('Shar Pei strabismus') and Wolfhound. The medial rectus muscle seems to be more commonly affected, resulting in esotropia, enophthalmos, visual impairment and even blindness (Scagliotti, 1999). Treatment during active inflammation can include immunomodulators and corticosteroids in immunosuppressive doses; after fibrosis has developed, surgical correction may be necessary.

Nerve supply to the extraocular muscles

Figure 15.17 shows the extraocular muscles, their actions and innervation.

Oculomotor (III): Different motor areas control movement of the eye and pupillary constriction and lens accommodation. Fibres from the oculomotor motor nucleus (rostral mesencephalon) innervate the dorsal, medial and ventral rectus muscles, the ventral oblique muscle and the levator palpebrae superioris. These muscles elevate, depress, cause extorsion (twist outward) and turn the globe nasally, and the levator palpebrae superioris elevates the upper eyelid. Interference with the parasympathetic component of the oculomotor nerve results in a fixed dilated pupil. When the general somatic efferent component of the nerve is affected there is a lateral and ventral strabismus (the 'down and out eye') and an upper eyelid ptosis. In some instances, dysfunction of the oculomotor nerve does not result in strabismus, but the eye is unable to move normally (Bagley, 1996).

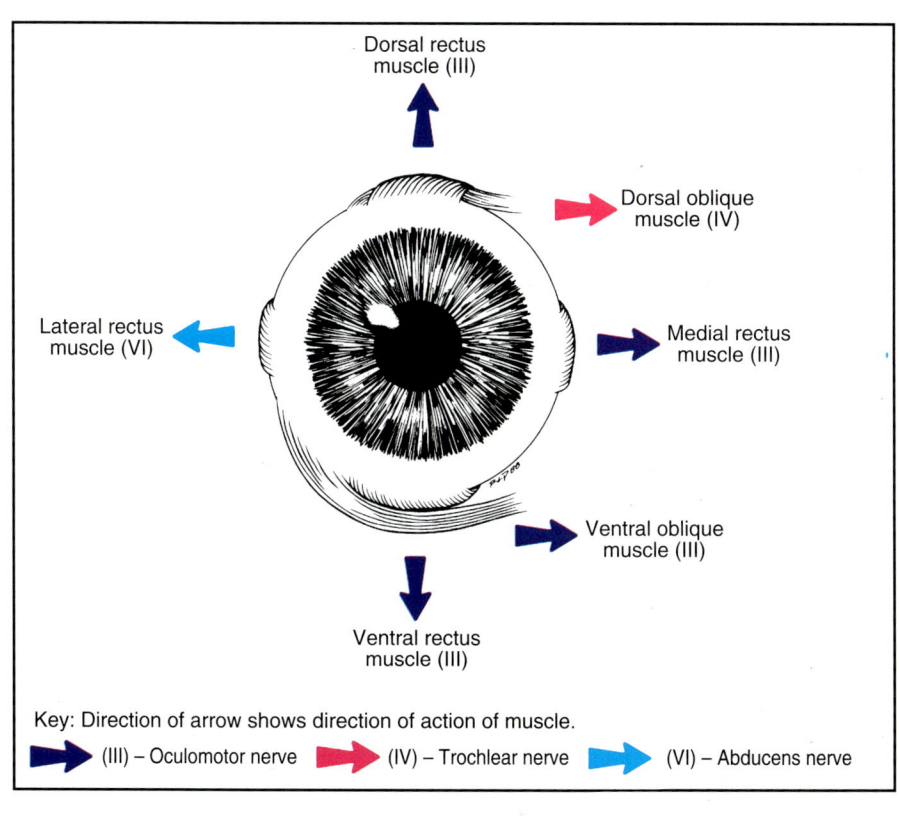

Figure 15.17 Diagrammatic anterior view of the right eye, showing extraocular muscles, their actions and innervation. Note that the retractor bulbi muscle (VI) is not shown – this muscle retracts the eyeball within the orbit. (Reproduced from the *BSAVA Manual of Small Animal Neurology*.)

Trochlear (IV): The trochlear nerve is unique because it is the only cranial nerve that exits via the dorsal aspect of the brainstem and also the only one that decussates 100%. It innervates the dorsal oblique muscle. This muscle forms a tendon, coursing rostrally and nasally, that passes through a groove in the trochlea, which is a cartilaginous plaque attached at the level of the nasal angle of the eye to the wall of the orbit. The tendon of the dorsal oblique muscle, after passing around the trochlea, deviates and courses temporally and attaches to the sclera under the tendon of insertion of the dorsal rectus muscle. Dorsal oblique contraction turns nasally (intorts) the dorsal portion of the globe. Lesions of either the trochlear nucleus or nerve paralyse the dorsal oblique muscle, resulting in rotation of the globe, with the dorsal portion turned laterally. Ophthalmoscopy may show the dorsal vein and arteriole deviated laterally, which is a very useful clue in species with a round pupil. In the cat it is easier to diagnose trochlear nerve (IV) lesions because the dorsal aspect of the vertical pupil is deviated laterally (temporally).

Abducens (VI): This innervates the retractor bulbi and lateral rectus muscles. These muscles retract and turn the globe temporally, respectively. Lesions of the abducens nerve result in a medially diverted globe (esotropia or convergent strabismus), which cannot be abducted or retracted.

Lesions on the floor of the skull involving a very vascularized area – the cavernous sinus – which encircles the pituitary fossa, can cause paralysis of all extraocular muscles because the oculomotor (III), trochlear (IV) and abducens (VI) nerves, the sympathetic innervation to the eye and the ophthalmic branch of the trigeminal nerve (V) course in this region prior to exiting the skull via the orbital fissure. The resulting complete ophthalmoplegia is also called cavernous sinus syndrome.

Disorders of eye movement

The coordination of eye movements is a complex mechanism, with inputs from the vestibular system, cerebellum and higher centres. Communication between the nuclei of the nerves and the extraocular muscles occurs via the medial longitudinal fasciculus (MLF) and helps coordinate the extraocular muscles. The vestibular system is involved in controlling eye movements and position as well as maintaining the position of the trunk and limbs in relation to the position or movement of the head (see Figure 15.6).

Abnormalities of nystagmus

- Abnormal nystagmus occurring when an animal's head is unrestrained is called 'spontaneous nystagmus'
- Nystagmus occurring when an animal's head is held in an abnormal position by the examiner is called 'positional nystagmus'.

Vestibular disease
Peripheral vestibular disease results in spontaneous horizontal nystagmus. The direction of the nystagmus (fast phase) is always opposite to the side of the peripheral lesion. The direction of the nystagmus does not change if the position of the animal's head is altered by the examiner. Other signs of vestibular disease such as head tilt, circling, rolling and loss of balance may also be present (Figure 15.18).

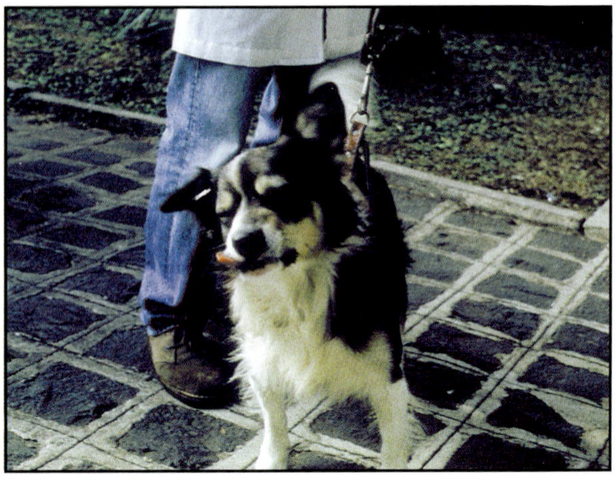

Figure 15.18 Peripheral vestibular disease: note the head tilt.

Vestibular disease may cause one eye to be deviated ventrally or ventrolaterally when the neck is extended. The ventrally deviated eye is usually on the side of the lesion (Thomas, 2000).

Central vestibular disease can cause a vertical or positional nystagmus (where the direction of nystagmus alters as the head's position is altered). In some instances the fast phase can be towards the side of the lesion (paradoxical vestibular syndrome). Other cranial nerve deficits may accompany central vestibular disease.

Cerebellar disease
Cerebellar disorders may result in nystagmus, this being a form of intention tremor of the extraocular muscles.

Congenital nystagmus
Congenital nystagmus may sometimes be observed in puppies or kittens and is manifested as continual fine oscillations of the globes.

- In Siamese cats it is thought to be associated with congenital abnormalities of the central visual pathways (see above)
- Congenital blindness may be accompanied by continuous, almost random, eye movements described as 'searching nystagmus'. The correct name for this is amaurotic nystagmus. If the potential for vision is later restored, these movements will remain
- A rotatory nystagmus is often seen in puppies that have microphthalmos and congenital cataracts, even if the lesions do not render them totally blind
- Nystagmus may develop in animals that lose their vision at a very early age, e.g. Abyssinian kittens with early-onset generalized progressive retinal atrophy

- Pendular nystagmus is usually due to congenital disorders (e.g. Siamese cats, Belgian Sheepdogs). In Belgian Sheepdogs it can be a clinical sign of an autosomal recessive trait characterized by a lack of decussation at the optic chiasma. All retinal ganglion cell axons in the affected animals extend directly into the ipsilateral optic tract (Hogan and Williams, 1995). Pendular nystagmus can also be seen in poisonings that cause diffuse body tremors and as part of 'shaker syndrome' (de Lahunta, 2002).

Disorders of blinking

The normal blink reflex is important for the wellbeing of the eye. A deficiency in blinking can result in corneal disease. Lack of a normal blink may result from lesions of the afferent (sensory) or efferent (motor) arms of the corneal or palpebral reflex (see Figure 15.5).

Sensory innervation of the eye

The ophthalmic division of the trigeminal (V) nerve supplies sensory innervation to the globe, the upper eyelid and the medial canthal region. Branches of the maxillary division of the trigeminal nerve supply the lateral parts of the upper eyelid (overlapping with the ophthalmic branch), the lower eyelid and surrounding skin. The trigeminal nerve transmits sensory impulses to the trigeminal nucleus in the brainstem. After synapsing, these impulses cross to the contralateral thalamic nuclei and from there to the cerebral cortex for conscious perception.

Corneal blink reflex

The corneal blink reflex is used to assess corneal sensation; the efferent arm of this reflex is via the facial (VII) nerve. Several attempts have been made to establish a method of quantitatively evaluating corneal sensation in animals. Corneal sensation can be assessed using a syringe filled with air to generate an air puff stimulus. For greater consistency a Cochet–Bonnet aesthesiometer can be used (Figure 15.19) with a relatively good degree of objectivity and repeatability (Brooks *et al.*, 2000). Canine dolichocephalic breeds are more sensitive to this stimulus than brachycephalic breeds. Also, the central cornea is the most sensitive region for the test (Barret *et al.*, 1991).

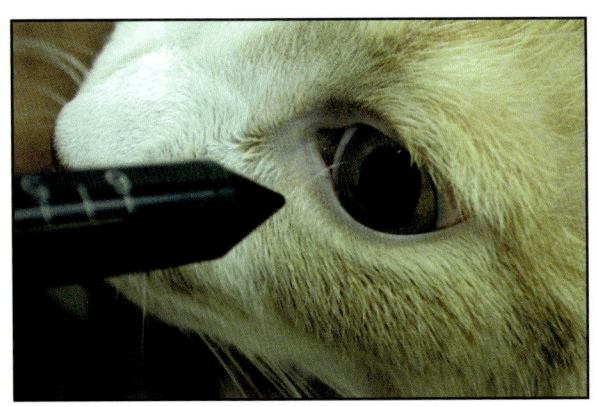

Figure 15.19 The Cochet–Bonnet aesthesiometer being used to evaluate corneal sensation.

Abnormalities due to sensory deficits

Denervation of sensory supply to the globe

- A neurotrophic keratopathy results from a sensory deficit of the cornea (see Chapter 8). This affects the cornea exposed within the interpalpebral fissure. Note that the menace reflex will cause the animal to blink if the eye is still visual
- Infranuclear lesions (i.e. between the sensory nerve endings and cells of the trigeminal nuclei) may result in total anaesthesia or partial anaesthesia. Hypoalgesia of the three branches of the trigeminal nerve due to a supranuclear lesion may be accompanied by supranuclear facial nerve palsy, due to the close proximity of thalamic nuclei and the internal capsule. Lesions of the trigeminal nerve may result from hydrocephalus, neoplasia, infection or skull fractures. Attempts should be made to identify the site and cause of the lesion and to treat it if possible. A neurotrophic keratopathy should be treated symptomatically, providing antibiotic cover and tear substitute treatment
- In the dog, tumours of the cranial nerves most often involve the trigeminal nerve (V) (Summers *et al.*, 1995).

Motor innervation of the eyelids

The facial nerve (VII) supplies the muscles of facial expression and carries parasympathetic nerves that innervate the lacrimal glands. It passes from the brain alongside the auditory nerve until it enters the facial canal that passes adjacent to the medial wall of the tympanic cavity. Fibres innervating the lacrimal gland pass via the major petrosal nerve and are given off just as the facial canal bends to become adjacent to the tympanic cavity. This close anatomical association between the facial nerve and the tympanic cavity is of clinical significance. The facial nerve emerges through the stylomastoid foramen and innervates the muscles of facial expression, including the orbicularis oculi muscle that effects blinking. The ability to blink may be checked by a number of reflexes: the menace response (see Figure 15.2) and dazzle reflex (see Figure 15.3) use the optic nerve (II) as the afferent pathway; the corneal or palpebral blink reflex uses the ophthalmic branch of the trigeminal nerve (V) as the afferent arm (see Figure 15.5).

Abnormalities due to motor deficits

Lesions of the facial nerve

Facial nerve paralysis results in an inability to blink. When the animal is stimulated to attempt to blink by the menace response test or corneal blink reflex, the globe is retracted and the third eyelid flicks across the cornea, but the upper and lower lids are incapable of closing the palpebral fissure. The cornea may be unaffected in cases where the parasympathetic supply to the lacrimal gland is spared and the third eyelid can adequately distribute the pre-ocular tear film. However, brachycephalic breeds with prominent globes may develop an exposure keratopathy because the third eyelid cannot pass completely across the cornea in these individuals; thus the pre-ocular tear film is not adequately spread. The cause of the facial nerve lesion, such as trauma, neoplasia, or otitis media, should be identified and treated if possible. Ocular treatment is not usually necessary unless a brachycephalic breed is affected or lacrimal function is impaired, in which case tear substitutes should be used.

Idiopathic facial paralysis
This condition can be unilateral or bilateral. Signs include drooping ears, drooling from the corner of the mouth, lip weakness, widening of palpebral fissure and weak or absent palpebral and corneal reflexes. Despite the absence of a confirmed association with otitis media–interna, animals with idiopathic facial weakness or paralysis frequently have vestibular signs. An association with hypothyroidism has been noted in some affected dogs. In idiopathic cases a comparison with Bell's palsy may be appropriate (Summers et al., 1995).

Hemifacial spasm
This is the result of increased motor activity of the facial nerve. It is characterized by the spontaneous onset of unilateral intermittent spasms of the orbicularis oculi muscle. It may, at first glance, be confused with facial nerve paralysis of the contralateral side. It has been reported in dogs with chronic otitis media (irritation of facial nerve) and following facial paralysis (Roberts and Vainisi, 1967; Parker et al., 1973). True hemifacial spasms should be differentiated from unilateral facial tics, tetanus, and focal epilepsy (Glaser, 1990).

Abnormalities of lacrimation

Tear production may be measured by the Schirmer tear test (see Chapters 1a and 6). Abnormalities of lacrimation are also dealt with in Chapter 6.

The tearing reflex
The afferent component of so-called reflex tearing is the trigeminal sensory stimulation from exposure of the eye to light, cold wind or other irritants; the efferent arm of this reflex is mediated by the preganglionic parasympathetic fibres that arise near the facial nucleus in the pontine tegmentum in a nuclear column ventral to the fourth ventricle. These fibres exit the brainstem and travel with the sensory root of the facial nerve and join the major petrosal nerve. The major petrosal nerve leaves the facial nerve within the facial canal in the medial wall of the middle ear cavity; the presynaptic fibres enter the pterygopalatine ganglion where they synapse with postganglionic fibres (Glaser, 1990). Then these latter fibres innervate the lacrimal gland by joining the zygomatic branch of the maxillary division of the trigeminal nerve.

Lesions of the afferent arm
Sensation conveyed from the cornea, conjunctiva and, to a certain extent, the nasal mucosa via the trigeminal nerve, acts as the afferent arm of the reflex to increase tear production. Lesions in this pathway are often overlooked as a potential cause of keratoconjunctivitis sicca (KCS). Lesions of the trigeminal nerve have been discussed above.

Lesions of the efferent arm
Pre-ganglionic parasympathetic fibres that arise near the facial nucleus in the pontine tegmentum mediate reflex tearing. These fibres travel with the initial portion of the facial nerve (VII). Therefore, lesions of the parasympathetic supply to the lacrimal gland are commonly accompanied by facial nerve (VII) lesions. The consequent denervation of the tear glands results in much reduced tear production and KCS. The lateral nasal gland, a serous secreting gland that keeps the nose moist, is innervated by a different branch of the facial nerve that separates at the level of the pterygopalatine ganglion. Therefore, KCS associated with a dry nose suggests a preorbital lesion, likely to be at the level of the petrous temporal bone (Smith, 2002). A neurological lesion should therefore be suspected, and treated if possible.

Topical tear substitutes and ointments can be used. Oral parasympathomimetics, such as 1% pilocarpine given in food twice a day (1–4 drops), may be of benefit because of denervation hypersensitivity of the tear-producing tissue. Topical cyclosporine treatment alone is usually of some help in these cases but often will not result in a satisfactory remission of the clinical signs because immune-mediated dacryoadenitis is not present. A parotid duct transposition is indicated if medical treatment fails to control the condition.

Paradoxical tearing
Paradoxical tearing (gustolacrimal reflex, 'crocodile tears') is the onset of excessive tearing while the patient is eating or anticipating a meal. It is called 'crocodile tears' after the myth that crocodiles cry while eating their prey. The afferent input is the stimulation of taste receptors. This phenomenon is the result of aberrant sprouting of salivary nerve fibres that gain access to the ipsilateral lacrimal glands. It has been reported in humans and in small animals (Glaser, 1990; Hacker, 1990). The condition is rare, usually unilateral, and may occur following facial palsies.

References and further reading

Ackerman L (1999) The genetic connection. In: *Ophthalmic Disorders*, ed. L. Ackerman, pp. 147–171. AAHA Press, Colorado

Bacon BA, Lepore F and Guillemot JP (1999) Binocular interactions and spatial disparity sensitivity in the superior colliculus of the Siamese cat. *Experimental Brain Research* **124**, 181–192

Bagley RS (1996) Recognition and localization of intracranial disease. *Veterinary Clinics of North America: Small Animal Practice* **26**, 711–733

Barlow CM and Root WS (1949) The ocular sympathetic path between the superior cervical ganglion and the orbit in the cat. *Journal of Comparative Neurology* **90**, 195–207

Barnett KC, Kelly DF and Singleton WM (1967) Retrobulbar and chiasmal meningioma in a dog. *Journal of Small Animal Practice* **8**, 391–394

Barret PM, Scagliotti RH, Merideth RE, Jackson PA and Alarcon FA (1991) Absolute corneal sensitivity and corneal trigeminal nerve anatomy in dogs. *Progress in Veterinary and Comparative Ophthalmology* **1**, 245–254

Bistner S, Rubin L, Cox TA and Condon WE (1970) Pharmacological diagnosis of Horner's syndrome in the dog. *Journal of the American Veterinary Medical Association* **157**, 1220–1224

Boydell P (2000) Idiopathic Horner syndrome in the Golden Retriever. *Journal of Neuroophthalmology* **20**, 288–290

Bradford CA (1999) Neuro-ophthalmology. In: *Basic Ophthalmology for Medical Students and Primary Care Residents, 3rd edn,* ed. CA Bradford, pp. 110–128. American Academy of Ophthalmology, San Francisco

Braund KG, Vandervelde M, Albert RA and Higgins RJ (1977) Central (post retinal) visual impairment in the dog – a clinical pathological study. *Journal of Small Animal Practice* **18**, 395–405

Brooks DE, Clark CK and Lester GD (2000) Cochet–Bonnet aesthesiometer-determined corneal sensitivity in neonatal foals and adult horses. *Veterinary Ophthalmology* **3**, 133–137

Davidson MG, Nasisse MP, Breitschwerdt EB, Thrall DE, Page RL, Jamieson VE and English RV (1991) Acute blindness associated with intracranial tumors in dogs and cats: eight cases (1984–1989). *Journal of the American Veterinary Medical Association* **199**, 755–758

de Lahunta A (1973) Small animal neuro-ophthalmology. *Veterinary Clinics of North America: Small Animal Practice* **3**, 491–501

de Lahunta A (1983) *Veterinary Neuroanatomy and Clinical Neurology, 2nd edn.* WB Saunders, Philadelphia

de Lahunta A (2002) Nystagmus. In: *Small Animal Ophthalmology Secrets,* ed. RC Riis, pp. 131–138. Hanley & Belfus, Philadelphia

de Lahunta A and Cummings JF (1967) Neuro-ophthalmological lesions as a cause of visual deficit in dogs and horses. *Journal of the American Veterinary Medical Association* **150**, 994–1011

Evinger C (1988) Extraocular motor nuclei: location, morphology and afferents. In: *Neuroanatomy of the oculomotor system, 1st edn,* ed. JA Buttner-Ennever, pp. 81–117. Elsevier, Amsterdam

Fischer CA and Jones GT (1972) Optic neuritis in dogs. *Journal of the American Veterinary Medical Association* **160**, 68–79

Glaser JS (1990) Neuro-ophthalmic examination: general considerations and special techniques. In: *Neuro-ophthalmology, 2nd edn,* ed. JS Glaser, pp. 37–60. Lippincott, Philadelphia

Goldfarb S and Swann PG (1984) Case report: idiopathic tonic pupil or Adie's syndrome in a dog. *Australian Veterinary Practice* **14**, 20

Gonzalez F and Perez R (1998) Neural mechanisms underlying stereoscopic vision. *Progress in Neurobiology* **55**, 191–224

Hacker DV (1990) Crocodile tears syndrome in a cat: case report. *Journal of the American Animal Hospital Association* **26**, 245–246

Hamilton HL and McLaughlin SA (2000) Diagnosis of blindness. In: *Kirks' Current Veterinary Therapy, XIII,* ed. JD Bonagura, pp.1038–1041. WB Saunders, Philadelphia

Hanson S, de Lahunta A and Slatter D (2001) Neuro-ophthalmology. In: *Fundamentals of Veterinary Ophthalmology,* ed. DH Slatter, pp. 457–495. WB Saunders, Philadelphia

Hoffmann KP, Ballas I and Wagner HJ (1984) Double labelling of retinofugal neurons in the cat: a study using anterograde transport of 3H-proline and horseradish peroxidase. *Experimental Brain Research* **53**, 420–430

Hoffmann KP and Fischer WH (2001) Directional effect of inactivation of the nucleus of the optic tract on optokinetic nystagmus in the cat. *Vision Research* **41**, 3389–3398

Hogan D and Williams RW (1995) Analysis of the retinas and optic nerves of achiasmatic Belgian sheepdogs. *Journal of Comparative Neurology* **352**, 367–380

Ichinohe N, Shoumura K and Takahashi H (1996) Quantitative electromicroscope study of the oculomotor parasympathetic neurons projecting to the ciliary ganglion in cats: comparison of the synaptic (axon-somatic and axo-proximal dendritic) organization of anterior-dorsal and ventral cell groups. *Anatomy and Embryology* (Berlin) **193**, 229–238

Jamieson PM, Scusamore CL, Ruppert CE, Mauchline S and Simpson JW (2002) Canine dysautonomia: two clinical cases. *Journal of Small Animal Practice* **43**, 22–26

King AS (1987) Clinical neurological tests: diagnostic exercises. In: *Physiological and Clinical Anatomy of the Domestic Mammals, 1st edn,* ed. AS King, pp. 220–244. Oxford University Press, Oxford

Konno S and Ohtsuka K (1997) Accommodation and pupilloconstriction areas in the cat midbrain. *Japanese Journal of Ophthalmology* **41**, 43–48

Lane I (2000) Diagnosis and management of urinary retention. *Veterinary Clinics of North America: Small Animal Practice* **30**, 25–57

Laties AM and Sprague JM (1966) The projection of optic fibers to the visual centers of the cat. *Journal of Comparative Neurology* **127**, 35–70

Loewy AD, Saper CB and Yamodis ND (1978) Re-evaluation of the efferent projections of the Edinger–Westphal nucleus in the cat. *Brain Research* **141**, 153–159

Moore MP, Bagley RS, Harrington ML and Gavin PR (1996) Intracranial tumors. *Veterinary Clinics of North America: Small Animal Practice* **26**, 759–777

Parker AJ, Cusick PK, Park RD and Small E (1973) Hemifacial spasms in a dog. *Veterinary Record* **93**, 514–516

Pu M (2000) Physiological response properties of cat retinal ganglion cells projecting to suprachiasmatic nucleus. *Journal of Biological Rhythms* **15**, 31–36

Roberts SR and Vainisi SJ (1967) Hemifacial spasm in dogs. *Journal of the American Veterinary Medical Association* **150**, 381–385

Roste GK and Dietrichs E (1988) Cerebellar cortical and nuclear afferents to the Edinger–Westphal nucleus in the cat. *Anatomy and Embryology* (Berlin) **178**, 59–65

Sayoko EM and Lichter PR (2001) Ocular pharmacology. In: *Goodman & Gilman's The Pharmacological Basis of Therapeutics, 10th edn,* ed. JG Hardman and LE Limbrid, pp. 1821–1848. McGraw-Hill, New York

Scagliotti RH (1980) Current concepts in veterinary neuro-ophthalmology. *Veterinary Clinics of North America: Small Animal Practice* **10**, 417–436

Scagliotti RH (1999) Comparative neuro-ophthalmology. In: *Veterinary Ophthalmology, 3rd edn,* ed. KN Gelatt, pp. 1307–1400. Lippincott, Williams & Wilkins, Philadelphia

Skerritt GC, Obwolo MJ and Squires RA (1986) Bilateral blindness in a dog due to invasion of the optic chiasma by a glioma. *Journal of Small Animal Practice* **27**, 97

Slatter DH and de Lahunta A (1990) Neurophthalmology. In: *Fundamentals of Veterinary Ophthalmology, 2nd edn,* ed. DH Slatter, p. 437. WB Saunders, Philadelphia

Smith JS (2002) Optic neuropathies. In: *Small Animal Ophthalmology Secrets,* ed RC Riis, pp.139–146. Hanley & Belfus, Philadelphia

Stiles J (1999) Ocular manifestation of systemic disease. The cat. In: *Veterinary Ophthalmology, 3rd edn,* ed. KN Gelatt, pp.1448–1473. Lippincott, Williams & Wilkins, Philadelphia

Summers B, Cummings J and de Lahunta A (1995) Autonomic nervous system. In: *Veterinary Neuropathology,* ed. B Summers *et al.,* pp. 469–481. Mosby-Year Book, St. Louis

Takada M, Itoh K, Yasui Y, Mitani A, Nomura S and Mizuno N (1984) Distribution of premotor neurons for orbicularis oculi motoneurons in the cat, with particular reference to possible pathways for blink reflex. *Neuroscience Letters* **50**, 251–255

Taylor SM (2000) Selected diseases of muscle and the neuromuscular junction. *Veterinary Clinics of North America: Small Animal Practice* **30**, 59–75

Thomas WB (2000) Vestibular dysfunction. *Veterinary Clinics of North America: Small Animal Practice* **30**, 1–24

Toyoshima K, Kawana E and Sakai H (1980) On the neuronal origin of the afferents to the ciliary ganglion in the cat. *Brain Research* **185**, 67–76

von Grunau MW and Rauschecker JP (1983) Natural strabismus in non-Siamese cats: lack of binocularity in the striate cortex. *Experimental Brain Research* **52**, 307–310

Wheeler SJ (1991) The nervous system. In: *Manual of Small Animal Oncology,* ed. RAS White, pp. 315–339. BSAVA Publications, Cheltenham

Williams JO, Garlick EC and Beard DC (1961) Glioma of the optic nerve of a dog. *Journal of the American Veterinary Medical Association* **138**, 377–378

16

Rabbits

David L. Williams

Introduction

The explosion of veterinary interest in the pet rabbit over the past few years has been paralleled by an increase in attention paid to the ophthalmic diseases of this species. Despite the fact that the rabbit eye is widely used in comparative research, the physiology and gross and microscopic anatomy differ substantially from that of other mammals, including humans. These differences result in significant variations in disease presentations from those seen in the dog and cat. This chapter will highlight those differences against the background of similarities between the eyes of the rabbit and other companion mammals.

The orbit

Orbital anatomy

The rabbit orbit is dissimilar from that of other mammals in several respects. The eyes are placed laterally, set widely apart, and project well beyond the orbital rim. In addition to opening into the cranial cavity, each optic foramen communicates directly with the opposite orbit through an opening approximately 5 mm wide; this anatomical feature has clinical significance, potentially enabling infection to pass from one orbit to the other in cases of orbital cellulitis or retrobulbar abscess. Two further important anatomical features of the rabbit orbit are the retrobulbar venous plexus (or 'orbital sinus') and the glands associated with the globe.

Orbital sinus

The retrobulbar venous plexus extends from the orbital apex to the globe equator and lies immediately internal to the periorbital membrane, effectively a 'second lining for the bony orbit' (Ruskell, 1964). The venous plexus communicates with several major veins. The reflex vein is the largest vessel draining the plexus; the apical group of small veins drains into the pterygoid sinus. A group of small veins connects the orbital venous plexus with the intracranial cavernous sinus, giving the potential for cerebral spread of orbital infection. Other veins draining to the orbital sinus are the anterior palpebral vein, the orbitotemporal vein and the superior ophthalmic vein. The orbital sinus is of clinical significance when enucleation or exenteration is undertaken, as it can be a source of significant bleeding.

Orbital glands

The glands occupying the orbit are very different from the analogous structures in the cat or dog.

- The lacrimal gland and an accessory lacrimal gland with orbital and retro-orbital lobes are situated dorsolaterally
- The third eyelid has a superficial (nictitans) gland and a deep gland. The nictitans gland is buried within the nictitating membrane and envelops the deep end of the cartilage of the nictitating membrane. The deep gland has a white dorsal lobe and a pink ventral lobe and is known as the Harderian gland. It is almost completely enveloped by the orbital venous sinus. The fascia of the Harderian gland is tightly attached to the fascia surrounding the extraocular muscles and to the base of the nictitating membrane.

Conditions of the orbit

Prolapse of the globe

Rabbits have very prominent globes, and relatively minor trauma, including poor restraining techniques, can result in prolapse of the globe.

Exophthalmos

Exophthalmos in the rabbit is most commonly due to a retrobulbar abscess; less common causes include neoplasia, impeded venous drainage from the orbit, and orbital vascular anomalies (Figure 16.1).

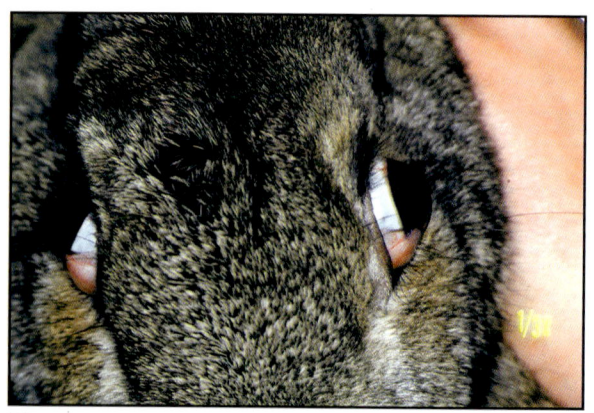

Figure 16.1 A rabbit with stress-related exophthalmos which was caused by an anterior thoracic mass compressing the anterior vena cava. (Courtesy of C. Gillespie.)

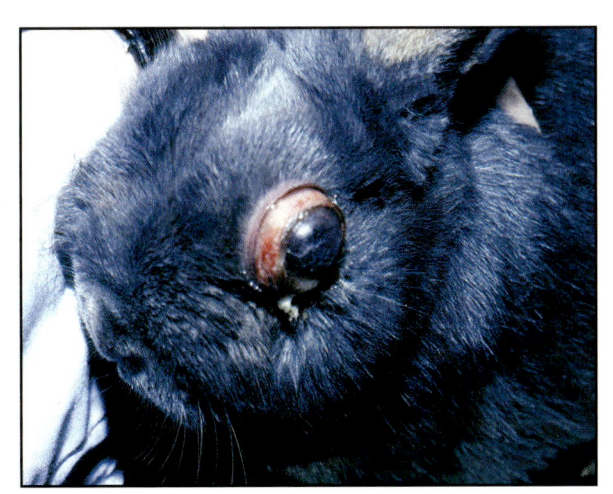

Retrobulbar abscess: Retrobulbar abscessation (Figure 16.2) is the commonest orbital disease of the rabbit. The majority of retrobulbar abscesses are related to dental disease; *Pasteurella multocida* has been implicated, though without firm evidence. Infected molar tooth roots that are retropulsed into the orbit can readily lead to an orbital abscess and cure is rare in such cases. The purulent discharge associated with a retrobulbar abscess is difficult, if not impossible, to evacuate completely and even after complete orbital exenteration the majority of chronic retrobulbar abscesses will recur. The use of antibiotic-impregnated beads in the orbit may be valuable, as has been reported for the treatment of dental abscesses in the rabbit. Calcium hydroxide paste, which is bactericidal as a result of its high pH, may be useful (Remeeus and Verbeek, 1995).

Figure 16.2 Retrobulbar abscess characterized by lagophthalmos and exophthalmos, and associated with *Pasteurella multocida* molar tooth root infection.

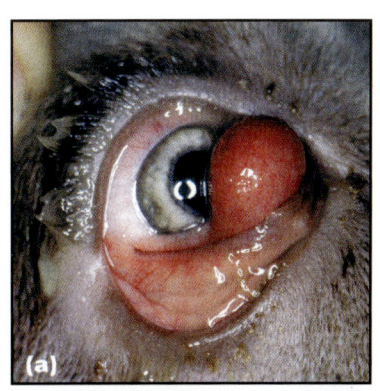

Figure 16.3 Orbital gland prolapses: (a) superficial nictitans gland; (b) Harderian gland.

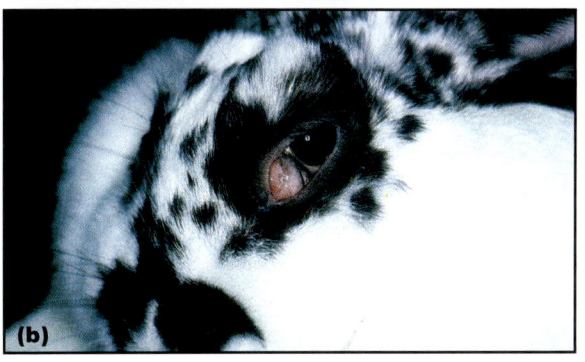

Orbital gland prolapse

Prolapse of the glands associated with the third eyelid is not common but has been reported (Roxburgh *et al.*, 1998; Janssens *et al.*, 1999). Given the anatomy, it might be expected that the prolapsed gland would invariably be the more superficial nictitans gland (Figure 16.3a), but it is usually the Harderian gland (Figure 16.3b) that is involved (Janssens *et al.*, 1999).

A mucosal pocket technique as described for the dog (Morgan *et al.*, 1993) can be used to effect repair (see Figure 5.46). Preservation of the gland may not be necessary to maintain tear production but the high vascularity of the gland means that excision may be accompanied by severe haemorrhage.

Enucleation

A transconjunctival approach to enucleation is preferred. With this technique the dissection can be made close to the globe, with each extraocular muscle being sectioned at its insertion on the sclera. The optic nerve and accompanying vessels are sectioned last. This approach minimizes the chance of causing serious bleeding by disrupting or damaging the orbital sinus.

Retrobulbar anaesthesia

Retrobulbar anaesthesia can be performed to allow lighter levels of general anaesthesia when enucleation, orbital surgery or intraocular surgery is undertaken. A needle is inserted at the dorsal border of the zygomatic arch and directed posteromedially to reach the superior orbital fissure; 0.5–1 ml of lignocaine (lidocaine) is injected. The nerves supplying the extraocular muscles and those for orbital nociception pass through the superior orbital fissure (Diesem, 1964). This procedure should be performed with care to avoid inadvertent penetration of the globe.

Eyelid and conjunctival diseases

Infectious conditions involving the eyelids often also involve the conjunctiva.

Blepharoconjunctivitis and conjunctivitis

Causes

Irritation: Conjunctivitis may be caused by irritation from dust arising from poor-quality hay or straw. Distichia and ectopic cilia have not been reported as causes of ocular irritation and inflammation in the rabbit, although single ectopic cilia unassociated with clinical signs are occasionally observed arising from the nictitating membrane.

Infection:

- *Haemophilus* spp. have been reported as a primary cause of conjunctivitis in the rabbit (Srivastava *et al.*, 1986) but other infectious agents are often isolated

- Blepharoconjunctivitis with mucopurulent ocular discharge and eyelid thickening and crusting has been reported associated with localized *Staphylococcus aureus* infection (Millichamp and Collins, 1986). Topical and parenteral gentamicin was curative
- Blepharitis and blepharoconjunctivitis in the rabbit may be associated with rabbit syphilis caused by the spirochaete *Treponema cuniculi*. *T. cuniculi* is transmitted to neonates by the genitally infected dam (Harkness and Wagner, 1989)
- Myxomatosis is most commonly seen in wild rabbits and is caused by the myxoma virus. Affected rabbits suffer from periocular swelling and a white purulent ocular discharge, probably as a result of secondary infections with bacteria such as *Staphylococcus* spp. or *Pasteurella* spp. (Figure 16.4). Animals that have been vaccinated may develop periorbital swelling associated with facial oedema when they encounter field strains of the virus.

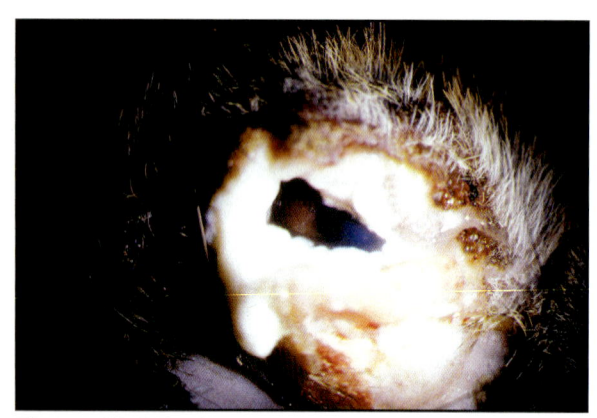

Figure 16.4 Purulent ocular discharge in a rabbit with myxomatosis.

Diagnosis and treatment

- Laboratory diagnostic techniques should include bacteriology and cytology using Giemsa and Gram stains. Gram staining of a conjunctival sample helps in the immediate choice of an appropriate antibiotic while awaiting confirmation from culture and sensitivity
- Diagnosis of rabbit syphilis is made by demonstrating the spirochaete on a conjunctival scrape, the prepared slide is best viewed with dark field illumination
- An autogenous vaccine has been suggested for the treatment of staphylococcal conjunctivitis (Hinton, 1977).

Eyelid tumours

Squamous cell carcinoma can mimic the clinical signs of treponemal blepharoconjunctivitis (Bagley and Lavach, 1985) but cytology should be diagnostic as neoplastic epithelial cells can be demonstrated when the cause is squamous cell carcinoma. Surgical excision is the current preferred treatment, although brachytherapy, if available, would be a radiotherapeutic option.

Fibrosarcoma is another possible tumour of the orbital and periobital region; exenteration, the only surgical option, is rarely curative.

Aberrant conjunctival overgrowth

Aberrant overgrowth of the conjunctiva to cover the cornea (Figure 16.5) is an unusual abnormality unique to the rabbit (Matros *et al.*, 1986; Bauck, 1989; Dupont *et al.*, 1995). The aetiology of the condition is unknown. While it may present as a congenital defect, it can also develop in adult animals.

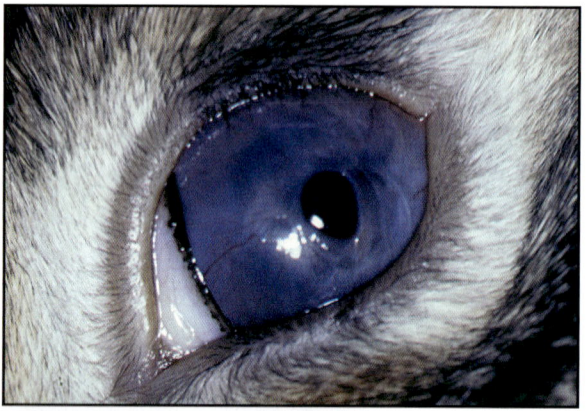

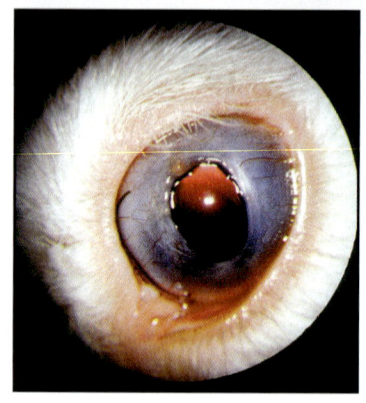

Figure 16.5 Two cases of aberrant overgrowth of limbal conjunctiva to cover the peripheral cornea, demonstrating the variation in extent of the overgrowth.

A fold of conjunctival tissue arises circumferentially from the limbus and grows over the cornea but is nonadherent. It appears as a thin annulus that covers a considerable portion of the ocular surface and in some cases can completely cover the cornea. Typically the condition recurs following simple surgical removal. Suturing the fold back to the sclera, or using topical cyclosporin after surgery, reduces the degree of recurrence so that permanent visual impairment is avoided. Histology of resected tissue shows no inflammatory changes, although one study demonstrated aberrant contractile elements in the leading edge of the conjunctiva (PE Miller, personal communication, 2001).

Lacrimal system

Tear production

There is a wide range in normal tear production as measured by the Schirmer 1 tear test. In a study by Abrams *et al.* (1990) of 142 apparently normal eyes, the average value was 5.3 ± 2.9 mm/min, with a range from 0 to 15 mm/min. Breed differences accounted for the wide variation in this study; while it might be supposed that larger breeds would have the higher readings, the study showed Netherland Dwarf rabbits to have an unusually high reading of 12.0 ± 2.5 mm/min. Given the breed and individual variation, if reduced tear production is suspected it is essential to compare tear production in a diseased eye with the normal fellow eye.

Tear drainage

The rabbit's nasolacrimal system is unusual in that there is only one ventrally placed lacrimal punctum which is located deep within the medial portion of the ventral conjunctival sac, at the base of the external surface of the third eyelid. The nasolacrimal duct takes a tortuous pathway from the lacrimal punctum through the lacrimal and maxillary bones and has two sharp bends associated with duct narrowing (Figure 16.6). The duct passes close to the roots of both molar and incisor teeth, emerging through the nasal mucosa (Burling et al., 1991).

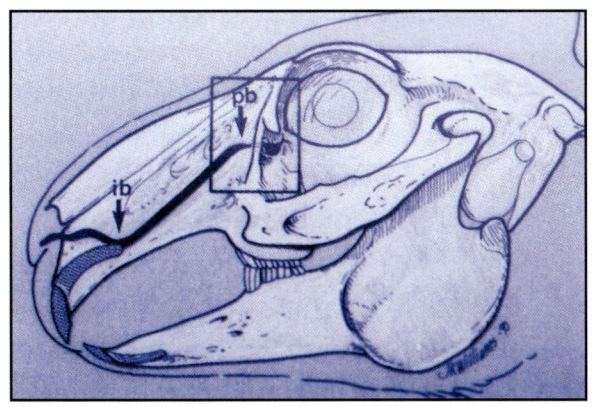

Figure 16.6 Tortuosity and narrowing of the nasolacrimal duct. ib = bend at incisor root, pb = proximal maxillary bend (Courtesy of T. Burling.)

Conditions of the lacrimal system

Keratoconjunctivitis sicca (KCS)

KCS causing frank ocular surface pathology does not appear to be common in the rabbit and, as noted above, normal rabbits can have very low tear production. Nevertheless, a Schirmer tear test should be performed as part of the basic diagnostic work-up for any case with ocular surface disease. It is possible that altered tear production, or other abnormality of the tear film components, may play a role in persistent corneal ulceration (see below). Although Schirmer tear test values may not be substantially reduced, treatment with tear replacement agents may benefit a high proportion of cases with persistent ulceration.

Nasolacrimal duct obstruction and dacryocystitis

Interference with nasolacrimal drainage and development of infections involving the nasolacrimal system are a common cause of ocular discharge in the rabbit.

Diagnosis and investigation: Ocular discharge is a frequent finding in rabbits, ranging from simple epiphora, mucoid and mucopurulent discharge (Figure 16.7a), to dense white purulent nasolacrimal emission (Figure 16.7b). A key feature in the investigation of such cases is defining whether the discharge merely signals a localized conjunctivitis or whether, as is most usual, it is the result of dacryocystitis. With dacryocystitis, mucopurulent material may be seen emerging from the lacrimal punctum or can be expressed by digital pressure over the medial canthal region (Figure 16.7c). Expressed material should be collected for bacterial culture and sensitivity testing.

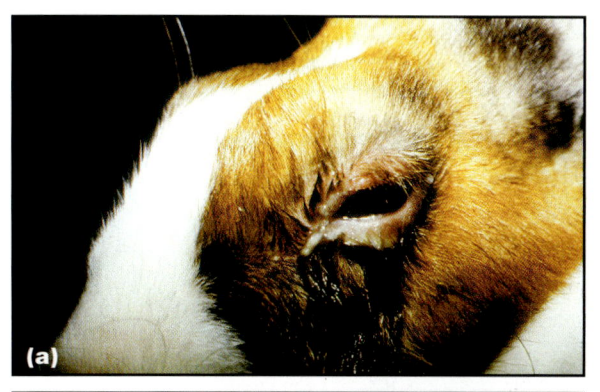

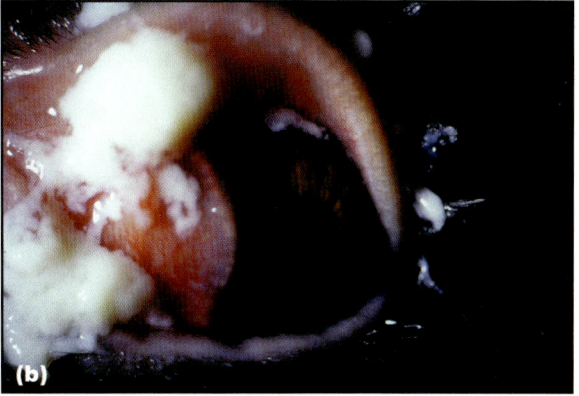

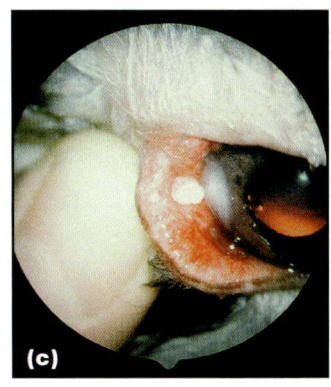

Figure 16.7 Dacryocystitis: (a) mucopurulent ocular discharge; (b) copious white nasolacrimal discharge; (c) purulent material expressed from the nasolacrimal punctum; note the accompanying corneal abscess. (Courtesy of SM Crispin.)

If any doubt remains, conjunctivitis and dacryocystitis can be differentiated by cannulation and irrigation of the nasolacrimal duct (Figure 16.8). Easy flushing, without the appearance of purulent material around the cannula, suggests that dacryocystitis is not present.

Radiography, including dacryocystorhinography (Figure 16.9), can be useful in the investigation of dacryocystitis. The nasolacrimal duct is cannulated

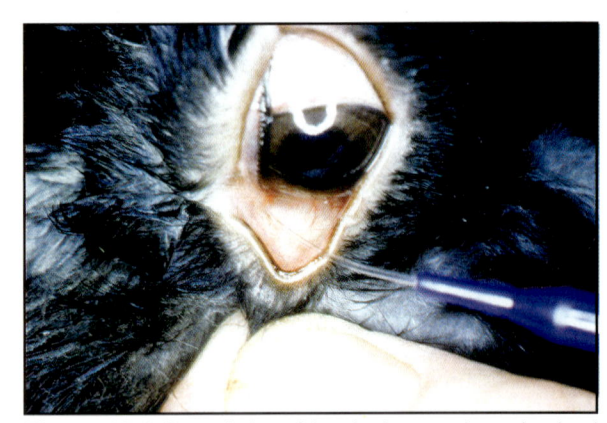

Figure 16.8 Cannulation of the single ventral nasolacrimal punctum. Digital pressure ventrally on the lower eyelid causes the lips of the punctum to 'pout', facilitating introduction of a 23 gauge nasolacrimal cannula.

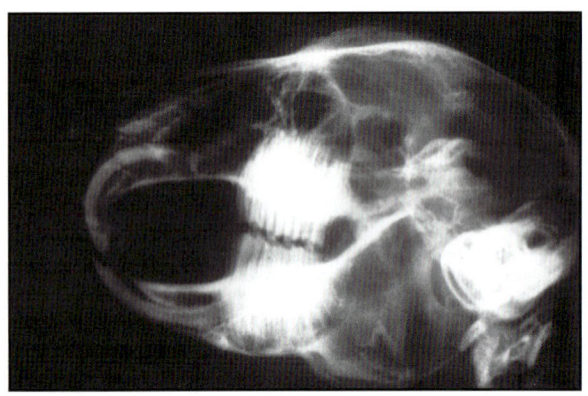

Figure 16.9 Dacryocystorhinography to show the nasolacrimal duct.

with a 23 gauge lacrimal cannula and 0.2 ml of non-ionic contrast medium injected. Radiography, utilising lateral and dorsoventral views, will delineate structural abnormalities of the duct and demonstrate the relationship between the duct and any dental pathology.

Causes: The normal rabbit nasolacrimal duct has specific portions where it suddenly narrows. These are potential sites for obstruction.

- Occasionally functional obstruction can be caused by sterile oil droplets of indeterminate origin; this results in epiphora (Figure 16.10) (Marini *et al.,* 1996)

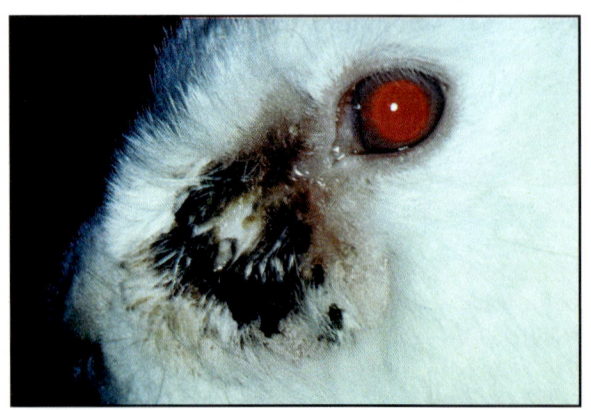

Figure 16.10 Epiphora with dermal scalding. (Courtesy of SM Crispin.)

- In dacryocystitis, infected purulent material causes the obstruction (Petersen-Jones and Carrington, 1988; Bauck, 1989)
- The close association between the nasolacrimal duct and the roots of incisors and molars means that tooth malocclusion and root retropulsion can contribute to duct obstruction
- The architectural changes in maxillary bones secondary to dietary metabolic bone disease probably also has an important part to play in nasolacrimal duct pathology. Nutritional hyperparathyroidism-related dental and facial bone abnormalities (Harcourt-Brown, 1996) are common, particularly in dwarf rabbits, and frequently result in nasolacrimal duct obstruction leading to dacryocystitis
- Bacterial infection also plays a role in dacryocystitis:
  - *Pasteurella multocida* is often considered to be the most common bacterial pathogen in the rabbit but a wide range of bacterial species may be isolated
  - Marini *et al.* (1996) showed a wide range of organisms, including *Neisseria* spp., *Moraxella* spp., *Bordetella* spp., *Pseudomonas* spp., *Streptococcus viridans* and *Oligella urethralis*, in the bacterial flora from rabbits affected by epiphora alone. Which organisms were pathogenic and which were part of the normal flora is not clear, since the same organisms were found in nasolacrimal flushes from unaffected rabbits. The most frequently isolated organism in an earlier study of dacryocystitis (Petersen-Jones and Carrington, 1988), *Pasteurella multocida*, was not detected
  - In a survey of staphylococcal disease in rabbits, over 60% had nasal exudate with conjunctivitis (Snyder *et al.,* 1976). In a more recent study (Cobb *et al.,* 1999) *Staphylococcus* spp. was isolated from 40% of rabbits with ocular infection, while *P. multocida* occurred in only 12%.

Treatment: Treatment of chronic dacryocystitis can be frustrating and there has been no critical evaluation of treatment regimens in the rabbit. While treatment of an early case through nasolacrimal irrigation with the appropriate antibiotic solution, with follow-up topical treatment, can be curative, a significant number of animals require long-term treatment. Some veterinary ophthalmologists consider that repeated flushing is indicated, while others suggest that in cases unresponsive to topical medication, lifelong systemic antibiotic treatment is the only means of controlling the problem. Enrofloxacin (5 mg/kg) delivered in the drinking water is probably the initial treatment of choice if this long-term approach is taken.

To flush the nasolacrimal duct, digital retraction is applied ventrally on the medial lower eyelid causing the lips of the punctum to 'pout', facilitating introduction of a 23 gauge nasolacrimal cannula (see Figure 16.8). The duct can be difficult to cannulate when there is concurrent severe conjunctivitis with a hyperaemic and hyperplastic conjunctiva (Figure 16.11).

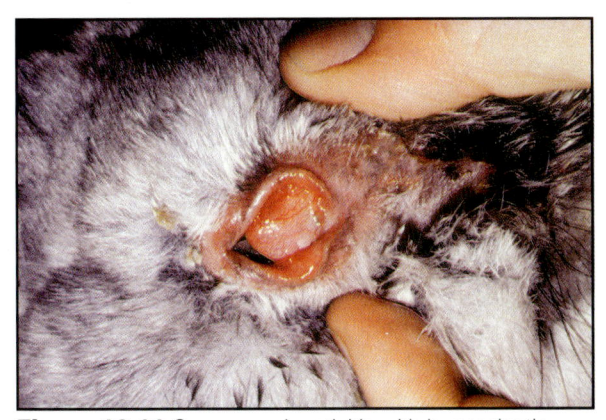

Figure 16.11 Severe conjunctivitis with hyperplastic conjunctiva can render duct cannulation difficult.

Cornea

Corneal dystrophies

Corneal epithelial dystrophy has been reported in the rabbit, presenting as peripheral areas of epithelial thinning and hyperplasia (Port and Dodd, 1983). Another report described plaque-like paracentral granular stippling with irregularly thickened epithelial basement membrane in American Dutch belted rabbits (Moore et al., 1987). Occasional sporadic conditions resembling epithelial dystrophy may be noted (Figure 16.12) but since 'dystrophy' refers to an inherited condition, in the absence of any affected relatives a definitive diagnosis is difficult.

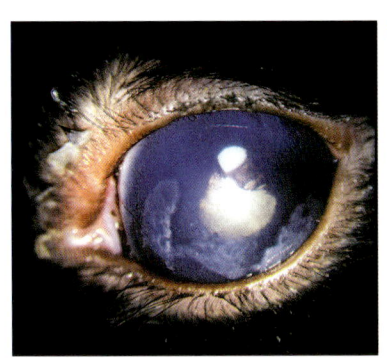

Figure 16.12 Epithelial pathology suggestive of corneal dystrophy in a Netherland Dwarf rabbit.

Lipid keratopathy

Lipid keratopathy has, not surprisingly for an obligate herbivore, been documented in rabbits experimentally fed cholesterol-rich diets to induce atherosclerosis (Fallon et al., 1988) and in rabbits fed a maintenance diet consisting of 10% fishmeal (Sebesteny et al., 1985). There are two case reports of ocular lipid deposition in pet rabbits fed high fat diets, one predominantly milk-based (Gelatt, 1977), the other rich in cheese and butter (Crispin, 1993).

Ulcerative keratitis

Persistent indolent superficial epithelial erosions occur (Figure 16.13), similar to those described in dogs (see Chapter 8). Debridement to remove all the non-adherent epithelium, with or without ocular surface protection with a 'bandage' contact lens, allows re-epithelialization in many cases. In others, grid keratotomy to achieve long-term epithelial stability is required (see Chapter 8). In a small number of rabbits epithelial healing appears to be defective to the extent that, even after debridement and grid keratotomy, epithelial healing does not occur. In such cases, a superficial keratectomy is required although care should be exercised, as the rabbit has a thinner cornea than the dog where this surgery is more regularly undertaken. Use of a Martinez corneal dissector or crescent knife is recommended.

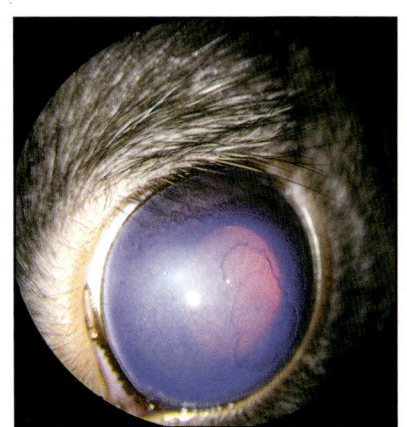

Figure 16.13 Recurrent erosion with devitalized non-adherent epithelial lip, similar to basement membrane epithelial dystrophy in, for example, the Boxer dog.

Deeper ulceration is often associated with stromal abscessation, with one potential cause being a partial-thickness penetrating injury from hay or straw shafts. The optimal therapeutic strategy for such stromal lesions involves removal of the majority of suppurative material under topical local or general anaesthesia. This allows collection of material for bacteriological investigation by cytology, culture and sensitivity testing. Frequent topical administration of an appropriate antibiotic for 2–3 weeks is usually effective, although a mild corneal opacity often persists at the site of previous ulceration.

Corneal oedema

Corneal oedema is a common feature of glaucoma (Figure 16.14); it may also be associated with indolent ulceration. Bullous keratopathy is a not infrequent complication of stromal oedema. When rupture of epithelial bullae occurs, causing recurrent superficial ulceration and pain, thermal keratoplasty (see Chapter 8) could be considered, but the thin cornea of the rabbit makes this a potentially dangerous procedure.

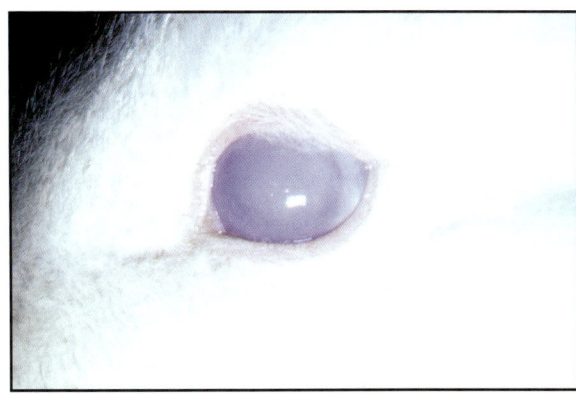

Figure 16.14 Glaucoma in a *bu/bu* New Zealand White rabbit.

Other non-ulcerative keratitis

White corneal inflammatory lesions similar to those of feline eosinophilic keratoconjunctivitis (see Chapter 8) are on occasion seen in the rabbit. Cytological examination may reveal eosinophils or a more generalized spectrum of inflammatory cells. In either case topical steroid treatment with prednisolone acetate two or three times daily can be efficacious and treatment is tapered off when the problem has resolved.

Uveal tract and lens

Uveitis

Uveitis in the rabbit may be caused by bacteria, presumed to be seeded into the eye during a septicaemic episode. Characteristic signs include flare or frank hypopyon and synechiae, and possibly also secondary cataract formation (Figure 16.15). Other cases are characterized by large iridal abscesses in eyes with frank panophthalmitis (Figure 16.16). A more common presentation is that of a solitary white mass with, or more often without, other more overt signs of intraocular inflammation (Figure 16.17). These cases were previously thought to be manifestations of *Pasteurella multocida* infection, but recently many have been shown to be a phacoclastic uveitis with a fascinating and unusual pathogenesis.

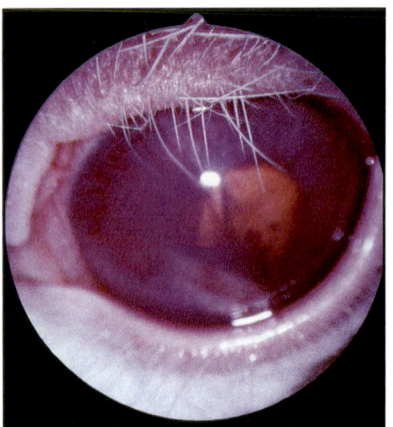

Figure 16.15 *Pasteurella multocida*-associated uveitis with posterior synechiae and cataract formation.

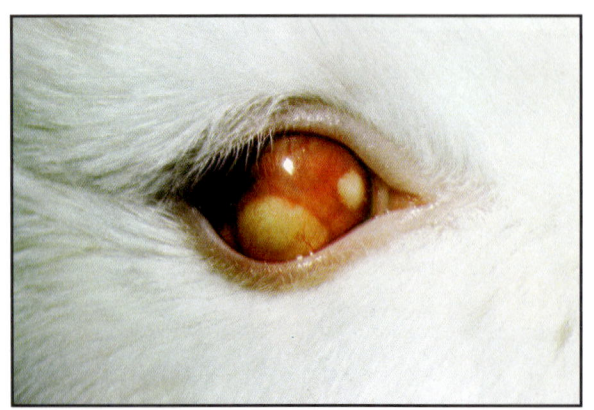

Figure 16.16 Intraocular abscessation and panophthalmitis associated with *Staphylococcus aureus*.

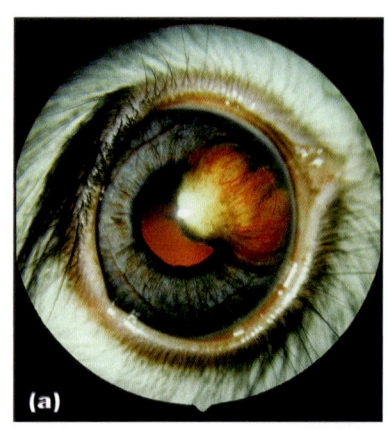

Figure 16.17 *Encephalitozoon cuniculi*-associated uveitis with an obvious vascular response in (a) but no such reaction in (b). (a: Courtesy of SM Crispin.)

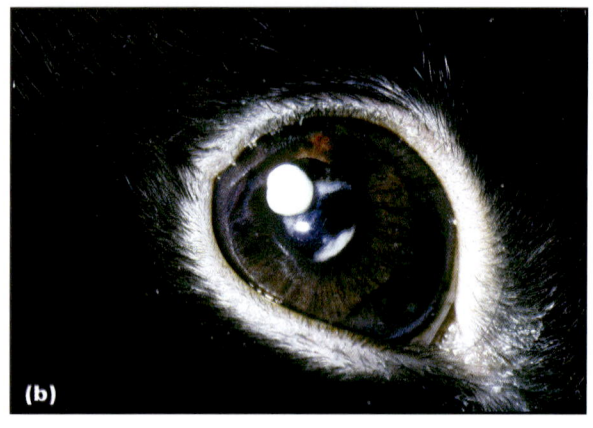

The microsporidian parasite *Encephalitozoon cuniculi* has for some time been known to cause cataract and lens capsule rupture in rabbits (Ashton *et al.*, 1976). It would appear that it enters the lens during development *in utero* and eventually leads to capsular rupture, with or without cataract. Release of lens material into the anterior chamber leads to a phacoclastic uveitis (Wolfer *et al.*, 1992). The only treatment for such an intraocular inflammation is lens removal, ideally by phacoemulsification. However, one case has been reported where albendazole at a dosage of 30 mg/kg orally every 24 hours over 4 weeks was effective in treating the parasitic infection, with concurrent topical steroid medication to reduce the associated inflammation (Stiles *et al.*, 1997).

Differentiating *Pasteurella/Staphyloccus*-associated uveitis from *Encephalitozoon cuniculi*-associated phacoclastic uveitis is very difficult. While paracentesis followed by bacteriology can give a definitive diagnosis, this is an invasive procedure and can result in exacerbation of the inflammatory process.

Phacoemulsification is the ideal treatment for *E. cuniculi*-associated phacoclastic uveitis. Topical anti-inflammatories (ketorolac) can suppress the inflammation sufficiently to prevent long-term sequelae. However, no long-term evaluation of different treatment modalities has been reported.

Glaucoma

Glaucoma is inherited in the New Zealand White (NZW) rabbit due to the recessive *bu* gene. This also occurs in pet rabbits of the NZW strain as well as in other white breeds. The inherited glaucoma in the

NZW rabbit has been well researched (McMaster, 1960; Hanna et al,. 1962; Lee, 1968). Intraocular pressure (IOP) in bu/bu homozygotes is normal (15–23 mmHg) early in life but at 1–3 months IOP rises to 26–48 mmHg (Kolker et al., 1963). The eyes become buphthalmic, with cloudy corneas (see Figure 16.14) but, while vision is lost, the eyes do not appear to be painful at this stage. This may be because of nociceptive nerve fibre damage occurring as the globe expands. Over the next several months IOP often returns to normal levels, since elevated IOP causes degeneration of the ciliary body which significantly reduces aqueous humour production. Affected eyes are characterized histologically by classical pectinate ligament dysplasia (Lee, 1968; Tesluk et al., 1982) (Figure 16.18). Medical treatment for this condition is rarely effective or necessary (Vareilles et al., 1980). The bu gene is known to be semilethal in heterozygote animals, with the production of small litters of unthrifty pups (Hanna et al., 1962).

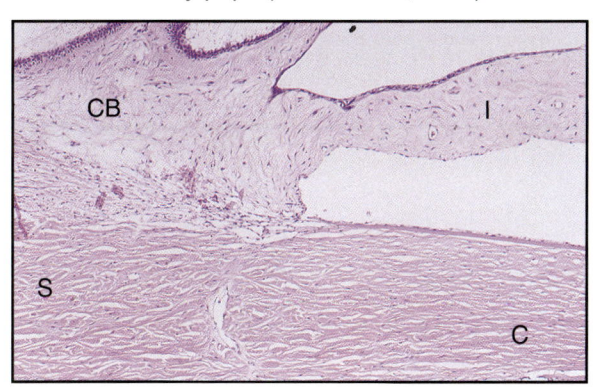

Figure 16.18 Histological appearance of dysplastic iridocorneal angle in a bu/bu affected glaucomatous rabbit. C = cornea, CB = ciliary body, I = iris, S = sclera.

Cataract

Lens opacity may be associated with E. cuniculi as noted earlier. It can be an inherited condition or can be secondary to trauma. The optimal treatment is photoemulsification but a significant complication is posterior capsular opacification, particularly severe in the rabbit.

Fundus

Anatomy of the posterior segment

The retinal blood supply in the rabbit is merangiotic, meaning that only a portion of the fundus is supplied by superficial retinal blood vessels. There is a horizontal band of nerve fibres, which are normally myelinated and thus appear white, with accompanying superficial retinal vasculature (Figure 16.19). Dorsal to this arrangement of vessels and myelinated nerve fibres is a horizontal band with densely packed photoreceptors that affords more detailed vision. This, combined with the lateral eye placement in this species, allows the rabbit to have a relatively high level of visual acuity in a band around the entire horizon, allowing it to readily identify advancing predators from any direction. The optic nerve head has a deep physiological pit.

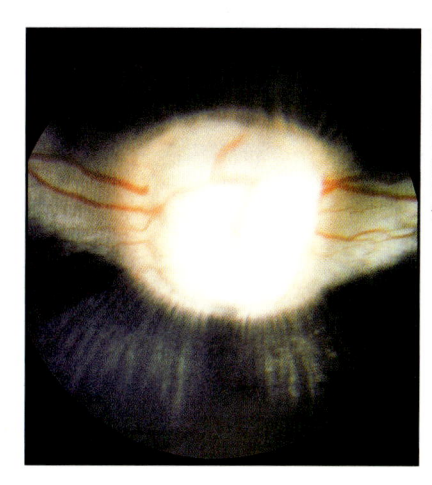

Figure 16.19 Optic nerve head with deep physiological pit in the normal merangiotic lagomorph fundus.

Posterior segment disease

It would appear that only one report exists of an inherited retinal degeneration in the rabbit (Reichenbach and Baar, 1985). The only two spontaneous posterior segment diseases commonly recognized in the rabbit are optic nerve coloboma and glaucomatous cupping of the optic disc. Optic nerve coloboma is an insignificant problem and appears not to cause visual disturbance but should be differentiated from the deep physiological pit in the centre of the optic disc.

References and further reading

Abrams KL, Brooks DE, Funk RS and Theran P (1990) Evaluation of Schirmer tear test in clinically normal rabbits. *American Journal of Veterinary Research* **51**, 1912–1913

Ashton N, Cook C and Clegg F (1976) Encephalitozoonosis (Nosematosis) causing bilateral cataract in a rabbit. *British Journal of Ophthalmology* **60**, 618–631

Bagley LH and Lavach D (1985) Ophthalmic diseases in rabbits. *Californian Veterinarian* **49**, 7–9

Bauck L (1989) Ophthalmic conditions in pet rabbits and rodents. *Compendium on Continuing Education for the Practicing Veterinarian* **11**, 258–268

Burling K, Murphy CJ, Curiel JS, Koblick P and Bellhorn RW (1991) Anatomy of the rabbit nasolacrimal duct and its clinical implications. *Progress in Veterinary and Comparative Ophthalmology* **1**, 33–40

Cobb MA, Payne B, Allen WM and Pott JM (1999) A survey of conjunctival flora in rabbits with clinical signs of superficial ocular infection. In: *Proceedings of the British Small Animal Veterinary Association Congress, April 1999, Birmingham UK*, p.250. BSAVA, Cheltenham

Crispin SM (1993) Ocular manifestations of hyperlipoproteinaemia. *Journal of Small Animal Practice* **34**, 500-506

Diesem CD (1964) The bony orbit. In: *The Rabbit in Eye Research*, ed. JH Prince, pp.545–547. Charles C Thomas, Springfield, IL

Dupont C, Carrier M and Gauvin J (1995) Bilateral precorneal membranous occlusion in a dwarf rabbit. *Journal of Small Exotic Animal Medicine* **3**, 41–44

Fallon MT, Reinhard MK, DaRif CA and Schwoeb TR (1988) Diagnostic exercise: eye lesions in a rabbit. *Laboratory Animal Science* **38**, 612–613

Gelatt GN (1977) Corneal lipidosis in a rabbit fed milk. *Journal of the American Veterinary Medical Association* **171**, 887–889

Hanna BL, Sawin PB and Sheppars LB (1962) Buphthalmia in the rabbit. *Journal of Heredity* **62**, 294–299

Harcourt-Brown F (1996) Calcium deficiency, diet and dental disease in pet rabbits. *Veterinary Record* **139**, 567–571

Harkness JE and Wagner JE (1989) *The Biology and Medicine of Rabbits and Rodents, 3rd edn*. Philadelphia, Lea and Febiger

Hinton M (1977) Treatment of purulent staphylococcal conjunctivitis in rabbits with autogenous vaccine. *Laboratory Animals* **11**, 163–164

Janssens G, Simoens P, Muylle S and Lauwers H (1999) Bilateral prolapse of the deep gland of the third eyelid in a rabbit: diagnosis and treatment. *Laboratory Animal Science* **49**, 105–109

Kolker AE, Moses RA, Constant MA and Becker B (1963) The development of glaucoma in rabbits. *Investigative Ophthalmology* **2**, 316–321

Lee PF (1968) Gonioscopic study of hereditary buphthalmia in rabbits. *Archives of Ophthalmology* **79**, 775–778

Marini RP, Foltz CJ, Kersten D, Batchelder M, Kaser W, Li X (1996) Microbiologic, radiographic and anatomic study of the nasolacrimal duct apparatus in the rabbit (*Oryctolagus cuniculus*). *Laboratory Animal Science* **46**, 656–662

Matros LE, Ansari MM and Van Pelt CS (1986) Eye anomaly in a dwarf rabbit. *Veterinary Medicine (Avian/Exotic Practice)* **3**, 13–14

McMaster PRB (1960) Decreased aqueous outflow in rabbits with hereditary buphthalmia. *Archives of Ophthalmology* **64**, 388–391

Millichamp NJ and Collins BR (1986) Blepharoconjunctivitis associated with *Staphylococcus aureus* in a rabbit. *Journal of the American Veterinary Medical Association* **189**, 1153–1154

Moore CP, Dubielzig R and Glaza SM (1987) Anterior corneal dystrophy of American Dutch belted rabbits: biomicroscopic and histopathological findings. *Veterinary Pathology* **24**, 28–33

Morgan RV, Duddy JM and McClurg K (1993) Prolapse of the gland of the third eyelid in dogs: a retrospective study of 89 cases (1980 to 1990). *Journal of the American Animal Hospital Association* **29**, 56–60

Petersen-Jones SM and Carrington SD (1988) *Pasteurella* dacryocystitis in rabbits. *Veterinary Record* **122**, 514–515

Port CD and Dodd DC (1983) Two cases of corneal epithelial dystrophy in rabbits. *Laboratory Animal Science* **33**, 587–588

Prince JH (1964) *The Rabbit in Eye Research*. Charles C Thomas, Springfield, IL

Reichenbach A and Baar U (1985) Retinitis pigmentosa-like tapetoretinal degeneration in a rabbit breed. *Documenta Ophthalmologica* **60**, 71–78

Remeeus P and Verbeek M (1995) The use of calcium hydroxide in the treatment of abscesses in the cheek of the rabbit resulting from a dental periapical disorder. *Journal of Veterinary Dentistry* **12**, 19–22

Roxburgh G, Boydell P and Genovese L (1998) Prolapse and hyperplasia of a third eyelid gland in 4 rabbits. *Journal of the British Association of Veterinary Ophthalmologists* **12**, 4

Ruskell GL (1964) Blood vessels of the orbit and globe. In: *The Rabbit in Eye Research*, ed. JH Prince, pp.545–547. Charles C Thomas, Springfield, IL

Sebesteny A, Sheraidah GAK and Trevam DJ (1985) Lipid keratopathy and atheromatosis in an SPF rabbit colony attributable to diet. *Laboratory Animals* **19**, 180–188

Snyder SB, Fox JG, Campell LH and Soave OA (1976) Disseminated staphylococcal disease in laboratory rabbits (*Oryctolagus cuniculus*). *Laboratory Animal Science* **26**, 86–88

Srivastava KK, Pick JR and Johnson PT (1986) Characterisation of a *Hemophilus* sp. isolated from a rabbit with conjunctivitis. *Laboratory Animals* **36**, 291–293

Stiles J, Didler E, Ritchie B, Greenacre C, Willis M and Martin C (1997) *Encephalitozoon cuniculi* in the lens of a rabbit with phacoclastic uveitis: conformation and treatment. *Veterinary and Comparative Ophthalmology* **7**, 233–238

Tesluk G, Peiffer RL and Brown D (1982) A clinical and pathological study of inherited glaucoma in New Zealand White rabbits. *Laboratory Animals* **16**, 234–239

Vareilles P, Coquet P and Lotti VJ (1980) Intraocular pressure responses to antiglaucoma agents in spontaneous buphthalmic rabbits. *Ophthalmology Research* **12**, 2296–2302

Williams DL (1999) Laboratory animal ophthalmology. In: *Veterinary Ophthalmology*, 3rd edn, ed. KN Gelatt, pp. 1209–1236. Lippincott, Williams and Wilkins, Philadelphia

Wolfer J, Grahn B and Wilcock B (1992) Spontaneous lens rupture in the rabbit. *Veterinary Pathology* **29**, 478–480

17

Exotic species

Martin P.C. Lawton

This chapter will consider ophthalmic conditions of:

- Primates
- Rodents
- Birds
- Reptiles
- Fish.

Only the more common conditions, or those differing significantly from conditions encountered in cats and dogs, are described.

Ophthalmic examination

The general approach to the ophthalmoscopic examination of exotic species should not differ from that for any domestic species. Many ocular conditions are common to all species.

Some exotic species may be dangerous to handle when conscious, and anaesthesia or sedation may be required. The majority of exotic animals have small eyes, so it is advantageous to use a magnifying loupe, slit-lamp biomicroscope or direct ophthalmoscope (with a +10 to +15 dioptre lens selected) for examination of the anterior segment. Examination without additional magnification could result in subtle changes being missed. Fundoscopy in all but the larger species is best achieved by indirect ophthalmoscopy with a 90 dioptre lens; this allows examination through a small (often undilated) pupil.

Primates

Although all primates in the UK, except marmosets (*Callithrix* spp.), are covered under the Dangerous Wild Animals Act 1976, they are nevertheless still kept as pets and may be presented to veterinary surgeons in practice for examination and treatment. For the safety of the ophthalmologist and veterinary staff, they are best sedated or anaesthetized unless an experienced handler is available. Ketamine is routinely used, although this in itself can lead to a drying of the cornea and a secondary keratitis.

Primates, except the nocturnal owl monkey or dourucouli (*Aotes trivirgatus*) have a fovea, which is a small avascular cone-rich area responsible for fine visual discrimination (Slatter, 1981).

Congenital conditions
Rhesus monkeys (*Macaca* spp.), in common with other primates, demonstrate a variety of developmental abnormalities (Acland, 1980), including colobomas of the iris and lens, subcapsular cataracts, persistent pupillary membrane and macular degeneration.

Ocular infections
Herpesvirus simiae infection of any primate, prenatal or postnatal, may result in neurological deficiency and visual impairment. This organism also has zoonotic potential.

Lens changes
As in other species, nuclear sclerosis of the lens is a common finding in the ageing non-human primate (Bellhorn, 1981).

Rodents

A variety of rodents are kept as pets. Rodents are also utilized in laboratories for toxicological studies and as experimental models, particularly for the understanding of ophthalmic pathology. Such studies have furthered knowledge of ophthalmic problems in pet rodents.

Examination is aided by correct handling. If rodents are restrained by the scruff of the neck, exophthalmos is likely, particularly in hamsters. This substantially alters the appearance of the conjunctiva, eyelids and, in some cases, cornea. The use of a short-acting gaseous anaesthetic such as isoflurane allows a thorough examination of the eyes to be performed and any necessary samples taken. This causes almost no stress to the rodent.

Mydriatics have a variable effect in rodents. Those with pigmented irises (e.g. Lister hooded rats) are more resistant to the effects of mydriatics, possibly because the drug binds to melanin in the iris, reducing its availability to the synaptic terminal. Repeated application of 10% phenylephrine three or four times within a 15-minute period usually achieves mydriasis (Kern, 1989).

Lacrimal apparatus and conjunctiva

Epiphora
Epiphora is associated with obstruction of the nasolacrimal duct as a result of malocclusion or overgrowth of the incisors. Corrective dentistry may treat this problem and prevent it from recurring.

Chromodacryorrhoea
Chromodacryorrhoea (red tears) is a common finding, especially in older rodents (Figure 17.1). It is caused by porphyrin secretion from the Harderian glands (Bauck, 1989). Infection with the coronavirus sialodacryoadenitis virus (SDAV) may also cause chromodacryorrhoea, often accompanied by other ocular problems, including blepharospasm, keratoconjunctivitis, megaloglobus and hyphaema. SDAV is highly contagious and spreads rapidly by aerosol, direct contact and fomite transmission. SDAV can also cause focal chorioretinopathy and secondary retinal degeneration.

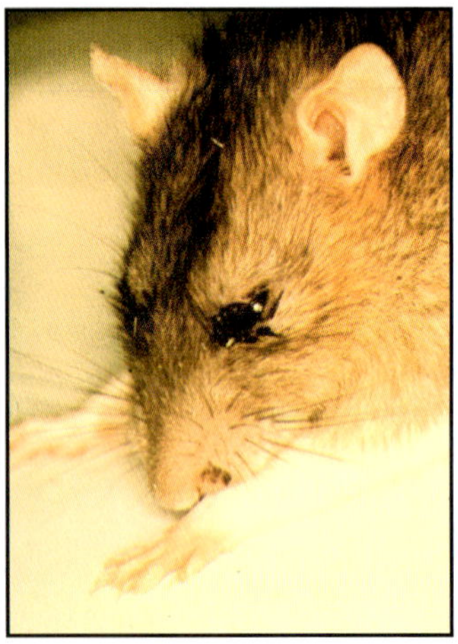

Figure 17.1 A rat with chromodacryorrhoea.

Conjunctivitis
Conjunctivitis is seen in rodents, especially hamsters, and the resulting exudate may result in the eyelids sticking together. This is often associated with the presence of sawdust bedding and is more common in old or debilitated hamsters that are no longer grooming themselves or that are dehydrated. Gentle bathing will open the eyelids, allowing treatment with topical antibiotic drops such as fusidic acid. Ointments should be avoided, as these tend to cause accumulation of further sawdust or bedding material. The bedding should be changed to newspaper and any underlying cause treated, if possible.

In common with cats and koalas (Canfield, 1987; Girjes et al., 1988), guinea pigs have been reported as being susceptible to chlamydial infection (Kern, 1989; Cherian and Magee, 1990). The condition is known as guinea pig inclusion conjunctivitis (GPIC). It is caused by *Chlamydophila caviae*. GPIC is a self-limiting disease. Initially, it presents as a mild serous ocular discharge that usually resolves in 3 or 4 weeks. *C. caviae* may also cause neonatal conjunctivitis (transmitted from the genital tracts of females).

Conjunctival foreign bodies
It is not uncommon to encounter seeds as foreign bodies in the conjunctiva of guinea pigs, especially if poor quality hay is used. Treatment involves flushing with Hartmann's solution, using a fine soft catheter. Once the foreign body has been removed, any infection should be treated topically with a suitable antibiotic (e.g. gentamicin).

Third eyelid
Prolapse of the nictitans gland occurs in gerbils. Surgical removal is indicated. Radiosurgery/electrosurgery should be employed to limit the possibility of fatal haemorrhage from the orbital venous sinus.

Cornea

Corneal dystrophy
Spontaneous inherited corneal dystrophy and stromal corneal degenerations have been reported in rats.

Trauma
The cornea can be damaged by fights or scratches (such as from hay or straw bedding). In most cases, topical treatment with a suitable antibiotic and removal of the possible cause is advised. Where the cornea has been lacerated, suturing of the cornea or placement of a third eyelid flap may be necessary, as well as antibiotic treatment. In guinea pigs, scarring of the cornea, without a previous history of trauma, is a common finding. This damage can often be associated with lipidosis, especially as guinea pigs are prone to obesity and fatty liver syndrome and often have abnormal lipid deposits in their blood vessels.

Ulceration
Corneal ulceration is quite common in pet rodents and can be confirmed by the application of topical fluorescein. Foreign bodies such as sawdust or hay bedding are a common cause, but ulceration can also result from fighting, for example, in male mice or chinchillas that are kept together. The conjunctival fornix of affected animals should be flushed to remove all foreign material and topical antibiotic drops provided. The cornea usually heals rapidly.

Lens

Cataract
Reversible lens opacities may develop during heavy sedation or anaesthesia (Bellhorn, 1973). These are thought to be associated with prolonged periods of non-blinking, resulting in the evaporation of fluid from the anterior chamber which, in turn, affects the transparency of the anterior lens.

Hereditary, dietary (sucrose) and drug-induced (e.g. streptozotocin) cataracts have all been reported in rats.

Cortical cataracts of suspected genetic origin have been reported in strains of Abyssinian and English short-haired guinea pigs (Kern, 1989). Cataracts are commonly found in older animals.

Retina
In most rodents the whole retina receives a direct blood supply from superficial retinal vessels and, like that of the dog and cat, is referred to as holangiotic. The guinea pig has a paurangiotic retinal blood supply (minute retinal vessels extending only a short distance from the disc).

Inherited retinopathy
Mice and rats have been found to show a variety of inherited retinal problems, including various retinal degenerations.

Phototoxic retinopathy

Phototoxic retinopathy is a common and important cause of degenerative retinal disease in rodents, particularly albino rats. Predisposing factors are photoperiodicity, illumination intensity and temperature. Even low intensities of light over a long period of time can produce changes in the retina. A thorough description has been given by Semple-Rowland and Dawson (1987).

Birds

The avian pupil responds poorly to changes in light intensity but it does constrict actively to aid accommodation, which may be further facilitated by compression of the protruding lens by the iris. A consensual light reflex does not occur in birds (Fox *et al.*, 1977) and slight anisocoria may be normal (Kern, 1997).

The iris musculature is predominantly striated, allowing voluntary control of pupil size (Walls, 1942). Therefore, mydriatics such as atropine or tropicamide, which act at smooth muscle neuromuscular junctions, do not dilate the pupil, even after repeated applications. Mydriasis is best achieved by general anaesthesia (especially using ketamine) or through the use of D-tubocurarine, either topically or injected into the anterior chamber. Several topical applications of a 3 mg/ml solution of D-tubocurarine over a 15-minute period has been reported as useful (Karpinski, 1986). Kern (1997) demonstrated that two applications of alcuronium chloride (5 mg/ml) 15 minutes apart can provide mydriasis for up to 3 hours, although its use was not without side effects, ranging from eyelid paralysis to hind limb paralysis.

The globe

The globe is very large in proportion to the size of the head, with the posterior segment being substantially larger than the anterior segment. Marked family differences in the shape of the eye occur. Kern (1997) describes three basic shapes of avian globes: flat (found in most birds), globose (found in diurnal raptors and crows) and tubular (found in owls).

Sunken eye disease

'Sunken eye disease' or enophthalmitis is seen in macaws (*Ara* spp.) secondary to sinusitis. This should not be confused with a lowered intraocular pressure due to anterior uveitis. Additionally, it should be noted that birds are unable to retract the globe because they have no retractor bulbi muscles (Kern, 1997). Birds with 'sunken eye disease' often have a copious mucopurulent nasal discharge in addition to the enophthalmos. This condition responds to treatment with antibiotics, combined with flushing of the sinuses. Flushing of the sinuses can be undertaken with Hartmann's solution and an appropriate antibiotic, either via the nostril cavities (with the head pointing downwards) or by intrasinus injection.

Globe rupture

Traumatic rupture of the eye does not result in collapse of the globe because of the presence of scleral ossicles. The cornea should be repaired, if possible; otherwise, support for healing from a third eyelid flap or conjunctival graft should be considered.

Enucleation

Indications for enucleation include severe trauma, neoplasia and endophthalmitis ± panophthalmitis. The technique is similar to that in mammals, except that the globe is often proportionately larger for the size of the head. A lateral canthotomy allows for better exposure (Murphy, 1987). Scissors are introduced between the globe and the orbit; the extraocular muscles and connective tissue and, eventually, the optic nerve are severed. Care must be taken when handling the globe, as traction on the optic nerve can cause damage to the optic chiasma, resulting in blindness in the contralateral eye.

Eyelids and periorbital tissues

The lower eyelid contains a semicircular fibrous plate that can make retraction and exposure of the ventral conjunctiva difficult. Eyelid neoplasia is rare.

Ankyloblepharon

Ankyloblepharon has been reported in cockatiels (*Nymphicus hollandicus*) (Buyukmihci *et al.*, 1990). Surgical attempts to reconstruct the palpebral fissures were unsuccessful, as the skin overlying the globe returned to the preoperative state, often within one month of surgery. Kern *et al.* (1985) also reported problems with attempted blepharoplasty of a partial upper eyelid agenesis in a peregrine falcon (*Falco peregrinus*).

Periorbital swellings

Swelling of the eyelids or periorbital structures are common, particularly in psittacine birds (Lawton, 1991). Swellings medial and ventromedial to the globe, often accompanied by a fibrinopurulent ocular discharge, are often the result of infraorbital sinus infection. The infraorbital sinus of birds is part of the cervicocephalic air sac system and is often involved in respiratory infections. Bacterial, viral and fungal infections have all been reported (Lawton, 1999a).

Periorbital swellings, usually without any ocular discharge, are often associated with hypovitaminosis A. This results in squamous cell metaplasia of the lacrimal gland system (Figure 17.2) and a build-up of

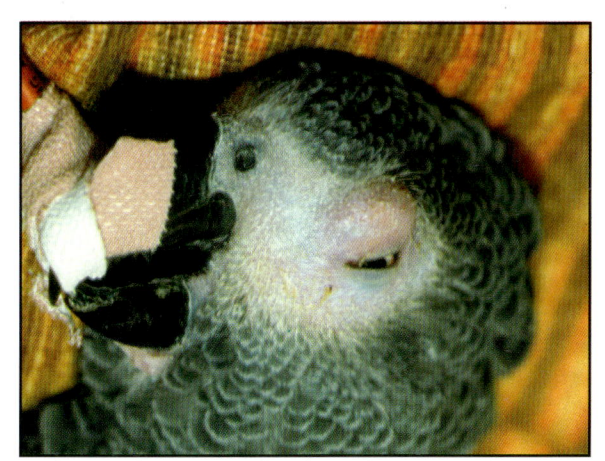

Figure 17.2 Squamous cell metaplasia of the lacrimal gland in an African grey parrot.

sterile inspissated pus (Lawton, 1988). Treatment involves surgical exploration of these masses under general anaesthesia, and the diet should be changed to one that provides adequate levels of vitamin A.

Viral blepharitis
Poxvirus infection can result in a mild proliferative lesion that may progress to a pseudotumour involving the eyelids. Poxvirus lesions generally develop 10–14 days after infection and start as a mild blepharitis. This is followed by a serous ocular discharge and swelling of the lids with the formation of dry crusty scabs that may completely seal the lids so that they are shut (Figure 17.3). Caseous masses of white fluid collect under the closed lids, leading to corneal oedema and ulceration, which may even progress to corneal perforation. The clinical illness lasts from 2–6 weeks in parrots (Karpinski and Clubb, 1986). The ocular lesions may precede a generalized infection. Poxvirus lesions respond poorly to treatment, and secondary bacterial infections should be controlled. Kern (1997) suggests that parenteral vitamin A (10,000–25,000 IU/300 g) may limit the severity of the disease if given early in its course.

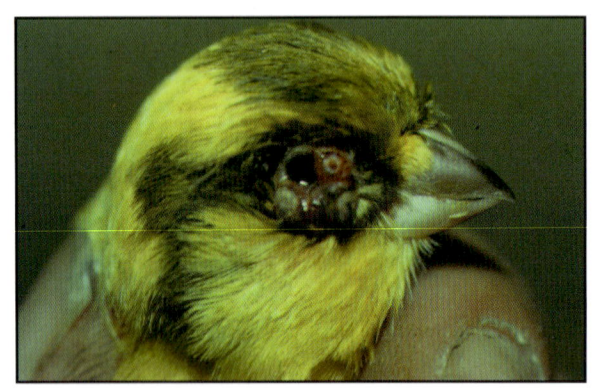

Figure 17.3 Poxvirus affecting the eyelids of a canary.

Parasitic blepharitis
Cnemidocoptes pillae (the cause of 'scaly face') can cause eyelid deformities as a result of the keratinous changes induced by the parasite (Figure 17.4). Treatment is with ivermectin at 200 μg/kg s.c. *Plasmodium* spp. have been reported as a cause of blepharitis in canaries and domestic poultry (Kern, 1997).

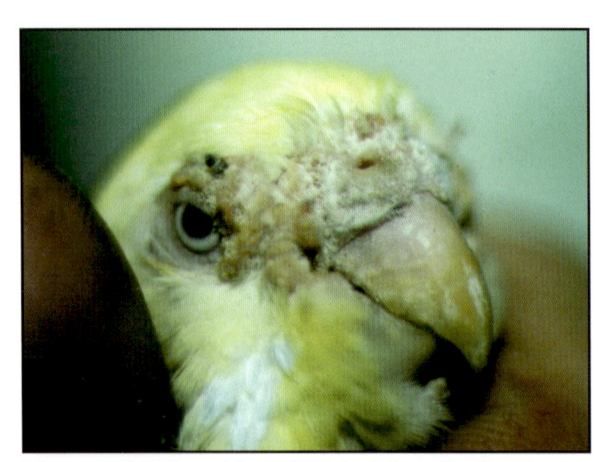

Figure 17.4 *Cnemidocoptes* infestation affecting the eyelids and cere of a budgerigar.

Trauma
Trauma to the eyelids is frequently encountered. If it is severe enough to damage the leading edge of the eyelid margin, repair should be performed under general anaesthesia using a fine (6-0) absorbable suture material.

Tear film
The Harderian gland is the major source of tears. Its duct opening can be seen as an extremely large opening in the conjunctiva at the medial canthus. A lacrimal gland is also present in all birds except penguins and owls, and is positioned inferotemporally to the globe. In budgerigars there also is a salt gland within the orbit, dorsomedial to the globe. This can result in salt precipitates forming around the eyelids, though they form more usually near the cere.

Keratoconjunctivitis sicca
Keratoconjunctivitis sicca (dry eye) occurs in birds, often as a result of lacrimal gland damage due to hypovitaminosis A (Lawton, 1991). It is characterized by a mucoid discharge on the eyelid margins and is confirmed by performing a Schirmer tear test with strips that have been cut down lengthways. The aqueous part of the tear film should be considered inadequate if it is less than 10 mm/min. Tear production may be improved by dietary changes and vitamin supplementation. Application of an artificial tear preparation, such as any used in dogs or cats but particularly the acetylcysteine/hypromellose combination is useful, especially if there is damage to the cornea.

Conjunctiva and cornea

Conjunctivitis and keratitis
Conjunctivitis and keratitis are common and may be accompanied by accumulations of inspissated pus, which cause swellings under either the upper or the lower eyelid. If the upper eyelid is affected, the pus is often found behind the third eyelid as well. Treatment involves removal of the pus by flushing the conjunctival fornix with Hartmann's solution via a fine flexible cannula. Cytology and bacteriology may be performed, although a suitable broad-spectrum antibiotic such as ciprofloxacin will often cure the condition.

Upper respiratory tract infections (viral and bacterial) are frequently associated with conjunctivitis.

Corneal ulceration
Corneal ulceration may be associated with trauma, infection, foreign bodies and dry eye.

Budgerigars (*Melopsitticus undulatus*) and cockatiels (*Nymphicus hollandicus*) kept on loose sand may experience problems if sand gets into the eye. Other foreign bodies encountered include grass awns, seed husks and gravel. Rubbing the face on the bottom of the cage tends to exacerbate the problem, because more irritant material gets into the eye. Treatment is by flushing out the foreign material with Hartmann's solution. A 5-day course of topical antibiotics (e.g. ciprofloxacin) may also be appropriate.

Severe corneal ulceration should be treated in a similar way as in mammals. For example, a third eyelid flap may be utilized (Figure 17.5). The third eyelid of birds is located in the dorsomedial fornix of the conjunctiva sac. Under general anaesthesia and with the aid of magnification, the third eyelid is pulled down and sutured to the ventrolateral bulbar conjunctiva with two small mattress sutures of 6-0 absorbable suture material. The flap is usually left in place for 2 weeks. Application of cyanoacrylate glue to the ulcer bed has also been described (Kern, 1997). In this procedure, it is important to hold the eyelids apart, dry the cornea and apply a thin film of cyanoacrylate, such as a drop on a tip of a 25 gauge needle, and allow it to dry before releasing the eyelids.

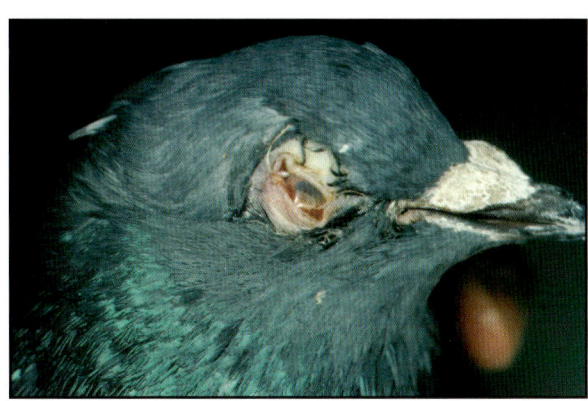

Figure 17.5 A third eyelid flap in a pigeon with corneal ulceration.

Anterior chamber and uvea

Iris colour in some species may be an indication of age or sex (Karpinksi and Clubb, 1986; Kern, 1997). Fledgling macaws have brown irises that fade to grey within the first year. Young Amazon parrots (*Amazona* spp.) have brown irises that become red/orange as they age. The irises of African grey parrots (*Psittacus erithacus*) change from a dark blue through to a grey or brown colour. Juvenile red-tailed hawks have yellow-grey irises that change to chocolate brown by 4 years of age. The irises of osprey (*Pandion* spp.) and kites (Accipitridae) are grey in nestlings, yellow in juveniles and orange in older birds, ending up as ruby-red by 5 years of age.

Many species of cockatoo (*Cacatua* spp.) show sexual dimorphism: adult males have dark brown to black irises, whereas adult females have red irises. The young of both sexes have brown irises.

Trauma

Trauma or penetrating injury can result in hyphaema, which often regresses within a few weeks. However, treatment with topical antibiotics and corticosteroids may often bring about resolution, provided there is no corneal ulceration.

Uveitis

Idiopathic recurrent uveitis is common in Macaws (Lawton, 1991). Treatment with topical corticosteroids and atropine brings temporary relief. The uveitis may not recur for several months but, ultimately, recurrent bouts result in secondary cataracts (Figure 17.6) and posterior synechiae. Chronic uveitis can result in ciliary

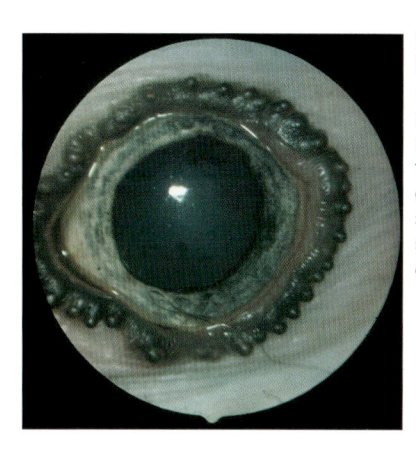

Figure 17.6 Chronic recurrent uveitis in a macaw. The iris is darkened and there is evidence of posterior synechiae and a secondary cataract.

body atrophy and phthisis bulbi (Kern, 1997), although shrinkage of the globe is limited by the presence of the scleral ossicles.

Lens

Cataract

Birds with cataracts often fail to feed properly. Cataracts are reported to occur frequently in raptors (Buyukmihci *et al.*, 1988), often associated with intraocular inflammation. However, they are also commonly noted in any aged bird. Resorption of the cataract with partial restoration of vision may occur in some cases. In others, lensectomy can be performed; however, due to the size and power of the lens, the vision of an aphakic bird is very poor. Therefore, surgery should only be contemplated in cases of bilateral cataract. The lens of birds is substantially softer than that of mammals, being mainly fluid, and, although phacoemulsification in birds has been described (Murphy and Riis, 1984), simple aspiration of the cataractous material without ultrasonic fragmentation will suffice. This may be performed through a small corneal incision.

Posterior segment

Many species with an anangiotic retina (lack of visible retinal blood vessel) have modified vessels protruding into the vitreous to supply nutrients and to remove metabolic wastes from the retina. In birds, this device is known as the pecten (Figure 17.7). The pecten is not just involved in nutritional support but also plays a part in elaboration of the intraocular fluids (Kern, 1997). On ocular movement, the pecten mechanically agitates the vitreous, facilitating fluid movement within the eye.

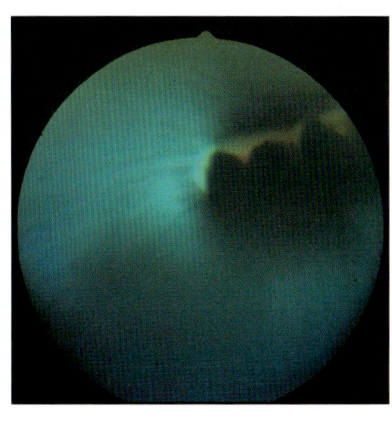

Figure 17.7 Pecten and fundus of an African grey parrot.

290 Exotic species

The avian optic disc is elongated and oval but is often hidden by the pecten. The majority of birds have one or two fovea(e), although these are absent in some waterbirds, most domestic birds and some ground dwellers, which usually only have an area centralis or visual streak. Monofoveal birds such as owls and swifts have a central fovea. Bifoveal birds include many passerines, hawks, eagles and other birds of prey; they have a principal central fovea and a secondary temporal one. In some species of hawk and eagles, these two fovea are connected by a ribbon-like area which can be visualized by ophthalmoscopy (Greenwood and Barnett, 1981). Colour vision is well developed and some birds can also see ultraviolet light which, it is now thought, may even allow them to distinguish sexes. In birds that were previously thought to be monomorphic, the feathers of males and females appear different under ultraviolet light, perhaps allowing the birds to distinguish the sexes.

Congenital conditions
Retinal dysplasia, optic nerve hypoplasia and various colobomatous defects have been associated with microphthalmos in raptors (Buyukmihci et al., 1988).

Trauma
Rupture of the pecten results in a massive haemorrhage into the vitreous and is encountered in casualty birds, especially kestrels and owls. This haemorrhage may regress over a period of several months, but a traction detachment of the retina may occur as the resulting clot contracts (Lawton, 1991).

Chorioretinitis
Chorioretinitis is common in owls. It may be associated with either nutritional deficiencies or toxoplasmosis (Greenwood and Barnett, 1981). Granulomatous inflammatory changes have been reported (Miller et al., 1988), and these may necessitate enucleation.

Retinal degenerations
Several retinal dystrophies have been reported in chickens. In one form, impaired vision was noticed at 3–8 weeks and resulted in a reduced pupillary light response (Curtis et al., 1987).

Reptiles

Reptiles, in common with birds, have striated muscle in the iris, allowing voluntary control of the pupil size. Millichamp and Jacobson (1986) used D-tubocurarine as a mydriatic in larger species of lizards or crocodilians. The injection of 0.05–0.1 ml via a 27–30 gauge needle into the anterior chamber resulted in mydriasis lasting from 30 minutes to several hours.

Reptiles have a rapid direct light response but no consensual light response.

Globe
The globe of most reptiles is almost spherical. Scleral ossicles (6–17) play an important part in accommodation in reptiles by changing the shape of the eye itself and, therefore, altering the distance between the cornea and fundus.

The ophid (snake) eye is the exception, in that it has no scleral ossicles or cartilage (Walls, 1942); it achieves accommodation by a combination of changing the shape of the lens and also moving the lens anteriorly or posteriorly (Davies, 1981). Movement of the eye is limited, except in chameleons, due to poor development of the rectus muscles, although the retractor bulbi muscle is well developed.

Congenital abnormalities
Microphthalmos is the most commonly reported congenital disorder and seems to be most common in snakes (Dupont and Murphy, 1998). It can often be mistaken for anophthalmos (very rare) unless histopathology is undertaken (Lawton, 1998a).

Eyelids
Snakes, some geckos and skinks (*Ablepharus* sp.) have fused upper and lower eyelids and, hence, no palpebral fissure. The fused eyelids form a transparent membrane known as the spectacle, brille or eyecap. Snakes and lizards (order Squamata) have a tertiary spectacle, which is mainly derived embryologically from the lower eyelid. Although it is a horny dry transparent eyescale, Millichamp et al. (1983) showed it to be highly vascular by using microsilicone injection. When the spectacle is inflamed, the vessels can be seen easily with the aid of magnification (Lawton, 1998b). Some lizards have a transparent lower eyelid, with reduced or absent scales. This allows vision through the closed eyelids while still providing protection to the eye from sand or grit (Duke-Elder, 1958).

Crocodilians, like humans, have a well developed tarsal plate (Millichamp and Jacobson, 1986); this may often become ossified (Dupont and Murphy, 1998).

Trauma
Trauma to the eyelids may occur in all species and is especially frequent in red-eared terrapins (*Trachemys scripta elegans*) as a result of feeding frenzy and fighting. Frye (1972) described damage to the eyelids in an iguana as a result of heatlamp burns and outlined a blepharoplasty technique for repair. The technique is essentially the same as that used for similar injuries in mammals.

Trauma to the spectacle of snakes, especially avulsion, is serious, as it can result in corneal desiccation due to a lack of continuity of the tear film (Figure 17.8)

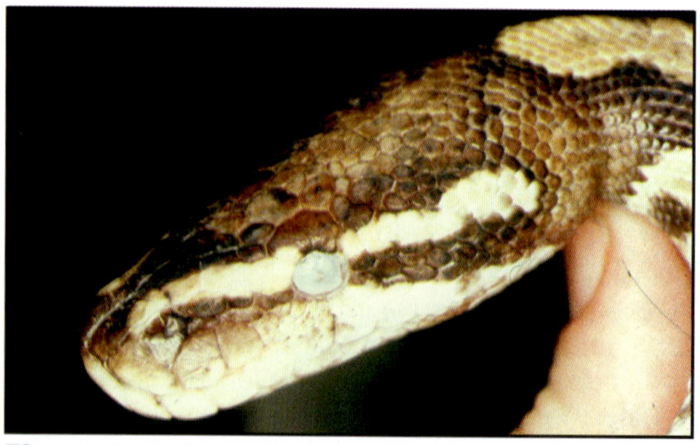

Figure 17.8 Desiccated eye following avulsion of the spectacle in a royal python.

and may ultimately result in loss of the eye (Lawton, 1998b). Treatment may be attempted with topical antibiotics and artificial tears, a cut-down soft contact lens or by transposing oral mucosa over the eye. Some success has recently been achieved by using porcine small intestinal submucosa (Lawton, unpublished data).

Blepharoedema
Blepharoedema is a common finding in reptiles and is often associated with hypovitaminosis A (see below).

Neoplasia
Neoplasia of the eyelids associated with viral infection has been reported in a number of species. These include a fibroma/papilloma in green sea turtles (*Chelonia mydas*), papillomas in green lizards (*Lacertilia* spp.; Figure 17.9) and papillomas associated with poxvirus in the speckled caiman (*Caiman crocodilus*) (Millichamp et al., 1983; Millichamp and Jacobson, 1986). In all these cases surgery may be attempted but because the tumours are associated with viruses recurrence is common.

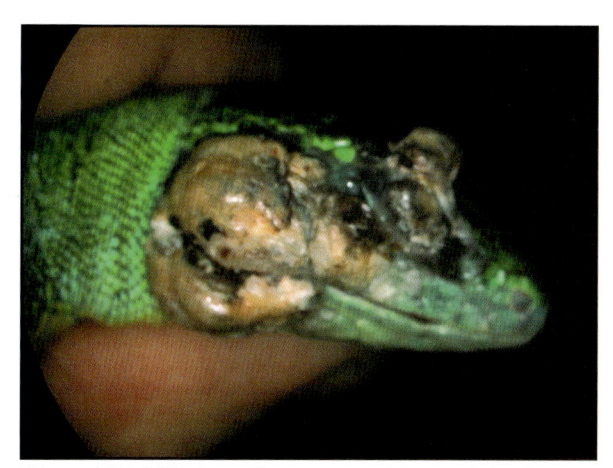

Figure 17.9 Viral papillomas around the eyelids of a European green lizard.

Retained spectacle
This is the most common ocular problem in snakes. It presents in the early stages as an indentation of the normally smooth spectacle, but the appearance becomes increasingly abnormal as there is a build-up of retained spectacles. The spectacle takes on a silver/white appearance due to the thick layer of dead skin and, in extreme cases, this will cause blindness. Diagnosis is aided with the use of magnification and, in particular, biomicroscopy. It arises because of a failure of the old spectacle to be shed during ecdysis (Lawton, 1992, 1998b, 1999b).

The retained spectacles may become secondarily infected, resulting in permanent blindness. Furthermore, temporary visual impairment may result from the retention of several spectacles.

Treatment involves soaking the retained spectacle to aid its removal. This is best done by using a wet cotton bud and rubbing from the medial and lateral canthi towards the centre of the spectacle. If the spectacle does not detach following gentle manipulation with a cotton bud, artificial tears (hypromellose) should be applied several times daily for a few days to soften the spectacle and then the technique should be repeated. Although Frye (1981) suggested using forceps or other instruments to remove a retained spectacle, this author considers that inexperienced operators could cause damage to, or even avulsion of, the underlying spectacle. If the retained spectacle cannot be removed easily, it is best to wait until the next slough and then to try again.

Third eye
In two suborders of Squamata, the Saura (lizards) and Rhyncocephalia (tuatara), there is a parietal eye (third eye). This is the remnant of the median eye, which was originally a paired visual organ on the roof of the head of provertebrates (Walls, 1942). Histologically, this is shown to have a neurological input and to contain a primitive retina and, in the case of the tuatara (*Sphenodon punctatus*), also a lens. The third eye is located in a hole below the parietal bone and, in the tuatara, the overlying scales are transparent. There is a relationship between the parietal eye, the pineal body and the habenular nucleus. The parietal eye is thought to play a role in hormone production and thermoregulation.

Tear film

Keratoconjunctivitis sicca
Keratoconjunctivitis sicca in reptiles (Figure 17.10) is most commonly due to changes in the lacrimal and Harderian glands associated with vitamin A deficiency (Elkan and Zwart, 1967). The deficiency also causes conjunctival and corneal epithelial metaplasia and hyperkeratosis. Early treatment can reverse these changes, but the more established the deficiency, the more likelihood there is of some permanent damage. Definitive diagnosis of dry eye is made using Schirmer tear test strips that have been cut down lengthways; if these show a reading of <3 mm/min, a positive diagnosis can be made. Treatment is similar to that employed in mammals, using artificial tear preparations and, when xerophthalmos is due to vitamin A deficiency, administration of vitamin A. A dose rate of 2000 IU/kg (s.c. or i.m.) on a weekly basis is advised (Lawton, 1997).

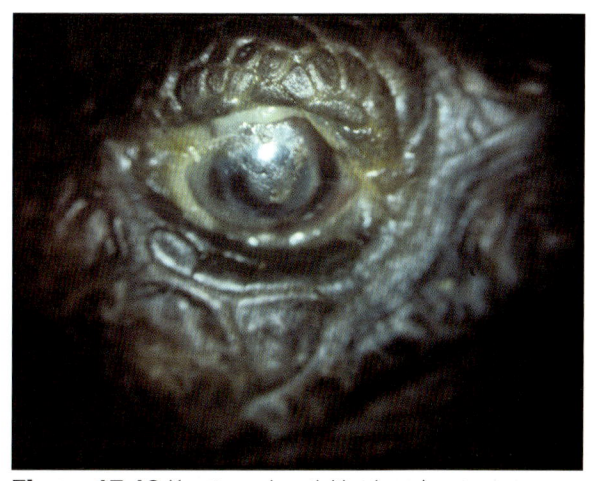

Figure 17.10 Keratoconjunctivitis sicca in a Mediterranean tortoise.

Impaired tear drainage

'Tear staining syndrome' is common in some species of tortoise (*Testudo* spp.) due to the lack of a functional nasolacrimal system (Lawton, 1997). The tears naturally spill over the eyelids and down the side of the face, eventually evaporating.

Blockage of the nasolacrimal system in snakes will result in accumulation of tears between the cornea and spectacle, resulting in an enlargement of the subspectacular space (Lawton, 1992). This can be differentiated from subspectacular abscesses because the fluid is clear. Patency of the snake's nasolacrimal drainage system may be investigated by injecting a small amount of fluorescein through the lateral canthus of the spectacle into the subspectacular space and then examining the mouth for signs of fluorescein drainage (Lawton, 1999b). Patency is usually restored by cannulation via the mouth. If this is not possible, conjunctivoralostomy may be performed to create a surgical fistula (Millichamp *et al.*, 1986). Under general anaesthesia, an incision is made through the spectacle and an 18 gauge needle passed between the inferior fornix of the subspectacular space and the roof of the mouth, emerging between the palatine and maxillary teeth. Fine (0.635 mm) sialastic tubing is threaded through the needle and left *in situ* for 1 month to maintain patency (Lawton, 1998b).

Conjunctiva

Foreign bodies

The presence of foreign bodies in the conjunctival fornix is often linked to environmental conditions. In tortoises, hay seeds are a common finding, especially in those that hibernate in hay. Lizards kept on peat or sand may occasionally get these materials into their eyes, resulting in blepharospasm (Lawton, 1997). Treatment involves the removal of the foreign body by grasping it with fine forceps, or by flushing it out with Hartmann's solution via a soft fine-gauge intravenous cannula. Any ulceration or abrasion of the cornea should be treated with topical antibiotics such as gentamicin or ciprofloxacin.

Conjunctivitis

This is a common problem but, because of the lack of lysosomes in the heterophils, a mucopurulent discharge is not seen. Infectious conjunctivitis usually results in caseous plaques that are often retained within the conjunctival fornix (Figure 17.11). The causative organism is usually opportunistic and of the Gram-negative family, Enterobactereacae; *Pseudomonas* spp. are especially common. The presence of these plaques can cause a foreign body reaction. In reptiles other than snakes presented with a closed eye, the conjunctival fornix should be flushed with Hartmann's solution via a fine soft cannula (24 gauge) or explored by using wetted endodontic paper points in order to remove any caseous plaques. Topical broad-spectrum antibiotics such as ciprofloxacin usually control the infection (Lawton, 1997).

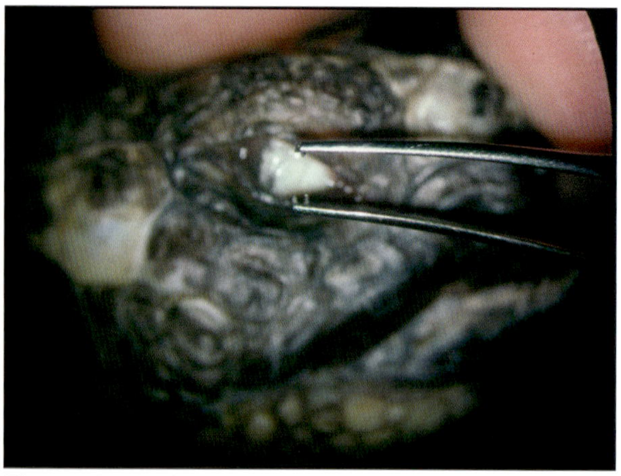

Figure 17.11 Caseous plaque in the conjunctival fornix of a Mediterranean tortoise.

Reptiles with vitamin A deficiency may develop caseous masses in the conjunctival fornix of similar appearance to those found in conjunctivitis. In this instance, however, the masses are associated with desquamated cells due to xerophthalmos (see above).

Conjunctivitis in snakes presents as a subspectacular abscess (Lawton, 1999b). The spectacle appears cloudy or white and may be distorted. These cases often result from stomatitis and ascending infection of the nasolacrimal duct, although haematogenous spread of systemic infection may occur. The condition may be unilateral or bilateral. Treatment involves cutting a small wedge through the spectacle at the lateral canthus and flushing the subspectacular space with Hartmann's solution daily (Figure 17.12). A swab should also be taken for culture and sensitivity. A suitable ophthalmic solution such as ciprofloxacin or gentamicin is applied after flushing. Depending on the culture and sensitivity results, systemic antibiotic treatment may also be required.

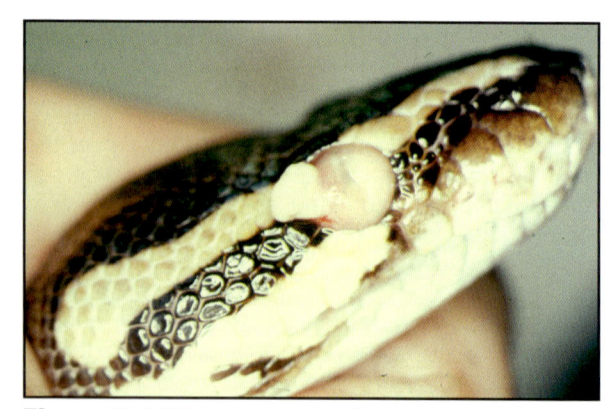

Figure 17.12 Subspectacular abscess in a royal python. The spectacle has been lanced laterally.

Cornea

The reptilian cornea is thin. There is no Bowman's layer, although Descemet's membrane is present in all reptiles except a few geckos (Duke-Elder, 1958).

Keratitis

Keratitis in tortoises associated with a white corneal mass may be the result of infection with *Moraxella,*

Pseudomonas or *Aeromonas* spp. (Lawton, 1997; Figure 17.13). Such keratitis is contagious and should be considered to be a 'herd' problem. Treatment consists of removal of the plaque from the cornea under general anaesthesia. Samples should be sent for culture and sensitivity. Topical treatment with a suitable antibiotic such as ciprofloxacin usually cures any infection.

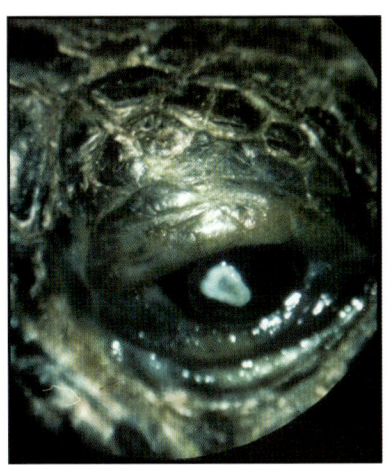

Figure 17.13 Bacterial keratitis in a Mediterranean tortoise.

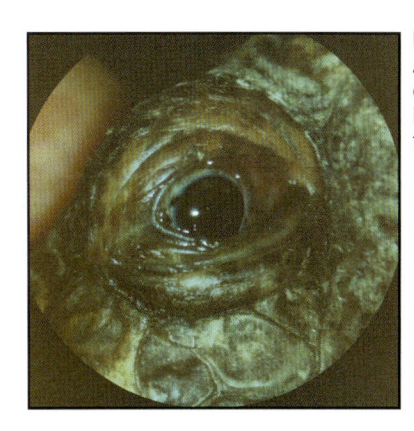

Figure 17.15 Arcus lipoides corneae in a Mediterranean tortoise.

Fungal keratitis occurs in snakes (Figure 17.14); if untreated, panophthalmitis may result, necessitating enucleation of the affected eye (Zwart *et al.*, 1973). Long-term administration of corticosteroids can predispose to fungal overgrowth. Diagnosis is made by demonstrating fungal hyphae on corneal scrapings. Treatment is with topical miconazole.

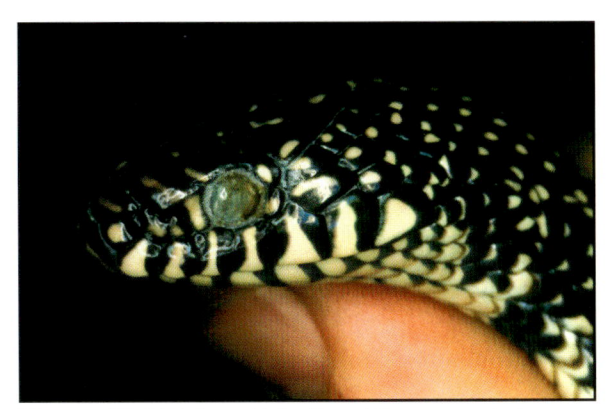

Figure 17.14 A fungal infection of the spectacle in a Florida king snake.

Corneal ulceration

Ulceration may be associated with foreign bodies or trauma, as in other species. Traumatic lacerations can be sutured with a fine suture material (8-0 or 10-0 Mersilene, Ethicon) and a course of topical antibiotic should also be provided. Severe ulcerations in chelonia and lizards may be treated by performing a third eyelid flap.

Arcus lipoides corneae

Arcus lipoides corneae is seen as a white infiltration of the peripheral cornea. This is most commonly seen in adult tortoises (Figure 17.15) and is considered part of the normal ageing process (Lawton, 1997).

Anterior chamber and uveal tract

Uveitis

Uveitis may result from trauma or infection (bacterial, fungal or viral) or may be associated with neoplasia. The clinical signs and treatment are similar to those in mammals.

Hyphaema and hypopyon may occur following exposure to freezing temperatures, due to hibernation in unsuitable conditions or unnatural environments; this is particularly noted in chelonians (Lawton, 1989; Figure 17.16). The resulting problems are a direct result of subnormal temperatures. The effects on the eyes are evident on emergence from hibernation. The owners often present such animals to the veterinary surgeon as they are anorexic, showing signs of blindness or, in extreme cases, showing CNS signs due to brain or liver damage, which is also caused from the freezing episodes. Cataracts (see below) may also be present.

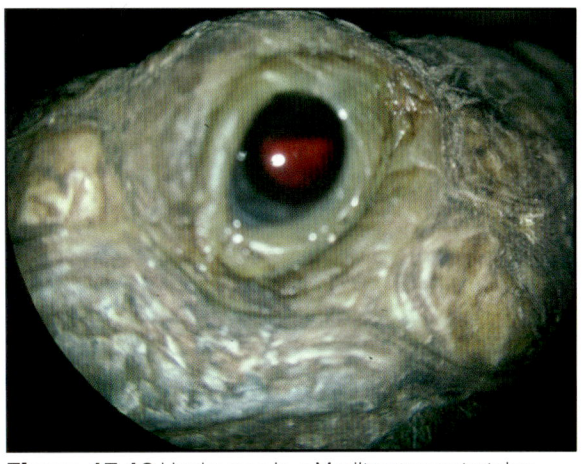

Figure 17.16 Hyphaema in a Mediterranean tortoise recently out of hibernation.

Lens

Cataract

As in all species, cataracts may occur for a variety of reasons. Cataracts in tortoises have been associated with freezing episodes (Lawton, 1989; Lawton and Stoakes, 1989). Duke-Elder (1958) reported that the chelonian lens is extremely soft and almost fluid-like in consistency. It is hypothesized that, because of this, they are particularly prone to damage from low temperatures. In some cases, these changes are reversible, although it may take up to 18 months for the lens to clear (Lawton and Stoakes, 1989). Cataract surgery in reptiles can be performed in a similar manner to that already described for birds.

Retina
Like birds, reptiles have an anangiotic retina containing both rods and cones. Nutrients are supplied and metabolic wastes removed by choroidal blood vessels or modified vessels protruding into the vitreous. Chelonians rely solely on choroidal blood vessels. In lizards a structure similar to the avian pecten is present, known as the conus papilaris. In snakes, there is a vascular network that overlies the retina, known as the membrana vasculosa retinae, which is a branching array of vessels from the choroid running into the posterior vitreous near the optic disc. In adult crocodilians the conus papilaris is functionless and is reduced to a glial pad with one or two capillaries that scarcely protrudes into the vitreous (Walls, 1942; Duke-Elder, 1958). In addition, crocodilians have a tapetum formed by guanine crystals.

Retinal damage and degeneration
Retinal damage associated with vitamin A deficiency, and following freezing episodes, has been reported in tortoises (Lawton, 1989). In certain circumstances, treatment with vitamin A (2000 IU/kg s.c. or i.m. at 7–14-day intervals for up to three occasions) may result in a clinical improvement.

Retinal degeneration has been reported in tokay geckos (*Gekko gecko*) (Bonney *et al.*, 1978; Schmidt and Toft, 1981), although it is also thought to be a sporadic finding in most reptile families (Millichamp and Jacobson, 1986).

Fish

Ophthalmological examination of pet fish is seldom undertaken. Cataracts and corneal lesions occur commonly and should be looked for during the routine clinical examination. Toxic, dietary or parasitic aetiologies should always be considered.

Cornea
Any chemicals added to the water should be considered as capable of having an effect on the eye. The actions of surfactants on the eyes of the carp family have been investigated (Kohbara *et al.*, 1987).

Transportation of fish may result in a high incidence of corneal opacity as a result of injury and corneal oedema (Ubels and Edelhauser, 1987). Corneal epithelial abrasions in fish are demonstrated by topical application of fluorescein dye when the fish are out of water. Anything that compromises the integrity of the corneal epithelium will result in oedema and opacity. In severe cases of damage to the corneal epithelium resulting in corneal oedema, cataracts may also develop, usually within 24 hours of the original damage. The oedema may persist for as long as 96 hours after the initial injury. Provided there are no complications, both cornea and lenses should regain normal transparency within 7 days (Ubels and Edelhouser, 1987). Elasmobranchs are an exception, for in these fish the corneal stroma does not swell, so opacity due to corneal oedema is not seen, and the presenting sign of corneal epithelial damage is cataract formation.

Lens

Cataract
Reversible cataracts in fish can result from osmotic changes. Most fish have a limited capacity to regulate their aqueous humour osmolarity and, therefore, a reduction in water osmolarity will cause the lens to become oedematous, giving it a cloudy appearance.

Parasites, such as various trematode species in trout and *Diplostomum spathaceum* in freshwater fish, cause cataracts by direct invasion of the lens by larvae. *Tylodeiphys podicipina* is specific to perch, where the metacercariae infect the eyes (Kennedy, 1987).

Retina

Retinoblastoma
Retinoblastoma, the most common intraocular tumour of children, has been reported in two species of fish (Reimschuessell *et al.*, 1989).

References

Acland GM (1980) Development anomalies. In: *The Eye in Veterinary Practice. Vol. 1: Extraocular diseases*, ed. JR Blogg, pp. 106–107. WB Saunders, Philadelphia

Bauck L (1989) Ophthalmic conditions in pet rabbits and rodents. *Compendium on Continuing Education for the Practicing Veterinarian* **11**, 258–266

Bellhorn RW (1973) Ophthalmological disorders of exotic and laboratory animals. *Veterinary Clinics of North America: Small Animal Practice* **3**, 345–355

Bellhorn RW (1981) Laboratory animal ophthalmology. In: *Textbook of Veterinary Ophthalmology*, ed. KN Gelatt, pp. 649–671. WB Saunders, Philadelphia

Bonney CH, Hartfiel DH and Schmidt RW (1978) *Klebsiella pneumoniae* infection with secondary hypopyon in Tokay gecko lizards. *Journal of the American Veterinary Medical Association* **173**, 1115–1116

Buyukmihci NC, Murphy CJ and Schulz T (1988) Developmental ocular disease of raptors. *Journal of Wildlife Diseases* **24**, 207–213

Buyukmihci NC, Murphy CJ, Paul-Murphy J, Hacker DB, Laratta LJ and Brooks DE (1990) Eyelid malformation in four cockatiels. *Journal of the American Veterinary Medical Association* **196**, 1490–1492

Canfield TJ (1987) A mortality survey of free-range koalas from the north coast of New South Wales. *Australian Veterinary Journal* **64**, 325–328

Cherian PV and Magee WE (1990) Monoclonal antibodies to *Chlamydia psittaci* guinea pig inclusion conjunctivitis (GPIC) strain. *Veterinary Microbiology* **22**, 43–51

Curtis PE, Baker JR, Curtis R and Johnston A (1987) Impaired vision in chickens associated with retinal defects. *Veterinary Record* **190**, 113–114

Davies PMC (1981) Anatomy and physiology. In: *Diseases of Reptilia, vol.1*, ed. JE Cooper and OF Jackson, pp. 9–73. Academic Press, London

Duke-Elder S (1958) The eyes of reptiles. In: *Systems of Ophthalmology, vol. 1: The Eye in Evolution*, pp. 353–395. Mosby, St. Louis

Dupont C and Murphy CJ (1998) Ocular disorders in reptiles. In: *The Biology, Husbandry and Health Care of Reptiles, Vol. III: Health Care of Reptiles*, ed. L Ackerman, pp. 735–746. TFH, Neptune City, NJ

Elkan E and Zwart P (1967) The ocular diseases of young terrapins caused by vitamin A deficiency. *Pathologia Veterinaria* **4**, 201–222

Fox R, Lehmkuhl SW and Bush RC (1977) Stereopsis in the falcon. *Science* **197**, 79–81

Frye FL (1972) Blepharoplasty in an iguana. *Veterinary Medicine and Small Animal Clinician* **67**, 1110–1111

Frye FL (1981) Traumatic and physical diseases. In: *Diseases of the Reptilia, Vol. 2,* ed. JE Cooper and OF Jackson, p.387. Academic Press, London

Girjes AA, Hugall AF, Timms P and Lavin MF (1988) Two distinct forms of *Chlamydia psittaci* associated with disease and infertility in *Phascolarctos cinereus* (koala). *Infection and Immunity* **56**, 1897–1900

Greenwood AG and Barnett KC (1981) The investigation of visual defects in raptors. In: *Recent Advances in the Study of Raptor Diseases,* ed. JE Cooper and AG Greenwood, pp.131–135. Chiron Publications, Keighley

Karpinski LG (1986) Ophthalmology. In: *Clinical Avian Medicine and Surgery, including Aviculture,* ed. GJ Harrison and LR Harrison, pp. 278–281. WB Saunders, Philadelphia

Karpinski LG and Clubb SL (1986) Clinical aspects of ophthalmology in caged birds. In: *Current Veterinary Therapy IX,* ed. RW Kirk, pp. 616–621. WB Saunders, Philadelphia

Kennedy CR (1987) Long term stability in the populations of the eye fluke *Tylodephys physpodicipina* (Digenea; diplostomatidae) in perch. *Journal of Fish Biology* **31**, 571–581

Kern TJ (1989) Ocular disorders of rabbits, rodents and ferrets. In: *Current Veterinary Therapy X,* ed. RW Kirk, pp. 681–685. WB Saunders, Philadelphia

Kern TJ (1997) Disorders of the special senses. In: *Avian Medicine and Surgery,* ed. RB Altman *et al.,* pp. 563–589. WB Saunders, Philadelphia

Kern TJ, Murphy CJ and Heck WR (1985) Partial upper eyelid ageneses in a peregrine falcon. *Journal of the American Veterinary Medical Association* **187**, 1207

Kohbara J, Murachl S and Namba K (1987) Ocular abnormalities in carp chronically exposed to various surfactants. *Nippon Suisan Gakka* **53**, 979–983

Lawton MPC (1988) Nutritional diseases. In: *Manual of Parrots, Budgerigars and Other Psittacine Birds,* ed. CJ Price, pp. 157–162. BSAVA Publications, Cheltenham

Lawton MPC (1989) Neurological problems of exotic species. In: *Manual of Small Animal Neurology,* ed. SJ Wheeler, pp. 233–247. BSAVA Publications, Cheltenham

Lawton MPC (1991) Avian ophthalmology. In: *Proceedings, 1st Conference of the European Committee of Avian Veterinarians,* ed. G Dorrestein, pp. 154–156. AAV, Vienna

Lawton MPC (1992) Ophthalmology. In: *Manual of Reptiles,* ed. PH Beynon *et al.,* pp. 157–169. BSAVA Publications, Cheltenham

Lawton MPC (1997) Common ophthalmic problems seen in Chelonia. In: *Proceedings, 4th Annual Conference of the Association of Reptilian and Amphibian Veterinarians, Texas,* ed. MW Frahm, pp.175–178. ARAV, Chester Heights, PA

Lawton MPC (1998a) Introduction to reptilian ophthalmology. In: *Proceedings, 5th Annual Conference of the Association of Reptilian and Amphibian Veterinarians, Kansas City, Missouri,* ed. MW Frahm, pp.115–118. ARAV, Chester Heights, PA

Lawton MPC (1998b) Disease of the spectacle. In: *Proceedings, 5th Annual Conference of the Association of Reptilian and Amphibian Veterinarians, Kansas City, Missouri,* ed. MW Frahm, pp.119–122. ARAV, Chester Heights, PA

Lawton MPC (1999a) Management of respiratory disease in psittacine birds. *Journal of Veterinary Postgraduate Clinical Study, In Practice* **21**(2), 76–88

Lawton MPC (1999b) *The Spectacle in Health and Disease.* RCVS Diploma of Zoological Medicine dissertation.

Lawton MPC and Stoakes LC (1989) Post hibernation blindness in tortoises (*Testudo* spp.). In: *Third International Colloquium on Pathology of Reptiles and Amphibians, Orlando, Florida,* ed. ER Jacobson, pp. 97–98. ARAV, Chester Heights, PA

Miller WW, Boosinger DR and Maslin WR (1988) Granulomatous uveitis in an owl. *Journal of the American Veterinary Medical Association* **193**, 365–366

Millichamp NJ and Jacobson ER (1986) Ophthalmic diseases of reptiles. In: *Current Veterinary Therapy IX,* ed. RW Kirk, pp. 621–624. WB Saunders, Philadelphia

Millichamp NJ, Jacobson ER and Woolf ED (1983) Diseases of the eye and ocular adnexae in reptiles. *Journal of the American Veterinary Medical Association* **183**, 1205–1212

Millichamp NJ, Jacobson ER and Dziezyc J (1986) Conjunctivoralostomy for the treatment of an occluded lacrimal duct in a blood python. *Journal of the American Veterinary Medical Association* **189**, 1136–1138

Murphy CJ (1987) Raptor ophthalmology. *Compendium on Continuing Education for the Practicing Veterinarian* **9**, 241–260

Murphy CJ and Riis RC (1984) Lens extraction by phacoemulsification in two raptors. *Journal of the American Veterinary Medical Association* **185**, 1403–1406

Reimschuessell R, Bennett RO, May EB and Lipsky MM (1989) Retinoblastoma in a porkfish (*Anisotremus virginicus linnaeus*) and a brown bullhead (*Lectalurus nebulosus lesueur*). *Journal of Comparative Pathology* **101**, 215–220

Schmidt RE and Toft JD (1981) Ophthalmic lesions in animals from a zoological collection. *Journal of Wildlife Diseases* **17**, 267–275

Semple-Rowland SL and Dawson WW (1987) Retinal cyclic light damage threshold for albino rats. *Laboratory Animal Science* **37**, 289–298

Slatter DH (1981) *Fundamentals of Veterinary Ophthalmology.* WB Saunders, Philadelphia

Ubels JL and Edelhauser HF (1987) Effects of corneal epithelial abrasion on corneal transparency, aqueous humour composition and lenses of fish. *Progressive Fish Culturist* **49**, 219–224

Walls GL (1942) The vertebrate eye and its adaptive radiation. *Cranbrook Institute of Science Bulletin* **19**, 607–640

Zwart P, Verwer MAJ, Devrles GA, Hermandiez-Nijhof EJ and Devries HW (1973) Fungal infection of the eyelids of the snake, *Epicrates chenchria maurus*: Enucleation under halothane narcosis. *Journal of Small Animal Practice* **14**, 773–779

Appendix 1

Differential diagnosis

Simon Petersen-Jones and Sheila Crispin

This Appendix considers the differential diagnosis of those presenting signs or owner's complaints where the primary lesion may be in one of a number of ocular or adnexal tissues. These cases require a thorough and logical approach if the primary lesion is to be identified.

The presentations included are:

- Canine 'wet' eye
- Acute canine red eye
- The painful eye in dogs and cats
- The opaque eye
- Sudden loss of vision
- Slowly progressive vision loss
- Congenital and early-onset poor vision/blindness.

Canine 'wet' eye

Condition	Key features
Unrelated to tear film	Aqueous leakage after penetrating and perforating injuries, post-surgical wound breakdown and wound dehiscence.
Excessive lacrimation	Associated with pain (see Painful eye).
Inadequate tear distribution	Note that ocular discomfort may be an accompanying feature of some of the conditions listed below: e.g. low-grade trauma from facial hair and lashes may be a feature of entropion, medial canthal hairs and nasal folds; discomfort from exposure keratopathy may be a feature of eyelid colobomas, ectropion and lagophthalmos. Conditions such as ectopic cilia and large eyelid masses impinging directly on the cornea will result in frank ocular pain.
Poor eyelid anatomy	Entropion. Ectropion. Complex combinations. Diagnosis made by simple observation of the eyelids in an unrestrained unsedated conscious animal.
Lash and hair abnormalities	Trichiasis, distichiasis, ectopic cilia. Medial canthal hairs, nasal folds. Diagnosis made from simple observation; magnification should be used when ectopic cilia are suspected.
Eyelid colobomas	Diagnosis made from simple observation.
Lagophthalmos	Diagnosis made by observing blink rate, adequacy of blink and examining eyelid/globe apposition (congruence).
Eyelid masses	Diagnosis made from simple observation of the eyelids, including movement of the mass on blinking.
Eyelid cicatrization	Diagnosis made from simple observation of the eyelids, including adequacy of blinking.
Inadequate tear drainage (epiphora)	
Congenital and developmental	Aplasia/hypoplasia of any portion of the drainage system. In dogs and cats, commonest abnormality is at proximal end of lacrimal drainage system. Related to conformational defects in breeds such as the Miniature and Toy Poodle and Bichon Frisé. Diagnosis made by direct visual inspection.
Acquired	Internal narrowing or blockage of lacrimal drainage system (e.g. foreign bodies, dacryocystitis). Discharge originates from lacrimal punctum and foreign bodies can often be seen lodged there. External pressure on lacrimal drainage system (e.g. dental disease, inflammatory and neoplastic sinus and nasal problems).

Acute canine red eye

Condition	Key features
Acute problems of globe and orbit	
Globe prolapse	Redness due to vascular congestion because of impeded venous return.
Endophthalmitis and panophthalmitis	Gross changes in intraocular appearance as well as hyperaemia of externally visible vessels ± neovascularization of the cornea.
Space-occupying lesions	Inflammatory (e.g. abscess/cellulitis) and neoplastic.
Acute conjunctivitis	Common. Uncomfortable rather than painful. Ocular discharge. Active hyperaemia of conjunctival vessels, usually affecting all the conjunctival surfaces (bulbar, palpebral and nictitating) as a diffuse superficial redness. Conjunctival vessels superficial and mobile. Conjunctival oedema (chemosis). No effect on intraocular structures. No effect on vision. Intraocular pressure (IOP) normal.
Acute keratitis	Relatively common, especially as a consequence of trauma. Pain, blepharospasm, photophobia and lacrimation. Active hyperaemia of the conjunctival vessels ± deeper vessels, depending on the depth of corneal involvement. Some form of corneal opacity will be present and ulceration may also be part of the presentation. Reflex uveitis may be present and the pupil may be more constricted (miotic) than that of an unaffected eye. May affect vision, depending upon the extent of corneal opacity and the degree of pain. IOP normal, except for deep keratitis with uveal involvement.
Acute anterior uveitis	Uncommon. Marked pain, blepharospasm, photophobia and lacrimation. Note that retraction of the globe may be a feature of ocular pain irrespective of cause – apparent enophthalmos. In early cases, there is active hyperaemia of conjunctival and deeper vessels, most marked immediately behind the limbus overlying the ciliary body (perilimbal hyperaemia). Later, the inflammation hyperaemia is more diffuse but only affects the globe. Subtle pancorneal oedema. Loss of anterior chamber clarity because of aqueous flare. Iris hyperaemic and swollen; fine detail lost. Pupil may be constricted and poorly responsive under a range of lighting conditions. Variable vision loss according to the severity of the inflammation (loss of vision is likely if panuveitis is present). IOP reduced.
Acute glaucoma	Uncommon but should always be ruled out in susceptible breeds, including terriers with lens luxation. Marked pain, blepharospasm, photophobia and lacrimation. Obvious congestion of conjunctival and episcleral vessels. Episcleral vessels wider than conjunctival vessels and arranged at 90 degrees to the limbus. Panstromal oedema if IOP >40 mmHg. Anterior chamber clear; iris detail normal. Pupil dilated, often widely, and usually unresponsive to light. Lens may be in situ, subluxated or luxated. Iridodonesis will be present if the lens has luxated or is subluxated. IOP raised. Vision loss to some extent parallels rise in IOP; when IOP >60 mmHg the eye may be blind.
Episcleritis	Uncommon. Non-painful to uncomfortable. Inflamed region may be nodular and localized, or diffuse. Active hyperaemia of conjunctival vessels and underlying episcleral vessels, localized or diffuse according to region affected. Mild corneal oedema or frank lipid deposition may be present; depth of corneal involvement is best guide to level of inflammation. Usually no effect on intraocular structures and no effect on vision.
Scleritis	Rare. Non-painful to painful. Inflamed area usually nodular, less commonly diffuse, but depth of inflammation makes boundaries difficult to define. Although overlying conjuctival and episcleral vessels are hyperaemic, the inflammation is based on the scleral vessels. Application of phenylephrine blanches superficial vessels and allows visualization of inflamed scleral vessels. Inflamed scleral vessels appear dark red, bluish red or almost purple and are immobile. Mild corneal oedema or frank lipid deposition may be present; depth of corneal involvement is best guide to level of inflammation. Low-grade uveitis may be present. Fundus examination may suggest thickening of the sclera posteriorly; ultrasonography is useful to confirm this. IOP normal or reduced. Vision ranges from unaffected to slightly impaired.
Retrobulbar abscess and orbital cellulitis	Reasonably common. Acute onset of ocular discomfort. Pyrexia may be present. Severe pain on attempting to open the mouth. Often marked congestion of the conjunctiva and a mucopurulent ocular discharge. Third eyelid prominent; exophthalmos may be present. Diffuse orbital swelling may be present when there is cellulitis.
Trauma	Common. Many possible ocular manifestations (e.g. contusion, laceration, perforation, blunt injury). Some injuries associated with foreign bodies. Redness usually relates to haemorrhage (see below) and bruising.
Ocular and intraocular haemorrhage	Common after trauma (e.g. subconjunctival, intraocular). Less common from other causes (e.g. developmental abnormalities such as collie eye anomaly and persistence of the primary vitreous, as well as clotting defects, neoplasia, systemic hypertension, chronic glaucoma). If haemorrhage prevents examination of intraocular structures, ultrasonography is necessary. Eye may be comfortable or acutely painful. IOP normal, decreased or increased.

The painful eye in dogs and cats

Ocular pain is typically associated with blepharospasm, excessive lacrimation and photophobia. Signs of ocular pain are often more subtle in cats than in dogs. Note that retraction of the globe may be a feature of ocular pain irrespective of cause – apparent enophthalmos – in the dog, but is less likely to be observed in the cat as the globe fits more closely into the orbit.

Condition	Key features
Globe/Orbital problems in which inflammation is the major abnormality	
Endophthalmitis	Uncommon. May follow penetrating injury. Can be occasional complication of intraocular surgery.
Abscess/cellulitis	Quite common (see Acute canine red eye). History of fighting helpful in the cat.
Traumatic injury and foreign bodies	Severe bruising, lacerations, blunt and penetrating injuries ± retained foreign bodies affecting the eye and adnexa (see Acute canine red eye). Long-haired dogs require careful examination, especially to ascertain extent of eyelid injuries.
Lash/hair problems	
Distichiasis	Common in the dog but often asymptomatic unless misdirected. A single misdirected lash is all that is needed to cause ocular pain. Visible on eyelid margin, usually arising from meibomian gland orifices; magnification helpful. Breed-related. Rare in the cat but when it occurs is usually associated with colobomatous eyelid defects.
Trichiasis	Common in certain dog breeds (e.g. English and American Cocker Spaniels), especially in older dogs with megalotrichiasis. Readily visible. Usually discomfort rather than frank pain.
Ectopic cilia	Uncommon in the dog. Invariably painful. Distichiasis may also be present. Cilia visible beneath the eyelid (usually the middle of the upper eyelid); magnification is helpful. Ulceration likely if presence of cilia missed. Extremely rare in the cat.
Nasal folds	Common and breed-related problem in the dog. Visible. Usually uncomfortable rather than painful.
Skin hair	In cats usually associated with colobomatous eyelid defects or eyelid surgery. In dogs usually associated with previous eyelid surgery. Diagnosis by simple observation.
Eyelid problems	
Entropion and any other eyelid defect in which eyelid turns inwards	Relatively common in the dog, but not always a cause of gross discomfort. Anatomical: Usually breed-related in the dog; site of entropion variable. Persian cats may have anatomical entropion involving the lower medial eyelid. Diagnosis by careful observation. Spastic: Less likely to be seen in the cat than the dog (anatomical differences of eyelid congruity and close orbital fit in the cat). An underlying cause (e.g. corneal ulcer) should be sought by careful examination.
Eyelid inflammation, swelling and masses	In both cats and dogs some forms of inflammatory eye disease, such as acute blepharoconjunctivitis, can be painful. Meibomianitis, chalazia and lipogranulomatous masses can cause discomfort by direct corneal contact. Pain can also be consequence of direct mechanical damage to the cornea from eyelid tumours. Benign neoplasia commonest in the dog. Squamous cell carcinoma in cats produces typical erosion of eyelid margins and is *not* associated with frank pain.
Acute dry eye	Quite common in the dog; less common in the cat. Lacklustre cornea ± corneal ulcer. Low or zero Schirmer tear test reading.
Conjunctivitis	Common. Usually irritation and discomfort rather than frank pain. Lacrimation/discharge, chemosis and active hyperaemia of conjunctival vessels. May be more severe with concurrent disease (e.g. chlamydiosis or FIV infection in the cat).
Ulcerative keratitis	Common. Usually painful. Redness and change of corneal appearance and fluorescein-positive area (see Acute canine red eye; substantially similar in the cat).
Acute anterior uveitis	Uncommon. Pain can be severe (see Acute canine red eye). Most cases of anterior uveitis in the cat, other than those caused by trauma, are chronic and not particularly painful.
Acute glaucoma	
Primary glaucoma	Uncommon in the dog and breed-related (see Acute canine red eye). Breed-related glaucoma very rare in the cat.
Secondary glaucoma	Reasonably common in the dog. Rare in the cat. In the dog, primary lens luxation is a common cause and is painful. In the cat, lens luxation does not necessarily result in glaucoma and the eye is uncomfortable rather than painful.
Scleritis and scleral infiltration	May be painful, especially if uveitis also present (see Acute canine red eye). In the cat lymphomatous infiltration can occur and is associated with pain and redness, although the conjunctiva is probably a commoner site

The opaque eye

Unless otherwise stated, the examples apply to both the dog and the cat.

Condition	Examples and features
Globe/orbit defects	Opacity may be result of multiple or single ocular defects. Extent of ocular involvement variable.
Congenital and developmental	Congenitally small eye (e.g. cystic eye, microphthalmos). Cornea: focal or diffuse opacities; depth of corneal involvement varies. Anterior segment dysgenesis (e.g. ppm attached to cornea ± lens). Lens: cataract (position and extent of opacity varies); variations in lens shape and size. Vitreous: persistence of primary vitreous, tunica vasculosa lentis, persistent hyperplastic primary vitreous. Vitreous and retina: vitreoretinal dysplasia, congenital non-attachment of retina.
Endophthalmitis/panophthalmitis	Gross opacity of the globe usually a feature.
Phthisis bulbi	End result of severe ocular insult; the eye is small and opaque.
Traumatic injury and foreign bodies	Many potential causes of opacity; that associated with chemical and thermal injury often the most spectacular. Corneal damage. Iris prolapse. Intraocular haemorrhage. Lens subluxation and luxation. Lens rupture. Cataract (delayed complication). Globe rupture/collapse.
Dry eye	Lacklustre cornea initially ± ulceration. Severe corneal changes in chronic cases (vascularization/pigmentation/xerosis).
Conjunctivitis	Ocular discharge.
Cornea	The hallmark of corneal disease is opacity (see Chapter 8 for a more complete list)
Dystrophies	Epithelial and endothelial dystrophies
Accumulations/infiltrates/deposits	Neurometabolic storage diseases. Florida keratopathy. Inflammatory cells. Lipid. Pigment. Calcium. Foreign bodies.
Neovascularization	Many possible causes (see Chapter 8).
Ulcerative keratitis	Many possible causes. Universally associated with a change of corneal appearance (see Chapter 8).
Non-ulcerative keratitis	Chronic superficial keratoconjunctivitis (pannus) in the dog. Proliferative keratoconjunctivitis, corneal sequestrum and chronic herpetic keratitis in the cat. Pigmentary keratitis: predisposing factors usually anatomical combined with anaesthetic cornea. Epithelial inclusion cyst in the dog. Corneal abscess.
Anterior chamber	Haemorrhage (see Acute canine red eye). Lipid: raised plasma triglyceride – turbid aqueous; raised chylomicrons – opaque (milk white), aqueous. Aqueous flare, keratic precipitates, mutton fat precipitates. Hypopyon. Neoplastic cells. Pigment. Lens (anterior luxation). Lens material (lens rupture).
Glaucoma	Acute: panstromal corneal oedema. Chronic: Haab's striae (breaks in Descemet's membrane), corneal vascularization, oedema, globe enlargement ± exposure keratopathy. Chronic glaucoma can be associated with intraocular haemorrhage. Lens may be subluxated or luxated.
Uveal tract	
Uveitis	Subtle panstromal oedema. Inflammatory cells and debris (posterior cornea, anterior chamber, anterior and posterior lens capsule, vitreous). Hyphaema may be a feature of severe inflammation. Miotic pupil, iris oedema and infiltration.
Uveal neoplasia	Hyphaema. Neoplastic cells. Iris infiltration
Lens	Trauma-induced changes (see earlier). Senile nuclear sclerosis. Cataract. Subluxation and luxation.
Vitreous	
Vitritis	Inflammatory cells: intermediate uveitis – pars planitis; more widespread – vitritis (hyalitis).
Endophthalmitis and panophthalmitis	Gross infiltration by inflammatory cells to frank pus.
Synchysis scintillans	Mainly cholesterol crystals.
Asteroid hyalosis	Calcium and lipid complexes.
Haemorrhage	For differential diagnosis see Acute canine red eye. When intraocular neoplasia is present, mass may be demonstrable by direct examination ± imaging techniques.
Intravitreal cysts	Cystic mass may be identified by direct examination ± imaging techniques.
Posterior luxation of lens	
Retina	Congenital and acquired (usually post-traumatic) vascular anomalies/abnormalities. Pre-retinal haemorrhage. Retinal detachment.

Sudden loss of vision

Vision loss associated with unilateral conditions may not be apparent to the owners. The presenting sign in some conditions may also include pain and altered appearance of the eye(s). Some animals with disease that causes a slow loss of vision present with a history of apparent sudden loss of vision. This may be because they have been coping with the slow loss of vision and the vision loss becomes obvious to the owners when the animal's environment is changed.

Condition	Key features
Trauma	Unilateral or bilateral. Signs of ocular damage or head injury apparent e.g. globe prolapse, red eye, loss of corneal integrity, hyphaema, retinal detachment. Ocular ultrasonography may be useful to assess extent of damage to globe where anterior segment lesions preclude direct visualization.
Acute onset of corneal opacity (e.g. oedema)	Unilateral or bilateral. Obvious corneal opacity.
Uveitis (anterior, posterior and panuveitis)	Unilateral or commonly bilateral. Anterior uveitis and panuveitis associated with red, painful or uncomfortable eye. Change in appearance: corneal oedema, aqueous turbidity, flare, hypopyon, hyphaema, miotic pupil. Posterior uveitis associated with active chorioretinitis lesions, retinal oedema, haemorrhage, detachment and possibly papillitis.
Glaucoma (see also Painful eye and Acute canine red eye)	Most commonly unilateral initially but other eye may be predisposed. May be primary angle closure or goniodysgenesis, or secondary to anterior lens luxation. Other secondary forms of glaucoma usually have a preceding history of ocular abnormality. Altered appearance of globe: corneal oedema, mid-dilated poorly responsive pupil. With anterior lens luxation, lens can be seen in anterior chamber. Uncommon in cats.
Diabetic cataract	Usually bilateral. Can have very rapid onset of cataract formation. Rapidly developing cataracts are often associated with a lens-induced uveitis that may cause a red eye and discomfort. Rare in the cat.
Intraocular haemorrhage	Unilateral or bilateral. May be due to trauma or coagulopathies. May also occur in animals with congenital/early-onset disease such as collie eye anomaly and persistent hyperplastic primary vitreous/persistent hyperplastic tunica vasculosa lentis.
Retinal detachment	Unilateral or sometimes bilateral. Usually total detachment if the eye is blind. Detached retina seen as a grey membrane with surface blood vessels in the vitreous. May be associated with posterior segment disease such as collie eye anomaly, retinal dysplasia, inflammatory or neoplastic disease. Systemic abnormalities such as hypertension should be considered and some instances are idiopathic.
Sudden acquired retinal degeneration (SARD) in the dog	Bilateral. Typically very rapid loss of vision but may be over a 1-week period. Middle-aged slightly obese bitches over-presented. Often a history of increased appetite and thirst. Pupillary light reflex may be absent or remarkably well retained. Fundus appears normal. Distinguish from central causes of sudden-onset blindness by electroretinogram (non-recordable in dogs with SARD).
Optic neuritis and retrobulbar neuritis	Often bilateral. When optic nerve head is involved it will appear abnormal, with swelling and haemorrhages. If retrobulbar portion of optic nerve inflamed, fundus examination is normal and electroretinogram is initially normal.
Intracranial lesions	Often bilateral. Neoplasia compressing optic chiasma (e.g. pituitary macroadenoma, meningioma) is second commonest cause (after SARD) of sudden-onset bilateral blindness where eye examination is unremarkable (except for reduced pupillary light reflexes). If ERG normal, CT or MRI indicated. Other central lesions (e.g. tentorial herniation, hydrocephalus) associated with additional neurological signs.
Consequence of hypoxia/anoxia (e.g. post-anaesthesia, cardiac arrest)	Commonest in cats following anaesthetic 'incidents'. Central vision loss often but not always accompanied by loss of pupillary light reflexes.
Feline ischaemic encephalopathy	Cerebral vascular infarction can lead to necrosis of the optic tracts or chiasma, leading to blindness with dilated non-responsive pupils. Other neurological deficits likely to be present.
Toxicity	Ivermectin toxicity in dogs can cause blindness ± other neurological signs. Collies particularly sensitive. Fluroquinolones (e.g. enrofloxacin) have been reported to induce irreversible panretinal degeneration in cats, even at a dose close to the recommended range.

Slowly progressive vision loss

Condition	Key features
Corneal oedema	Commonly bilateral. Progressive development of corneal oedema due to endothelial dysfunction. Commoner in dogs. May be primary endothelial dystrophy, endothelial cell damage due to inflammation, glaucoma, lens luxation, intraocular surgery, or drug toxicities (e.g. tocainide).
Keratitis	Commonly bilateral. Many possible causes, e.g. severe keratoconjunctivitis sicca, pannus (chronic superficial keratitis), pigmentary keratitis.
Chronic uveitis	Unilateral or bilateral. Red eye, ocular discomfort and altered appearance of the eye apparent and more likely to be the presenting signs rather than the vision loss.
Chronic glaucoma	Unilateral or bilateral. Occasionally dogs will be seen with apparent chronic open angle glaucoma that present with vision deterioration and altered globe appearance. Some canine secondary glaucomas and feline glaucomas may also present with vision loss rather than ocular pain, e.g. secondary to chronic uveitis, neoplasia in all species, and ocular melanosis of Cairn Terriers.
Cataract formation	Unilateral or bilateral. Obvious change in appearance of the eye(s) prior to signs of vision loss.
Progressive retinal atrophy	Bilateral. Typically there is initial loss of vision under dim lighting conditions. Breed-related problem. Commonest in dogs, but some forms occur in cats. Age at onset and rate of progression varies between the forms. Typical fundus lesions – generalized retinal thinning manifest as tapetal hyper-reflectivity and attenuation of the superficial retinal vessels.
Retinal pigment epithelial dystrophy	Bilateral. Breed-related problem. Characteristic fundus changes occur long before vision loss is apparent. Check serum Vitamin E levels.
Dietary deficiencies (e.g. taurine in cats, Vitamin E in dogs)	Feline central retinal degeneration (e.g. due to taurine deficiency) can, in the most severe cases, lead to panretinal degeneration. However, in most instances characteristic fundus lesions are present but vision loss is not apparent. Vitamin E deficiency leads to a retinopathy identical in appearance to retinal pigment epithelial dystrophy.
Chorioretinitis	Inflammatory lesions of the posterior segment can lead to a progressive loss of vision. Ophthalmoscopic changes ranging from retinal detachment, to posterior segment haemorrhage, to a retinal degeneration may be seen on ophthalmoscopy. The more severe cases may present as a sudden loss of vision; others have a more gradual progression.
Central lesions	Space-occupying lesions impinging on the optic chiasma may cause bilateral vision loss. Lesions elsewhere involving the central visual pathways may cause unilateral blindness or loss of vision that is worse in one eye than the other.
Lysosomal storage disease	Ceroid lipofuscinosis may be associated with blindness as well as lipopigment accumulation in neurons (including the retina). Fucosidosis and globoid cell leucodystrophy may cause blindness, usually in the later stages of the diseases.

Congenital and early-onset poor vision/blindness

Condition	Key features
Gross ocular malformation	Usually bilateral but may be unilateral. Examples include: anophthalmos (absence of eye); and microphthalmos with accompanying abnormalities (e.g. persistent pupillary membrane, cataract, retinal dysplasia). Gross abnormalities should be obvious.
Abnormal persistence of embryonic vasculature	Usually bilateral but may be unilateral. Extensive persistent pupillary membrane (ppm), or ppm associated with corneal opacity or cataract may impair vision. Persistent hyperplastic primary vitreous and persistent tunica vasculosa lentis (PHPV/PHTVL) can be associated with congenital vision loss; if secondary cataracts progress or intralenticular or intraocular haemorrhage occurs there may be deterioration of residual vision. PHPV/PHTVL may be unilateral or more frequently bilateral; inherited in Dobermann and Staffordshire Bull Terrier.
Cataracts	Usually bilateral but may be unilateral. Commoner in dogs than in cats. Congenital cataracts hereditary in some breeds, e.g. Miniature Schnauzer.
Congenital glaucoma	Usually bilateral. Rare; may be seen in cats and dogs. Leads to gross globe enlargement because the globe of young animals is easily stretched.
Early-onset progressive retinal atrophy	Bilateral. Early-onset forms described in cats (Abyssinian) and dogs (Irish Setter, Cardigan Welsh Corgi, Norwegian Elkhound). Typically initial night blindness demonstrable at a few weeks of age; slower loss of daytime vision. Typical fundus changes and ERG changes.
Retinal dysplasia	Bilateral. Environmental causes possible in cats and dogs (radiation, certain infections); inherited in some breeds of dog. Total retinal dysplasia is manifest as retinal non-attachment or early retinal detachment with other developmental ocular abnormalities. Geographic retinal dysplasia may result in total retinal detachment and blindness or large areas of retinal degeneration.
Collie eye anomaly	Collie breeds affected. Disease is bilateral; blindness, when it occurs, is usually unilateral. Most affected dogs have no obvious vision problems but some have retinal detachment or intraocular haemorrhage. Blinding lesions more likely to develop in younger dogs with more severe lesions (e.g. large colobomas).
Hydrocephalus	Bilateral vision loss. Can result in poor vision and other neurological signs.
Portosystemic shunts	After feeding when neurological signs are present affected animals may appear blind.

Appendix 2

Ophthalmological emergencies and referrals

Sheila Crispin

Ophthalmological emergencies

An emergency is an unexpected occurrence requiring immediate action. In all the examples listed below prompt and correct management will offer the best chance of full recovery at least cost to the client. The management options may include referral to a specialist veterinary ophthalmologist if the facilities of the practice are inadequate, or the expertise of the staff is insufficient to cope with the problem.

- Globe prolapse (commonest in dogs)
- Retrobulbar abscess and orbital cellulitis (all species, but commonest in dogs)
- Foreign bodies
- Gross trauma to globe and/or adnexa
- Deep or complicated ulceration, including descemetocoele
- Chemical injuries and liquefactive stromal necrosis (all species)
- Acute uveitis (mainly dogs)
- Acute glaucoma (mainly dogs)
- Sudden loss of vision (all species)
- Sudden onset of ocular pain (all species)

Referral of ophthalmic cases

The list given below should not be regarded as either obligatory or exhaustive, especially as the level of expertise in ophthalmology will vary from practice to practice. Referral should always be considered as one of the management options for difficult cases and the art of referral lies in recognizing not only which cases to refer, but how and when to refer them.

A letter of referral should set out the reason for referral, any information of relevance to the problem, the results of investigations, and any treatment that has been given. It is discourteous and usually unhelpful to send computer print-outs of the patient's life history and even worse to send no information whatsoever.

Problems that may require urgent or emergency referral are signified by an asterisk (*) in the list below and in these cases brief details (including treatment) can be given to the receptionist at the time of making the appointment, or faxed through, or sent with the client.

- Orbital neoplasia and complex adnexal and intraocular neoplasia
- Endophthalmitis and panophthalmitis
- Complicated blunt and penetrating trauma, including complex foreign bodies*
- Complex eyelid problems and those animals which have had previous eyelid surgery
- Deep corneal ulcers and penetrating corneal injuries*
- Liquefactive stromal necrosis including alkali burns*
- Corneal problems requiring keratectomy or keratoplasty
- Acute glaucoma*
- Lens luxation in the dog* and other species
- Cataract surgery (dogs with diabetic cataracts should be referred as early as possible)
- Acute canine* uveitis; uveitis where the aetiology is complex or not obvious
- Sudden blindness*
- Unexplained ocular pain or redness (urgency of referral depends upon the degree of pain)

Appendix 3
Eye schemes and hereditary eye disease

Sheila Crispin and Simon Petersen-Jones

Historically, eye schemes for the identification of canine inherited eye disease have been based on examination of the eye coupled with pedigree analysis and, less commonly, test mating. Experimental studies have been crucial in providing the scientific evidence on which such eye schemes are based. DNA testing for genetic eye disease is a powerful addition to the armoury and in Sweden, for example, the Kennel Club has a DNA testing and control scheme in operation.

In the last few years there has been a move towards harmonization of eye schemes in different countries, with the aim of providing an internationally acceptable certificate and there is a great willingness to seek common ground in the assessment, diagnosis, recording and publication of ocular disease in the dog. The Hereditary Defects Committee of the WSAVA (World Small Animal Veterinary Association) has suggested that an international certificate could be used alongside the certificates of each existing national scheme, thus facilitating data sharing while avoiding difficulties of standardization. The ultimate aim, however, is to have a single computer-readable international certificate; an international working party is currently engaged in reviewing eye schemes and hereditary eye disease on a country-by-country basis.

Hereditary Eye Scheme Certification in Europe

BVA/KC/ISDS Eye Scheme
The British Veterinary Association/Kennel Club/International Sheep Dog Society (BVA/KC/ISDS) Eye Scheme operates in the UK and has been in existence for some 30 years. Royal College of Veterinary Surgeons (RCVS) certificate or diploma holders, who have been assessed for the type of work involved, perform BVA/KC/ISDS eye examinations. The BVA/KC/ISDS Eye Scheme is primarily concerned with the examination of the eyes of dogs for inherited eye disease, but also includes a general examination of the eye and adnexa. Certificates of eye examination are issued in respect of inherited conditions of the eye only and not for inherited conditions of the adnexa. The results are published by the Kennel Club or, for ISDS-registered Border Collies, by the ISDS.

This scheme also enables breeders to screen litters of puppies, up to the age of 12 weeks, for congenital and early onset disease. Although DNA testing is available for a number of inherited eye conditions, such testing does not form part of the scheme, unlike the long established Eye Scheme administered by the Swedish Kennel Club. The British Veterinary Association publishes annually, on behalf of the BVA/KC/ISDS, a pamphlet on the canine eye conditions that are certified, as well as those that are under investigation. Further information on the Canine Health Schemes can be found on the BVA and the Kennel Club websites: http://www.bva.co.uk and http://www.the-kennel-club.org.uk

ECVO Eye Scheme
The Eye Scheme of the European College of Veterinary Ophthalmologists (ECVO) is relatively recent and has so far been adopted by the Netherlands, Norway, Denmark, Finland, Germany and Switzerland. Other European countries will undoubtedly adopt this scheme and the Kennel Club in England has announced recently that it will recognize results issued under the ECVO Scheme. Eye panellists issuing ECVO certificates are usually practising diplomates of the ECVO, although there is also a parallel track of assessed Eye Scheme examiners. The scheme is in part modelled on the BVA/KC/ISDS Scheme, with both certification of individual dogs and litter screening of puppies offered under the scheme. Accurate identification of the dog being examined is an important aspect of ECVO certification.

Hereditary Eye Scheme Certification in the USA

Canine hereditary eye disease certification in the USA is run by the Canine Eye Registration Foundation (CERF). This organization was founded by a group of concerned owners and breeders of pure-bred dogs who 'recognized that the quality of their dogs' lives were being affected by heritable eye disease'. The organization aims to 'accomplish the goal of elimination of heritable eye disease in all pure-bred dogs by forming a centralised, national registry'.

A CERF eye examination must be performed by an ophthalmologist board certified by the American College of Veterinary Ophthalmologists (ACVO). The examination findings are recorded on a computer readable form and if the tested dog is found free of eye disease the owner may apply to register the dog with CERF. CERF gathers data on all animals that undergo a CERF eye examination but only registers the dogs certified free of heritable eye diseases. The ACVO Genetics Committee publishes a booklet with lists of known or suspected hereditary eye disease in pure-bred dogs with breeder recommendations (e.g. 'don't breed' or 'breeding left to breeder's discretion'). This booklet is updated regularly.

More details about CERF are available at the following website: http://www.vmdb.org/cerf.html

Index

Abducens nerve, 272
Abnormal pigment deposition *see* Ocular melanosis
Abyssinian cats
   nystagmus, 272
   progressive retinal degeneration, 249–50
Accessory optic system, 263
Accommodation reflex, 264
Acetazolamide, 33
   glaucoma, 197, 198
Acetylpromazine, 34
Acid injuries, 144
Acute bullous keratopathy in cats, 153
Acyclovir, 53
Adenocarcinoma, 176
Adie's syndrome, 270
Adrenergic agents, 57
α-Adrenergic agonists, 198
β-Adrenergic blockers, 198
Aeromonas spp., 293
Afghan Hounds, crystalline stromal dystrophy, 138
African grey parrots, iris, 289
Akitas *see* Japanese Akitas
Alaskan Malamutes, cataract, 211, 212
Albendazole, 282
Albinism, 163–4
Alkali injuries, 144
Amazon parrots, iris, 289
American Cocker Spaniels
   cataract, 211
   corneal endothelial dystrophies, 139
   distichiasis, 88
   episcleritis, 157
   generalized progressive retinal atrophy, 236
   primary glaucoma, 193
Aminoglycosides, 51
Amlodipine, 199, 254
Amoxycillin/clavulanic acid, 52
Amphotericin B, 53
Anaemia, 232
Anaemic retinopathy, 250
Anaesthetic plan, 34
Analgesia, 30–1
   anti-inflammatory drugs, 30–1
   local anaesthetics, 30
   opioids, 31
Angiostrongylus vasorum
   uveitis, 170
   in vitreous, 224
Aniridia, 164
Anisocoria, 267–70
   afferent fibre lesions, 267
   causes, 367
   efferent pathway lesions, 267
   Horner's syndrome, 268–70
   intracranial disease, 270
   sympathetic innervation, 268

Ankyloblepharon
   birds, 287
   cats, 101
   dogs, 80
Anophthalmos, 68
Anterior chamber, 185
   birds, 289
Anterior scleritis, 158
Anterior segment dysgenesis, 164–5
Anterior uveal trauma
   cats, 181
   dogs, 173–4
      blunt ocular trauma, 174
      foreign bodies, 174
      penetrating injuries, 173–4
Anti-allergic drugs, 55
Anti-glaucoma drugs, 55–7
   adrenergic agents, 57
   carbonic anhydrase inhibitors, 56
   osmotic diuretics, 56
   parasympathomimetics, 56
   prostaglandin analogues, 56
Anti-inflammatory drugs, 30–1, 53–4
   corticosteroids, 33, 53–4
   topical glucocorticoids, 54
   non-steroidal anti-inflammatory drugs (NSAIDs), 30–1, 54–5
Antibacterials, 51–3
   aminoglycosides, 51
   fluoroquinolones, 51–2
   β-lactam antibiotics, 51
   lincosamides, 51
   macrolides, 51
   sulphonamides, 51
   tetracyclines, 51
Anticollagenases, 58–9
Antifibrotic agents, 59
Antifungals, 53
Antivirals, 53
Aphakia, 207
Applanation tonometers, 187
Apraclonidine, 198
Aqueous, 185
Aqueous outflow, 185–6
Arcus lipoides corneae
   cats, 153
   dogs, 147
   reptiles, 293
Area centralis in cats, 247
Arteriovenous shunts, 67
Aspirates, 24
Asteroid hyalosis, 222, 299
Atracurium, 34
Atropine, 198
Australian Cattle Dogs, generalized progressive retinal atrophy, 236
Australian Shepherd Dogs
   cataract, 212
   collie eye anomaly, 232
Azathioprine, 55
Azithromycin, 52

Bacitracin, 52, 53
Bacterial blepharitis, 103
Bacterial uveitis
   cats, 179
   dogs, 169
Bacteriology, 27
Barraquer cilia forceps, 37
Barraquer wire eyelid speculum, 37
Bartonellosis, 179
Basenjis, persistent pupillary membrane, 165
Basset Hounds, primary glaucoma, 193
Beagles, crystalline stromal dystrophy, 138
Bedlington Terriers, vitreoretinal dysplasia, 222
Behavioural tests, 228
Belgian Shepherd Dogs
   cataract, 211
   pendular nystagmus, 273
Bergmeister's papilla, 219, 221, 231
Betamethasone, 54
Betaxolol, 197
Bichon Frisé
   cataract, 212
   epiphora, 115
Binocular indirect ophthalmoscopy, 7–8
Biomicroscopy
   high-frequency ultrasound, 20
   slit lamp, 10
Biopsy, 24–5
   conjunctiva, 25
   cornea and orbit, 25
   eyelid, 25
Birds, 287–90
   anterior chamber and uveal tract, 289
   conjunctiva and cornea, 288–9
      conjunctivitis and keratitis, 288
      corneal ulceration, 288–9
   eyelids and periorbital tissues, 287–8
      parasitic blepharitis, 288
      trauma, 288
      viral blepharitis, 288
   globe, 287
   lens, 289
   posterior segment, 289–90
      chorioretinitis, 290
      congenital conditions, 290
      retinal degeneration, 290
      trauma, 290
   tear film, 288
Birman cats
   corneal sequestration, 152
   dermoid, 156
Bishop–Harmon tissue forceps, 37
Blastomyces dermatitidis, 253, 266
Blastomycosis, 253
Blepharitis
   birds, 288
   cats, 103
   dogs, 91–4
      chronic bacterial, 93

following parotid duct
transposition, 94
immune-mediated, 93–4
seborrhoeic, 94
rabbits, 278
Blepharoconjunctivitis in rabbits, 277–8
Blepharoedema in reptiles, 290
Blinking disorders, 273–4
motor deficits, 273–4
sensory deficits, 273
Blood pressure
and intraocular pressure, 32
see also Systemic hypertension
Blood-filled eye, 76
Bloodhounds, cataract, 212
Blue eye, 135, 168
Blue-smoke Persian cats, Chédiak–Higashi syndrome, 164
Bone lysis, 14
Border Collies
cataract, 212
collie eye anomaly, 232
lens luxation, 194, 215
Border Terriers, cataract, 212
Bordetella spp., 280
Borrelia burgdorferi, 169
Boston Terriers
cataract, 210, 211
corneal endothelial dystrophies, 139
Bouvier des Flandres, primary glaucoma, 193
Boxers
corneal endothelial dystrophies, 139
epithelial basement membrane dystrophy, 136
Branhamella spp., 51
Briards
progressive retinal degeneration, 236
retinal dystrophy, 238
Brinzolamide drops, 197, 198
Bromovinyldeoxuridine, 53
Brown–Adson tissue forceps, 37
Brucellosis, 169
Bruch's membrane, 163
Budgerigars, corneal ulceration, 288
Buphthalmos, 69, 190–1
Bupivacaine, 58
Buprenorphine, 34
Burmese cats
dermoid, 156
fundus, 247
hypertriglyceridaemia, 181

Cairn Terriers, ocular melanosis, 165, 196
Calcium hydroxide, 144, 145
Calcium keratopathy in dogs, 148
Canaliculitis, 117–19
clinical signs, 118
diagnosis, 118
treatment, 118–19
Candida albicans, 253
Canine herpesvirus, 168
Carbonic anhydrase inhibitors, 33, 56, 198
Cardigan Welsh Corgis, generalized progressive retinal atrophy, 236
Castroviejo eyelid speculum, 37, 38
Castroviejo fixation forceps, 37
Cataract, 301
birds, 289
cats, 216
dogs, 208–14
capsular, 207
classification by aetiology, 210–13
classification by age of onset, 208–9
classification by stage of development, 209–10

congenital, 208
hereditary, 210–12
hypermature, 209–10
immature, 209
incipient, 209
intumescent, 209
juvenile, 209
mature, 209
metabolic, 213
Morgagnian, 210
senile, 209, 213
toxic/dietary, 213
traumatic, 212
treatment, 213–14
fish, 294
and glaucoma, 190, 192
rabbits, 283
reptiles, 293–4
rodents, 286
ultrasonography, 18–19
Cats
arcus lipoides corneae, 153
blepharitis, 103
calicivirus, 131
choroid, 247
choriocapillaris, 247
tapetum, 247
conjunctiva
conjunctivitis, 130–2
epibulbar dermoid, 129
neoplasia, 133
symblepharon, 132
trauma and foreign bodies, 133
corneal disease, 148–51
absence/microcornea/megalocornea, 148
acquired conditions, 149–51
acute bullous keratopathy, 153
corneal dystrophies, 149
corneal opacity, 148
developmental, 148
eosinophilic keratoconjunctivitis, 153
exposure keratopathy, 153
Florida keratopathy, 153
keratitis, 149–51
lipid deposition, 153
lipid keratopathy, 153
neurometabolic disease, 148
neurotrophic keratopathy, 153
corneal foreign bodies, 152
corneal sequestration, 152
corneal trauma, 151
dry eye, 119–20
dysautonomia, 120
keratoconjunctivitis sicca, 119–20
lipid abnormalities, 119
mucin abnormality, 120
epibulbar dermoid, 129
epiphora, 121
eyelid conditions, 101–4
ankyloblepharon, 101
associated with cilia, 103
blepharitis, 103
coloboma, 101–2
dermoid, 102
ectropion, 102
entropion, 102
eosinophilic plaques, 103
neoplasia, 103
symblepharon, 102
third eyelid, 103–4
fundus, 247–56
acquired diseases, 248–55
anatomy and physiology, 247
developmental diseases, 248
glaucoma, 201–2
aetiology, 201–2

clinical signs, 202
therapy, 202
herpesvirus, 130–1
lacrimal system, 119–22
lens conditions, 216–17
acquired, 216–17
cataract, 216
congenital, 216
lens luxation, 216–17
retinal detachment, 248, 253–4
inflammatory, 253–4
non-inflammatory, 253
retinal dysplasia, 248
ulcerative keratitis, 149–50
aetiology, 149
clinical findings, 149–50
treatment, 150
uveal tract abnormalities, 177–83
anterior uveal trauma, 181
foreign bodies, 181
lipaemic aqueous, 181
uveal neoplasia, 182–3
uveitis, 177–81, 225
vitreous anomalies, 225–6
acquired, 225–6
chronic feline uveitis, 225
congenital, 225
vitreal haemorrhage, 225–6
wet eye, 119
see also Feline
Cavalier King Charles Spaniels
cataract, 211, 212
crystalline stromal dystrophy, 137–8
keratoconjunctivitis sicca, 112
retinal dysplasia, 235
Cavernous sinus syndrome, 272
Central blindness, 262–7
causes, 262
central visual pathways, 263–4
cerebellar lesions, 266–7
diagnosis, 262–3
lesions of LGN, optic radiation or occipital cortex, 266
optic chiasma lesions, 266
optic nerve lesions, 265–6
post-chiasmal optic trace lesions, 266
Central visual pathways, 263–4
accommodation reflex, 264
optic tract projections, 263–4
pupillary light reflex see Pupillary light reflex
Cephalexin, 52
Cephalosporins, 51
Cerebellar lesions, 266–7
Chalazia, 92–3
Chédiak–Higashi syndrome, 164
Chemical cauterants, 137
Chemical injury
dogs, 144–5
acid injuries, 144
alkali injuries, 144
emergency treatment, 145
subsequent treatment, 145
Chesapeake Bay Retrievers
cataract, 211
generalized progressive retinal atrophy, 236
Chihuahuas, corneal endothelial dystrophies, 139
Chlamydophila spp., 26, 27, 51, 52
Chlamydophila caviae, 286
Chlamydophila felis, 131–2
Chloramphenicol, 52, 53
Chlortetracycline, 53
Choriocapillaris, 228
Chorioretinitis, 240–1, 301
birds, 290
causes, 240

clinical and pathological features, 240–1
management, 241
treatment, 241
Choroid
    cats, 247
        choriocapillaris, 247
        tapetum, 247
    dogs
        anatomy and physiology, 163, 228
        choriocapillaris, 228
        suprachoroidea, 228
Chow-Chows
    entropion, 82
    uveodermatological syndrome, 171
Chromodacryorrhoea in rodents, 286
Chronic superficial keratoconjunctivitis in dogs, 143–4
Chylomicronaemia, 175, 242
Cicatricial entropion, 83
Cilia forceps, 37
Ciliary body, 185
    anatomy and physiology, 163
    pharmacological ablation, 200
Ciliary body adenoma, 176
Ciliary cleft, 185
Ciliary flush, 135
Ciliary processes, 185
Ciprofloxacin, 53, 288
Clindamycin, 52, 252
Close direct ophthalmoscopy, 6–7
Clumber Spaniels, diamond eye, 83
Cnemidocoptes pillae, 288
Coagulopathies, 241
Coccidioides immitis, 253
Cockatiels
    ankyloblepharon, 287
    corneal ulceration, 288
Cockatoos, iris, 289
Colibri corneal utility forceps, 37
Collie eye anomaly, 156, 221, 232–3
    clinical and pathological features, 232–3
    heritability and disease control, 233
Coloboma, 164
    cats
        eyelid, 101–2
        optic nerve, 248
    dogs
        eyelid, 80
        lens, 207
        optic nerve, 243
Colourpoint cats, corneal sequestration, 152
Computed tomography, 20–1
    appearance of scans, 20–1
    detection of neoplasia, 21
    guidance for diagnostic tests, 21
    indications, 21
    orbit, 62
    reformatted images, 21
Conjunctiva, 124–33
    anatomy, 44, 124
    birds, 288–9
    cats
        conjunctivitis, 130–2
        epibulbar dermoid, 129
        neoplasia, 133
        symblepharon, 132
        trauma and foreign bodies, 133
    dogs
        conjunctivitis, 125–7
        epibulbar dermoid, 124–5
        foreign bodies, 128
        neoplasia, 128–9
        symblepharon, 127
        systemic disorders with conjunctival involvement, 129
        trauma, 127–8
    embryology, 124
    pathology, 124
    physiology, 124
    rabbits, aberrant overgrowth, 278
    reptiles, 292
Conjunctival biopsy, 25
Conjunctival scrapings, 23–4
Conjunctival swabs, 23
Conjunctivitis, 124, 298, 299
    birds, 288
    cats, 130–2
        aetiology, 130–1
        Chlamydophila felis, 131–2
        feline calicivirus, 131
        Mycoplasma, 132
    dogs, 125–7, 297
        aetiology, 126
        clinical signs, 125–6
        diagnosis, 127
        history, 125
        treatment, 127
    rabbits, 277–8
    reptiles, 292
    rodents, 286
    see also Conjunctiva
Contrast orbitography, 15
Cornea, 134–54
    Descemet's membrane, 134, 135
    embryology, anatomy and physiology, 134
    endothelial damage, 135
    epithelial damage, 135
    oedema, 135
    pigmentation, 135
    response to injury, 135
    stroma, 134
    stromal damage, 135
    ulceration *see* Corneal ulceration
    vascularization, 135
    wound healing, 135
    see also Corneal disease
Corneal anatomy, 44
Corneal arcus *see* Arcus lipoides corneae
Corneal biopsy, 25
Corneal blink reflex, 260–1, 273
Corneal disease
    cats, 148–51
        absence/microcornea/megalocornea, 148
        acquired conditions, 149–51
        acute bullous keratopathy, 153
        corneal dystrophies, 149
        corneal opacity, 148
        developmental, 148
        eosinophilic keratoconjunctivitis, 153
        exposure keratopathy, 153
        Florida keratopathy, 153
        keratitis, 149–51
        lipid deposition, 153
        neurometabolic disease, 148
        neurotrophic keratopathy, 153
    dogs, 135–45
        absence/microcornea/megalocornea, 136
        acquired conditions, 136–48
        calcium keratopathy, 148
        corneal opacity, 136
        dermoid, 136
        developmental conditions, 136
        epithelial inclusion cyst, 148
        Florida keratopathy, 148
        investigation, 136
        keratitis, 140–4
    fish, 294
    rabbits, 281–2
        corneal dystrophy, 281
        corneal oedema, 281
        lipid keratopathy, 281
        non-ulcerative keratitis, 282
        ulcerative keratitis, 281
    reptiles, 292–3
        arcus lipoides corneae, 293
        corneal ulceration, 293
        keratitis, 292–3
    rodents, 286
Corneal dystrophies, 299
    cats, 149
    dogs, 136–40
        crystalline stromal dystrophy, 138–9
        endothelial dystrophies, 139–40
        epithelial dystrophies, 136–8
    rabbits, 281
    rodents, 286
Corneal endothelial dystrophies, 139–40
    pathology, 139
    treatment, 140
Corneal foreign bodies
    cats, 152
    dogs, 146, 147
Corneal lipidoses in dogs, 146–7
Corneal neoplasia in dogs, 148
Corneal neovascularization, 190
Corneal oedema, 300, 301
    in glaucoma, 188–9
    rabbits, 281
Corneal opacity
    cats, 148
    dogs, 136
Corneal scrapings, 23–4
Corneal sequestration in cats, 152
Corneal swabs, 23
Corneal trauma, 145–6, 151
    cats, 151
    dogs, 145–6
        blunt trauma, 145
        chemical injury, 144–5
        penetrating trauma, 145–6
        thermal injury, 144
        uveitis, 171
    rodents, 286
Corneal ulceration, 190
    birds, 288–9
    reptiles, 293
    rodents, 286
Corneal vascularization, 189
Corneoscleral limbus, 155
Correctopia, 164
Corticosteroids, 33, 53–4
    uveitis, 172
Cranial sinus venography, 15
Crocodile tears, 274
Cryptococcosis, 253
Cryptococcus neoformans, 253, 266
Cryptophthalmos, 68
Crystalline stromal dystrophy, 137–8
    clinical findings, 138–9
    pathology, 139
    treatment, 139
Cyclo-oxygenase, 30
Cyclocryotherapy, 200
Cycloplegics, 57
Cyclosporin, 55
Cysts
    epithelial inclusion, 148
    iridociliary, 166
    nasolacrimal, 119
    uveal, 165, 224
Cytobrush, 24
Cytology, 25–6
Cytotoxic drugs in uveitis, 173

Dachshunds, corneal endothelial dystrophies, 139

Feline immunodeficiency virus, 178–9, 251
Feline infectious peritonitis, 177–8, 251
Feline ischaemic encephalopathy, 300
Feline leukaemia virus, 178, 251
Fentanyl, 34
Fibrinolytics, 59
Fibrosarcoma, 176
Fibrosing strabismus, 271
Field Spaniels, cataract, 212
Filtration angle, 185
Fish, 294
Flat-coated Retrievers
  distichiasis, 88
  ectopic cilia, 89
  primary glaucoma, 193
Florida keratopathy
  cats, 153
  dogs, 148
Fluorescein, 9–10
  angiography, 9–10, 229
  break-up time, 108, 138
  in ulcerative keratitis, 140
  lacrimal dysfunction, 107
  Seidel test, 145
Fluorescein drainage test, 108
Fluorescein test for nasal patency, 9
Fluorometholone, 54
Fluoroquinolones, 51–2
5-Fluorouracil, 59
Flurbiprofen sodium, 55
Focal illumination, 1, 5
Follicular hypertrophy, 124
Foreign bodies, 298
  conjunctiva
    dogs, 128
    reptiles, 292
    rodents, 286
  cornea, 146, 147, 152
  nasolacrimal system, 117
  uveal tract, 174, 181
  vitreous, 223–4
Fossa hyaloidea, 220
Fox Terriers, lens luxation, 215
French Bulldogs, cataract, 212
Frontal sinus
  fractures of, 71
  radiography, 14
Fundus, canine, 227–46
  acquired disease of the retina, 235–42
    chorioretinitis, 240–1
    generalized progressive retinal atrophy, 235–7
    neoplasia, 242
    neuronal ceroid-lipofuscinoses, 242
    photic retinopathy, 242
    retinal detachment, 238–40
    retinal dystrophy in Briard dogs, 238
    retinal pigment epithelial dystrophy, 237–8
    retinal vascular disease, 241–2
    sudden acquired retinal degeneration, 238
    vitamin E deficiency, 242
  acquired diseases of optic disc and optic nerve, 243–5
    optic atrophy, 245
    optic nerve neoplasia, 244
    optic neuritis, 243–4
    papilloedema, 243
  choroid, 227–8
  congenital abnormalities of optic nerve, 243
  developmental lesions, 232–5
    collie eye anomaly, 156, 221, 232–3
    retinal dysplasia, 234–5

investigations, 228–30
  behavioural tests, 228
  electroretinogram, 229
  fluorescein angiography, 229
  molecular genetic tests, 229–30
  ophthalmoscopy, 228
  reflexes, 228
  ultrasonography, 228
ophthalmoscopic abnormalities, 232
ophthalmoscopic features, 230–2
  non-tapetal fundus, 230–1
  optic disc, 231
  retinal vasculature, 231–2
  tapetal fundus, 230
retina, 227–8
Fundus, feline, 247–56
  acquired diseases, 248–54
    anaemic retinopathy, 250
    inflammatory, 251–3
    inherited enzyme deficiencies, 250–1
    lipaemia retinalis, 255
    non-inflammatory, 249–51
    optic nerve lesions, 255
    parasitic, 252
    progressive retinal degeneration, 249–50
    quinolone-associated retinopathy, 250
    retinal detachments, 253–4
    systemic fungal, 252–3
    taurine deficiency/feline central retinal degeneration, 249
    viral, 251–2
  anatomy and physiology, 247
  developmental diseases, 248
Fundus, rabbits, 283
Fusidic acid, 53

Geckos, fused eyelids, 290
Generalized progressive retinal atrophy, 235–7
  breed incidence and disease control, 236
  clinical features, 235–6
  early diagnosis, 236–7
  molecular genetics, 237
Genetic assessment, 28–9
  marker alleles, 28–9
  specific mutations, 28
Gentamicin, 53
German Shepherd Dogs
  cataract, 211
  chronic superficial keratoconjunctivitis, 143
  pseudopapilloedema, 231
Giant Schnauzers, cataract, 212
Glaucoma, 76, 185–203, 297, 298, 299, 300, 301
  acute, 188–90
  cats, 201–2
    aetiology, 201–2
    clinical signs, 202
    therapy, 202
  chronic, 190–3
  classification and causes, 193–6
  clinical signs, 188–93
    corneal changes, 191
    corneal oedema, 188–9
    corneal vascularization, 189
    episcleral congestion, 189
    equatorial staphyloma, 191
    globe enlargement, 190
    intraocular haemorrhage, 192
    lens changes, 191–2
    mydriasis, 189
    optic disc cupping, 192–3
    pain, 188

phthisis bulbi, 193
retinal and optic nerve atrophy, 193
vision loss, 189–90
control of intraocular pressure, 185–6
diagnosis, 186–8
  gonioscopy, 187–8
  tonometry, 186–7
medical treatment, 197–9
  α-adrenergic agents, 198
  β-adrenergic blockers, 198
  atropine, 198
  carbonic anhydrase inhibitors, 198
  miotics, 198
  neuroprotection, 199
  osmotic diuretics, 197
  prophylactic, 199
  prostaglandin analogues, 198
  tissue plasminogen activator, 198
primary, 193–4
  acute 'closed-angle', 193–4
  chronic 'open-angle', 194
  goniodysgenesis, 193–4
rabbits, 282–3
secondary, 194–6
  intraocular haemorrhage, 196
  lens pathology, 196
  neoplasia, 195–6
  ocular melanosis, 196
  primary lens luxation, 194
  uveitis, 195
  vitreous prolapse, 196
surgical treatment, 199–201
  increasing aqueous outflow, 200–1
  lens extraction, 199
  reduction of aqueous production, 199–200
Globe
  birds, 287
  blunt trauma, 72–3
  enlargement, 190
  immobilization of, 34
  opaque eye, 299
  pathological examination, 76–7
  penetrating trauma, 71–2
  prolapse of, 69–70, 297
  rabbits, 276
  reptiles, 290
  see also Orbit
Glucocorticoids, topical, 54
Glycerol, 197
Glycosaminoglycans, 134
Golden Retrievers
  cataract, 208, 210, 211, 212
  episcleritis, 157
  fibrosing strabismus, 271
  generalized progressive retinal atrophy, 236
  immune-mediated uveitis, 171
  iridociliary cysts, 166
  primary glaucoma, 193
  pseudopapilloedema, 231
  retinal dysplasia, 235
  uveitis, 195
Goniolenses, 3
Gonioscopy, 187–8
Gramicidin, 52
Granulomatous meningoencephalitis, 177
Great Danes
  iridociliary cysts, 166
  primary glaucoma, 193
Green lizards, eyelid neoplasia, 291
Green sea turtles, eyelid neoplasia, 290–1
Greenland Dogs, cataract, 212
Griffon Bruxellois, cataract, 212
Gustolacrimal reflex, 274

Haab's striae, 190, 191
Haemangiosarcoma, 176
Haemophilus spp., 277
Haemorrhage
   intraocular, 192, 196
   retinal, 232
   vitreal, 222–3, 225–6
Halothane, 34
Handling of patients, 31
Hemifacial spasm, 274
Hereditary Eye Scheme Certification
   Europe, 303
   USA, 303–4
Herpesvirus simiae, 285
Herpetic keratitis in cats, 150–1
   aetiology, 150
   clinical findings, 150–1
      clinical course, 151
      diagnosis, 151
      treatment, 151
      vaccination, 151
Heterochromia, 163
Himalayan cats
   esotropia, 270
   fundus, 247
Hippus, 270
Histiocytoma, 95
Histiocytosis, 177
Histology, 25–6
Histoplasma capsulatum, 253, 266
Histoplasmosis, 253
History, 4
Hordeolum, 91–2
Horner's syndrome, 67, 268–70
   causes, 269
   clinical features, 268–9
   diagnosis and differentiation, 269–70
Hyalocytes, 220
Hyaloideocapsular ligament, 220
Hydrocephalus, 301
Hydrocortisone, 54
Hydrophthalmos, 190–1
Hydroxyamphetamine, 269
Hyperlipoproteinaemia, 232
Hyperviscosity syndrome, 232, 241
   and retinal detachment in cats, 254
Hyphaema
   cats, 177, 178
   reptiles, 293
Hypocalcaemia, and cataracts, 213
Hypopyon
   cats, 177, 179, 181
   dogs, 169, 171
   reptiles, 293

Idiopathic facial paralysis, 274
Idiopathic lymphocytic-plasmacytic uveitis in cats, 180–1
Idoxuridine, 53
Immobilization of globe, 34
Immune-mediated blepharitis, 93–4
Immune-mediated keratitis in dogs, 143–4
Immune-mediated uveitis, 171–2
Impression cytology, 24
Indirect ophthalmoscopy, 2–3, 7–8, 214
   binocular, 7–8
   monocular, 8
Infectious canine hepatitis, 168
Infectious cyclic thrombocytopenia, 168
Infectious uveitis
   cats, 177–80
      bacterial, 179
      mycotic, 179
      parasitic, 179–80
      viral, 177–9
   dogs, 168–71
      bacterial, 169
      mycotic, 169–70
      parasitic, 170–1
      rickettsial, 168–9
      viral, 168
Inherited enzyme deficiencies in cats, 250–1
Instruments for surgery, 36–41
   care of, 40–1
   Desmarres chalazion clamp, 38
   disposable materials and drapes, 40
   eyelid specula, 37–8
   Jaeger eyelid plate, 38
   needle holders, 39
   scalpels and blades, 38
   scissors, 38–9
   suture material, 39–40
   suture needles, 40
   tissue and cilia forceps, 37
Interferon, 53
Intracranial disease, pupil abnormalities, 270
Intraocular haemorrhage, 190, 192, 196, 297, 300
Intraocular infection, 73–4
Intraocular melanoma, 76
Intraocular pressure, 31–2
   blood pressure, 32
   direct pressure on globe, 32
   drugs, 32
   endotracheal intubation, 32
   measurement, 214
   normal variations, 186
   physiological control of, 185–6
   venous pressure, 31–2
   ventilation, 32
   see also Systemic hypertension
Iridociliary cysts in dogs, 166
Iridocorneal angle, 185
Iridocyclitis, 167
Iridocytes, 247
Iridodenesis, 215
Iris, 185
   anatomy and physiology, 162
   atrophy, 190
   hypoplasia, 164
Iris atrophy in dogs, 165–6
Iris bombé, 195
Iris pigmentation
   cats, 177
   dogs, 165
Irish Setters, generalized progressive retinal atrophy, 236
Irish Wolfhounds, generalized progressive retinal atrophy, 236
Iritis, 167
Irrigating solutions, 58
Isoflurane, 34

Jack Russell Terriers, lens luxation, 215
Jaeger eyelid plate, 38
Japanese Akitas
   fibrosing strabismus, 271
   generalized progressive retinal atrophy, 236
   immune-mediated uveitis, 171
   uveodermatological syndrome, 172
Juvenile pyoderma, 93

Keratinocytes, 134
Keratitis
   birds, 288
   cats, 149–51
      deep corneal ulceration, 150
      herpetic keratitis, 150–1
      mycobacterial keratitis, 151
      mycotic keratitis, 151
      superficial corneal ulceration, 150
      ulcerative keratitis, 149–50
   dogs, 140–4, 297
      descemetocoele, 143
      immune-mediated, 143–4
      punctate, 143
      ulcerative, 140–3
   reptiles, 292–3
Keratoconjunctivitis sicca, 274
   birds, 288
   cats, 119–20
   dogs, 112–13
   rabbits, 279
   reptiles, 291
Keratomalacia in dogs, 144
Ketamine, 34
Ketoconazole, 53
Ketorolac trometamol, 55

Laboratory investigations, 23–9
   cytological and histological assessment, 25–6
   genetic assessment, 28–9
   microbiological assessment, 26–8
   sample collection and handling, 23–5
Labrador Retrievers
   cataract, 208, 210, 211
   generalized progressive retinal atrophy, 236
   iris melanoma, 176
   primary glaucoma, 193
   retinal dysplasia, 234, 235
   short-limbed dwarfism, 235
Lacrimal cannulae, 3
Lacrimal puncta, 106
Lacrimal punctal aplasia, 114–15
Lacrimal sac, 106
Lacrimal system, 105–23
   abnormalities of lacrimation, 274
   anatomy and physiology, 105–7
   assessment of surface damage, 107
   cats
      anatomy, 119
      distribution problems, 120
      excretory problems, 121–2
      secretory problems, 119–20
   dogs
      acquired conditions, 116–19
      distribution problems, 113–14
      excretory problems, 114–16
      secretory problems, 110–13
   rabbits, 278–81
      dacryocystitis, 279–81
      keratoconjunctivitis sicca, 279
      nasolacrimal duct obstruction, 279–81
      tear drainage, 279
      tear production, 278–9
   rodents, 285–6
      chromodacryorrhoea, 286
      conjunctival foreign bodies, 286
      conjunctivitis, 286
      epiphora, 285
   tear drainage tests, 108–9
   tear production tests, 107–8
   tear stability tests, 108
β-Lactam antibiotics, 51
Lagophthalmos, 296
Lancashire Heelers
   cataract, 212
   collie eye anomaly, 232
Large Munsterlanders, cataract, 211
Laser cyclophotocoagulation, 199–200
Latanoprost drops, 197, 198
Lateral geniculate nucleus, 263
   lesions affecting, 266
Leishmania donovani chagasi, 170
Leishmania donovani infantum, 170
Leishmaniasis, 170

Lens, 204–18
 adult, 205–6
 birds, 289
 blood supply, 205
 cats, 216–17
  acquired conditions, 216–17
  cataract, 216
  congenital conditions, 216
  lens luxation, 216–17, 299
 dogs, 207–16
  acquired conditions, 208–16
  aphakia, 207
  cataract, 208, 208–14
  congenital conditions, 207–8
  lens coloboma, 207
  lens luxation, 215–16, 299
  microphakia, 207
  nuclear sclerosis, 208
  persistent pupillary membrane, 207
  PHTVL/PHPV, 207–8
 embryology, anatomy and physiology, 204–6
 examination, 206
  distant direct ophthalmoscopy, 206
  magnification, 206
  pupillary dilation, 206
  slit lamp biomicroscopy, 214
  transillumination, 206
  ultrasonography, 18–19
  see also Ocular examination
 fish, 294
 primates, 285
 reptiles, 293–4
 rodents, 286
Lens coloboma, 207
Lens extraction, 199
Lens luxation, 191–2, 194–5
 cats, 216–17
 dogs, 215–16
Lens rupture, 72
Lens subluxation, 190, 191–2
Lenticonus, 221
Lentiglobus, 221
Leonbergers, cataract, 212
Leptospirosis, 169
Levobunolol, 197
LGN see Lateral geniculate nucleus
Lhasa Apsos, keratoconjunctivitis sicca, 112
Lignocaine, 34, 58
Lipaemia retinalis
 cats, 255
 dogs, 242
Lipaemic aqueous
 cats, 181
 dogs, 175
Lipid keratopathy
 cats, 153
 dogs, 147
 rabbits, 281
Local anaesthetics, 30, 58
 injectable, 58
 topical, 58
Lyme disease, 169
Lymphoma
 cats, 183
 dogs, 176
Lysosomal storage disease, 301

Macaws, enophthalmitis, 287
Macropalpebral fissure, 80–1
Magnetic resonance imaging, 21–2
 indications, 22
 orbit, 62
 resolution and contrast, 21–2
Magnification, 1
Maltese Terriers, epiphora, 115

Mannitol, 33, 197
Marbofloxacin, 52
Marcus–Gunn pupil, 265
Masticatory myositis, 66
Mastiffs, entropion in, 82
Maze test, 257
Medial canthal entropion, 83
Megacornea
 cats, 148
 dogs, 136
Megoestrol acetate, 55
Meibomianitis, 92, 130
Melanocytoma, 159–60
Melanoma
 eyelid, 95
 intraocular, 76
 uveal tract, 175–6, 182
Menace response, 258, 259
Methazolamide, 197, 198
Metipranolol, 197
Metronidazole, 52
Meyerhoefer chalazion curette, 39
Microbiology, 26–8
 culture and susceptibility testing, 27
 direct microscopic examination, 26
 polymerase chain reaction, 27–8
 serology, 28
Microcornea
 cats, 148
 dogs, 136
Micropalpebral fissure, 82
Microphakia, 207
Microphthalmos
 dogs, 68–9
 reptiles, 290
Micropunctum, 115
Midazolam, 34
Mill Hill cats, strabismus, 270
Miniature Bull Terriers, lens luxation, 215
Miniature Dachshunds, dermoid, 156
Miniature Longhaired Dachshunds, generalized progressive retinal atrophy, 236
Miniature Poodles
 epiphora, 115
 generalized progressive retinal atrophy, 236, 237
 optic nerve hypoplasia, 243
Miniature Schnauzers
 cataract, 208, 211
 generalized progressive retinal atrophy, 236
Miniature Smooth-haired Dachshunds, generalized progressive retinal atrophy, 236
Miosis, 268
Miotics, 198
Mitomycin C, 59
Mittendorf's dot, 210, 219
Monitoring of patients, 34–5
Monocular indirect ophthalmoscopy, 8
Monocytic ehrlichiosis, 168
Moraxella spp., 292–3
Mucin abnormality
 cats, 120
 dogs, 113
Mucinomimetics, 58
Müller cells, 219, 228
Mycobacterial keratitis in cats, 151
Mycobacterial uveitis in cats, 179
Mycology, 27
Mycoplasma spp., 26, 27, 51, 52, 132
Mycotic keratitis in cats, 151
Mycotic uveitis
 cats, 179
 dogs, 169–70
Mydriasis, 5
 in glaucoma, 189

Mydriatic cycloplegics, 173
Mydriatics, 57
Myiasis, 171
Myxomatosis, 278

Nanophthalmos, 68
Nasolacrimal duct, 106–7
 obstruction in rabbits, 279–81
Nasolacrimal system, 44, 79
 dogs, 116–19
  acquired obstructions, 116–17
  canaliculitis and dacryocystitis, 117–19
  foreign bodies, 117
  neoplasia and cysts, 119
  traumatic damage, 116
Necrotizing scleritis, 158
Neisseria spp., 280
Neomycin, 53
Neoplasia
 computed tomography, 21
 conjunctiva, 128–9, 133
 eyelid
  cats, 103
  dogs, 94–7
  rabbits, 278
  reptiles, 290–1
 fundus, 242, 254
 and glaucoma, 195–6
 nictitating membrane, 100–1, 104
 optic nerve, 244
 orbit, 14, 63–6, 67
 sclera, 159–60
 uveal tract, 175–7, 182–3
 uveitis associated with, 172
 vitreous, 224
Neospora caninum, 170
Neuro-ophthalmology, 257–75
 abnormalities of eye position and movement, 270–3
  nystagmus, 272–3
  strabismus, 270–2
 abnormalities of lacrimation, 275
 anisocoria, 267–70
  afferent pathway lesions, 267
  causes, 267
  efferent pathway lesions, 267
  Horner's syndrome, 268–70
  intracranial disease, 270
  sympathetic innervation of eye, 268
 central blindness, 262–7
  causes, 262
  central visual pathways, 263–4
  cerebellar lesions, 266–7
  diagnosis, 262–8
  lesions of LGN, optic radiation or occipital cortex, 266
  optic chiasma lesions, 266
  optic nerve lesions, 265–6
  post-chiasmal optic lesions, 266
 clinical tests, 257–62
  corneal and palpebral reflexes, 260–1
  dazzle reflex, 258, 259
  ophthalmoscopy, 260
  optokinetic nystagmus, 261–2
  pupillary light reflex and 'swinging flashlight' test, 258, 260
  reflex pupillary dilatation, 260
  swinging flashlight test, 5, 258, 260
  tests of vision, 257–8
  vestibular nystagmus, 261
 disorders of blinking, 273–4
  motor deficits, 273–4
  motor innervation of eyelids, 273

Index 313

sensory deficits, 273
sensory innervation of eye, 273
problem-orientated approach, 262
Neuronal ceroid-lipofuscinoses, 242
Neurotrophic keratopathy
  cats, 153
  dogs, 147
Nictitating membrane, 44, 79–80
  cats, 103–4
    neoplasia of, 104
    prolapse of gland, 103
    protrusion of, 103
    scrolling, 103
  dogs, 97–101
    foreign bodies behind, 100
    inflammation, 99
    neoplasia of, 100–1
    prolapse of gland, 99
    protrusion of, 101
    scrolling, 97–9
    trauma, 100
  rodents, 286
Nocturnal owl monkey, 285
Nodular episclerokeratitis, 157–8
Non-steroidal anti-inflammatory drugs, 30–1, 54–5
  uveitis, 173
Non-tapetal fundus, 230–1
Norwegian Buhunds, cataract, 211
Norwegian Elkhounds
  cataract, 211
  generalized progressive retinal atrophy, 236
  primary glaucoma, 194
Nuclear (senile) sclerosis, 6
Nyctalopia, 235
Nystagmus, 272–3
  amaurotic, 272
  cerebellar disease, 272
  congenital, 272–3
  optokinetic, 261
  pendular, 261, 273
  positional, 272
  searching, 272
  spontaneous, 272
  vestibular, 261
  vestibular disease, 272

Occipital cortex, lesions affecting, 266
Ocular centesis, 11
Ocular haemorrhage, 297
Ocular imaging, 13–22
  computed tomography, 20–1
  cross-sectional imaging, 15–20
  magnetic resonance imaging, 21–2
  radiography, 14–15
  ultrasonography, 10, 15–20
Ocular melanosis, 160, 165, 196
Ocular pain, 298
Oculocardiac reflex, 32–3
Oculomotor nerve, 271
Old English Sheepdogs
  cataract, 208, 211, 212
  persistent pupillary membrane, 165
Oligella urethralis, 280
Opaque eye, 76, 299
Ophthalmia neonatorum, 80
Ophthalmic examination, 1–12
  darkened room with focal illumination and magnification, 5
  electroretinography, 11
  equipment, 1–3
  exotic species, 285
  fluorescein, 9–10
  globe, 76–7
  indirect ophthalmoscopy, 7–8
  microscopic, 26

normal illumination without instruments, 4–5
ocular centesis, 11
ocular ultrasonography, 10
ophthalmoscopy, 6–7
orbit, 61–2
penlight, 5
protocol, 3–12
retinal photography, 12
retinoscopy, 11
rose bengal, 10
Schirmer tear test, 8, 107–8, 214, 274, 279
signalment and history, 4
slit lamp biomicroscopy, 10
specular microscopy, 11
tear drainage system, 10, 108
testing vision, 4–5
Ophthalmic surgery
  anatomy and physiology, 43–4
  immobilization of globe, 34
  instrumentation, 36–41
  patient and surgeon positioning, 42
  sterile preparation, 42–3
  tissue separation, 45–6
  tissue stabilization, 44–5
  tissue uniting, 46–9
Ophthalmomyiasis interna posterior, 252
Ophthalmoscopy, 6–8, 260
  fundus disorders, 228
  see also Direct ophthalmoscopy; Indirect ophthalmoscopy
Opioids, 31
Optic atrophy, 245
Optic chiasma lesions, 266
Optic disc/optic nerve head
  birds, 290
  cats, 247
  dogs, 231
    acquired diseases, 243–5
    optic atrophy, 245
    papilloedema, 243
Optic disc cupping, 190, 192–3
Optic nerve atrophy, 190, 193
Optic nerve coloboma
  cats, 248
  dogs, 243
Optic nerve lesions, 265–6
  cats, 255
  dogs
    acquired diseases, 243–5
    congenital abnormalities, 243
    hypoplasia, 243
    neoplasia, 244
    optic atrophy, 245
    optic neuritis, 243–4
  Marcus–Gunn pupil, 265
Optic neuritis, 243–4, 266, 300
  clinical features, 243
  diagnosis, 243–4
  management, 244
Optic radiation, lesions affecting, 266
Optokinetic nystagmus, 261
Ora ciliaris retinae
  cats, 247
  dogs, 227
Orbit, 60–77
  anatomy, 43, 60
  clinical examination, 61–2
  clinical signs of disease, 60–1
  diagnostic imaging, 62
  differential diagnosis, 60–1
  diseases of
    active retraction of painful eye, 67
    arteriovenous shunts, 67
    atrophy of orbital tissues, 67
    blunt trauma to globe, 72–3
    buphthalmos, 69

enophthalmos, 67
exophthalmos, 62–7
extraocular polymyositis, 66–7
Horner's syndrome, 67
intraocular infection, 73–4
masticatory myositis, 66
microphthalmos, 68
orbital trauma, 70–1
penetrating trauma to globe, 71–2
phthisis bulbi, 68–9
prolapse of globe, 69–70
retrobulbar abscessation/cellulitis, 62–3
small or recessed eye, 67–9
temporomandibular osteopathy, 67
zygomatic salivary gland mucocoele, 67
enucleation, 74–5, 201, 277, 287
evisceration and implant, 75–6
investigation of disease, 61–2
pathological examination of globe, 76–7
rabbits, 276–7
  anatomy, 276
  enucleation, 277
  exophthalmos, 276–7
  orbital gland prolapse, 277
  orbital glands, 276
  prolapse of globe, 276
Orbital biopsy, 25
Orbital cellulitis, 62–3, 297, 298
Orbital glands in rabbits, 276
Orbital neoplasia, 14, 63–6, 67
  further investigation, 64–5
  history and clinical signs, 64
  management, 65
  pathogenesis, 63
  surgical treatment, 65–6
Orbital sinus in rabbits, 276
Orbital trauma, 70–1
Osmotic diuretics, 56, 197
  see also individual drugs
Ospreys, iris, 289
Osteosarcoma, 176
Otoscope, 5
Oxymorphone, 34

Pain, 30–1
Palpebral conjunctiva, 78
Palpebral ligaments, 79
Palpebral reflex, 260–1
Pancuronium, 34
Pannus, 143–4
Panophthalmitis, 297, 299
Papilloedema, 243
Papilloma, 94
Papillons, generalized progressive retinal atrophy, 236
Paradoxical tearing, 274
Paradoxical vestibular syndrome, 272
Parasitic blepharitis, 103
Parasitic infection of vitreous, 224
Parasitic uveitis
  cats, 179–80
  dogs, 170–1
Parasympathomimetics, 56
Pasteurella spp., 52, 278
Pasteurella multocida, 51, 149, 169, 179, 181, 277, 280
Pavementing, 236
Pecten, 290
Pectinate ligament, 185, 193
Pembroke Welsh Corgis
  epithelial basement membrane dystrophy, 136
  persistent pupillary membrane, 165
Pendular nystagmus, 261

Penetrating keratoplasty, 140
Penicillins, 51
Penlight examination, 5
Pentobarbitone, 34
Peregrine falcons, ankyloblepharon, 287
Periocular hair, clipping of, 43
Periorbital swelling in birds, 287–8
Peripheral anterior synechiae, 194, 195
Persian cats
    corneal sequestration, 152
    entropion, 102
Persistent hyaloid artery, 220–1
Persistent hyperplastic primary vitreous/
    persistent hyperplastic tunica
        vasculosa lentis
    cats, 248
    dogs, 207–8, 221–2
Persistent pupillary membrane, 164–5, 207
Persistent tunica vasculosa lentis, 221
Phacoclastic uveitis, 171
Phacodonesis, 215
Phacoemulsification, 213
Phaeochromocytoma, 176
Phenol red thread test, 108
Phenylephrine, 269–70
Photic retinopathy, 242
Photoreceptors, 247
Phototoxic retinopathy, 286
Phthisis bulbi, 68–9, 190, 193
PHTVL/PHPV see Persistent
    hyperplastic primary vitreous/
    persistent hyperplastic tunica
    vasculosa lentis
Physostigmine, 267
Pigmentary glaucoma see Ocular
    melanosis
Pilocarpine, 197, 198, 267
Plain film radiography, 14
Plasmodium spp., 288
Poliosis, 171
Polyarteritis nodosa in cats, 181
Polymerase chain reaction, 27–8
Polymixin B, 52, 53
Posterior scleritis, 158
Pre-iridal fibrovascular membranes in
    dogs, 165
Pre-ocular tear film, 105–7
    birds, 288
    cats
        distribution problems, 120
        excretory problems, 121–2
    distribution, 106
    dogs
        distribution problems, 113–14
        excretory problems, 114–16
    excretion, 106–7
    reptiles, 291–2
    secretion, 105–6
Prednisolone, 54
Preoperative evaluation, 33
Pretectum, 263
Primates, 285
Progressive retinal atrophy, 249, 301
Progressive retinal degeneration, 249–50
Progressive rod–cone degeneration, 237
Propofol, 34
Propracaine, 34
Prostaglandin analogues, 56
Proteus spp., 51, 52
Prototheca wickerhamii, 169
Prototheca zopfii, 169
Protothecosis, 169
Proxymetacaine, 58
Pseudomonas spp., 51, 52, 280, 292, 293
Pseudomonas aeruginosa, 9, 51, 141, 142
Pseudopapilloedema, 231
Ptosis, 87

Pulse oximetry, 35
Punctate keratitis, dogs, 143
Pupil, 185
Pupil size, 162
    abnormalities of see Anisocoria
Pupillary escape, 260
Pupillary light reflex, 206, 228, 258, 260, 263
    afferent and efferent lesions, 266, 267
    neuronal pathway, 264
Purkinje image, 4

Rabbits, 276–84
    cornea, 281–3
        corneal dystrophies, 281
        corneal oedema, 281
        lipid keratopathy, 281
        non-ulcerative keratitis, 281
        ulcerative keratitis, 281
    eyelid and conjunctival diseases, 277–8
        aberrant conjunctival overgrowth, 278
        blepharoconjunctivitis and
            conjunctivitis, 277–8
        eyelid tumours, 278
    fundus, 283
    lacrimal system, 278–81
        keratoconjunctivitis sicca, 279
        nasolacrimal duct obstruction
            and dacryocystitis, 279–81
        tear drainage, 279
        tear production, 278–9
    orbit, 276–7
        anatomy, 276
        enucleation, 277
        exophthalmos, 276–7
        orbital gland prolapse, 277
        orbital glands, 276
        orbital sinus, 276
        prolapse, 276
    uveal tract and lens, 282–3
        cataract, 283
        glaucoma, 282–3
        uveitis, 282
Radiography, 14–15
    bone lysis, 14
    contrast orbitography, 15
    contrast techniques, 15
    cranial sinus venography, 15
    dacryocystography, 15
    dental disease, 14
    frontal sinuses, 14
    orbit, 62
    orbital neoplasia, 14
    plain film, 14
    sialography of zygomatic salivary
        gland, 15
Red eye, 4, 297
Red-eared terrapins, eyelid trauma, 290
Referral, 302
Reflex pupillary dilation, 260
Reflex uveitis, 168
Reptiles, 290–4
    anterior chamber and uveal tract, 293
    conjunctiva, 292
    cornea, 292–3
        arcus lipoides corneae, 293
        corneal ulceration, 293
        keratitis, 292–3
    eyelids, 290–1
        blepharoedema, 290
        neoplasia, 290–1
        retained spectacle, 291
        trauma, 290
    globe, 290
    lens, 293–4
    retina, 294

    tear film, 291–2
        impaired tear drainage, 292
        keratoconjunctivitis sicca, 291
    third eye, 291
Retained spectacle in snakes, 291
Retina
    anatomy and physiology, 227–8
    fish, 294
    ganglion cell layer, 228
    haemorrhage, 232
    inner limiting membrane, 228
    inner nuclear layer, 228
    inner plexiform layer, 228
    outer limiting membrane, 228
    outer nuclear layer, 228
    outer plexiform layer, 228
    photoreceptor layer, 227
    reptiles, 294
    rodents, 286–7
    vasculature, 231–2
        changes in, 232
Retinal degeneration
    birds, 290
    reptiles, 294
Retinal detachment, 300
    cats, 248, 253–4
        inflammatory, 253–4
        'morning glory', 253
        non-inflammatory, 253
    dogs, 238–40
        classification, 239–40
        clinical features, 239
        exudative/serous, 239
        pathological features, 238
        rhegmatogenous, 239
        solid, 239
        traction, 239
Retinal dysplasia, 301
    cats, 248
    dogs, 234–5
        clinical features, 234
        diagnostic problems, 235
        heritability and disease control, 235
Retinal nerve atrophy, 190, 193
Retinal photography, 12
Retinal pigment epithelial dystrophy, 237–8, 301
    clinical features, 237
    management, 238
    pathological features, 237
Retinal pigment epithelium, 247
Retinal vascular disease, 241–2
    coagulopathies, 241
    diabetic retinopathy, 241–2
    hyperviscosity syndrome, 241
    lipaemia retinalis, 242
    systemic hypertension, 241
Retinoblastoma in fish, 294
Retinopathy
    anaemic, 250
    diabetic, 232, 241–2
    enrofloxacin-associated, 52, 250
    photic, 242
    rodents
        inherited, 286
        phototoxic, 286
Retinoscopy, 11
Retrobulbar abscess, 62–3, 297
    rabbits, 277
Retrobulbar anaesthesia, 277
Retrobulbar block, 34
Retrobulbar cellulitis, 62–3
Rhabdomyosarcoma, 176
Rhesus monkeys, 285
Rickettsia spp., 51
Rickettsia rickettsii, 168
Rickettsial uveitis, 168–9
Rocky Mountain spotted fever, 168

Rodents, 285–7
    cornea, 286
    lacrimal apparatus and conjunctiva,
        285–6
        chromodacryorrhoea, 286
        conjunctival foreign bodies, 286
        conjunctivitis, 286
        epiphora, 285
    lens, 286
    retina, 286–7
        inherited retinopathy, 286
        phototoxic retinopathy, 287
    third eyelid, 286
Rose bengal, 10
    lacrimal dysfunction, 107
Rostral (anterior) colliculus, 263–4
Rottweilers
    cataract, 211, 212
    entropion, 82
Rough Collies
    cataract, 212
    collie eye anomaly, 232
    crystalline stromal dystrophy, 137–8
    generalized progressive retinal
        atrophy, 236
    microphthalmos in, 68

St Bernards
    dermoid, 156
    diamond eye, 83
Salmonella spp., 51
Samoyeds
    crystalline stromal dystrophy, 138
    immune-mediated uveitis, 171
    primary glaucoma, 193
    retinal dysplasia, 234
    uveodermatological syndrome, 171
Sample collection and handling, 23–5
    aspirates, 24
    biopsy, 24–5
    conjunctival and corneal swabs, 23
    cytobrushes, 24
    eyelid, conjunctival and corneal
        scrapings, 23–4
    impression cytology, 24
Schiøtz tonometer, 186–7
Schirmer I test, 8
Schirmer II test, 8
Schirmer tear test, 8, 107–8, 214, 274, 279
Sclera, 247
    acquired abnormalities, 157–9
        abscess, 159
        degenerative diseases, 161
        inflammatory diseases, 157–9
        neoplastic disease, 159–60
        ocular melanosis, 160
        scleritis, 158
        traumatic diseases, 160–1
        ulcerative limbal keratitis, 159
    anatomy, 155
    developmental abnormalities, 156–7
        congenital staphyloma with
            ectasia, 156
        dermoid, 156
        sclerocornea, 156–7
        thin sclera, 156
    vasculature, 155
Scleral thinning, 151
Scleral trephination and peripheral
    iridectomy, 200
Scleral venous circulation, 185
Scleritis, 158, 297, 298
Sclerocornea, 156–7
Scleromalacia perforans, 158
Scottish Terriers, temporomandibular
    osteopathy, 67
Sealyham Terriers
    lens luxation, 215

vitreoretinal dysplasia, 222
Sebaceous adenocarcinoma, 95
Sebaceous adenoma, 94
Seborrhoeic blepharitis, 94
Seidel test, 145
Seminoma, 176
Senile entropion, 83
Serology, 28
Sevoflurane, 34
Shar Peis
    entropion, 82
    fibrosing strabismus, 271
    lens luxation, 194, 215
Shetland Sheepdogs
    collie eye anomaly, 232
    crystalline stromal dystrophy, 138
    epithelial dystrophy, 138
    immune-mediated uveitis, 171
Shih Tsus, keratoconjunctivitis sicca, 112
Shotgun pellet injury, 71
Sialodacryoadenitis virus, 286
Sialography of zygomatic salivary gland,
    15
Siamese cats
    corneal sequestration, 152
    esotropia, 270
    fundus, 247
    pendular nystagmus, 273
    progressive retinal degeneration, 250
Siberian Huskies
    cataract, 211
    crystalline stromal dystrophy, 138
    generalized progressive retinal
        atrophy, 235
    immune-mediated uveitis, 171
    primary glaucoma, 193
Skinks, fused eyelids, 290
Slit lamp biomicroscopy, 10, 214
Smooth Collies, collie eye anomaly, 232
Snakes
    conjunctivitis, 292
    fungal keratitis, 293
    fused eyelids, 290
    nasolacrimal blockage, 292
    retained spectacle, 291
Spastic entropion, 83
Spastic pupil syndrome, 270
Speckled caiman, eyelid neoplasia, 291
Specular microscopy, 11
Squint *see* Strabismus
Stabilizers and preservatives, 51
Staffordshire Bull Terriers
    cataract, 210, 211
    PHTVL/PHPV, 221
Standard Poodles, cataract, 211, 212
Staphylococcus spp., 26, 278
Staphylococcus aureus, 278
Staphyloma, 156
Stars of Winslow, 163, 230
Stereopsis, 270
Stevens tenotomy scissors, 39
Strabismus, 270–2
    congenital, 270
    extraocular polymositis, 271
    fibrosing, 271
    traumatic, 271
Streptococcus spp., 26
Streptococcus viridans, 280
Stroma, 134
    damage, 135
Stye, 91–2
Subalbinism, 163–4
Subalbinotic fundi in cats, 247
Subconjunctival granuloma, 159
Sudden acquired retinal degeneration,
    238, 300
Sudden loss of vision, 300
Sulphonamides, 51

Sunken eye disease in birds, 287
Superficial fungal blepharitis, 103
Superficial keratectomy, 137
Superficial keratotomy, 137
Suprachiasmatic nucleus, 263
Suprachoroidea, 228
Surgery *see* Ophthalmic surgery
Susceptibility testing, 27
Suture material, 39–40
Suture needles, 40
Swinging flashlight test, 5, 258, 260
Symblepharon, 102–3, 161
    cats, 132
    dogs, 127
Synchysis scintillans, 222, 223, 299
Synechiae in dogs, 166
Syneresis, 222
Systemic hypertension
    and retinal detachment in cats, 253–4
    and retinal vascular changes, 232,
        241

Tapetal reflex, 6
Tapetum
    cats, 247
    dogs
        hyperreflectivity, 232
        tapetal fundus, 230
Taurine deficiency in cats, 249, 301
Tear drainage, 107
    inadequate *see* Epiphora
    rabbits, 279
    reptiles, 292
Tear drainage system, cannulation of, 10
Tear drainage tests, 108–9
    cannulation and irrigation, 109
    dacrocystorhinography, 109
    direct examination, 108
    fibreoptic illumination, 109
    fluorescein drainage test, 108
Tear film *see* Pre-ocular tear film
Tear production tests, 8, 107–8
    in rabbits, 278–9
Tear stability tests, 108
Tear staining syndrome in reptiles, 292
Tear substitutes, 57–8
    aqueous, 57
    lipid-based, 58
    mucinomimetics, 58
Tearing reflex, 274
Temporomandibular osteopathy, 67
Tetracyclines, 51
Thermal injury in dogs, 144
Thiopentone, 34
Third eye in reptiles, 291
Third eyelid *see* Nictitating membrane
Tibetan Spaniels
    epiphora, 115
    generalized progressive retinal
        atrophy, 236
Tibetan Terriers
    cataract, 212
    generalized progressive retinal
        atrophy, 236
    lens luxation, 215
Timolol, 197
Tissue forceps, 37
Tissue plasminogen activator, 198
Tokay geckos, retinal degeneration, 294
Tonometers, 3
Tonometry, 186–7, 195
    applanation tonometers, 187
    digital, 186
    Schiotz tonometer, 186–7
Topical drugs, 51
Tortoises
    keratitis, 292
    tear staining syndrome, 292

Toxocara canis, 224
Toxoplasma gondii, 51, 170, 179, 252, 262, 266
Toxoplasmosis
    cats, 179–80
    dogs, 170
Toy Poodles
    epiphora, 115
    generalized progressive retinal atrophy, 236, 237
    optic nerve hypoplasia, 243
TPA, see tissue plasminogen activator
Trabecular meshwork, 185
Transilluminator, 206
Transmissable venereal tumour, 176
Trauma, 300
    anterior uveal, 173–4, 181
    conjunctival, 127–8, 133
    corneal, 145–6, 151
    eyelid, 288
    globe, 71–3
    lens, 216, 212
    nasolacrimal system, 116
    nictitating membrane, 100
    orbit, 70–1
    scleral, 160–1
    uveal tract, 173–4, 180
Treponema cuniculi, 278
Trichiasis, 298
Trifluorothymidine, 53
Trochlear nerve, 272
Tropical canine pancytopenia, 168
Tylodeiphys podicipina, 294

Ulcerative keratitis, 298, 299
    cats, 149–50
        causes, 149
        clinical findings, 149–50
        treatment, 150
    dogs, 140–3
        causes, 140
        clinical findings, 140
        diagnosis, 140
        management, 140–3
    rabbits, 281
Ulcerative limbal keratitis, 159
Ultrasonography, 10, 15–20
    abnormalities, 17–20
    anterior view, 16
    cataract, 18–19
    fundus disorders, 228
    high-frequency ultrasound biomicroscopy, 20
    hyperechoic, 17, 18, 19
    hypoechoic, 17, 19
    image production and display, 15–16
    intraocular disease, 17
    membranous lesions, 17–18
    multiple point-like echoes, 17
    orbit, 62
    posterior view, 16–17
    retrobulbar disease, 19–20
    technique, 16
Uveal cysts, 165, 224
Uveal melanoma, 195
Uveal tract, 162–84
    choroid, 163
    ciliary body, 163
    developmental anomalies, 163–5
        aniridia and iris hypoplasia, 164

        anterior segment dysgenesis, 164–5
        deficiencies of pigmentation, 163–4
        uveal cysts, 165
    iris, 162
Uveal tract abnormalities
    birds, 289
    cats, 177–83
        anterior uveal trauma, 181
        foreign bodies, 181
        lipaemic aqueous, 181
        uveal neoplasia, 182–3
        uveitis, 177–81, 225
    dogs, 165–77
        anterior uveal trauma, 173–5
        ectropion uveae, 165
        iridociliary cysts, 166
        iris atrophy, 165–6
        iris pigmentation, 165
        lipaemic aqueous, 175
        pre-iridal fibrovascular membranes, 165
        synechiae, 166
        uveal neoplasia, 175–7
        uveitis, 167–73
    rabbits, 282–3
        glaucoma, 282–3
        uveitis, 282
    reptiles, 293
Uveitis, 298, 299, 300, 301
    birds, 289
    cats, 177–81, 225
        causes, 177
        idiopathic, 180–1
        immune-mediated, 178–9
        infectious, 177–80
        lens damage, 180
        neoplasia-associated, 180
        trauma-associated, 180
    dogs, 167–73, 297
        causes, 168
        clinical features, 167
        corneal insult, 171
        diagnosis, 167
        immune-mediated, 171–2
        infectious, 168–71
        lens damage, 171
        neoplasia-associated, 172
        reflex, 168
        toxicity-associated, 171
        treatment, 172–3
    and glaucoma, 195
    rabbits, 282
    reptiles, 293
Uveodermatological syndrome, 171, 172

Venous pressure, 31–2
Ventilation, 32
Ventral lateral geniculate nucleus, 264
Vestibular nystagmus, 261
Vidarabine, 53
Viral uveitis
    cats, 177–8
    dogs, 168
Virology, 27
Vision loss
    congenital and early onset, 301
    slowly progressive, 301
    sudden, 300

Vision tests, 4–5, 257–8
    dazzle reflex, 258, 259
    maze test, 257
    menace response, 258, 259
    visual tracking, 257
Visual tracking, 257
Visually evoked potentials, 11
Vitamin E deficiency in dogs, 242, 301
Vitiligo, 171
Vitreal haemorrhage
    cats, 225–6
    dogs, 222–3
Vitreal herniation, 224
Vitreal prolapse, 196, 224
Vitrectomy, 225
Vitreoretinal dysplasia, 222
Vitreous, 219–26
    acquired conditions in cats, 225–6
        chronic feline uveitis, 225
        vitreal haemorrhage, 225–6
    acquired conditions in dogs, 222–4
        asteroid hyalosis, 222
        cysts, 224
        foreign bodies, 223–4
        neoplasia, 224
        parasites, 224
        prolapse and herniation, 224
        synchysis scintillans, 222
        syneresis, 222
        vitreal haemorrhage, 222–3
        vitritis, 223
    anatomy, physiology and biochemistry, 219–20
    cellular elements, 220
    congenital anomalies in cats, 225
    congenital anomalies in dogs, 220–2
        persistent hyaloid artery, 220–1
        persistent tunica vasculosa lentis, 220–1
        PHTVL/PHPV, 221–2
        vitreoretinal dysplasia, 222
    embryology, 219
    light transmission, 220
    matrix, 220
    therapeutic intravitreal injection, 225
    vitrectomy, 225
Vitreous base, 220
Vitreous gel, 220
Vitritis, 223, 299
Vitrosin, 219, 220

Welsh Springer Spaniels
    cataract, 211
    distichiasis, 88
    primary glaucoma, 193, 194
Welsh Terriers, primary glaucoma, 193
West Highland White Terriers
    cataract, 208, 212
    keratoconjunctivitis sicca, 112
    temporomandibular osteopathy, 67
Westcott tenotomy scissors, 39
Wet eye
    cats, 119
    dogs, 110, 296

Yorkshire Terriers, cataract, 212

Zygomatic arch, fractures of, 71
Zygomatic salivary gland mucocoele, 67